Inflammatory Mechanisms in Allergic Diseases

CLINICAL ALLERGY AND IMMUNOLOGY

Series Editors

MICHAEL A. KALINER, M.D.

Medical Director
Institute for Asthma and Allergy
Washington, D.C.

RICHARD F. LOCKEY, M.D.

Professor of Medicine, Pediatrics, and Public Health
Joy McCann Culverhouse Professor of Allergy and Immunology
Director, Division of Allergy and Immunology
University of South Florida College of Medicine
and James A. Haley Veterans Hospital
Tampa, Florida

1. Sinusitis: Pathophysiology and Treatment, *edited by Howard M. Druce*
2. Eosinophils in Allergy and Inflammation, *edited by Gerald J. Gleich and A. Barry Kay*
3. Molecular and Cellular Biology of the Allergic Response, *edited by Arnold I. Levinson and Yvonne Paterson*
4. Neuropeptides in Respiratory Medicine, *edited by Michael A. Kaliner, Peter J. Barnes, Gert H. H. Kunkel, and James N. Baraniuk*
5. Provocation Testing in Clinical Practice, *edited by Sheldon L. Spector*
6. Mast Cell Proteases in Immunology and Biology, *edited by George H. Caughey*
7. Histamine and H_1-Receptor Antagonists in Allergic Disease, *edited by F. Estelle R. Simons*
8. Immunopharmacology of Allergic Diseases, *edited by Robert G. Townley and Devendra K. Agrawal*
9. Indoor Air Pollution and Health, *edited by Emil J. Bardana, Jr., and Anthony Montanaro*
10. Genetics of Allergy and Asthma: Methods for Investigative Studies, *edited by Malcolm N. Blumenthal and Bengt Björkstén*
11. Allergic and Respiratory Disease in Sports Medicine, *edited by John M. Weiler*
12. Allergens and Allergen Immunotherapy: Second Edition, Revised and Expanded, *edited by Richard F. Lockey and Samuel C. Bukantz*
13. Emergency Asthma, *edited by Barry E. Brenner*
14. Food Hypersensitivity and Adverse Reactions, *edited by Marianne Frieri and Brett Kettelhut*
15. Diagnostic Testing of Allergic Disease, *edited by Stephen F. Kemp and Richard F. Lockey*
16. Inflammatory Mechanisms in Allergic Diseases, *edited by Burton Zweiman and Lawrence B. Schwartz*

ADDITIONAL VOLUMES IN PREPARATION

Histamine and H_1-Antagonists in Allergic Disease: Second Edition, Revised and Expanded, *edited by Estelle R. Simons*

Inflammatory Mechanisms in Allergic Diseases

edited by

Burton Zweiman
University of Pennsylvania School of Medicine
Philadelphia, Pennsylvania

Lawrence B. Schwartz
Virginia Commonwealth University
Richmond, Virginia

MARCEL DEKKER

MARCEL DEKKER, INC. NEW YORK • BASEL

ISBN: 0-8247-0540-8

This book is printed on acid-free paper.

Headquarters
Marcel Dekker, Inc.
270 Madison Avenue, New York, NY 10016
tel: 212-696-9000; fax: 212-685-4540

Eastern Hemisphere Distribution
Marcel Dekker AG
Hutgasse 4, Postfach 812, CH-4001 Basel, Switzerland
tel: 41-61-261-8482; fax: 41-61-261-8896

World Wide Web
http://www.dekker.com

The publisher offers discounts on this book when ordered in bulk quantities. For more information, write to Special Sales/Professional Marketing at the headquarters address above.

Current printing (last digit):
10 9 8 7 6 5 4 3 2 1

PRINTED IN THE UNITED STATES OF AMERICA

Introduction

Inflammatory Mechanisms in Allergic Diseases is a real winner. First, it is edited by two outstanding clinicians/scientists, Burt Zweiman and Lawrence B. Schwartz; second, the authors of the chapters represent a ''who's who'' in the field of allergic inflammation. It should be a welcome addition to the libraries of all physicians.

The concept of allergic inflammation is undergoing change. Whereas immediate hypersensitivity, as defined by the classic IgE–mast cell interaction, continues to play a major role in allergic inflammation, many other mechanisms are also active in the causation of a variety of different allergic and immunological diseases, all for too long attributed primarily to this one mechanism. Recognition of the complexity of the allergic inflammation is really the nuts and bolts of this book.

Not only are the various cells, inflammatory mediators, and cytokines involved in allergic inflammation covered extensively, but so too are the various inflammatory mechanisms as they relate to certain allergic diseases—for example, nasal polyposis, sinusitis, atopic dermatitis, urticaria, and vasculitis.

Part Four describes various treatment modalities currently available as well as some that are still in development. Genetically engineered allergen derivatives are a topic of discussion, as are anti-IgE antibody therapy and DNA immunomodulation of asthma. Traditional subcutaneous allergen immunotherapy is also discussed.

All in all, this book is required reading for any trainee or physician in the field of allergy and immunology as well as for physicians who want to update themselves in a field that affects up to 20% of the individuals seen in general practice clinics.

Michael A. Kaliner
Richard F. Lockey

Preface

It is now generally recognized that most allergic diseases are not simply due to an immediate immune reaction involving the rapid release of mediators such as histamine. Rather, the clinical manifestations are often the end result of a complex inflammatory process involving several cellular and humoral participants.

Therefore, incisive reviews of the nature and roles of each of the major participants in allergic reactions should be of great interest and importance to both investigators and clinicians.

A major objective of this book is to provide such reviews. An introductory chapter sets the scene with an overview of the milieu of allergic inflammatory reactions. This is followed by in-depth reviews of the functions in such reactions by individual components such as mast cells, eosinophils, basophils, epithelial cells, the major mediators, and cytokines.

However, it is now recognized that the expression of allergic reactions may not be the same in all organ systems. Therefore, another major objective of this book is to describe current knowledge about allergic inflammation in disorders such as asthma, atopic dermatitis, urticaria, and anaphylaxis, facilitating the understanding of both similarities and differences in the patterns of allergic reactivity in different organ systems. In this way, this book differs from existing texts or monographs that deal with allergic inflammation in a particular organ system.

Following these chapters is a section containing brief reviews of the therapy for allergic disorders and asthma, based on the knowledge described previously in the text. The book ends with an attempt to put the major findings given earlier into perspective for the physician who treats patients with allergic disorders and to point out possible future avenues of investigation.

Burton Zweiman
Lawrence B. Schwartz

Contents

Contributors

Nabih I. Abdou, M.D., Ph.D. Clinical Professor of Medicine, University of Missouri School of Medicine, and Center of Rheumatology, Allergy, and Immunology, Department of Medicine, St. Luke's Hospital, Kansas City, Missouri

Daniel C. Adelman, M.D. Associate Adjunct Professor, Department of Medicine, University of California at San Francisco, San Francisco, California

Rafeul Alam, M.D., Ph.D. Professor and Director, Division of Allergy and Immunology, Department of Internal Medicine, University of Texas Medical Branch, Galveston, Texas

Pedro C. Avila, M.D. Assistant Clinical Professor, Departments of Medicine and Pediatrics, University of California at San Francisco, San Francisco, California

Zuhair K. Ballas, M.D. Professor and Director, Division of Allergy-Immunology, Department of Internal Medicine, University of Iowa College of Medicine, Iowa City, Iowa

James N. Baraniuk, M.D. Associate Professor, Department of Medicine, Georgetown University, Washington, D.C.

Leonard Bielory, M.D., F.A.C.P., F.A.A.A.A.I., F.A.C.A.A.I. Director, Asthma and Allergy Research Center, Associate Professor of Medicine, Pediatrics, and Ophthalmology, and Codirector, Immuno-ophthalmology Service, UMDNJ–New Jersey Medical School, Newark, New Jersey

Bruce S. Bochner, M.D. Professor, Division of Allergy and Clinical Immunology, Department of Medicine, Johns Hopkins University School of Medicine, Baltimore, Maryland

Sergio Bonini, M.D. Professor of Allergology and Clinical Immunology, Second University of Naples, and Institute of Experimental Medicine, Italian National Research Council (CNR), Rome, Italy

Stefano Bonini, M.D. Associate Professor, Department of Ophthalmology, University of Rome Tor Vergata, Rome, Italy

Agnes Bugajska-Schretter, Ph.D Vienna General Hospital (AKH) and Department of Medical and Clinical Chemistry, University of Vienna Medical School, Vienna, Austria

William W. Busse, M.D. Professor and Head, Allergy and Immunology Section, Department of Medicine, University of Wisconsin Medical School, Madison, Wisconsin

Pandora E. Christie, M.D. Senior Fellow, Allergy Section, Department of Medicine, University of Washington, Seattle, Washington

Kelly L. Davenpeck, Ph.D. Research Assistant Professor, Division of Cardiology, Department of Medicine, Thomas Jefferson University, Philadelphia, Pennsylvania

Stephen R. Durham, M.D., F.R.C.P. Professor of Allergy and Respiratory Medicine, Imperial College School of Medicine, National Heart & Lung Institute, and Royal Brompton Hospital, London, England

Mark S. Dykewicz, M.D. Associate Professor and Director of Training Program in Allergy and Immunology, Division of Allergy and Immunology, Department of Internal Medicine, St. Louis University School of Medicine, St. Louis, Missouri

Saju S. Eapen, M.D. Fellow, Allergy and Immunology Section, Department of Medicine, University of Wisconsin Medical School, Madison, Wisconsin

Margit Focke-Tejkl, Ph.D. Vienna General Hospital (AKH) and Department of Pathophysiology, University of Vienna Medical School, Vienna, Austria

Malcolm Watson Greaves, M.D., Ph.D., F.R.C.P. Emeritus Professor, University of London, and St. John's Institute of Dermatology, St. Thomas Hospital, London, England

Paul A. Greenberger, M.D. Professor, Division of Allergy-Immunology, Department of Medicine, Northwestern University Medical School, Chicago, Illinois

Rebecca S. Gruchalla, M.D., Ph.D. Associate Professor and Chief, Division of Allergy and Immunology, Department of Internal Medicine, The University of Texas Southwestern Medical Center at Dallas, Dallas, Texas

William R. Henderson, Jr., M.D. Professor and Head, Allergy Section, Department of Medicine, University of Washington, Seattle, Washington

Gita Kampen, M.S. Laboratory of Medical Allergology, National University Hospital, Copenhagen, Denmark

A. Barry Kay, Ph.D., F.R.C.P., F.R.S.C. Professor and Academic Head, Department of Allergy and Clinical Immunology, Imperial College School of Medicine, National Heart & Lung Institute, London, England

Jeffrey L. Kishiyama, M.D. Assistant Clinical Professor, Department of Medicine, University of California at San Francisco, San Francisco, California

Joel N. Kline, M.D. Associate Professor, Division of Pulmonary, Critical Care and Occupational Medicine, Department of Internal Medicine, University of Iowa College of Medicine, Iowa City, Iowa

Dietrich Kraft, M.D. Vienna General Hospital (AKH) and Professor, Department of Pathophysiology, University of Vienna Medical School, Vienna, Austria

Donald Y. M. Leung, M.D., Ph.D. Professor and Head, Division of Pediatric Allergy-Immunology, National Jewish Medical and Research Center, Denver, Colorado

Donald MacGlashan, Jr., M.D., Ph.D. Professor, Division of Allergy and Clinical Immunology, Department of Medicine, Johns Hopkins University School of Medicine, Baltimore, Maryland

Janet M. Oliver, Ph.D. Regents Professor, Department of Pathology, University of New Mexico Health Sciences Center, Albuquerque, New Mexico

Peck Y. Ong, M.D. Division of Allergy and Immunology, National Jewish Medical and Research Center, Denver, Colorado

Yong-Jin Park, M.D. Assistant Professor of Medicine, Department of Otolaryngology, The Catholic University of Korea, and St. Vincent's Hospital, Suwon, Korea

Clive R. Roberts, Ph.D. Associate Professor, Faculties of Dentistry and Medicine, The University of British Columbia, Vancouver, British Columbia, Canada

Douglas S. Robinson, M.A., M.D., F.R.C.P. Senior Lecturer, Department of Allergy and Clinical Immunology, Imperial College School of Medicine, National Heart & Lung Institute, London, England

Sergio Romagnani, M.D. Professor, Department of Internal Medicine, University of Florence, Florence, Italy

R. Robert Schellenberg, M.D., F.R.C.P.C. Professor, Faculty of Medicine, The University of British Columbia, Vancouver, British Columbia, Canada

Lawrence B. Schwartz, M.D., Ph.D. Professor, Department of Internal Medicine, Virginia Commonwealth University, Richmond, Virginia

Raymond G. Slavin, M.D. Professor and Director, Division of Allergy and Immunology, Department of Internal Medicine, St. Louis University School of Medicine, St. Louis, Missouri

Roland Solensky, M.D. Fellow, Division of Allergy and Immunology, Department of Internal Medicine, The University of Texas Southwestern Medical Center at Dallas, Dallas, Texas

Susanne Spitzauer, M.D. Vienna General Hospital (AKH) and Professor, Department of Medical and Clinical Chemistry, University of Vienna Medical School, Vienna, Austria

Ines Swoboda, Ph.D. Vienna General Hospital (AKH) and Department of Medical and Clinical Chemistry, University of Vienna Medical School, Vienna, Austria

Anna Twardosz, M.D. Vienna General Hospital (AKH) and Department of Pulmology, Internal Medicine IV, University of Vienna Medical School, Vienna, Austria

Rudolf Valenta, M.D. Vienna General Hospital (AKH) and Professor, Department of Pathophysiology, University of Vienna Medical School, Vienna, Austria

Eva-Maria Varga, M.D. Division of Respiratory and Allergic Disease, Department of Pediatrics, Klinische Abteilung für Pädiatrische Pulmonologie und Allergologie, Universitätsklinik für Kinder- und Jugendheilkunde, Graz, Austria

Donata Vercelli, M.D. Associate Professor, Department of Cell Biology and Anatomy, and Associate Research Scientist, Respiratory Sciences Center, University of Arizona, Tucson, Arizona

Susanne Vrtala, Ph.D. Vienna General Hospital (AKH) and Department of Pathophysiology, Vienna General Hospital (AKH), Vienna, Austria

David C. Walker, M.A., Ph.D. Associate Professor, Department of Pathology and Laboratory Medicine, The University of British Columbia, Vancouver, British Columbia, Canada

Andrew J. Wardlaw, Ph.D., F.R.C.P. Professor, Department of Respiratory Medicine, Institute for Lung Health, University of Leicester, Leicester, England

Bridget S. Wilson, Ph.D. Assistant Professor, Department of Pathology, University of New Mexico Health Sciences Center, Albuquerque, New Mexico

Burton Zweiman, M.D. Professor of Medicine and Neurology, Division of Pulmonary, Allergy, and Critical Care Medicine, Department of Medicine, University of Pennsylvania School of Medicine, Philadelphia, Pennsylvania

1

Introduction

BURTON ZWEIMAN

University of Pennsylvania School of Medicine, Philadelphia, Pennsylvania

1 WHAT IS ALLERGIC INFLAMMATION?

The major evolution in our thinking about the pathogenesis of allergic diseases is now well recognized by investigators and clinicians. Allergic diseases were traditionally considered to be the result of immediate reactions involving the effects of mediators released from activated mast cells. It is now well established that allergic reactions are often not just an immediate event, but a continuing process involving a complex inflammatory response, affected by genetic, environmental, and internal control factors. Investigations to date by many groups have revealed the presence of numerous cellular and humoral proinflammatory agents in the sites of allergic diseases. Yet, the role of each of these components in the pathogenesis of allergic diseases is still not completely defined. Some of the persisting questions under current active investigation include

1. What is the relative contribution of individual humoral and cellular inflammatory components in the pathogenesis of allergic diseases?
2. How do these participants interact?
3. What is the pathogenic relation of the ‘‘immediate-phase’’ to the ‘‘late-phase’’ component of allergic reactions?
4. What are the precise mechanisms underlying the various therapeutic approaches in allergic disease?

The overall objective of this text is to enhance our understanding related to these questions. Part Two includes the individual inflammatory components relevant to allergic inflammation. Part Three includes reviews of the inflammatory pathways involved in diseases in which allergic mechanisms are thought to be at least partially responsible. Part Four deals with the effect on allergic inflammation of several therapeutic approaches, both traditional and recently developed. We will end this text with brief concluding remarks attempting to put the foregoing discussions into perspective. To achieve this objective, we have enlisted the participation of colleagues who are at the cutting edge of these areas. We believe that this text will considerably enhance your understanding of allergic inflammation and its role in human disease.

2

Mast Cells and Basophils

LAWRENCE B. SCHWARTZ

Virginia Commonwealth University, Richmond, Virginia

1 INTRODUCTION

Mast cells and basophils are generally recognized as the principal cell types to initiate IgE-dependent immediate hypersensitivity reactions (type I), and more recently as a cell that also might contribute to innate and acquired immunity and to tissue remodeling (Fig. 1). Experimental allergen challenges of an IgE-sensitized host reveals two phases of the subsequent immediate hypersensitivity reaction. The early phase of the IgE-dependent reactions (5–30 min postchallenge), depending on the target tissue and distribution of allergen, involves local edema, smooth-muscle contraction, vasodilation, and increased permeability of postcapillary venules. The late phase of an immediate hypersensitivity reaction (4–12 hr postchallenge) involves the recruitment and activation of basophils, eosinophils, and other cell types. These late reactions can persist for at least 2 days in the challenged lower airway, but eventually appear to completely resolve. In contrast, chronic allergic inflammation results from prolonged allergen exposure and may provoke changes in the target tissue that resolve much more slowly, if at all.

Mast cells occupy sentinel positions in tissues where noxious substances might attempt entry and immediate-type hypersensitivity reactions typically begin. These cells are most concentrated at sites in the lamina propria around the upper and lower airways, conjunctiva, dermis, gastrointestinal mucosa, and perivascular tissues. Elegant studies in mice have indicated a role for mast cells in resistance to gram-negative bacteria by non–IgE-dependent production of tumor necrosis factor (TNF)-α when bacteria come into contact with mast cells. Also, roles for mast cells in classic Arthus immune–complex-type reactions and in antigen-processing and presentation processes have been reported primarily in mice. Whether these capabilities have been conserved during evolution is still uncertain. For example, the expression of FcγRIII receptors, through which activating

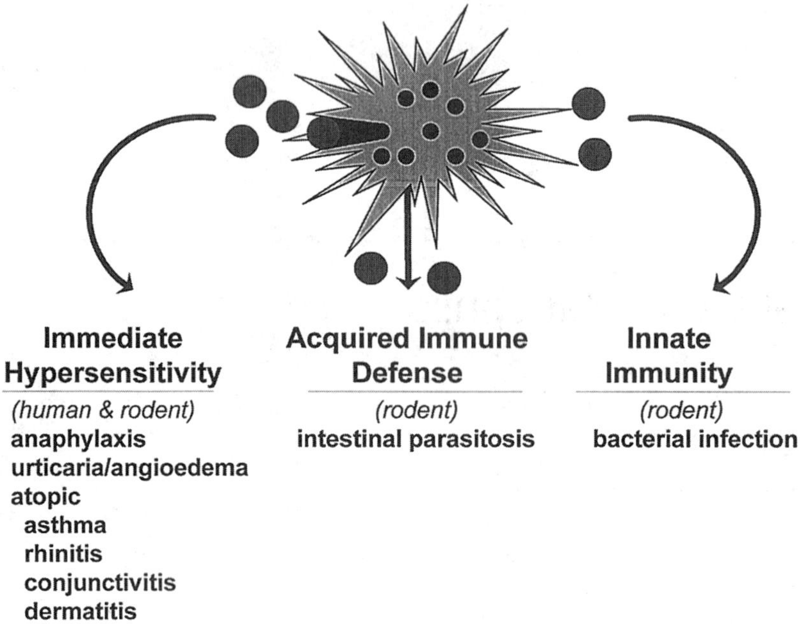

Figure 1 Immunological effector roles of mast cells and basophils: mast cells and basophils are the primary effector cells in immediate hypersensitivity reactions, but also may participate in innate immune defense and in immunity against certain parasites.

signals can be transmitted, is well-documented for murine mast cells, but has not been observed in human mast cells and, thereby, may limit participation of human mast cells in IgG-dependent immune-complex reactions.

Basophils normally reside in the circulation, but enter tissues at sites of inflammation, particularly during the late phase of IgE-mediated immediate hypersensitivity reactions and during the early phase of cell-mediated delayed-type hypersensitivity reactions. Mast cells and basophils are the only two cell types that constitutively express substantial quantities of the high-affinity, tetrameric receptor for IgE (FcεRI), and store histamine in their secretory granules. These two cell types are distinguished from one another through pathways for growth, differentiation, and survival; patterns of cell surface adhesion, cytokine, and chemokine receptors; responses to non–IgE-dependent agonists; secretory granule proteoglycans and proteases; and cell morphologies. For example, nuclei of peripheral blood basophils have deeply divided lobes, whereas those of mast cells in normal tissues are rounded.

Mast cells in human tissues have been divided into two major types based on the protease content of their secretory granules. Those with tryptase, together with chymase, carboxypeptidase, and cathepsin G, are called MC_{TC} cells; those with only tryptase are called MC_T cells. These two phenotypes of mast cells have been studied by electron (Fig. 2) and light microscopy (Fig. 3). In Figure 2 mast cells and basophils (see Fig. 2A, D, G) and their respective secretory granules (see Fig. 2B, C, E, F, and H) are visualized. Also, immunogold labeling with antichymase and antitryptase monoclonal antibodies (MAbs) (see Fig. 2B, E) illustrates the protease phenotypes just described, whereas the

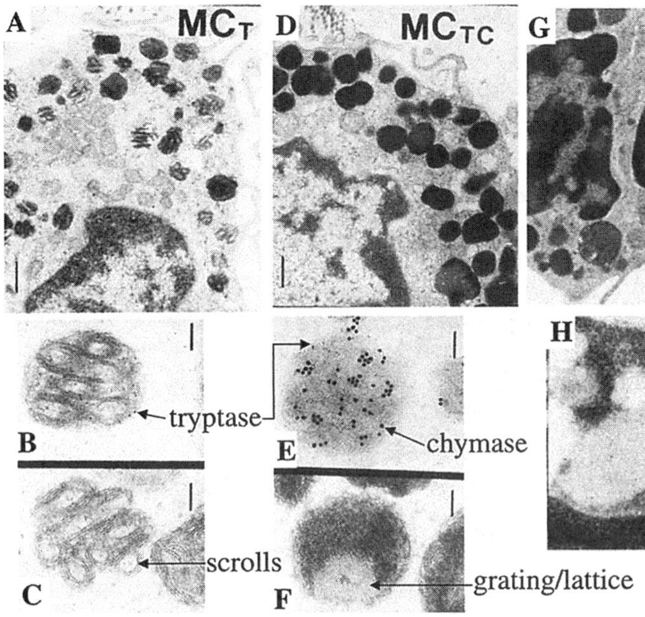

Figure 2 Ultrastructure of mast cells and basophils: (A) Electron micrographs of an MC_T cell; (B) an MC_T secretory granule incubated with antitryptase and antichymase antibodies linked with small (5-nm) and large (15-nm) gold particles, respectively, but labeled only by the small particles; (C) an MC_T secretory granule not subjected to labeling, and showing multiple complete scrolls; (D) an MC_{TC} cell; (E) an MC_{TC} secretory granule treated as in B, but labeled by both large and small gold particles; (F) an MC_{TC} secretory granule not subjected to labeling and showing a grating/lattice substructure; (G) a peripheral blood basophil; (H) basophil secretory granules labeled with 2D7 MAb linked to gold particles. Bars in A, D, and G indicate a 1-μm length; those in B, C, E, F, and H indicate a 0.1-μm length.

scroll-rich (see Fig. 2C) and grating/lattice (see Fig. 2F) substructures serve to further characterize these cells. Localization of a potential marker of basophils to secretory granules also is shown (see Fig. 2H) (see following). As shown in Figure 3, MC_{TC} cells are the predominant mast cell type in normal (see Fig. 3A) and urticaria pigmentosa (see Fig. 3B) skin and in small bowel submucosa (see Fig. 3G), whereas MC_T cells are the predominant type found in the normal airway (see Fig. 3C–E) and appear to be selectively recruited near the surface of the airway during seasonal allergic disease (see Fig. 3F). Of possible interest is the selective attenuation in numbers of MC_T cells in the small bowel of patients with end-stage immunodeficiency diseases (see Fig. 3H). Mast cells from different tissues, irrespective of their protease phenotype, may exhibit functional differences in their response to non–IgE-dependent activators and pharmacological modulators of activation. The selected participation of basophils and different types of mast cells in various clinical conditions, as well as the duration, intensity, and tissue distribution of a particular response, will depend on various characteristics of the agonist, immunological sensitivity of the host, the target tissue involved, and any underlying pathology. This chapter will focus on human mast cells and basophils, because of their obvious relevance to human disease.

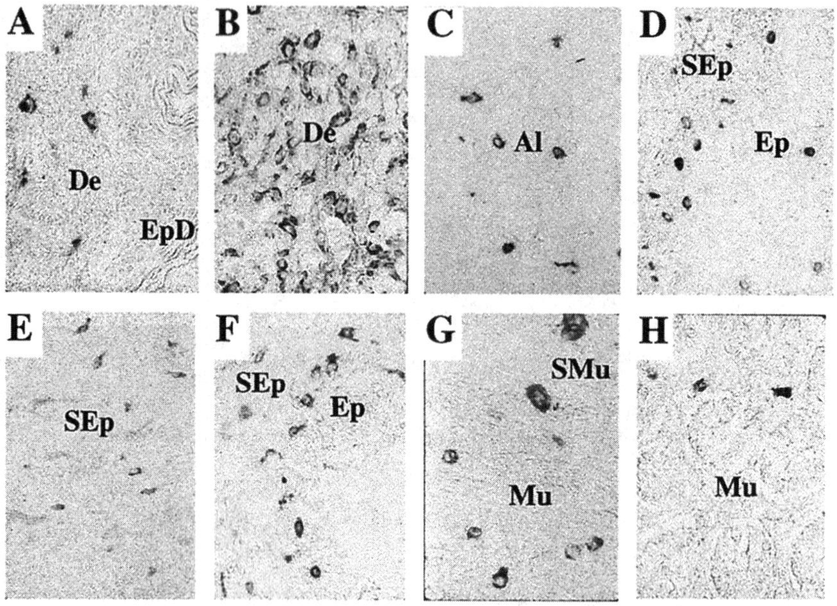

Figure 3 MC_T and MC_{TC} types of human mast cells in various tissues. Sections from tissues fixed in Carnoy's fluid were labeled first with biotinylated antichymase MAb and peroxidase–streptavidin; then with alkaline phosphatase-conjugated antitryptase MAb. The reddish-brown dye deposited on chymase-positive cells blocks subsequent labeling with antitryptase, permitting the MC_{TC} type of mast cell to be identified. Those cells without chymase are labeled with antibody against tryptase and stain blue, identifying them as the MC_T type of mast cell. Shown in this black and white photomicrograph are (A) mast cells from normal skin (all MC_{TC}); (B) skin from an urticaria pigmentosa lesion (all MC_{TC}); (C) alveolar wall (all MC_T); (D) bronchus (arrows show MC_{TC} cells, remaining dark cells are MC_T); (E) nasal mucosa (arrows show MC_{TC} cells, remaining dark cells are MC_T); (F) nasal mucosa from a subject with active seasonal allergic rhinitis (arrows show MC_{TC} cells, remaining dark cells are MC_T); (G) small intestine (arrows show MC_{TC} cells, remaining dark cells are MC_T); and (H) small intestine from a subject with end-stage severe combined immunodeficiency disease (all mast cells brown). Dermis (De) and epidermis (EpD) of skin, alveolar wall (Al), epithelium (Ep) and subepithelium (SEp) in the airway and mucosa (Mu) and submucosa (SMu) of small intestine are so labeled.

2 GROWTH AND DIFFERENTIATION OF MAST CELLS

Both mast cells and basophils originate from hematopoietic stem cells, as outlined in Figure 4. Basophils, similar to most myeloid cells, complete their differentiation in the bone marrow and then enter the circulation. In contrast, a cell destined to reside in peripheral tissues as a mast cell will leave the bone marrow as an immature progenitor, probably with multipotential capabilities, enter a peripheral tissue still without secretory granules and cell surface FcεRI, and then complete their differentiation to a mast cell. Basophils develop largely under the influence of interleukin (IL)-3, a process that is augmented by transforming growth factor (TGF)-β. Mast cells differentiate under the influence of stem cell factor (SCF) (1–3), the ligand for Kit, a product of the c-*kit* proto-oncogene. IL-3 has little if any influence on the differentiation of human mast cells other than to expand the pool of hematopoietic progenitor cells, in contrast with rodent mast cells for which

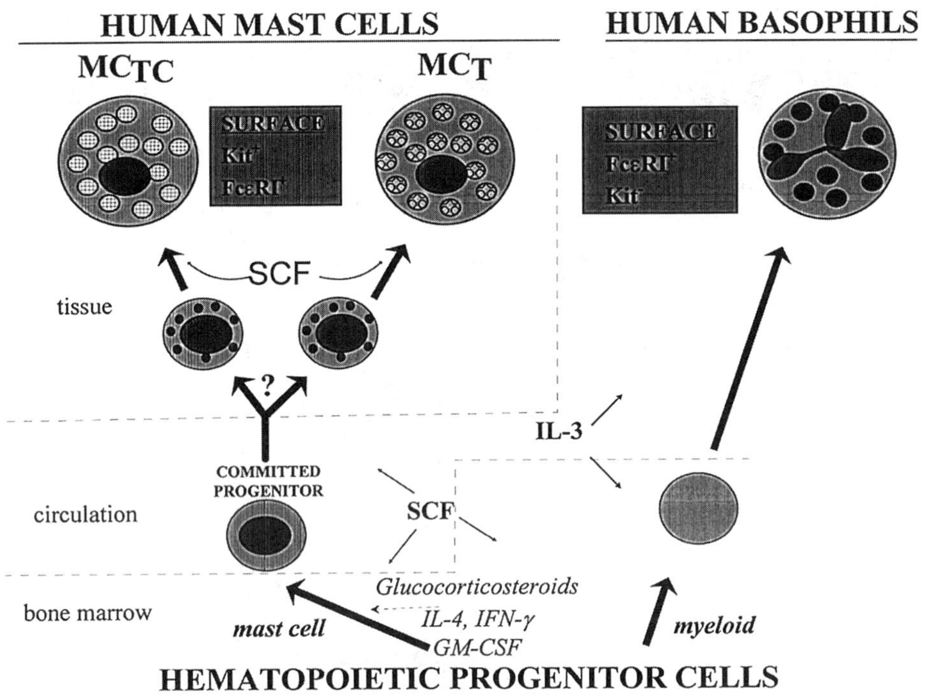

Figure 4 Differentiation of human mast cells and basophils: hematopoietic progenitor cells give rise to both mast cells and basophils, but the growth factors involved and the sites where maturation occurs differ between these two cell types.

IL-3 is an important growth and differentiation factor in vitro. In vivo, IL-$3^{-/-}$ mice have normal basal levels of mast cells and basophils, but fail to increase intestinal levels of mast cells or blood basophils during parasitic infection (4). Mast cell progenitors identified in human peripheral blood have been distinguished from basophils, monocytes, or other leukocytes by patterns of the detected cell surface molecules (5). Also, multipotential precursors isolated from cord blood or peripheral blood that are either positive for CD34 and CD38 (6), or for CD34, CD13, and Kit (7) give rise to pure mast cell colonies along with other pure or mixed lineage colonies, principally monocytic, implying a distinct myeloid lineage for mast cells. However, controversy has arisen with the report that peripheral blood metachromatic cells can exhibit both mast cell (tryptase, chymase, carboxypeptidase, and Kit) and basophil (polymorphonuclear; PMN) characteristics during drug hypersensitivity and asthmatic reactions (8). These findings need to be confirmed before criteria previously employed to distinguish mast cells from basophils are revised.

Conditions that influence the selective development or recruitment of MC_{TC} and MC_T cells are not yet understood. The expression of CXCR2 on HMC-1 cells and relatively mature cord blood-derived mast cells (9,10) and CCR3 and 5 and CXCR2 and 4 on developing cord blood-derived mast cells suggest potential chemokine-dependent pathways of mast cell recruitment. Unlike other myelocytes that stop expressing Kit as they mature, mast cells express increasing amounts of Kit as they develop. Thus, SCF exerts various effects on mast cells throughout their development, including differentiation, survival, chemotaxis, activation, and priming. The effects on differentiation and survival are particu-

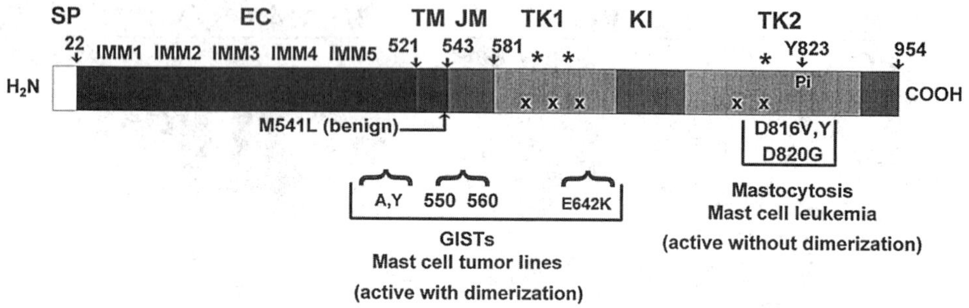

Figure 5 Mutations in the gene encoding Kit: various extracellular, transmembrane, and intracellular domains are shown, along with the sites of inactivating mutations, and activating mutations that enhance SCF-independent tyrosine kinase activity either by facilitating dimerization or by directly affecting the catalytic domain. x, inactivating autosomal dominant point mutations, which along with frameshift mutations, are associated with human piebaldism; *, catalytic triad residues; GIST, gastrointestinal stromal tumor; SP, signal peptide; EC, extracellular; TM, transmembrane; JM, juxtamembrane; TK, tyrosine kinase; KI, kinase insert.

larly evident in certain strains of mice with inactivating mutations either in Kit or in SCF, both of which result in a profound mast cell deficiency. Removal of SCF from mast cells in mice, and presumably humans (11), results in apoptosis. As illustrated in Figure 5, certain gain of function mutations in human Kit (12) and, less commonly, loss of function mutations in Kit (13), are associated with systemic mastocytosis, perhaps indicating that there are factors other than Kit involved in this condition. On the other hand, a different group of activating Kit mutations is associated with intestinal stromal cell tumors in which interstitial cells of Cajal are transformed (14). Of potential interest is the observation that TGF-β inhibits the ability of SCF to rescue murine mast cells from apoptosis (15).

Why mast cells fail to develop in the bone marrow, where SCF clearly affects the development of other cell types, is an enigma. Either the bone marrow microenvironment lacks an accessory factor present in peripheral sites, or the microenvironment contains additional factors that are not permissive for mast cell development. The latter seems to be partly true, because both granulocyte–monocyte colony-stimulating factor (GM-CSF) and IL-4 appear to diminish SCF-dependent development of mast cells from progenitors in vitro, but have little effect on more mature mast cells. The ability of IL-4 to down-regulate expression of Kit may help explain the ability of this cytokine to attenuate mast cell development under some circumstances. However, IL-4 exhibits several effects on mast cells, including induction of surface FcεRI on fetal liver-derived (16) and cord blood-derived (17) mast cells, proliferation of intestinal mast cells (18), and apoptosis of cord blood-derived mast cells (19). Glucocorticosteroids inhibit mast cell development in vitro, whereas mature mast cells are relatively resistant to these agents. IL-6 also has pleiotropic effects on developing human mast cells, including both attenuation (20) and enhancement (21) of mast cell numbers, and blocking of IL-4–mediated apoptosis (19). Both IL-4 and IL-6 can enhance the percentage of mast cells expressing chymase (20,22).

Two experiments suggest that MC_{TC} and MC_T cells develop among distinct pathways. First, in humans with inherited combined immunodeficiency disease and in those with acquired immunodeficiency syndrome (AIDS), marked and selective decreases in MC_T cell concentrations occur in the bowel, whereas the concentration and distribution of MC_{TC} cells are unaffected (23). This suggests that the appearance in tissues of MC_T

cells is dependent on functional T lymphocytes, and that MC_{TC} cell development proceeds independently. Second, immature MC_T cells contain granules with complete scrolls and tryptase alone, whereas MC_{TC} cells have granules with electron-dense cores surrounded by a less–electron-dense matrix and tryptase, together with chymase (24). Thus, commitment to a particular mast cell type in vivo appears to occur by the time granules begin to form.

3 ACTIVATION AND REGULATED SECRETION

Immunological activation of mast cells and basophils typically begins when IgE bound to the high-affinity Fcε receptor (FcεR1; $K_a = 10^9\ M^{-1}$) is cross-linked by multivalent allergen (Fig. 6). The complete FcεR1 receptor is composed of four subunits, $\alpha\beta\gamma_2$, which appear to float on the cell surface in lipid-based domains called rafts (25). The α-chain contains the extracellular IgE-binding domain. The β- and two disulfide-linked γ-chains are located primarily in the membrane and cytoplasmic domains. The γ-chains are also present in the CD16 and FcγRIII receptors of natural killer cells and may substitute for the T-cell receptor ζ-chain.

Regulated secretion by mast cells and basophils also may be induced by non-immunological agonists. Multivalent lectins, such as bivalent concanavalin A, cross-link membrane FcεRI or IgE. Calcium ionophores activate by translocating calcium. Basic biomolecules, such as compound 48/80, C3a, C5a, morphine, codeine, mellitin, eosino-

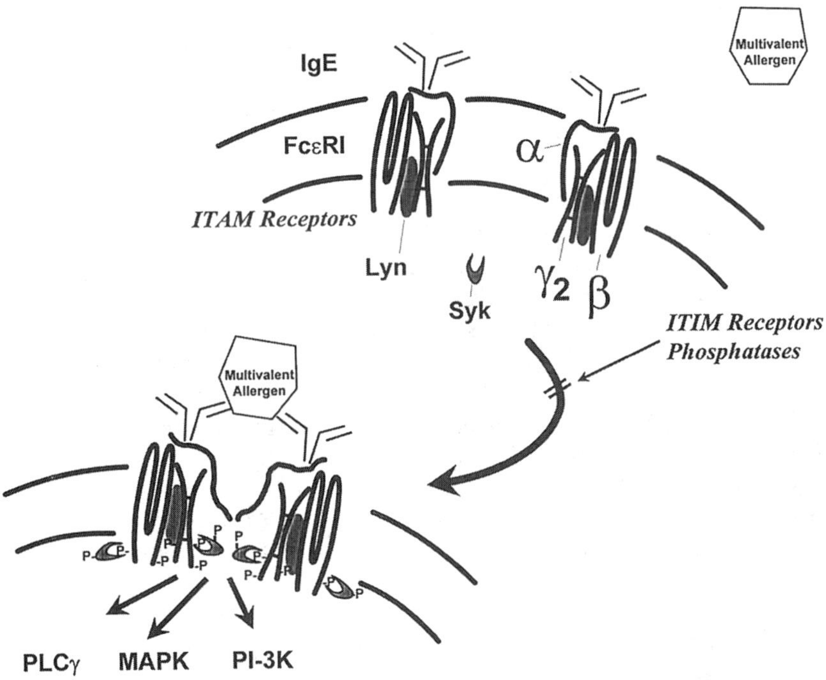

Figure 6 Initial biochemical events of mast cell and basophil activation following cross-linking of FcεRI: activation of Lyn TK, and recruitment of Syk TK to ITAMs signal up-regulation of PLCγ, MAPK, and PI-3K pathways, whereas phosphatases recruited to ITIMs down-regulate the process.

phil-derived major basic protein, and various neuropeptides, such as substance P, vasoactive intestinal peptide (VIP), somatostatin, and calcitonin gene-related protein (CGRP), activate human mast cells derived from skin, but are inactive against mast cells derived from most other tissues. In contrast, basophils respond to C5a and C3a, but not to the neuropeptides, compound 48/80, morphine, and codeine. Heart mast cells respond to C5a, but not to substance P (26). The desArg derivatives of C3a and C5a are inactive on skin mast cells, but still show limited agonist activity against basophils. Whether these basic peptides activate mast cells and basophils by stereospecific receptor interactions, or by ionic perturbations of membrane components is unclear (27). Basophils can also be activated as well as primed to better respond to antigen by IL-3, an interleukin that does not affect human mast cell activation. Differences in the secretory response between mast cells isolated from different tissues may partly relate to microenvironmental influences. For example, the RBL rat mucosal mast cell line reversibly acquires responsiveness to substance P when cocultured with 3T3 fibroblasts without otherwise changing its phenotype. Basophils, similar to eosinophils, but in contrast with mast cells, express surface FcαR, and can be activated by an IgA-dependent pathway (28,29). The peptide f-Met-Leu-Phe (FMLP) activates human basophils, but not mast cells. Human immunodeficiency virus (HIV)-1 gp120 activates IgE-armed basophils to secrete IL-4 and IL-13 (30), of possible interest to immediate hypersensitivity reactions commonly observed in HIV-infected individuals. Immunological activation of mast cells can be enhanced by adenosine (31), possibly through the adenosine A2b receptor in humans (32). In contrast, mediator release from human basophils is inhibited by adenosine. Also, ATP can enhance mediator release from activated mast cells by binding to the P2Y surface purinoreceptor expressed on human lung-derived mast cells (33).

Various histamine-releasing factors derived from monocytes, lymphocytes, platelets, and neutrophils that are of potential clinical significance have also been described. The protein termed p23, for example, has IgE-dependent histamine-, cytokine-, and LTC_4-releasing activity on basophils, an effect on mast cells being uncertain (34,35). Chemokines, initially discovered because of their abilities to attract predominantly monocytes or neutrophils, include potent basophil histamine-releasing and attracting agents (36). Active chemokines include monocyte chemotactic protein (MCP)-1 to -4 (CCL2, CCL8, CCL7, CCL13); RANTES (CCL5); monocyte inflammatory peptide (MIP)-1α (CCL3) and -1β (CCL4); eotaxin (CCL11) and eotaxin-2 (CCL24); and ecalectin. Most of these chemokines affect eosinophils as well as basophils. The presence of the chemokine receptor, CCR3, on basophils and eosinophils dovetails with the cellular specificity of these CC class chemokines (37). However, a further level of complexity was revealed for MCP-1, which, when intact, preferentially activates basophils over eosinophils, but after the N-terminal amino acid is removed, preferentially activates eosinophils over basophils. In contrast to the effects of these chemokines on basophils, mast cell mediator release appears to be unaffected (38,39), even though human mast cells express CCR3 (10,40). However, human mast cells appear to be capable of producing both MCP-1 and MIP-1α (41,42), suggesting a mechanism in which basophils may be recruited to, and activated at, tissue sites of mast cell activation. The differences between basophils and mast cells relative to their non–IgE-mediated pathways of activation, in theory, could lead to the activation of one cell type in the absence of the other.

Pharmacological responsiveness of mast cells also varies depending on the tissue source and differs from that of basophils. Cromolyn sodium (disodium cromoglycate) and nedocromil—each used for the treatment of allergic asthma, rhinitis, and conjunctivitis—at high concentrations are weak inhibitors of lung-derived mast cells, but not those from skin and intestine. β-Adrenoceptor agonists, at concentrations theoretically achievable on the airway surface with inhaled medication, produce 10–50% inhibition of IgE-dependent histamine release in vitro from dispersed human lung mast cells, whereas generation of leukotriene-C_4 (LTC_4) and prostaglandin-D_2 (PGD_2) is inhibited to a greater extent. Cyclosporin A and Tacrolimus (FK 506) produce rapid and long-lasting inhibition of IgE-dependent histamine release from human basophils and skin- and lung-derived mast cells. Sirolimus (rapamycin) interferes with the inhibitory activity of FK 506 by competing for the same FK-binding protein, but by itself does not inhibit mast cell or basophil activation. Dexamethasone in vitro inhibits mediator secretion by human basophils, but not by human lung-derived mast cells. In vivo, local instillation of nasal glucocorticosteroids diminished mediator release during the immediate response to nasal allergen challenge, perhaps owing to the capacity for local steroids to diminish mast cell concentrations, as demonstrated in the synovium (43), skin (44), and rectal mucosa (45), or to the prevention of the superficial migration of mast cells that apparently occurs in atopic subjects during the allergy season (46,47).

Mast cells undergo regulated exocytosis when FcεRI (α,β,γ_2) molecules are dimerized by multivalent antigen or antireceptor antibody. The earliest biochemical events involved in signal transduction after FcεRI aggregation involve phosphorylation of the β- and γ-chains of the high-affinity receptor. Phosphorylation of tyrosines in membrane proteins often occurs on a special motif consisting of six conserved amino acids (two Tyr residues) distributed over a 26-amino–acid stretch called an immunoreceptor tyrosine activation motif (ITAM). These ITAMs associate with Src-family protein tyrosine kinases (PTKs) such as Lyn. Activation of these PTKs lead to the phosphorylation of Tyr residues in the ITAMs and then activation of downstream effector molecules. ITAMs are found on both the γ- and β-subunits, and these two subunits are phosphorylated within seconds after receptor cross-linking, and dephosphorylated almost immediately on disruption of the receptor aggregates. The PTK Lyn associates with the β- and γ-chains, when the cells are at rest, and initiates phosphorylation of these chains after receptor aggregation (48). The presence of the β-chain, although not essential for surface receptor expression or signal transduction, markedly amplifies phosphorylation of the γ-chains and signal transduction, increasing the magnitude of the host response (49,50). Phosphorylation of these sites increases the affinity of the cytoplasmic PTK, Syk, for these chains. Syk is then phosphorylated by Lyn and possibly by itself and is required for mast cell activation (51–53). Human basophils also require Syk for IgE-dependent signal transduction, because individuals with low expression of Syk in their basophils are nonreleasors to FcεRI cross-linking, a process that can be reversed by IL-3, which induces Syk expression and return of releasability (54). These early events also are regulated by signal regulatory proteins (SIRPs) that contain ITIMs (immunotyrosine inhibition motifs), such as SIRPα, which is expressed in human mast cells and has been shown in mice to act in part by recruiting SH2-bearing protein tyrosine phosphatases (SHP-1 and -2) that dephosphorylate ITAMs on FcεRI-β and -γ, thereby down-regulating signal transduction and mediator release (55). CD45, a protein tyrosine phosphatase, promotes mediator release because mast cells from mice that are deficient in this enzyme do not exhibit IgE-dependent activation (56). Phosphorylated Syk then recruits other signal transduction molecules, such as Btk in mice, although perhaps not in human mast cells (57). Defective Btk in mice attenuates degranulation and cytokine production by activated mast cells as well as the anaphylactic response of the animal (58,59). SLP-76, an adapter protein known to be a substrate for both ZAP-70 and Syk, when knockedout of mice, results in mast cells that can undergo phosphorylation of Syk with FcεRI cross-linking, but do not release mediators (60). The activation signal is transmitted to pathways involving PLCγ, MAP kinase, protein kinase C, and PI-3 kinase.

Degranulation is associated with activation of small G proteins that cause actin polymerization and actin relocalization (61,62). Metabolism of phospholipids, which mostly reside in secretory granules, occurs early during the secretory response, is necessary for the later secretion of lipid mediators, and may be important for regulated secretion to ensue. Generation of inositol 1,3,4-triphosphate (IP_3) and diacylglycerol after FcεRI receptor aggregation occurs and results in release of calcium from the endoplasmic reticulum. This, in turn, stimulates calcium-dependent isoforms of protein kinase C, and may directly facilitate fusion of lipid bilayers as exocytosis proceeds. A cytoplasmic calcium sensor called synaptotagamin II also influences exocytosis by mast cells (63).

4 MEDIATORS

Mediators secreted by activated mast cells and basophils can be divided into those stored in secretory granules before cell activation, and those that are newly generated after an activation signal. The former include histamine, proteoglycans, and proteases; the latter include metabolites of arachidonic acid, cytokines, and chemokines, as summarized in Figure 7.

4.1 Biogenic Amine(s)

4.1.1 Histamine

Histamine is the sole biogenic amine in human mast cells and basophils. Histamine (β-imidazolylethylamine) is formed from histidine by histidine decarboxylase (Fig. 8). Hista-

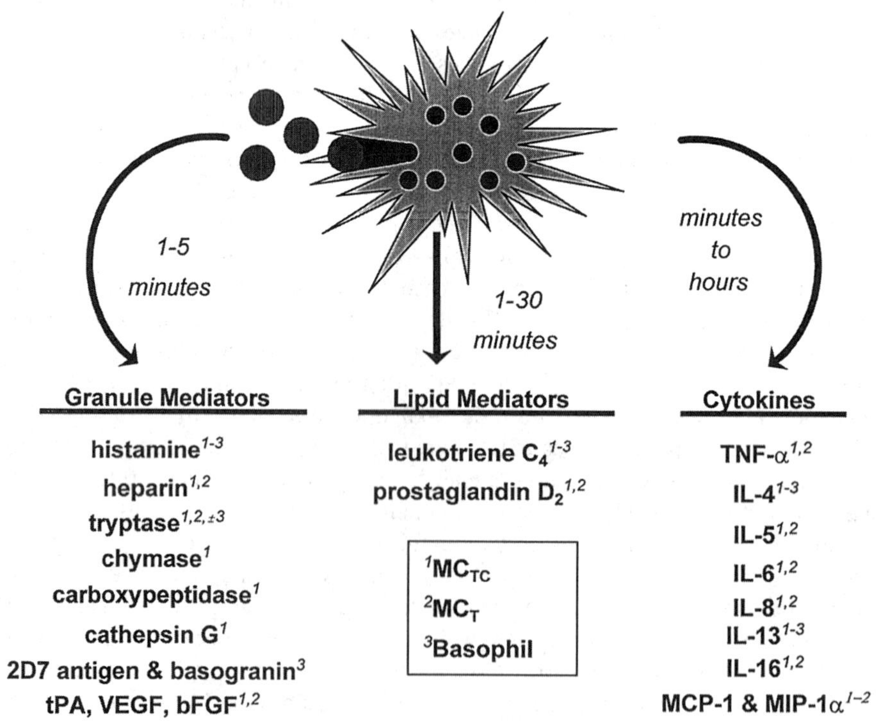

Figure 7 Mediators of activated mast cells and basophils.

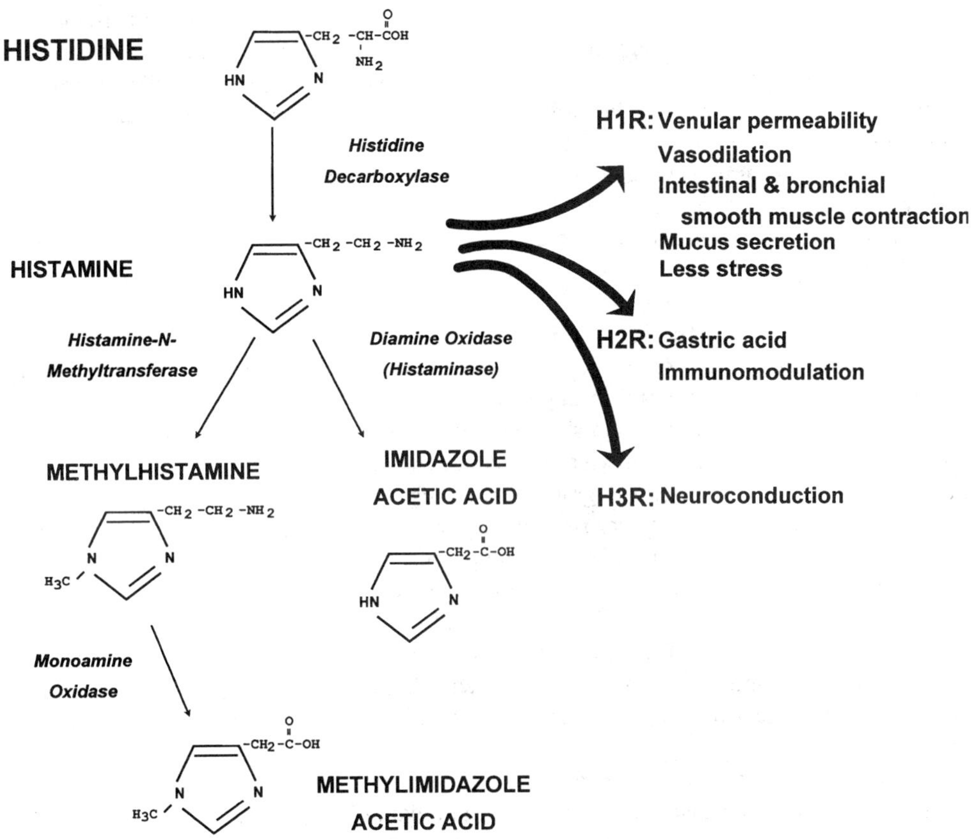

Figure 8 Histamine synthesis and metabolism.

mine is then stored in secretory granules. Histamine is the only preformed mediator of human mast cells with direct potent vasoactive and smooth-muscle spasmogenic effects. With degranulation histamine is released and diffuses rapidly. Extracellular histamine is metabolized within minutes of release, suggesting that it is destined to act quickly and locally. Human mast cells and basophils contain 1–3 pg of histamine per cell. Histamine concentrations of about 0.1 M are estimated to exist inside secretory granules; whereas concentrations of about 2 nM exist in plasma. The amount of histamine present in circulating basophils, if released, could raise plasma histamine levels about 500-fold, so great care must be exercised to avoid disrupting basophils when collecting blood for a plasma histamine determination. Histamine levels in samples obtained from sites outside of the circulation reflect local rates of production and removal. Elevated levels of histamine in plasma or urine are detected after anaphylactic reactions to allergens or radiocontrast dyes and in a portion of subjects with mastocytosis, consistent with mast cell and or basophil involvement. However, in subjects in septic shock and in those with an attack of hereditary angioedema, histamine levels are not elevated, consistent with a lack of involvement of these cells.

Histamine exerts its biological and pathobiological effects through its interaction with cell-specific receptors designated H_1, H_2, and H_3, which initially were defined with the recognition of specific agonists and antagonists. H_1 (64) and H_2 (65) receptors each have seven regions predicted to span the plasma membrane, and are G protein-coupled receptors. H_1 receptors are blocked by chlorpheniramine; H_2 receptors are blocked by cimetidine; and H_3 receptors are blocked by thioperamide. Examples of receptor specific agonists include 2-methylhistamine at H_1 receptors, dimaprit at H_2 receptors, and α-methylhistamine at H_3 receptors.

Effects of histamine (see Fig. 8) mediated by H_1 receptors include enhanced permeability of postcapillary venules, vasodilation, contraction of bronchial and gastrointestinal smooth muscle, and increased mucus secretion at mucosal sites. Increased vasopermeability will facilitate the tissue deposition of factors from plasma that may be important for tissue growth and repair, and of foreign material or immune complexes that result in tissue inflammation. Histamine, by an H_1–receptor-dependent mechanism in rodents, also activates endothelial cells to transfer P-selectin from internal Weibel–Palade bodies to the cell surface, where neutrophil rolling is thereby enhanced (66,67). $H_1R^{-/-}$ mice exhibit modest neurological alterations, but show no developmental abnormalities (68). H_2 receptor agonists stimulate gastric acid secretion by parietal cells. H_2 agonists also inhibit secretion by cytotoxic lymphocytes and granulocytes; augment suppression by T lymphocytes; enhance epithelial permeability across human airways; stimulate chemokinesis of neutrophils and eosinophils and expression of eosinophil C3b receptors; and activate endothelial cells to release a potent inhibitor of platelet aggregation, prostacyclin (PGI_2). Stimulation of H_3 receptors affect neurotransmitter release and histamine formation in the central and peripheral nervous system. They are postulated, but not proved to be involved in crosstalk between mast cells and peripheral nerves. Bronchial hyperreactivity in atopics with asthma to irritant stimuli may be partly mediated by histamine-mediated neurogenic hyperexcitability.

The combined effects of H_1– and H_2–receptor-mediated activities of histamine are required for the full expression of vasoactivity. For example, the ''triple response'' caused by an intradermal injection of histamine—namely, a central erythema within seconds (histamine arteriolar vasodilation), followed by circumferential erythema (axon reflex vasodilation mediated by neuropeptides) and a central weal (histamine vasopermeability, edema) peaking at about 15 min—is mostly blocked by H_1 receptor antagonists, but is completely blocked only with a combination of H_1 and H_2 receptor antagonists (69). Analogous results have been observed for the tachycardia, widened pulse pressure, diastolic hypotension, flushing, and headaches resulting from intravenous infusion of histamine (70).

4.2 Proteoglycans

4.2.1 Heparin and Chondroitin Sulfates E and A

The presence of highly sulfated proteoglycans in secretory granules of mast cells and basophils results in metachromasia when these cells are stained with basic dyes. Proteoglycans are composed of glycosaminoglycan side chains (repeating unbranched disaccharide units of a uronic acid and hexosamine moieties that are variably sulfated) covalently linked to a single-chain protein core by a specific trisaccharide–protein linkage region consisting of-Gal-Gal-Xyl-Ser. The intracellular proteoglycans of concern to mast cells are heparin and chondroitin sulfate E. Chondroitin sulfate A is the predominant type in human basophils and eosinophils. Among bone marrow-derived cells, heparin is selectively expressed by mast cells, and resides in the secretory granules of all mature mast cells (71). Glial cells are also capable of producing heparin (72). When mast cells are activated to degranulate, heparin proteoglycan is exocytosed along with other granule constituents in a complex with positively charged proteases likely to include tryptase and chymase.

The characteristic disaccharide units of heparin, chondroitin sulfate E and chondroitin sulfate A are shown in Figure 9. The average number of sulfate residues per respective disaccharide is 2.5, 1.5, and 1.0. The characteristic susceptibility of heparin to nitrous acid is due to attack at the *N*-sulfate residue; chondroitin sulfates lack this residue and are resistant to nitrous acid.

The same peptide core is associated with heparin and chondroitin sulfate proteoglycans, and both proteoglycan types may reside in the same cell, even on the same peptide core. In humans the core protein is 17,600 Da and contains a glycosaminoglycan attachment region of 18 amino acids, where two to three glycosaminoglycans of about 20,000 Da are attached. The attachment region is rich in alternating Ser-Gly residues, and the gene is located on chromosome 10.

The biological functions of endogenous mast cell proteoglycans are somewhat speculative. These proteoglycans bind to histamine, neutral proteases, and acid hydrolases at the acidic pH inside mast cell secretory granules and may facilitate processing of the enzymes as well as uptake and packaging of these mediators into the secretory granules. The stabilizing effect of heparin and, to a lesser degree, chondroitin sulfate E, on human tryptase activity may be crucial for the full expression of mast cell-mediated events. Heparin and chondroitin sulfate E (to a smaller extent) express anticoagulant, anticomplement,

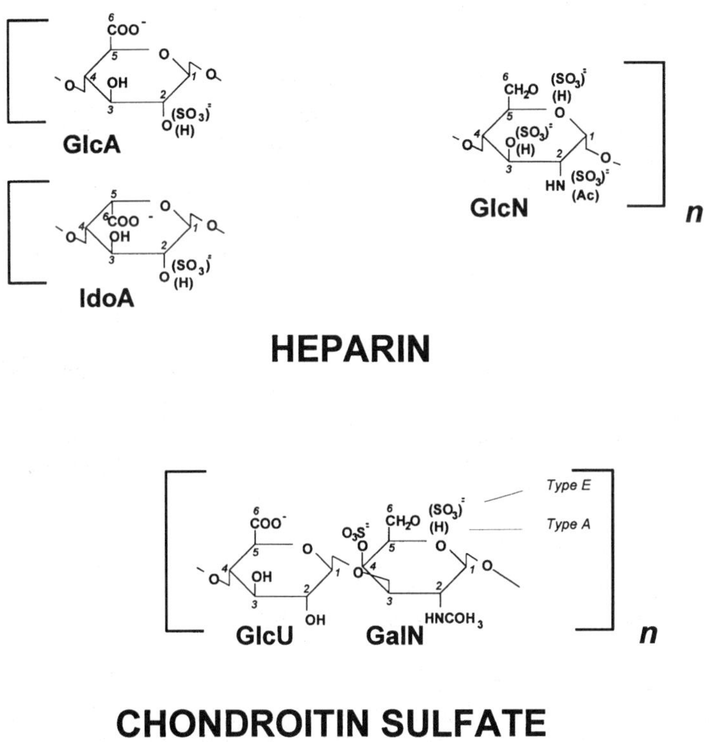

Figure 9 Structures of the disaccharides characteristic of heparin and chondroitin sulfate glycosaminoglycans.

antikallikrein, and Hageman factor autoactivation activities. Heparin neutralizes the ability of eosinophil-derived major basic protein to kill schistosomula and enhances the binding of fibronectin to collagen. Heparin protects and facilitates basic fibroblast growth factor activity, which appears to reside in cutaneous mast cells (73), and modulates the cell adhesion properties of matrix proteins, such as vitronectin, fibronectin, and laminin. Binding of heparin to L- and P-selectins inhibits inflammation (74), perhaps by blocking leukocyte rolling. The anticoagulant activities of human and commercial porcine heparin are similar and depend on a specific pentasaccharide sequence. However, when heparin is saturated with tryptase and other mast cell proteases, these activities may be attenuated. Disrupting the gene encoding glucosaminyl *N*-deacetylase/*N*-sulfotransferase-2 (NDST-2) (75,76) in mice yields mast cells containing oversulfated chondroitin sulfate and undersulfated heparin. Only those mast cells that normally produce heparin in mice were affected (the so-called connective tissue-type mast cell). These mouse mast cells exhibited large vacuolated granules that were deficient in histamine and protease activities, but coagulation-related problems were not noted.

4.3 Proteases

Proteases are enzymes that cleave peptide bonds, and certain ones are the dominant protein components of secretory granules in human and rodent mast cells. Basophils, compared with mast cells, are deficient in the secretory granules' protease activity. Some of these enzymes serve as selective markers that distinguish mast cells from other cell types, including basophils, and different mast cell subpopulations from one another.

4.3.1 Tryptase

Trypsin-like activity was first associated with human mast cells by histoenzymatic stains (77–79). Abundant and releasable trypsin-like activity was found in human lung-derived mast cells in 1981 (80), followed by purification to homogeneity of the enzyme, accounting for more than 90% of this activity, which was named tryptase (81). The enzyme was a tetramer that spontaneously and irreversibly reverted to inactive monomers at neutral pH in a physiological salt solution unless stabilized by heparin or dextran sulfate (82,83). In 1998, the crystal structure of lung-derived tryptase was solved (84), confirming the tetrameric structure and the length of the heparin-binding groove previously predicted (82). Two heparin grooves per tetramer were found, each spanning the two adjacent subunits bound to one another only through weak hydrophobic interactions. All of the active sites faced into the small, central pore of the planar tetramer, thereby restricting inhibitor (and substrate) access (85). Because tryptase is selectively concentrated in mast cell secretory granules, it has also been studied as a clinical marker of mast cell-mediated diseases.

Different Human Mast Cell Tryptases

Several cDNAs for human tryptase have been cloned (86). Tryptase genes are clustered on the short arm of human chromosome 16 (87,88). They have been divided into two types, α-tryptase and β-tryptase, and several subtypes, each encoding a 30-amino acid leader and 245-amino acid catalytic portions. α-Tryptases show approximately 90% sequence identity with β-tryptases. Defining differences appear to include R^{-3} and G^{215} in β-tryptases and Q^{-3} and D^{215} in α-tryptases. The αI- and αII- tryptases and βI-, βII-, βIII-tryptases show at least 98% identity within types. Each of these tryptase genes is organized into six exons and five introns. By comparison mouse mast cell tryptases mMCP-6 and mMCP-7 (89,90), syntenic on mouse chromosome 17, have amino acid sequences 71% identical with one another, each of which shows about 75% sequence identity and an exon–intron organization similar to the human enzymes. Human α- and β-tryptases are more closely related to one another than to known nonhuman tryptases (91). Although some ambiguity still remains in the number of tryptase genes per human haploid chromosome, at least one or two of the three β-tryptase subtypes, at least one of the two α-tryptase subtypes, and one pseudotryptase gene appear to reside on human chromosome 16.

Confusion arose when the term tryptase was applied to other trypsin-like serine proteases that are not closely related to tryptase. These include trypsin-like enzymes in natural killer (NK) and cytotoxic T cells (NK-tryptases) (92–94), a MOLT-4 Th cell line (tryptase TL_2) (95), and lung Clara cells (tryptase Clara) (96). However, these enzymes do not show sufficient sequence homology or comparable biochemical properties to include them in the mast cell tryptase family described in the foregoing, and they also reside in distinct genetic loci. A family of serine protease genes has been cloned near the tryptase locus on human chromosome 16 and mouse chromosome 17, and they are referred to as transmembrane tryptases because of a predicted transmembrane region near the C-terminus and trypsin-like substrate specificity (97). Again, these enzyme appear to be biochemically and immunologically distinct from α- and β-tryptases. Herein the term tryptase will be used only for the α- and β-tryptases of human mast cells.

Processing of Tryptase Precursors

Purified recombinant αI-protryptase and βII-protryptase were used to study processing to the active enzyme(s) (98,99). No pathway for processing α_I-protryptase was found. βII-Protryptase was processed in two proteolytic steps. First, autocatalytic intermolecular cleavage at R^{-3} occurred optimally at acidic pH and in the presence of heparin (or dextran sulfate). Second, the remaining Pro′ dipeptide was removed by dipeptidyl peptidase I (DPPI), a cysteine peptidase, with an acidic pH optimum, found in most hematopoietic cells. The mature peptide spontaneously formed enzymatically active tetramers, a process that seemed to require heparin or dextran sulfate. This novel processing mechanism might explain why tryptase and heparin are coexpressed in human mast cells, and in mast cells of many other species. In humans, this mechanism predicts that processing of any β-tryptase in a cell without heparin and DPPI would be suboptimal. With αI-protryptase, the presence of Q^{-3} precludes optimal autocatalytic processing. Failure to process αI-protryptase to αI-pro′ tryptase might explain why human mast cells appear to spontaneously secrete α-protryptase, whereas βII-tryptase is stored in their secretory granules. Without a mechanism for processing αI (or αII)-protryptase, this protein will remain enzymatically inactive. Recombinant human αI- protryptase, with an enterokinase peptide cleavage site inserted next to the mature portion, was processed in vitro to a catalytically active enzyme (100), bypassing the need for a natural processing step. The resultant α-tryptase exhibited relatively little enzymatic activity against small synthetic substrates, and no fibrinogen-cleaving activity. Thus, a biological-processing mechanism for α-protryptase is still undefined, although removal of the pro-α peptide could result in an enzyme with limited proteolytic activity. Whether this human protein is simply a mistake of evolution without function, undergoes processing by an alternative pathway to an active form, or has a biological activity that does not require enzymatic activity remains to be understood.

Two studies in mice assessed the impact of heparin on processing of mouse tryptases by disrupting the gene encoding glucosaminyl *N*-deacetylase/*N*-sulfotransferase-2 (NDST-2) (75,76), leaving oversulfated chondroitin sulfate and partially sulfated heparin still present. Only those mast cells that normally produce heparin were affected, and they exhibited large vacuolated granules. In one study these cells were markedly deficient in histamine and in chymase and tryptase enzymatic activities (75), suggesting that processing of certain mouse chymases and mouse tryptases were suboptimal in the absence of heparin.

Tryptase Regulation

The quantity of catalytically active tryptase per mast cell (10–35 pg) (101) is dramatically higher than the levels of proteases found in other cell types, such as neutrophils (~1–3 pg of elastase and of cathepsin G per cell). What regulates tryptase activity after its release into the extracellular milieu is uncertain, because the enzyme is resistant to classic biological inhibitors of serine proteases (85). Regulation was postulated to occur by dissociation of the enzyme from heparin by basic proteins, such as antithrombin III (85), but this is slow and incomplete, providing an unsatisfactory mechanism for regulating catalytic activity.

A new possibility was raised after it was observed that lung and βII-tryptases degraded fibrinogen about 50-fold faster at pH 6 than at 7.4 (102). A similar acidic pH optimum was noted for processing of βII-protryptase (98) and for cleavage of low molecular weight kininogen (103) by lung-derived tryptase. Release of β-tryptase at sites of acidic pH (airway mucosal surface, foci of inflammation and areas of poor vascularity (e.g., solid tumor margins and wound healing sites), might be optimal for the enzyme, whereas diffusion away from such sites would result in reduced proteolytic activity. Such a mechanism would tend to limit the activity of β-tryptase to its local tissue site of release.

Catalytically active, tetrameric tryptase loses enzymatic activity and converts to monomers at neutral pH and physiological ionic strength in the absence of a stabilizing molecule such as heparin. Placing inactive tryptase monomers (formed at neutral pH) into an acidic environment leads to the complete reassociation of these monomers into a catalytically active tetramer (104). Thus, at the acidic pH optimum for proteolysis, β-tryptase catalytic activity is stabilized, and inactive tryptase monomers theoretically could reassociate into catalytically active tetramers.

Biological Activities of Tryptase

The biological activity(ies) of enzymatically active tryptase are not obvious from the involvement of mast cells in diseases such as mastocytosis, anaphylaxis, urticaria, and asthma. The most relevant biological substrate(s) of tryptase remain uncertain, although many potential ones have been evaluated, primarily in vitro. Predicted biological outcomes might include anticoagulation, fibrosis and fibrolysis, kinin generation and destruction, cell surface PAR-2 activation, enhancement of vasopermeability, angiogenesis, inflammation, and airway smooth-muscle hyperreactivity. Showing the importance of these potential activities in vivo remains a challenge. The emerging availability of pharmacological inhibitors of tryptase, and preliminary studies suggesting they attenuate the bronchial response to an allergen challenge may facilitate identification of the most important biological substrates.

4.3.2 Chymase

Chymase is one of two principal enzymes accounting for the chymotrypsin-like activity present in human cutaneous mast cells. The enzyme was purified from human skin (105), and the corresponding gene cloned and localized to human chromosome 14 (106). Chymase was selectively localized to a subpopulation of mast cells by enzymatic (107) and immunohistochemical techniques (108). Dispersed MC_{TC} cells obtained from skin contain approximately 4.5 pg of chymase per mast cell.

Human chymase is a monomer of 30,000 Da, for which the crystal structure has been solved (109). Its chymotryptic substrate specificity prefers the motif nX-P-[F,Y,W]-Y-Y, where n is 6 or more, X is any amino acid, and Y is any amino acid except P (110). Similar to tryptase, chymase is a serine esterase that is stored fully active in mast cell secretory granules, presumably bound to heparin or chondroitin sulfate E. Heparin facilitates processing of prochymase to active chymase by dipeptidyl peptidase I (111), and either attracts or repulses potential chymase substrates based on ionic forces (112). Unlike tryptase, chymase stability is not substantially affected by heparin and its activity is inhibited by classic biological inhibitors of serine proteases, such as α_1-antichymotrypsin, α_1-protease inhibitor, and α_2-macroglobulin (113). Neither chymotrypsin-like enzymatic activity nor chymase mRNA were detected in lung-derived MC_T cells (114).

Potential biological activities of chymase, similar to those of tryptase, are based on in vitro observations. Chymase is a potent activator of angiotensin I, inactivates bradykinin and PAR-1 receptors (115), and attacks the lamina lucida of the basement membrane at the dermal–epidermal junction of human skin. The potential importance of angiotensin II generation by mast cell chymase in humans is of great interest. Chymase potently stimulates mucus production from glandular cells in vitro (116), suggesting a similar role in asthma and allergic rhinitis, where release of chymase in proximity to glandular tissue might be involved in the state of hypersecretion. Biologically active Kit can be released from the cell surface by chymase (117). Processing of type I procollagen by chymase to collagen-like fibrils has been demonstrated in vitro (118), and may relate to the finding of chymase-containing mast cells at sites of fibrosis in places such as rheumatoid synovium.

4.3.3 Cathepsin G

Human mast cell cathepsin G, similar to chymase, is a serine class neutral protease with chymotryptic substrate specificity that is found in mast cells as well as in neutrophils and monocytes. The enzyme resides with chymase in MC_{TC} cells (119) and exhibits a molecular weight of 30,000. Similar to chymase, it stimulates glandular secretions (116), which is of possible importance in allergic asthma and rhinitis.

4.3.4 Mast Cell Carboxypeptidase

Human mast cell carboxypeptidase resides with chymase and cathepsin G in secretory granules of MC_{TC} cells (120). Stored fully active, when released it cleaves the C-terminal His^9–Leu^{10} bond of angiotensin I and behaves as a zinc-dependent exopeptidase. Human mast cells dispersed from skin contain 5–16 pg of carboxypeptidase per cell. Human mast cell carboxypeptidase is a monomer with a molecular weight of 34,500 (121). Based on analysis of the cDNA-derived amino acid sequence and gene structure (122), the human enzyme is more homologous with human pancreatic carboxypeptidase B than A, but the catalytic site is more homologous with human pancreatic carboxypeptidase A, as are its substrate specificities for C-terminal Phe and Leu residues.

4.3.5 Other Proteases and Enzymes

Tissue-type plasminogen activator has been identified in tissue-derived mast cells (123), potentially complementing mast cell antithrombotic and anticoagulant activities with the fibrinolytic properties of this protease. Matrix metalloprotease-9, a gelatinase, has been identified in cord blood-derived mast cells (124). Studies in dog mast cells suggest that SCF increases expression, whereas TGF-β down-regulates expression of progelatinase B (125), whereas in mice, SCF down-regulates MMP-9 (126). Thus, external agents may influence the fibrolytic versus fibrotic capabilities of this cell type. Mast cells also concentrate various acid hydrolases in their secretory granules, perhaps reflecting the lysosomal origin of this organelle, including β-galactosidase, aryl sulfatase, and β-hexosaminidase, the latter enzyme serving as a marker to evaluate degranulation of dispersed preparations of mast cells (80).

4.4 Lipids

Human mast cells that are dispersed and purified from lung incorporate exogenous arachidonic acid into neutral lipids and phospholipids, and store these lipids in membranes and cytoplasmic lipid bodies. Liberation of the arachidonic acid destined for oxidative metabolism, as shown in mice, is dependent on cytosolic phospholipase A_2 (127). In general, oxidation of arachidonic acid occurs through the cyclooxygenase (COX) pathway to prostaglandins (PGs) and thromboxanes (TXs), or the 5-, 12-, or 15-lipoxygenase (LO) pathways to monohydroxyl fatty acids, leukotrienes (LTs) that include both LTB_4, and the sulfidopeptides LTC_4, LTD_4, and LTE_4 (*slow-reacting substances of anaphylaxis*; SRS-A), and lipoxins. Platelet-activating factor, made by acetylating the lysophospholipid remaining after arachidonic acid departs, has not been shown to be a major secretory product of human mast cells and basophils. The major eicosanoid products secreted by activated mast cells and basophils are summarized in Figure 7.

Dispersed and purified preparations of human mast cells obtained from lung, skin, and intestine, on activation, produce PGD_2 (PGD synthase-dependent) and LTC_4 (LTC synthase-dependent) in weight ratios of approximately 5:1. Smaller amounts of LTB_4 isomers are also produced. Ratios of these metabolites cannot be used to distinguish MC_T from MC_{TC} cell activation. In contrast, peripheral blood basophils obtained from normal human subjects, when activated, synthesize LTC_4, but no PGD_2. However, cells other than mast cells and basophils produce PGD_2 (e.g., platelets and certain antigen-presenting cells) and LTC_4 (e.g., eosinophils). Thus, when these products are detected in a complex biological milieu, there may be ambiguity as to their cell source. Also, both leukotriene and prostaglandin production by activated mast cells can be blocked without altering release of granule mediators and cytokines.

The biological importance of mast cell-derived products of arachidonic acid has gained support with the advent of inhibitors of 5-lipoxygenase and the cysLT1 receptor (128) for LTD_4, both of which are helpful in atopic and in aspirin-induced asthma, each condition also involving activation of mast cells and eosinophils, another major source of LTC_4. Of potential clinical interest was the finding that dexamethasone can upregulate 5-LO levels and LTC_4 production by HMC-1 cells in vitro (129). A metabolite of PGD_2 is elevated in the urine of patients with active systemic mastocytosis. The importance of PGD_2 production in the subgroup of these patients with recurrent hypotensive episodes was suggested when administration of aspirin inhibited generation of the PGD_2 metabolite and led to clinical improvement (130). PGD_2 is produced by mast cells during both the immediate and late phases of immediate hypersensitivity reactions. COX-1 is responsible for PGD_2 produced during the early phase, COX-2 during the late phase (131,132). The ability of PGD_2 to activate human eosinophils (133) and to play a role during induction of allergic airway disease in mice (134) suggest its potential importance in human allergic diseases at sites of mast cell-dependent inflammation.

4.5 Cytokines and Chemokines

Human mast cells and basophils, when activated, produce a diverse array of cytokines and chemokines. These include TNF-α, ILs-3, 4, 5, 6, 8, 10, 13, and 16, lymphotactin, MCP-1, TGF-β_1 and MIP-1α by mast cells, and at least IL-4 and IL-13 by basophils. In some cases cytokines may be stored in secretory granules and released with other preformed mediators. Mast cells have been noted as the dominant IL-4$^+$ cell in allergic nasal mucosa (135) and the dominant IL-4$^+$ cell in allergen-challenged peripheral blood cells (PBCs) (136). Cytokines also can be newly generated and released hours after mast cells or basophils are activated. These cytokines serve to recruit and activate other cell types, thereby amplifying the host response during immediate hypersensitivity events. For example, endothelial cells are activated to recruit eosinophils and other cell types during the late-phase response of immediate hypersensitivity reactions. Mast cells can thereby be involved in sustaining allergic inflammation hours after granule exocytosis is finished.

5 BIOLOGY AND PATHOBIOLOGY OF HUMAN MAST CELLS

5.1 Clinical Markers of Mast Cells and Basophils

The involvement of mast cells and basophils in human diseases can be addressed in terms of both cell numbers and cell activation. Antibodies developed against cell-specific surface or granule components provide an immunohistological means for detecting these cells in tissues with greater sensitivity and specificity than classic dye-based histological stains. Moreover, immunoassays for cell-specific, releasable, and preformed granule mediators provide a more precise measure of either local or systemic activation of a particular cell type than is possible by either clinical criteria or documentation of antigen-specific IgE in an antigen-challenged subject.

The most selective surface marker phenotype for all human mast cells are the coexpression of high levels of Kit and FcεRI. This pattern can be readily demonstrated on dispersed mast cells by flow cytometry, but this method is technically more difficult to perform on tissue sections by immunohistochemistry. Tryptase is a granule marker selective for all human mast cells; the more than 100-fold smaller amounts present in basophils provide an adequate differential for distinguishing these two cell types from one another. MAbs against chymase and mast cell carboxypeptidase serve to identify the MC_{TC}-type mast cell, because no other cell type has been clearly shown to express these products in sufficient quantity to be confused with mast cells. No specific marker for the MC_T-type mast cell has been identified.

Most MAbs against human tryptase recognize both α- and β-tryptase products, whereas one MAb called G5 (linear epitope) recognizes β-tryptase but not α-protryptase. This is of clinical relevance because α-protryptase appears to be continuously secreted by human mast cells, levels in blood thereby serving as a measure of mast cell number. In contrast, β-tryptase is stored in secretory granules and is released only during granule exocytosis, levels thereby serving as a measure of mast cell activation. Immunoassays using G5 preferentially measure β-tryptase, those using other antitryptase MAbs (e.g., B12 [conformational epitope] and G4 [linear epitope]) measure total (α- plus β-) tryptase

Table 1 Characteristics of Immunoassays for Different Forms of Human Tryptase Measured in Serum

Clinical condition	β-Tryptase (ng/mL)	Total tryptase (α- and β-tryptases) (ng/mL)	Total/β-tryptase ratio (β-tryptase ≥ 1 ng/mL)
Normal	<1	1–15	NA
Systemic anaphylaxis (within 4 hr of onset)	≥1	↑ over baseline	≤10
Systemic mastocytosis (nonacute interval)	Varies	≥20	≥20

(137–139). The current immunoassay available commercially for total tryptase (B12 capture or G4 detection) has a lower limit of detection in serum of about 0.5 ng/mL, but detects tryptase in nearly all normal subjects (mean of 5 ng/mL; range 1–15 ng/mL). The immunoassay used for β-tryptase has a detection sensitivity of approximately 1 ng/mL in serum, and does not detect any tryptase in normal serum. Characteristics of these immunoassays for serum tryptase are summarized in Table 1.

Although an $Fc\varepsilon RI^+/Kit^-$ surface phenotype or $Fc\varepsilon RI^+$/tryptase$^-$ surface/granule phenotype have been considered to selectively represent basophils, the abilities of activated monocytes, eosinophils, and antigen-presenting cells, such as Langerhans cells, to express FcεRI make this consideration problematic, particularly at sites of inflammation (140). Two MAbs (141,142) that recognize components of basophil secretory granules, but do not label other cell types, including mast cells and eosinophils, identify basophils in tissues by immunohistochemisty. The respective antigens are called 2D7 antigen and basogranin, and may lead to the development of precise assays for assessing basophil activation that occurs in vivo.

Following are discussions of mast cells and basophils in several atopic and nonatopic conditions. These conditions are not inclusive, because involvement of these cells in atherosclerosis, blood pressure regulation, and a wide array of inflammatory disorders throughout the body have been reported.

5.2 Systemic Anaphylaxis

β-Tryptase levels in serum or plasma are elevated in most subjects with systemic anaphylaxis of sufficient severity to result in hypotension (143). β-Tryptase is released from mast cells in parallel with histamine (80), but diffuses more slowly than histamine, presumably owing to its association with the macromolecular protease:proteoglycan complex. During insect sting-induced anaphylaxis, β-tryptase levels in the circulation are maximal 15–120 min after the sting, whereas histamine levels peak at about 5 min and decline to baseline by 15–30 min (144,145). Peak β-tryptase levels decline with a half-life of 1.5–2.5 hr. The practical consequence of these different time courses is that plasma samples for histamine levels must be obtained within 15 min of the onset of such reactions, whereas those for β-tryptase levels can be obtained up to several hours after the reaction began, depending on its severity. In insect–sting-induced systemic anaphylaxis, the ratios of total tryptase to β-tryptase were less than 6 in 16 of 17 subjects; being 23 in the 1 outlier (138). Thus, when β-tryptase is detectable in serum, a total to β-tryptase ratio of 10 or less suggests systemic anaphylaxis. Mast cells also have been implicated in anaphylactic reactions to cyclooxygenase inhibitors by finding elevated levels of β-tryptase in blood (144,146). Whether COX-2-selective agents will activate mast cells in such subjects is unresolved.

β-Tryptase levels also have been used to investigate hypotensive episodes occurring during induction of general anesthesia with thiopentone and suxamethonium (147). One subject had an elevated level of β-tryptase associated with a finding of IgE against thiopentone, consistent with mast cell activation. The other subject had neither an elevated level of β-tryptase nor antigen-specific IgE, suggesting mast cells were not involved. A related case report of a hypotensive reaction to thiopental in which plasma histamine was elevated 10 min after the onset of hypotension, but no elevation of β-tryptase was detected at 45 min (148), suggests basophil, not mast cell, activation.

β-Tryptase levels in serum were determined in possible cases of fatal systemic anaphylaxis within 24 hr of death in 19 victims (149). Elevated levels (>10 ng/mL) appeared in 9 of 9 patients after Hymenoptera stings, 6 of 8 after food, and 2 of 2 to parenteral diagnostic or therapeutic agents. Levels were less than 5 ng/mL in 57 sequential sera collected postmortem from six control subjects. In general, β-tryptase levels were dramatically higher after parenteral, rather than oral, introduction of the allergen, in spite of a fatal outcome in each case. In cases of clinical anaphylaxis with a normal level of β-tryptase, pathogenetic mechanisms without mast cell activation should be considered. These might include basophil activation or complement anaphylatoxin generation.

Anaphylaxis has been postulated as a cause of the sudden infant death syndrome (SIDS), but neither allergen sensitivity nor mast cell activation had been shown (150–152). Elevated postmortem levels of β-tryptase in victims of SIDS were then reported in two studies that included comparable groups of victims of explained deaths (153,154), and in one study without an explained-death control group (155). Another study failed to find an increase in postmortem tryptase levels in a SIDS group compared with explained-death controls (156). Although no significant associations between antigen-specific IgE and β-tryptase levels were found in any of these studies, mast cell activation appears to be occurring in the SIDS group in three of the four studies, perhaps by a non–IgE-dependent mechanism. Increased numbers of eosinophils in lung tissue examined from SIDS infants (157), but no increase in tissue mast cells (154) also have been noted. Apnea as a manifestation of systemic anaphylaxis occurred in an infant with underlying systemic mastocytosis (158), and may reflect a different pathophysiological response in infants than in adults to systemic mast cell activation that is relevant to the subgroup of SIDS subjects with elevated levels of β-tryptase. However, no evidence for underlying systemic mastocytosis has emerged in SIDS. Mast cell-dependent anaphylaxis as one cause of SIDS will need to be considered further.

Against the diagnostic specificity of postmortem β-tryptase levels is a study that found elevated levels of β-tryptase (>10 ng/mL) in 5 of 49 cases thought to be nonanaphylactic deaths (158a). One was a salicylate overdose (23 ng/mL). Because mast cell activation occurs with anaphylactic and airway hypersensitivity reactions to cyclooxygenase inhibitors, this subject could have been aspirin-sensitive. Another had a diagnosis of atherosclerotic coronary vascular disease (33 ng of β-tryptase per milliliter) as did ten other subjects with levels less than 5 ng/mL. Details on drugs received near the time of death, particularly those that might activate mast cells, such as morphine, were unavailable. Three died of multiple trauma (20, 24, 106 ng of β-tryptase/mL). Thus, a careful consideration of the events near the time of death may be needed to fully interpret postmortem levels of β-tryptase.

5.3 Systemic Mastocytosis

Systemic mastocytosis is associated with mast cell hyperplasia in skin lesions (urticaria pigmentosa), liver, spleen, lymph nodes, and bone marrow (159). The disorder is subdivided into those with indolent mastocytosis, systemic mastocytosis associated with a hematological disorder, and aggressive systemic mastocytosis (160). Activating mutations of Kit appear to be associated with systemic or persistent disease (12,161). The gold standard for the diagnosis of mastocytosis is a tissue biopsy showing a pathological increase in the number of mast cells. However, in skin there is no precise mast cell concentration that defines cutaneous mastocytosis. In bone marrow biopsies, paratrabecular collections of spindle-shaped mast cells intermixed with fibroblasts, mononuclear cells, and eosinophils are characteristic of systemic mastocytosis (159,162). Such cells typically remain in the bone marrow environment, because granulated mast cells are rarely detected in the circulation. Mast cells in lesions of peripheral tissues presumably contain mast cells that mature in those tissue. However, characteristic lesions in the bone marrow are not always evident. Also, tryptase immunostaining may provide a more sensitive and specific marker of mastocytosis in bone marrow biopsy specimens than classic histochemical or histoenzymatic stains (163), suggesting false-negative readings in some cases subjected to a standard analysis of the biopsy. There is no precise mast cell concentration in bone marrow biopsies or aspirates now in use to distinguish mastocytosis from normal tissue. Because biopsy criteria for diagnosing systemic mastocytosis are not precise, and a biopsy could miss disease present at other sites, the relative value of α-protryptase levels in the workup of suspected systemic mastocytosis should be considered.

In a study of tryptase levels in subjects with biopsy-diagnosed mastocytosis, most of those with systemic mastocytosis (35 of 42), indicated by a bone marrow biopsy, had levels of total tryptase higher than 20 ng/mL and ratios of total tryptase to β-tryptase higher than 20 (139). Normal subjects ($n = 55$) had total tryptase levels less than 14 ng/mL (138). This suggested a specificity greater than 98%, and a sensitivity of 83% for total tryptase levels, when compared with a bone marrow biopsy. However, among the seven subjects with systemic mastocytosis and a serum total tryptase level below 20 ng/mL, all had total tryptase levels between 10 and 20 ng/mL; three had ambiguous bone marrow readings; and another had the bone marrow biopsy performed 5 years before the serum sample was collected. Most subjects with local cutaneous mast cell disease (10 of 13) had levels similar to normal controls (1–11 ng/mL; ratios $\leq$ 11). Among the three subjects with serum total tryptase levels above this range, one was an infant with diffuse cutaneous mastocytosis; and another had no bone marrow biopsy performed. The indolent group with urticaria pigmentosa and no evidence of systemic involvement had levels of total tryptase in the normal range. Thus, the level of total tryptase appears to distinguish those with local versus systemic disease. However, the absolute level of total tryptase did not predict clinical severity, suggesting that factors other than the mast cell burden alone are important. These might include the magnitude and frequency of mast cell activation events, the sites of mast cell hyperplasia, or the tissue response to mast cell mediators.

Daily subcutaneous injections of SCF over a 2-week interval in human volunteers with metastatic cancer produced marked increases in total tryptase levels, whereas those of β-tryptase remained undetectable, suggesting iatrogenic systemic mastocytosis (164). Levels returned to baseline within 1–2 weeks of discontinuation of SCF in the absence of signs of immediate hypersensitivity. Presumably, mast cells underwent apoptosis when excessive SCF was withdrawn, because there were no immediate hypersensitivity reactions associated with the decline in total tryptase levels.

Levels of total tryptase should be useful in evaluating therapies designed to reduce the mast cell burden in patients with systemic mastocytosis. Three subjects with this disorder were treated with 4–5 × 10^6 U/day m^2 of α-interferon for at least 12 months (164). Overall clinical status did not improve and total tryptase levels were unchanged, indicating no reduction in the mast cell burden.

Anaphylactic or anaphylactoid reactions may be a presenting manifestation of systemic mastocytosis. For example, in subjects who experienced anaphylaxis to insect stings, but were later found to be without venom-specific IgE, elevated total tryptase levels were found that suggested underlying mastocytosis was present and predisposed them to these anaphylactoid reactions (165,166). A previous report of tryptase levels in experimental insect sting-induced anaphylaxis found a total tryptase level higher than 10 ng/mL before the sting challenge in 5 of the 17 subjects who later developed severe anaphylactic reactions with higher levels of β-tryptase (138). These elevated baseline levels varied from 11 to 18 ng/mL. Whether tryptase levels in this range will prove to be an important risk factor for severe anaphylaxis needs further evaluation.

A retrospective analysis of the clinical value of an elevated level of total tryptase (≥20 ng/mL) with a normal or low (≤5 ng/mL) level of β-tryptase, using samples received in a diagnostic immunology laboratory over a 3.5-year period was performed (158). Among the 79 specimens that qualified, 52 patients were successfully evaluated, including 30 with clinically suspected systemic anaphylaxis, and 22 with clinically suspected systemic mastocytosis. Three hypotheses emerged. First, total tryptase serum levels are a better reflection of the total mast cell burden than focal tissue biopsies and, thereby, serve as a more sensitive and specific screening test for systemic mastocytosis. This is because the prevalence of positive biopsies for systemic mastocytosis increased as the level of total tryptase increased (100% positive biopsies if total tryptase >75 ng/mL, 50% positive biopsies if total tryptase levels were 20–75 ng/mL). Second, an elevated body burden of mast cells may spontaneously reverse, suggesting that follow-up total tryptase levels may have prognostic value. Third, anaphylaxis may be a presenting manifestation of systemic mastocytosis or mast cell hyperplasia, and that some adult subjects with apparent systemic mastocytosis, based on an elevated total tryptase level, may have transient disease.

Whether those subjects with a tryptase level from 20 to 75 ng/mL and a negative biopsy truly had systemic mastocytosis that was missed by a focal biopsy bears further consideration. One possibility is that total tryptase levels in this range may not always reflect an elevated mast cell burden. For example, if the output of α-protryptase per mast cell increases, or the rate of removal of α-protryptase from the circulation diminishes, higher levels of total tryptase would result. However, whether either of these two scenarios is biologically relevant remains to be clarified. Another possibility is that markedly elevated levels of basophils could lead to elevated levels of total tryptase. α-Tryptase mRNA is the predominant tryptase transcript in normal peripheral blood basophils, although tryptase mRNA and protein levels in basophils are much lower than in mast cells (114,167). At present, the primary determinant of α-protryptase levels appears to be the total body burden of mast cells.

Another consideration is whether an elevated mast cell burden is a permanent condition. Many, if not all, subjects diagnosed with systemic mastocytosis carry somatic mutations in Kit (12,168–170). Once such a mutation forms in an appropriate hematopoietic cell, one could predict that mast cell development and survival would increase (171), leading to a chronically increased mast cell burden, somewhat analogous to the outcome of exogenously administered SCF. However, in the latter instance, withdrawal of exogenous SCF permits the total tryptase level, and presumably the mast cell burden, to return to baseline. Another example of inducible mast cell hyperplasia, this time in rodent lungs, is one in which mast cell hyperplasia is associated with virus infection (172–174). Children with urticaria pigmentosa often experience spontaneous remission of their skin lesions with time. Thus, it is possible that transient elevations of SCF or of other putative mast cell growth factors could lead to a transient mast cell hyperplasia without involving somatic mutations of Kit. A predictive marker for persistence or remission would be clinically useful. Whether the respective presence or absence of the somatic Kit mutations associated with systemic mastocytosis (175,176) will serve this role is an issue for future research. Also, clinical trials aimed at reducing the mast cell burden need appropriate placebo control arms to take into account that even in adults an elevated mast cell burden may occasionally spontaneously decline.

5.4 Cutaneous Allergic Reactions

In studies of cutaneous allergic reactions using the skin chamber system, histamine levels are maximal by 30 min after allergen challenge, β-tryptase at about 60 min (177). Because β-tryptase and histamine are released together with degranulation, this delayed appearance of β-tryptase most likely reflects slower diffusion of β-tryptase (which is released as a complex with proteoglycan) through the cutaneous tissue. If the allergen challenge is interrupted by replacement of the fluid with buffer alone after the first hour, β-tryptase and histamine levels decline back to unstimulated levels within 4 h; in spite of an influx of leukocytes, including a few basophils, after the first hour. Of clinical interest is the observation that grass pollen immunotherapy administered to sensitive subjects results in declines both in skin test reactivity and in cutaneous mast cell concentrations (178).

A clinically apparent late response along with a greater recruitment of inflammatory cells occurs with a continuous allergen challenge over several hours in the skin chamber system. Nevertheless, β-tryptase levels return to baseline as before (179). In contrast, histamine levels decline to a modestly elevated level after the first hour of allergen and remain elevated for at least 6 hr of continuous challenge. Glucocorticosteroid pretreatment has no effect on β-tryptase and histamine levels during the immediate response to allergen, nor on codeine-induced release of β-tryptase and histamine, but completely blocks the persistent appearance of histamine (180). Direct evidence to support basophil involvement was provided by staining biopsies obtained after 6 hr of allergen challenge with a basophil-specific MAb (181,182). Basophils were abundant in and around blood vessels of antigen-challenged sites, but not at buffer-challenged sites, even though few if any metachromatic cells were associated with these areas. The findings indicate that basophils enter these sites through blood vessels, encounter allergen and a chemokine–interleukin-rich environment, and are strongly activated.

In contrast to urticaria induced by cutaneous allergen injection, most patients with idiopathic urticaria exhibit no concomitant late-phase reaction and a minimal cellular infiltrate. Mast cell hyperplasia is not apparent at lesional sites (183). In vivo, autoantibodies against FcεRIα (184) and against IgE (185) in subjects with idiopathic urticaria have been detected, suggesting an autoimmune etiology in some patients with this disorder. However, these autoantibodies alone do not explain the tissue specificity of these diseases for mast cells in skin which, in turn, might be explained by complement anaphylatoxin generated at these sites, because C5a activates mast cells from skin, but not those from lungs (186).

5.5 Rhinitis

In sensitive subjects, mediator levels in nasal lavage fluid following an allergen challenge indicate mast cells degranulate during the early phase of the response, whereas eosinophils and possibly basophils degranulate during the late phase. Accordingly, β-tryptase, histamine, and prostaglandin D_2 are elevated during the early response, but only histamine during the late response (187–190). Mast cell degranulation appears to be an ongoing process during seasonal allergic rhinitis, because β-tryptase levels in nasal fluid are elevated in-season, and return to baseline out-of-season (191). Mast cells, predominantly of the MC_T type, increase in number in the superficial nasal mucosa and epithelium during active seasonal allergic rhinitis (46,192). As in asthma, whether this represents a selective migration of MC_T cells from the deeper mucosa or selective recruitment and development of MC_T cells to this site is unknown. Nevertheless, inhaled allergen will have less of a distance to travel before encountering epithelial mast cells, which may partly account for the clinical hyperresponsiveness to inhaled aeroallergens noted during the allergy season. Drugs that prevent the appearance of epithelial mast cells, such as glucocorticosteroids (193), should reduce this seasonal hyperresponsiveness. Also, using basophil- and mast cell-specific MAbs, grass pollen immunotherapy reduced the seasonal increase in epithelial basophils, but did not affect total mast cell numbers (194).

5.6 Asthma

Mast cell activation appears to be a constitutive signature characteristic of the inflammatory process involved in asthma, whereas increased numbers of mast cells can be found in airway epithelium (195), but not in the subepithelium (196,197). Basophil numbers after an allergen challenge, using basophil-specific MAbs, are substantially elevated in sputum and in asthmatic airway tissue, but still appear to be much fewer than the numbers of eosinophils (182,198,199). Evidence for ongoing mast cell activation in well-controlled asthmatics includes elevated levels of histamine (200), tryptase (201), and PGD_2 (202) in bronchoalveolar lavage (BAL) fluid, mast cells with morphological characteristics of activation in bronchial biopsies (197), and by airway hyperresponsiveness to inhaled adenosine (203–205). Adenosine-dependent activation of asthmatic mast cells can be deduced because adenosine-induced bronchospasm is significantly inhibited by pretreatment with an H_1 antihistamine (204) and occurs with elevated levels of histamine, tryptase, and PGD_2 in bronchoalveolar lavage fluid (BALF) (144).

The early and late response to endobronchial challenge of atopic subjects without asthma (206) revealed a dose–response increase in tryptase levels in BALF 12 min after allergen challenge, but a return to baseline levels by 48 hr (Table 2). In contrast, eosinophil numbers and mediators were negligible early and markedly elevated late. Histamine levels were markedly elevated at 12 min, and, although diminished at 48 hr, were still higher than at baseline. These data suggest that after a single allergen challenge mast cell degranulation occurs early, but not late, and that the recruitment and activation of eosinophils, and possibly basophils, occurs during the late response. In addition, rhinovirus infection in atopic rhinitis patients results in increased amounts of tryptase and histamine being released after bronchial allergen challenge and the appearance of a late-phase response

Table 2 Mast Cell Activation in Asthma

Challenge condition	Tryptase in airway fluid
Atopic asthma	
Baseline	+
Early phase to allergen	++
Late phase to allergen	+
Early phase to adenosine	++
Aspirin	++
Exercise	+
Atopy without asthma	
Baseline	−
Early phase to allergen	+
Late phase to allergen	−

of pulmonary function, suggesting that virus infection may augment the mast cell response to allergen (207).

Mast cell involvement has been assessed in exercise-induced asthma (208,209). Before and approximately 30 min after exercise, levels of histamine, tryptase, PGD_2, and LTC_4, measured in the BAL fluid of atopic subjects with exercise-induced asthma did not increase, indicating that no activation of mast cells above baseline occurred with exercise. However, pharmacological studies with antihistamines or leukotriene antagonists attenuate exercise-induced bronchospasm, suggesting mast cell involvement. A possible unifying hypothesis is that elevated baseline levels of histamine and leukotrienes lower the threshold for neuronal activation, and that antagonists of these mediators raise this threshold, thereby attenuating the irritant response to exercise. Consequently, activation of mast cells by exercise beyond that which is present at baseline would not be necessary to evoke the observed bronchospastic response.

Mast cell activation appears to be involved in the immediate response to oral aspirin challenge of sensitive subjects, because aspirin challenge of sensitive asthmatics results in elevated tryptase levels in blood among those with a strong clinical response (210), and in nasal fluid among nearly all clinical responders (211). In the latter study, inhibition of 5-lipoxygenase before aspirin challenge not only attenuated nasal symptoms and levels of leukotriene, but also attenuated the elevation in tryptase levels, suggesting an unanticipated effect on mast cell activation. Thus, mast cells seem to be involved in immediate-type aspirin-induced respiratory reactions.

5.7 Arthritis

Possible roles for mast cell involvement in arthritis are well documented (212). Mast cell hyperplasia has been noted in rheumatoid synovium (not osteoarthitis synovium), which often is observed near sites of cartilage erosion (213). These findings may relate to expression of SCF by synovial fibroblasts (214). Increased numbers of the MC_T type of mast cell are seen in association with mononuclear infiltrates; increased MC_{TC} cells are seen with fibrosis (215,216). In this light, the in vitro observations that tryptase can stimulate fibroblasts to increase production of procollagen (217,218), while chymase can process procollagen to collagen fibrils (118), suggests a concerted action of these proteases toward fibrosis. Mast cells free in synovial fluid are occasionally observed. Suppression of mast cell hyperplasia occurs after intrasynovial injection of glucocorticosteroid, but not after treatment with low-dose methotrexate. IgE rheumatoid factors have been observed in synovial fluid capable of activating mast cells in vitro. However, astemizole, a potent antihistamine, did not affect the clinical course of rheumatoid arthritis, suggesting that if mast cells are involved, released histamine has little effect on the disease. Released tryptase may affect cartilage and bone turnover and synovial fibrosis. In synovial fluid taken from subjects with various arthritides, including osteoarthritis, rheumatoid arthritis, and acute gout, levels of tryptase did not correlate with a particular pathogenic etiology or with the degree of complement activation, although lower levels of tryptase were found more often in fluids with higher levels of C3a. Whether tryptase levels in synovial fluid accurately reflect levels of mast cell activation in synovial tissue is unclear. Larger volumes of synovial fluid, faster rates of exchange of soluble proteins across vascular surfaces, and higher turnover rates in inflamed tissue may obscure higher production rates of tryptase at such sites. However, synovial-derived mast cells express C5aR (CD88) (219), and thus might be activated at sites of complement activation. Thus, a better understanding of the mechanism of mast cell involvement in synovial inflammation is needed.

5.8 Fibrosis

Remodeling of the airway of chronic asthmatics results in irreversible losses of airflow and is characterized by fibrosis in and around the peribronchial–bronchiolar basement membrane (220). Involvement of mast cells in fibrotic disorders has been suggested based on the observation that increased numbers of mast cells appear in conditions characterized by fibrosis, such as fibrotic lung diseases (221–224), neurofibromatosis (225,226), and keloids (227). In scleroderma lung, mast cell numbers or activation may correlate with the level of pulmonary impairment, as judged by chest x-ray films (228). Although mast cell numbers in scleroderma skin are not elevated, the cells often appear fragmented (229), perhaps reflecting a cytotoxic factor. Whether mast cells are recruited into sites of fibrosis as innocent bystanders, or are actively involved in causing either fibrosis or fibrolysis is unresolved.

Experimentally, bidirectional effects have been noted between mast cells and fibroblasts. Fibroblasts can support the differentiation and survival of mast cells in vitro, at least partly related to their production of SCF. The production of SCF mRNA and protein from a schwanoma cell line derived from a patient with neurofibromatosis could explain the hyperplasia of mast cells observed at lesional sites in this disorder (230). β-Tryptase from human mast cells enhances proliferation of fibroblasts (210) and the production of type I procollagen (217,218), as does chymase (231). The ability of purified tryptase to activate latent collagenase derived from rheumatoid synovium (232), appears to contrast with the fibrogenic activity caused by fibroblast stimulation. However, the copresence of chymase may shift the fibrolytic–fibrogenic balance toward fibrosis, because this enzyme also can directly convert type I procollagen to collagen fibrils (118). In mice, production of TGF-β and TNF-α by mast cells is associated with increased collagen production by neighboring fibroblasts (233). Human mast cells can produce these cytokines as well as bFGF and VEGF (234,235).

REFERENCES

1. Irani AA, Nilsson G, Miettinen U, Craig SC, Ashman LK, Ishizaka T, Zsebo KM, Schwartz LB. Recombinant human stem cell factor stimulates differentiation of mast cells from dispersed human fetal liver cells. Blood 1992; 80:3009–3021.

2. Mitsui H, Furitsu T, Dvorak AM, Irani AA, Schwartz LB, Inagaki N, Takei M, Ishizaka K, Zsebo KM, Gillis S, Ishizaka T. Development of human mast cells from umbilical cord blood cells by recombinant human and murine c-*kit* ligand. Proc Natl Acad Sci USA 1993; 90: 735–739.
3. Valent P, Spanblöchl E, Sperr WR, Sillaber C, Zsebo KM, Agis H, Strobl H, Geissler K, Bettelheim P, Lechner K. Induction of differentiation of human mast cells from bone marrow and peripheral blood mononuclear cells by recombinant human stem cell factor/*kit*-ligand in long-term culture. Blood 1992; 80:2237–2245.
4. Lantz CS, Boesiger J, Song CH, Mach N, Kobayashi T, Mulligan RC, Nawa Y, Dranoff G, Galli SJ. Role for interleukin-3 in mast-cell and basophil development and in immunity to parasites. Nature 1998; 392:90–93.
5. Valent P. The phenotype of human eosinophils, basophils, and mast cells. J Allergy Clin Immunol 1994; 94(suppl):1177–1183.
6. Kempuraj D, Saito H, Kaneko A, Fukagawa K, Nakayama M, Toru H, Tomikawa M, Tachimoto H, Ebisawa M, Akasawa A, Miyagi T, Kimura H, Nakajima T, Tsuji K, Nakahata T. Characterization of mast cell-committed progenitors present in human umbilical cord blood. Blood 1999; 93:3338–3346.
7. Kirshenbaum AS, Goff JP, Semere T, Foster B, Scott LM, Metcalfe DD. Demonstration that human mast cells arise from a progenitor cell population that is CD34(+), c-*kit*(+), and expresses aminopeptidase N (CD13). Blood 1999; 94:2333–2342.
8. Li LX, Li Y, Reddel SW, Cherrian M, Friend DS, Stevens RL, Krilis SA. Identification of basophilic cells that express mast cell granule proteases in the peripheral blood of asthma, allergy, and drug-reactive patients. J Immunol 1998; 161:5079–5086.
9. Nilsson G, Mikovits JA, Metcalfe DD, Taub DD. Mast cell migratory response to interleukin-8 is mediated through interaction with chemokine receptor CXCR2/interleukin-8RB. Blood 1999; 93:2791–2797.
10. Ochi H, Hirani WM, Yuan Q, Friend DS, Austen KF, Boyce JA. T helper cell type 2 cytokine-mediated comitogenic responses and CCR3 expression during differentiation of human mast cells in vitro. J Exp Med 1999; 190:267–280.
11. Nilsson G, Miettinen U, Ishizaka T, Ashman LK, Irani AM, Schwartz LB. Interleukin-4 inhibits the expression of Kit and tryptase during stem cell factor-dependent development of human mast cells from fetal liver cells. Blood 1994; 84:1519–1527.
12. Nagata H, Worobec AS, Oh CK, Tannenbaum S, Suzuki Y, Metcalfe DD. Identification of a point mutation in the catalytic domain of the proto-oncogene c-*kit* in peripheral blood mononuclear cells of patients who have mastocytosis with an associated hematologic disorder. Proc Natl Acad Sci USA 1995; 92:10560–10564.
13. Longley BJ Jr, Metcalfe DD, Tharp M, Wang XM, Tyrrell L, Lu SZ, Heitjan D, Ma YS. Activating and dominant inactivating c-*KIT* catalytic domain mutations in distinct clinical forms of human mastocytosis. Proc Natl Acad Sci USA 1999; 96:1609–1614.
14. Hirota S, Isozaki K, Moriyama Y, Hashimoto K, Nishida T, Ishiguro S, Kawano K, Hanada M, Kurata A, Takeda M, Tunio GM, Matsuzawa Y, Kanakura Y, Shinomura Y, Kitamura Y. Gain-of-function mutations of c-*kit* in human gastrointestinal stromal tumors. Science 1998; 279:577–580.
15. Mekori YA, Metcalfe DD. Transforming growth factor-β prevents stem cell factor-mediated rescue of mast cells from apoptosis after IL-3 deprivation. J Immunol 1994; 153:2194–2203.
16. Xia HZ, Du ZM, Craig S, Klisch G, Noben–Trauth N, Kochan JP, Huff TH, Irani AM, Schwartz LB. Effect of recombinant human IL-4 on tryptase, chymase, and Fc_ϵ receptor type I expression in recombinant human stem cell factor-dependent fetal liver-derived human mast cells. J Immunol 1997; 159:2911–2921.
17. Yamaguchi M, Sayama K, Yano K, Lantz CS, Noben–Trauth N, Ra C, Costa JJ, Galli SJ. IgE enhances Fcε receptor I expression and IgE-dependent release of histamine and lipid mediators from human umbilical cord blood-derived mast cells: synergistic effect of IL-4

and IgE on human mast cell Fcε receptor I expression and mediator release. J Immunol 1999; 162:5455–5465.

18. Bischoff SC, Sellge G, Lorentz A, Sebald W, Raab R, Manns MP. IL-4 enhances proliferation and mediator release in mature human mast cells. Proc Natl Acad Sci USA 1999; 96:8080–8085.
19. Oskeritzian CA, Wang Z, Kochan JP, Grimes M, Du Z, Chang HW, Grant S, Schwartz LB. Recombinant human (rh)IL-4-mediated apoptosis and recombinant human IL-6-mediated protection of recombinant human stem cell factor-dependent human mast cells derived from cord blood mononuclear cell progenitors. J Immunol 1999; 163:5105–5115.
20. Kinoshita T, Sawai N, Hidaka E, Yamashita T, Koike K. Interleukin-6 directly modulates stem cell factor-dependent development of human mast cells derived from CD34(+) cord blood cells. Blood 1999; 94:496–508.
21. Saito H, Ebisawa M, Tachimoto H, Shichijo M, Fukagawa K, Matsumoto K, Iikura Y, Awaji T, Tsujimoto G, Yanagida M, Uzumaki H, Takahashi G, Tsuji K, Nakahata T. Selective growth of human mast cell induced by *Steel* factor, IL-6, and prostaglandin E_2 from cord blood mononuclear cells. J Immunol 1996; 157:343–350.
22. Toru H, Eguchi M, Matsumoto R, Yanagida M, Yata J, Nakahata T. Interleukin-4 promotes the development of tryptase and chymase double-positive human mast cells accompanied by cell maturation. Blood 1998; 91:187–195.
23. Irani AM, Craig SS, DeBlois G, Elson CO, Schechter NM, Schwartz LB. Deficiency of the tryptase-positive, chymase-negative mast cell type in gastrointestinal mucosa of patients with defective T lymphocyte function. J Immunol 1987; 138:4381–4386.
24. Craig SS, Schechter NM, Schwartz LB. Ultrastructural analysis of maturing human T and TC mast cells in situ. Lab Invest 1989; 60:147–157.
25. Baird B, Sheets ED, Holowka D. How does the plasma membrane participate in cellular signaling by receptors for immunoglobulin E? Biophys Chem 1999; 82:109–119.
26. Sperr WR, Bankl HC, Mundigler G, Klappacher G, Grosschmidt K, Agis H, Simon P, Laufer P, Imhof M, Radaszkiewicz T, Glogar D, Lechner K, Valent P. The human cardiac mast cell: localization, isolation, phenotype, and functional characterization. Blood 1994; 84: 3876–3884.
27. Mousli M, Hugli TE, Landry Y, Bronner C. Peptidergic pathway in human skin and rat peritoneal mast cell activation. Immunopharmacology 1994; 27:1–11.
28. Iikura M, Yamaguchi M, Fujisawa T, Miyamasu M, Takaishi T, Morita Y, Iwase T, Moro I, Yamamoto K, Hirai K. Secretory IgA induces degranulation of IL-3-primed basophils. J Immunol 1998; 161:1510–1515.
29. Iikura M, Yamaguchi M, Miyamasu M, Morita Y, Iwase T, Moro I, Yamamoto K, Hirai K. Secretory IgA-mediated basophil activation. Biochem Biophys Res Commun 1999; 264:575–579.
30. Patella V, Florio G, Petraroli A, Marone G. HIV-1 gp120 induces IL-4 and IL-13 release from human Fc epsilon RI+ cells through interaction with the V(H)3 region of IgE. J Immunol 2000; 164:589–595.
31. Peachell PT, Lichtenstein LM, Schleimer RP. Differential regulation of human basophil and lung mast cell function by adenosine. J Pharmacol Exp Ther 1991; 256:717–726.
32. Feoktistov I, Biaggioni I. Pharmacological characterization of adenosine A_{2B} receptors—studies in human mast cells co-expressing A_{2A} and A_{2B} adenosine receptor subtypes. Biochem Pharmacol 1998; 55:627–633.
33. Schulman ES, Glaum MC, Post T, Wang YH, Raible DG, Mohanty J, Butterfield JH, Pelleg A. ATP modulates anti-IgE-induced release of histamine from human lung mast cells. Am J Respir Cell Mol Biol 1999; 20:530–537.
34. MacDonald SM, Rafnar T, Langdon J, Lichtenstein LM. Molecular identification of an IgE-dependent histamine-releasing factor. Science 1995; 269:688–690.
35. Schroeder JT, Lichtenstein LM, MacDonald SM. Recombinant histamine-releasing factor

enhances IgE-dependent IL-4 and IL-13 secretion by human basophils. J Immunol 1997; 159:447–452.

36. Baggiolini M, Uguccioni M, Loetscher P. Chemokines and chemokine receptors in allergic inflammation. In: Marone G, Lichtenstein LM, Austen KF, Holgate ST, Kay AB, eds. Asthma and Allergic Diseases. Physiology, Immunopharmacology and Treatment. London: Academic Press 1998:157–167.
37. Uguccioni M, Mackay CR, Ochensberger B, Loetscher P, Rhis S, LaRosa GJ, Rao P, Ponath PD, Baggiolini M, Dahinden CA. High expression of the chemokine receptor CCR3 in human blood basophils. Role in activation by eotaxin, MCP-4, and other chemokines. J Clin Invest 1997; 100:1137–1143.
38. Hartmann K, Beiglböck F, Czarnetzki BM, Zuberbier T. Effect of CC chemokines on mediator release from human skin mast cells and basophils. Int Arch Allergy Immunol 1995; 108: 224–230.
39. Silverstein MD, Reed CE, O'Connell EJ, Melton LJ III, O'Fallon WM, Yunginger JW. Long-term survival of a cohort of community residents with asthma. N Engl J Med 1994; 331: 1537–1541.
40. Romagnani P, De Paulis A, Beltrame C, Annunziato F, Dente V, Maggi E, Romagnani S, Marone G. Tryptase–chymase double-positive human mast cells express the eotaxin receptor CCR3 and are attracted by CCR3-binding chemokines. Am J Pathol 1999; 155:1195–1204.
41. Baghestanian M, Hofbauer R, Kiener HP, Bankl HC, Wimazal F, Willheim M, Scheiner O, Füreder W, Müller MR, Bevec D, Lechner K, Valent P. The c-*kit* ligand stem cell factor and anti-IgE promote expression of monocyte chemoattractant protein-1 in human lung mast cells. Blood 1997; 90:4438–4449.
42. Yano K, Yamaguchi M, De Mora F, Lantz CS, Butterfield JH, Costa JJ, Galli SJ. Production of macrophage inflammatory protein-1α by human mast cells: increased anti-IgE-dependent secretion after IgE-dependent enhancement of mast cell IgE-binding ability. Lab Invest 1997; 77:185–193.
43. Malone DG, Wilder RL, Saavedra–Delgado AM, Metcalfe DD. Mast cell numbers in rheumatoid synovial tissues. Correlations with quantitative measures of lymphotic infiltration and modulation by anti-inflammatory therapy. Arthritis Rheum 1987; 30:130–137.
44. Lavker RM, Schechter NM. Cutaneous mast cell depletion results from topical corticosteroid usage. J Immunol 1985; 135:2368–2373.
45. Goldsmith P, McGarity B, Walls AF, Church MK, Millward–Sadler GH, Robertson DAF. Corticosteroid treatment reduces mast cell numbers in inflammatory bowel disease. Dig Dis Sci 1990; 35:1409–1413.
46. Bentley AM, Jacobson MR, Cumberworth V, Barkans JR, Moqbel R, Schwartz LB, Irani A–MA, Kay AB, Durham SR. Immunohistology of the nasal mucosa in seasonal allergic rhinitis: increases in activated eosinophils and epithelial mast cells. J Allergy Clin Immunol 1992; 89:877–883.
47. Enerbäck L, Pipkorn U, Granerus G. Intraepithelial migration of nasal mucosal mast cells in hay fever. Int Arch Allergy Appl Immunol 1986; 80:44–51.
48. Wilson BS, Kapp N, Lee RJ, Pfeiffer JR, Martinez AM, Platt Y, Letourneur F, Oliver JM. Distinct functions of the FcεR1 gamma andβ subunits in the control of FcεR1-mediated tyrosine kinase activation and signaling responses in RBL-2H3 mast cells. J Biol Chem 1995; 270:4013–4022.
49. Dombrowicz D, Lin SQ, Flamand V, Brini AT, Koller BH, Kinet JP. Allergy-associated FcRβ is a molecular amplifier of IgE- and IgG-mediated in vivo responses. Immunity 1998; 8:517–529.
50. Lin SQ, Cicala C, Scharenberg AM, Kinet JP. The FcεRIβ subunit functions as an amplifier of Fc_{ε}RIgamma-mediated cell activation signals. Cell 1996; 85:985–995.
51. Oliver JM, Burg DL, Wilson BS, McLaughlin JL, Geahlen RL. Inhibition of mast cell FcεR1-mediated signaling and effector function by the Syk-selective inhibitor, piceatannol. J Biol Chem 1994; 269:29697–29703.

52. Rivera VM, Brugge JS. Clustering of Syk is sufficient to induce tyrosine phosphorylation and release of allergic mediators from rat basophilic leukemia cells. Mol Cell Biol 1995; 15:1582–1590.
53. Vallé A, Kinet J–P. *N*-Acetyl-L-cysteine inhibits antigen-mediated Syk, but not Lyn tyrosine kinase activation in mast cells. FEBS Lett 1995; 357:41–44.
54. Kepley CL, Youssef L, Andrews RP, Wilson BS, Oliver JM. Syk deficiency in nonreleaser basophils. J Allergy Clin Immunol 1999; 104:279–284.
55. Lienard H, Bruhns P, Malbec O, Fridman WH, Daeron M. Signal regulatory proteins negatively regulate immunoreceptor-dependent cell activation. J Biol Chem 1999; 274:32493–32499.
56. Berger SA, Mak TW, Paige CJ. Leukocyte common antigen (CD45) is required for immunoglobulin E-mediated degranulation of mast cells. J Exp Med 1994; 180:471–476.
57. Suzuki H, Takei M, Yanagida M, Nakahata T, Kawakami T, Fukamachi H. Early and late events in FcεRI signal transduction in human cultured mast cells. J Immunol 1997; 159: 5881–5888.
58. Hata D, Kawakami Y, Inagaki N, Lantz CS, Kitamura T, Khan WN, Maeda–Yamamoto M, Miura T, Han W, Hartman SE, Yao L, Nagai H, Goldfeld AE, Alt FW, Galli SJ, Witte ON, Kawakami T. Involvement of Bruton's tyrosine kinase in FcεRI-dependent mast cell degranulation and cytokine production. J Exp Med 1998; 187:1235–1247.
59. Setoguchi R, Kinashi T, Sagara H, Hirosawa K, Takatsu K. Defective degranulation and calcium mobilization of bone-marrow derived mast cells from Xid and Btk-deficient mice. Immunol Lett 1998; 64:109–118.
60. Pivniouk VI, Martin TR, Lu–Kuo JM, Katz HR, Oettgen HC, Geha RS. SLP-76 deficiency impairs signaling via the high-affinity IgE receptor in mast cells. J Clin Invest 1999; 103: 1737–1743.
61. Frigeri L, Apgar JR. The role of actin microfilaments in the down-regulation of the degranulation response in RBL-2H3 mast cells. J Immunol 1999; 162:2243–2250.
62. Sullivan R, Price LS, Koffer A. Rho controls cortical F-actin disassembly in addition to, but independently of, secretion in mast cells. J Biol Chem 1999; 274:38140–38146.
63. Baram D, Adachi R, Medalia O, Tuvim M, Dickey BF, Mekori YA, Sagi–Eisenberg R. Synaptotagmin II negatively regulates Ca^{2+}-triggered exocytosis of lysosomes in mast cells. J Exp Med 1999; 189:1649–1657.
64. Yamauchi K, Sato R, Tanno Y, Ohkawara Y, Maeyama K, Watanabe T, Satoh K, Yoshizawa M, Shibahara S, Takishima T. Nucleotide sequence of the cDNA encoding L-histidine decarboxylase derived from human basophilic leukemia cell line, KU-812-F. Nucleic Acids Res 1990; 18:5891.
65. Gantz I, Schaffer M, DelValle J, Logsdon C, Campbell V, Uhler M, Yamada T. Molecular cloning of a gene encoding the histamine H_2 receptor [published erratum appears in Proc Natl Acad Sci USA 1991 Jul; 88(13):5937]. Proc Natl Acad Sci USA 1991; 88:429–433.
66. Asako H, Kurose I, Wolf R, DeFrees S, Zheng ZL, Phillips ML, Paulson JC, Granger DN. Role of H_1 receptors and P-selectin in histamine-induced leukocyte rolling and adhesion in postcapillary venules. J Clin Invest 1994; 93:1508–1515.
67. Kubes P, Kanwar S. Histamine induces leukocyte rolling in post-capillary venules. A P-selectin-mediated event. J Immunol 1994; 152:3570–3577.
68. Inoue I, Yanai K, Kitamura D, Taniuchi I, Kobayashi T, Niimura K, Watanabe T, Watanabe T. Impaired locomotor activity and exploratory behavior in mice lacking histamine H_1 receptors. Proc Natl Acad Sci USA 1996; 93:13316–13320.
69. Robertson I, Greaves MW. Responses of human skin blood vessels to synthetic histamine analogues. Br J Clin Pharmacol 1978; 5:319.
70. Kaliner M, Shelhamer JH, Ottesen EA. Effects of infused histamine: correlation of plasma histamine levels and symptoms. J Allergy Clin Immunol 1982; 69:283–289.

71. Craig SS, Irani A–MA, Metcalfe DD, Schwartz LB. Ultrastructural localization of heparin to human mast cells of the MC_{TC} and MC_T types by labeling with antithrombin III-gold. Lab Invest 1993; 69:552–561.
72. Stringer SE, Mayer–Proschel M, Kalyani A, Rao M, Gallagher JT. Heparin is a unique marker of progenitors in the glial cell lineage. J Biol Chem 1999; 274:25455–25460.
73. Reed JA, Albino AP, McNutt NS. Human cutaneous mast cells express basic fibroblast growth factor. Lab Invest 1995; 72:215–222.
74. Nelson RM, Cecconi O, Roberts WG, Aruffo A, Linhardt RJ, Bevilacqua MP. Heparin oligosaccharides bind L- and P-selectin and inhibit acute inflammation. Blood 1993; 82:3253–3258.
75. Forsberg E, Pejler G, Ringvall M, Lunderius C, Tomasini–Johansson B, Kusche–Gullberg M, Eriksson I, Ledin J, Hellman L, Kjellen L. Abnormal mast cells in mice deficient in a heparin-synthesizing enzyme. Nature 1999; 400:773–776.
76. Humphries DE, Wong GW, Friend DS, Gurish MF, Qiu WT, Huang CF, Sharpe AH, Stevens RL. Heparin is essential for the storage of specific granule proteases in mast cells. Nature 1999; 400:769–772.
77. Chiu H, Lagunoff D. Histochemical comparison of vertebrate mast cells. Histochem J 1972; 4:135–144.
78. Glenner GC, Cohen LA. Histochemical demonstration of species-specific trypsin-like enzyme in mast cells. Nature 1960; 185:846–847.
79. Hopsu VK, Glenner GG. A histochemical enzyme kinetic system applied to the trypsin-like amidase and esterase activity in human mast cells. J Cell Biol 1963; 17:503–510.
80. Schwartz LB, Lewis RA, Seldin D, Austen KF. Acid hydrolases and tryptase from secretory granules of dispersed human lung mast cells. J Immunol 1981; 126:1290–1294.
81. Schwartz LB, Lewis RA, Austen KF. Tryptase from human pulmonary mast cells. Purification and characterization. J Biol Chem 1981; 256:11939–11943.
82. Alter SC, Metcalfe DD, Bradford TR, Schwartz LB. Regulation of human mast cell tryptase. Effects of enzyme concentration, ionic strength and the structure and negative charge density of polysaccharides. Biochem J 1987; 248:821–827.
83. Schwartz LB, Bradford TR. Regulation of tryptase from human lung mast cells by heparin. Stabilization of the active tetramer. J Biol Chem 1986; 261:7372–7379.
84. Pereira PJ, Bergner A, Macedo–Ribeiro S, Huber R, Matschiner G, Fritz H, Sommerhoff CP, Bode W. Human β-tryptase is a ring-like tetramer with active sites facing a central pore. Nature 1998; 392:306–311.
85. Alter SC, Kramps JA, Janoff A, Schwartz LB. Interactions of human mast cell tryptase with biological protease inhibitors. Arch Biochem Biophys 1990; 276:26–31.
86. Miller JS, Westin EH, Schwartz LB. Cloning and characterization of complementary DNA for human tryptase. J Clin Invest 1989; 84:1188–1195.
87. Miller JS, Moxley G, Schwartz LB. Cloning and characterization of a second complementary DNA for human tryptase. J Clin Invest 1990; 86:864–870.
88. Pallaoro M, Fejzo MS, Shayesteh L, Blount JL, Caughey GH. Characterization of genes encoding known and novel human mast cell tryptases on chromosome 16p13.3. J Biol Chem 1999; 274:3355–3362.
89. Reynolds DS, Gurley DS, Austen KF, Serafin WE. Cloning of the cDNA and gene of mouse mast cell protease-6. Transcription by progenitor mast cells and mast cells of the connective tissue subclass. J Biol Chem 1991; 266:3847–3853.
90. McNeil HP, Reynolds DS, Schiller V, Ghildyal N, Gurley DS, Austen KF, Stevens RL. Isolation, characterization, and transcription of the gene encoding mouse mast cell protease 7. Proc Natl Acad Sci USA 1992; 89:11174–11178.
91. Caughey GH. Mast cell chymases and tryptases: phylogeny, family relations, and biogenesis. In: Caughey GH, ed. Mast Cell Proteases in Immunology and Biology. New York: Marcel Dekker, Inc. 1995:305–329.

92. Baker E, Sayers TJ, Sutherland GR, Smyth MJ. The genes encoding NK cell granule serine proteases, human tryptase-2 (*TRYP2*) and human granzyme A (*HFSP*), both map to chromosome 5q11-q12 and define a new locus for cytotoxic lymphocyte granule tryptases. Immunogenetics 1994; 40:235–237.
93. Hudig D, Allison NJ, Kam CM, Powers JC. Selective isocoumarin serine protease inhibitors block RNK-16 lymphocyte granule-mediated cytolysis. Mol Immunol 1989; 26:793–798.
94. Sayers TJ, Lloyd AR, McVicar DW, O'Connor MD, Kelly JM, Carter CRD, Wiltrout TA, Wiltrout RH, Smyth MJ. Cloning and expression of a second human natural killer cell granule tryptase, HNK-Tryp-2/granzyme 3. J Leukoc Biol 1996; 59:763–768.
95. Kido H, Fukutomi A, Katunuma N. A novel membrane-bound serine esterase in human $T4^+$ lymphocytes immunologically reactive with antibody inhibiting syncytia induced by HIV-1. Purification and characterization. J Biol Chem 1990; 265:21979–21985.
96. Kido H, Yokogoshi Y, Sakai K, Tashiro M, Kishino Y, Fukutomi A, Katunuma N. Isolation and characterization of a novel trypsin-like protease found in rat bronchiolar epithelial Clara cells. A possible activator of the viral fusion glycoprotein. J Biol Chem 1992; 267:13573–13579.
97. Wong GW, Tang YZ, Stevens RL. Cloning of the human homolog of mouse transmembrane tryptase. Int Arch Allergy Immunol 1999; 118:419–421.
98. Sakai K, Ren S, Schwartz LB. A novel heparin-dependent processing pathway for human tryptase: autocatalysis followed by activation with dipeptidyl peptidase I. J Clin Invest 1996; 97:988–995.
99. Sakai K, Long SD, Pettit DAD, Cabral GA, Schwartz LB. Expression and purification of recombinant human tryptase in a baculovirus system. Protein Express Purif 1996; 7:67–73.
100. Huang C, Li L, Krilis SA, Chanasyk K, Tang Y, Li Z, Hunt JE, Stevens RL. Human tryptases alpha and beta/II are functionally distinct due, in part, to a single amino acid difference in one of the surface loops that forms the substrate-binding cleft. J Biol Chem 1999; 274:19670–19676.
101. Schwartz LB, Irani AMA, Roller K, Castells C, Schechter NM. Quantitation of histamine, tryptase and chymase in dispersed human T and TC mast cells. J Immunol 1987; 138:2611–2615.
102. Ren S, Lawson AE, Carr M, Baumgarten CM, Schwartz LB. Human tryptase fibrinogenolysis is optimal at acidic pH and generates anticoagulant fragments in the presence of the anti-tryptase monoclonal antibody B12. J Immunol 1997; 159:3540–3548.
103. Proud D, Siekierski ES, Bailey GS. Identification of human lung mast cell kininogenase as tryptase and relevance of tryptase kininogenase activity. Biochem Pharmacol 1988; 37:1473–1480.
104. Ren S, Sakai K, Schwartz LB. Regulation of human mast cell β-tryptase: conversion of inactive monomer to active tetramer at acid pH. J Immunol 1998; 160:4561–4569.
105. Schechter NM, Fraki JE, Geesin JC, Lazarus GS. Human skin chymotryptic protease. Isolation and relation to cathepsin G and rat mast cell proteinase. J Biol Chem 1983; 258:2973–2978.
106. Caughey GH, Zerweck EH, Vanderslice P. Structure, chromosomal assignment, and deduced amino acid sequence of a human gene for mast cell chymase. J Biol Chem 1991; 266:12956–12963.
107. Osman IA, Garrett JR, Smith RE. Enzyme histochemical discrimination between tryptase and chymase in mast cells of human gut. J Histochem Cytochem 1989; 37:415–421.
108. Irani AA, Schechter NM, Craig SS, DeBlois G, Schwartz LB. Two types of human mast cells that have distinct neutral protease compositions. Proc Natl Acad Sci USA 1986; 83:4464–4468.
109. Huber R, Bode W, Schechter NM, Strobl S. The 2.2 Å crystal structure of human chymase in complex with succinyl-Ala-Ala-Pro-Phe-chloromethylketone: structural explanation for its dipeptidyl carboxypeptidase specificity. J Mol Biol 1999; 286:163–173.

110. Kinoshita A, Urata H, Bumpus FM, Husain A. Multiple determinants for the high substrate specificity of an angiotensin II-forming chymase from the human heart. J Biol Chem 1991; 266:19192–19197.
111. Murakami M, Karnik SS, Husain A. Human prochymase activation. A novel role for heparin in zymogen processing. J Biol Chem 1995; 270:2218–2223.
112. Pejler G, Sadler JE. Mechanism by which heparin proteoglycan modulates mast cell chymase activity. Biochemistry 1999; 38:12187–12195.
113. Walter M, Sutton RM, Schechter NM. Highly efficient inhibition of human chymase by alpha(2)-macroglobulin. Arch Biochem Biophys 1999; 368:276–284.
114. Xia H–Z, Kepley CL, Sakai K, Chelliah J, Irani A–MA, Schwartz LB. Quantitation of tryptase, chymase, $Fc_{\varepsilon}RI\alpha$, and Fc_{ε}RIgamma mRNAs in human mast cells and basophils by competitive reverse transcription–polymerase chain reaction. J Immunol 1995; 154:5472–5480.
115. Schechter NM, Brass LF, Lavker RM, Jensen PJ. Reaction of mast cell proteases tryptase and chymase with protease activated receptors (PARs) on keratinocytes and fibroblasts. J Cell Physiol 1998; 176:365–373.
116. Sommerhoff CP, Fang KC, Nadel JA, Caughey GH. Classical second messengers are not involved in proteinase-induced degranulation of airway gland cells. Am J Physiol 1996; 271: L796–L803.
117. Longley BJ, Tyrrell L, Ma YS, Williams DA, Halaban R, Langley K, Lu HS, Schechter NM. Chymase cleavage of stem cell factor yields a bioactive, soluble product. Proc Natl Acad Sci USA 1997; 94:9017–9021.
118. Kofford MW, Schwartz LB, Schechter NM, Yager DR, Diegelmann RF, Graham MF. Cleavage of type I procollagen by human mast cell chymase initiates collagen fibril formation and generates a unique carboxyl-terminal propeptide. J Biol Chem 1997; 272:7127–7131.
119. Schechter NM, Irani A–MA, Sprows JL, Abernethy J, Wintroub B, Schwartz LB. Identification of a cathepsin G-like proteinase in the MC_{TC} type of human mast cell. J Immunol 1990; 145:2652–2661.
120. Irani A–MA, Goldstein SM, Wintroub BU, Bradford T, Schwartz LB. Human mast cell carboxypeptidase: selective localization to MC_{TC} cells. J Immunol 1991; 147:247–253.
121. Goldstein SM, Kaempfer CE, Kealey JT, Wintroub BU. Human mast cell carboxypeptidase: purification and characterization. J Clin Invest 1989; 83:1630–1636.
122. Reynolds DS, Gurley DS, Stevens RL, Sugarbaker DJ, Austen KF, Serafin WE. Cloning of cDNAs that encode human mast cell carboxypeptidase A, and comparison of the protein with mouse mast cell carboxypeptidase A and rat pancreatic carboxypeptidases. Proc Natl Acad Sci USA 1989; 86:9480–9484.
123. Sillalber C, Baghestanian M, Bevec D, Willheim M, Agis H, Kapiotis S, Füreder W, Bankl HC, Kiener HP, Speiser W, Binder BR, Lechner K, Valent P. The mast cell as site of tissue-type plasminogen activator expression and fibrinolysis. J Immunol 1999; 162:1032–1041.
124. Kanbe N, Tanaka A, Kanbe M, Itakura A, Kurosawa M, Matsuda H. Human mast cells produce matrix metalloproteinase 9. Eur J Immunol 1999; 29:2645–2649.
125. Fang KC, Wolters PJ, Steinhoff M, Bidgol A, Blount JL, Caughey GH. Mast cell expression of gelatinases A and B is regulated by *kit* ligand and TGF-β. J Immunol 1999; 162:5528–5535.
126. Tanaka A, Arai K, Kitamura Y, Matsuda H. Matrix metalloproteinase-9 production, a newly identified function of mast cell progenitors, is downregulated by c-*kit* receptor activation. Blood 1999; 94:2390–2395.
127. Fujishima H, Mejia ROS, Bingham CO III, Lam BK, Sapirstein A, Bonventre JV, Austen KF, Arm JP. Cytosolic phospholipase A_2 is essential for both the immediate and the delayed phases of eicosanoid generation in mouse bone marrow-derived mast cells. Proc Natl Acad Sci USA 1999; 96:4803–4807.
128. Lynch KR, O'Neill GP, Liu Q, Im DS, Sawyer N, Metters KM, Coulombe N, Abramovitz M, Figueroa DJ, Zeng Z, Connolly BM, Bai C, Austin CP, Chateauneuf A, Stocco R, Greig

GM, Kargman S, Hooks SB, Hosfield E, Williams DL Jr, Ford–Hutchinson AW, Caskey CT, Evans JF. Characterization of the human cysteinyl leukotriene CysLT1 receptor. Nature 1999; 399:789–793.

129. Colamorea T, Di Paola R, Macchia F, Guerrese MC, Tursi A, Butterfield JH, Caiaffa MF, Haeggstrom JZ, Macchia L. 5-Lipoxygenase upregulation by dexamethasone in human mast cells. Biochem Biophys Res Commun 1999; 265:617–624.
130. Roberts LJ II, Sweetman BJ, Lewis RA, Austen KF, Oates JA. Increased production of prostaglandin D_2 in patients with systemic mastocytosis. N Engl J Med 1980; 303:1400–1404.
131. Murakami M, Bingham CO III, Matsumoto R, Austen KF, Arm JP. IgE-dependent activation of cytokine-primed mouse cultured mast cells induces a delayed phase of prostaglandin D_2 generation via prostaglandin endoperoxide synthase-2. J Immunol 1995; 155:4445–4453.
132. Underhill DM, Ozinsky A, Hajjar AM, Stevens A, Wilson CB, Bassetti M, Aderem A. The Toll-like receptor 2 is recruited to macrophage phagosomes and discriminates between pathogens. Nature 1999; 401:811–815.
133. Raible DG, Schulman ES, DiMuzio J, Cardillo R, Post TJ. Mast cell mediators prostaglandin-D_2 and histamine activate human eosinophils. J Immunol 1992; 148:3536–3542.
134. Matsuoka T, Hirata M, Tanaka H, Takahashi Y, Murata T, Kabashima K, Sugimoto Y, Kobayashi T, Ushikubi F, Aze Y, Eguchi N, Urade Y, Yoshida N, Kimura K, Mizoguchi A, Honda Y, Nagai H, Narumiya S. Prostaglandin D(2) as a mediator of allergic asthma. Science 2000; 287:2013–2017.
135. Wang M, Saxon A, Diaz–Sanchez D. Early IL-4 production driving T_h2 differentiation in a human in vivo allergic model is mast cell derived. Clin Immunol Immunopathol 1999; 90: 47–54.
136. Devouassoux G, Foster B, Scott LM, Metcalfe DD, Prussin C. Frequency and characterization of antigen-specific IL-4- and IL-13-producing basophils and T cells in peripheral blood of healthy and asthmatic subjects. J Allergy Clin Immunol 1999; 104:811–819.
137. Enander I, Matsson P, Nystrand J, Andersson A–S, Eklund E, Bradford TR, Schwartz LB. A new radioimmunoassay for human mast cell tryptase using monoclonal antibodies. J Immunol Methods 1991; 138:39–46.
138. Schwartz LB, Bradford TR, Rouse C, Irani A–M, Rasp G, Van der Zwan JK, Van Der Linden P–WG. Development of a new, more sensitive immunoassay for human tryptase: use in systemic anaphylaxis. J Clin Immunol 1994; 14:190–204.
139. Schwartz LB, Sakai K, Bradford TR, Ren SL, Zweiman B, Worobec AS, Metcalfe DD. The α form of human tryptase is the predominant type present in blood at baseline in normal subjects and is elevated in those with systemic mastocytosis. J Clin Invest 1995; 96:2702–2710.
140. Rajakulasingam K, Durham SR, O'Brien F, Humbert M, Barata LT, Reece L, Kay AB, Grant JA. Enhanced expression of high-affinity IgE receptor ($Fc_{\varepsilon}RI$) a chain in human allergen-induced rhinitis with co-localization to mast cells, macrophages, eosinophils, and dendritic cells. J Allergy Clin Immunol 1997; 100:78–86.
141. Kepley CL, Craig SS, Schwartz LB. Identification and partial characterization of a unique marker for human basophils. J Immunol 1995; 154:6548–6555.
142. McEuen AR, Buckley MG, Compton SJ, Walls AF. Development and characterization of a monoclonal antibody specific for human basophils and the identification of a unique secretory product of basophil activation. Lab Invest 1999; 79:27–38.
143. Schwartz LB, Metcalfe DD, Miller JS, Earl H, Sullivan T. Tryptase levels as an indicator of mast-cell activation in systemic anaphylaxis and mastocytosis. N Engl J Med 1987; 316: 1622–1626.
144. Schwartz LB, Yunginger JW, Miller JS, Bokhari R, Dull D. The time course of appearance and disappearance of human mast cell tryptase in the circulation after anaphylaxis. J Clin Invest 1989; 83:1551–1555.

145. Van der Linden P–WG, Hack CE, Poortman J, Vivié–Kipp YC, Struyvenberg A, Van der Zwan JK. Insect-sting challenge in 138 patients: relation between clinical severity of anaphylaxis and mast cell activation. J Allergy Clin Immunol 1992; 90:110–118.
146. Silvers WS, Essember LJ, Williams PB, Selner JC, Dolen WK. Anaphylaxis due to diclofenac sodium (Voltaren): evidence of mast cell mediator release. Immunol Allergy Pract 1991; 13: 193–196.
147. Matsson P, Enander I, Andersson A–S, Nystrand J, Schwartz L, Watkins J. Evaluation of mast cell activation (tryptase) in two patients suffering from drug-induced hypotensoid reactions. Agents Actions 1991; 33:218–220.
148. Sprung J, Schoenwald PK, Schwartz LB. Cardiovascular collapse due to thiopental-induced histamine release. Anesthesiology 1997; 86:1006–1007.
149. Yunginger JW, Nelson DR, Squillace DL, Jones RT, Holley KE, Hyma BA, Biedrzycki L, Sweeney KG, Sturner WQ, Schwartz LB. Laboratory investigation of deaths due to anaphylaxis. J Forensic Sci 1991; 36:857–865.
150. Coombs RR, McLaughlan P. The enigma of cot death: is the modified-anaphylaxis hypothesis an explanation for some cases? Lancet 1982; 1:1388–1389.
151. Coombs RRA, Holgate ST. Allergy and cot death: with special focus on allergic sensitivity to cows' milk and anaphylaxis. Clin Exp Allergy 1990; 20:359–366.
152. Parish WE, Barrett AM, Coombs RRA, Gunther M, Camps FE. Hypersensitivity to milk and sudden death in infancy. Lancet 1960; 2:1106–1110.
153. Holgate ST, Walters C, Walls AF, Lawrence S, Shell DJ, Variend S, Fleming PJ, Berry PJ, Gilbert RE, Robinson C. The anaphylaxis hypothesis of sudden infant death syndrome (SIDS): mast cell degranulation in cot death revealed by elevated concentrations of tryptase in serum. Clin Exp Allergy 1994; 24:1115–1122.
154. Platt MS, Yunginger JW, Sekula–Perlman A, Irani AA, Schwartz LB. Involvement of mast cells in sudden infant death syndrome. J Allergy Clin Immunol 1994; 94:250–256.
155. Edston E, Gidlund E, Wickman M, Ribbing H, Hage–Hamsten M. Increased mast cell tryptase in sudden infant death—anaphylaxis, hypoxia or artefact? Clin Exp Allergy 1999; 29: 1648–1654.
156. Hagan LL, Goetz DW, Revercomb CH, Garriott J. Sudden infant death syndrome: a search for allergen hypersensitivity. Ann Allergy Asthma Immunol 1998; 80:227–231.
157. Howat WJ, Moore IE, Judd M, Roche WR. Pulmonary immunopathology of sudden infant death syndrome. Lancet 1994; 343:1390–1392.
158. Kanthawatana S, Carias K, Arnaout R, Hu J, Irani AM, Schwartz LB. The potential clinical utility of serum alpha-protryptase levels. J Allergy Clin Immunol 1999; 103:1092–1099.
158a. Randall B, Butts J, Halsey JF. Elevated postmortem tryptase in the absence of anaphylaxis. J Forensic Sci 1995; 40:208–211.
159. Travis WD, Li C–Y, Bergstralh EJ, Yam LT, Swee RG. Systemic mast cell disease. Analysis of 58 cases and literature review. Medicine (Baltimore) 1988; 67:345–368.
160. Metcalfe DD. Classification and diagnosis of mastocytosis: current status. J Invest Dermatol 1991; 96:2S–4S.
161. Longley BJ, Tyrrell L, Lu SZ, Ma YS, Langley K, Ding TG, Duffy T, Jacobs P, Tang LH, Modlin I. Somatic c-*KIT* activating mutation in urticaria pigmentosa and aggressive mastocytosis: establishment of clonality in a human mast cell neoplasm. Nat Genet 1996; 12:312–314.
162. Kettelhut BV, Parker RI, Travis WD, Metcalfe DD. Hematopathology of the bone marrow in pediatric cutaneous mastocytosis: a study of 17 patients. Am J Clin Pathol 1989; 91:558–562.
163. Horny HP, Sillaber C, Menke D, Kaiserling E, Wehrmann M, Stehberger B, Chott A, Lechner K, Lennert K, Valent P. Diagnostic value of immunostaining for tryptase in patients with mastocytosis. Am J Surg Pathol 1998; 22:1132–1140.
164. Worobec AS, Kirshenbaum AS, Schwartz LB, Metcalfe DD. Treatment of three patients with systemic mastocytosis with interferon alpha-2b. Leuk Lymphoma 1996; 22:501–508.

165. Kors JW, van Doormaal JJ, de Monchy JGR. Anaphylactoid shock following Hymenoptera sting as a presenting symptom of systemic mastocytosis. J Intern Med 1993; 233:255–258.
166. Fricker M, Helbling A, Schwartz L, Muller U. Hymenoptera sting anaphylaxis and urticaria pigmentosa: clinical findings and results of venom immunotherapy in ten patients [see comments]. J Allergy Clin Immunol 1997; 100:11–15.
167. Castells MC, Irani AM, Schwartz LB. Evaluation of human peripheral blood leukocytes for mast cell tryptase. J Immunol 1987; 138:2184–2189.
168. Nagata H, Worobec AS, Semere T, Metcalfe DD. Elevated expression of the proto-oncogene c-*kit* in patients with mastocytosis. Leukemia 1998; 12:175–181.
169. Shah PY, Sharma V, Worobec AS, Metcalfe DD, Zwick DC. Congenital bullous mastocytosis with myeloproliferative disorder and c-*kit* mutation. J Am Acad Dermatol 1998; 39:119–121.
170. Nagata H, Okada T, Worobec AS, Semere T, Metcalfe DD. c-*kit* Mutation in a population of patients with mastocytosis. Int Arch Allergy Immunol 1997; 113:184–186.
171. Kitayama H, Tsujimura T, Matsumura I, Oritani K, Ikeda H, Ishikawa J, Okabe M, Suzuki M, Yamamura K, Matsuzawa Y, Kitamura Y, Kanakura Y. Neoplastic transformation of normal hematopoietic cells by constitutively activating mutations of c-*kit* receptor tyrosine kinase. Blood 1996; 88:995–1004.
172. Castleman WL, Owens SB, Brundage–Anguish LJ. Acute and persistent alterations in pulmonary inflammatory cells and airway mast cells induced by Sendai virus infection in neonatal rats. [published erratum appears in Vet Pathol 1989 Mar; 26(2):187]. Vet Pathol 1989; 26: 18–25.
173. Castleman WL, Sorkness RL, Lemanske RF Jr, McAllister PK. Viral bronchiolitis during early life induces increased numbers of bronchiolar mast cells and airway hyperresponsiveness. Am J Pathol 1990; 137:821–831.
174. Sorden SD, Castleman WL. Virus-induced increases in bronchiolar mast cells in Brown Norway rats are associated with both local mast cell proliferation and increases in blood mast cell precursors. Lab Invest 1995; 73:197–204.
175. Furitsu T, Tsujimura T, Tono T, Ikeda H, Kitayama H, Koshimizu U, Sugahara H, Butterfield JH, Ashman LK, Kanayama Y, Matsuzawa Y, Kitamura Y, Kanakura Y. Identification of mutations in the coding sequence of the proto-oncogene c-*kit* in a human mast cell leukemia cell line causing ligand-independent activation of c-*kit* product. J Clin Invest 1993; 92:1736–1744.
176. Nagata H, Worobec AS, Oh CK, Chowdhury BA, Tannenbaum S, Suzuki Y, Metcalfe DD. Identification of a point mutation in the catalytic domain of the protooncogene c-*kit* in peripheral blood mononuclear cells of patients who have mastocytosis with an associated hematologic disorder. Proc Natl Acad Sci USA 1995; 92:10560–10564.
177. Schwartz LB, Atkins PC, Bradford TR, Fleekop P, Shalit M, Zweiman B. Release of tryptase together with histamine during the immediate cutaneous response to allergen. J Allergy Clin Immunol 1987; 80:850–855.
178. Durham SR, Varney VA, Gaga M, Jacobson MR, Varga EM, Frew AJ, Kay AB. Grass pollen immunotherapy decreases the number of mast cells in the skin. Clin Exp Allergy 1999; 29: 1490–1496.
179. Shalit M, Schwartz LB, Golzar N, von Allman C, Valenzano M, Fleekop P, Atkins PC, Zweiman B. Release of histamine and tryptase in vivo after prolonged cutaneous challenge with allergen in humans. J Immunol 1988; 141:821–826.
180. Shalit M, Schwartz LB, von Allmen C, Atkins PC, Lavker RM, Zweiman B. Release of histamine and tryptase during continuous and interrupted cutaneous challenge with allergen in humans. J Allergy Clin Immunol 1990; 86:117–125.
181. Irani AM, Huang C, Xia HZ, Kepley C, Nafie A, Fouda ED, Craig S, Zweiman B, Schwartz LB. Immunohistochemical detection of human basophils in late-phase skin reactions. J Allergy Clin Immunol 1998; 101:354–362.

182. Macfarlane AJ, Kon OM, Smith SJ, Zeibecoglou K, Khan LN, Barata LT, McEuen AR, Buckley MG, Walls AF, Meng Q, Humbert M, Barnes NC, Robinson DS, Ying S, Kay AB. Basophils, eosinophils, and mast cells in atopic and nonatopic asthma and in late-phase allergic reactions in the lung and skin. J Allergy Clin Immunol 2000; 105:99–107.
183. Smith CH, Kepley C, Schwartz LB, Lee TH. Mast cell number and phenotype in chronic idiopathic urticaria. J Allergy Clin Immunol 1995; 96:360–364.
184. Hide M, Francis DM, Grattan CE, Hakimi J, Kochan JP, Greaves MW. Autoantibodies against the high-affinity IgE receptor as a cause of histamine release in chronic urticaria. N Engl J Med 1993; 328:1599–1604.
185. Gruber BL, Baeza ML, Marchese MJ, Agnello V, Kaplan AP. Prevalence and functional role of anti-IgE autoantibodies in urticarial syndromes. J Invest Dermatol 1988; 90:213–217.
186. Ferrer M, Nakazawa K, Kaplan AP. Complement dependence of histamine release in chronic urticaria. J Allergy Clin Immunol 1999; 104:169–172.
187. Castells M, Schwartz LB. Tryptase levels in nasal-lavage fluid as an indicator of the immediate allergic response. J Allergy Clin Immunol 1988; 82:348–355.
188. Naclerio RM, Meier HL, Kagey–Sobotka A, Adkinson NF, Meyers DA, Norman PS, Lichtenstein LM. Mediator release after nasal airway challenge with allergen. Am Rev Respir Dis 1983; 128:597.
189. Naclerio RM, Proud D, Togias AG. Inflammatory mediators in late antigen-induced rhinitis. N Engl J Med 1985; 313:65.
190. Naclerio RM, Hubbard W, Lichtenstein LM, Kagey–Sobotka A, Proud D. Origin of late phase histamine release. J Allergy Clin Immunol 1996; 98:721–723.
191. Rasp G, Hochstrasser K. Tryptase in nasal fluid is a useful marker of allergic rhinitis. Allergy 1993; 48:72–74.
192. Varney VA, Jacobson MR, Sudderick RM, Robinson DS, Irani AA, Schwartz LB, Mackay IS, Kay AB, Durham SR. Immunohistology of the nasal mucosa following allergen-induced rhinitis. Am Rev Respir Dis 1992; 146:170–176.
193. Jacobson MR, Juliusson S, Lowhagen O, Balder B, Kay AB, Durham SR. Effect of topical corticosteroids on seasonal increases in epithelial eosinophils and mast cells in allergic rhinitis: a comparison of nasal brush and biopsy methods. Clin Exp Allergy 1999; 29:1347–1355.
194. Wilson DR, Irani A–M, Walker SM, Baran M, Jacobson MR, Schwartz LB, Durham SR. Grass pollen immunotherapy reduces seasonal increases in epithelial basophils but not mast cells. J Allergy Clin Immunol 2000; 105:211.
195. Gibson PG, Allen CJ, Yang JP, Wong BJO, Dolovich J, Denburg J, Hargreave FE. Intraepithelial mast cells in allergic and nonallergic asthma: assessment using bronchial brushings. Am Rev Respir Dis 1993; 148:80–86.
196. Bradley BL, Azzawi M, Jacobson M, Assoufi B, Collins JV, Irani A–MA, Schwartz LB, Durham SR, Jeffery PK, Kay AB. Eosinophils, T-lymphocytes, mast cells, neutrophils, and macrophages in bronchial biopsy specimens from atopic subjects with asthma: comparison with biopsy specimens from atopic subjects without asthma and normal control subjects and relationship to bronchial hyperresponsiveness. J Allergy Clin Immunol 1991; 88:661–674.
197. Djukanovic R, Wilson JW, Britten KM, Wilson SJ, Walls AF, Roche WR, Howarth PH, Holgate ST. Quantitation of mast cells and eosinophils in the bronchial mucosa of symptomatic atopic asthmatics and healthy control subjects using immunohistochemistry. Am Rev Respir Dis 1990; 142:863–871.
198. Gauvreau GM, Lee J, Watson RM, Irani A–M, Schwartz LB, O'Byrne PM. Increased numbers of both airway basophils and mast cells after allergen inhalation in atopic asthmatics. J Allergy Clin Immunol 2000; 105:1149.
199. Irani A–M, Nouri–Aria KT, Jacobson MR, Varga EM, Till SJ, Durham SR, Schwartz LB. Basophil, eosinophil and IL-4 mRNA-positive cell numbers increase in the bronchial mucosa of atopic asthmatics 24 h after segmental bronchial allergen challenge. J Allergy Clin Immunol 2000; 105:827.

200. Casale TB, Wood D, Richerson HB, Zehr B, Zavala D, Hunninghake GW. Direct evidence of a role for mast cells in the pathogenesis of antigen-induced bronchoconstriction. J Clin Invest 1987; 80:1507–1511.
201. Wenzel SE, Fowler AA 3d, Schwartz LB. Activation of pulmonary mast cells by bronchoalveolar allergen challenge. In vivo release of histamine and tryptase in atopic subjects with and without asthma. Am Rev Respir Dis 1988; 137:1002–1008.
202. Liu MC, Bleecker ER, Lichtenstein LM, Kagey–Sobotka A, Niv Y, McLemore TL, Permutt S, Proud D, Hubbard WC. Evidence for elevated levels of histamine, prostaglandin D_2, and other bronchoconstricting prostaglandins in the airways of subjects with mild asthma. Am Rev Respir Dis 1990; 142:126–132.
203. Cushley MJ, Tattersfield AE, Holgate ST. Adenosine-induced bronchoconstriction in asthma. Antagonism by theophylline. Am Rev Respir Dis 1984; 129:380–384.
204. Rafferty P, Beasley CR, Holgate ST. The contribution of histamine to bronchoconstriction produced by inhaled allergen and adenosine 5′-monophosphate in asthma. Am Rev Respir Dis 1987; 136:369–373.
205. Polosa R, Ng WH, Crimi N, Vancheri C, Holgate ST, Church MK, Mistretta A. Release of mast-cell-derived mediators after endobronchial adenosine challenge in asthma. Am J Respir Crit Care Med 1995; 151:624–629.
206. Sedgwick JB, Calhoun WJ, Gleich GJ, Kita H, Abrams JS, Schwartz LB, Volovitz B, Ben–Jacob M, Busse WW. Localized airway eosinophil response to bronchial segmental antigen challenge. Am Rev Respir Dis 1990; 141:A934.
207. Calhoun WJ, Swensen CA, Dick EC, Schwartz LB, Lemanske RF Jr, Busse WW. Experimental rhinovirus 16 infection potentiates histamine release following antigen bronchoprovocation in allergic subjects. Am Rev Respir Dis 1991; 144:1267–1273.
208. Broide DH, Eisman S, Ramsdell JW, Ferguson P, Schwartz LB, Wasserman SI. Airway levels of mast cell-derived mediators in exercise-induced asthma. Am Rev Respir Dis 1990; 141:563–568.
209. Jarjour NN, Calhoun WJ, Stevens CA, Salisbury SM. Exercise-induced asthma is not associated with mast cell activation or airway inflammation. J Allergy Clin Immunol 1992; 89: 60–68.
210. Bosso JV, Schwartz LB, Stevenson DD. Tryptase and histamine release during aspirin-induced respiratory reactions. J Allergy Clin Immunol 1991; 88:830–837.
211. Fischer AR, Rosenberg MA, Lilly CM, Callery JC, Rubin P, Cohn J, White MV, Igarashi Y, Kaliner MA, Drazen JM, Israel E. Direct evidence for a role of the mast cell in the nasal response to aspirin in aspirin-sensitive asthma. J Allergy Clin Immunol 1994; 94:1046–1056.
212. Mican JM, Metcalfe DD. Arthritis and mast cell activation. J Allergy Clin Immunol 1990; 86(suppl):677–683.
213. Wasserman SI. The mast cell and synovial inflammation. Or, what's a nice cell like you doing in a joint like this? Arthritis Rheum 1984; 27:841–844.
214. Ceponis A, Konttinen YT, Takagi M, Xu JW, Sorsa T, Matucci–Cerinic M, Santavirta S, Bankl HC, Valent P. Expression of stem cell factor (SCF) and SCF receptor (c-*kit*) in synovial membrane in arthritis: correlation with synovial mast cell hyperplasia and inflammation. J Rheumatol 1998; 25:2304–2314.
215. Gotis–Graham I, Smith MD, Parker A, McNeil HP. Synovial mast cell responses during clinical improvement in early rheumatoid arthritis. Ann Rheum Dis 1998; 57:664–671.
216. Gotis–Graham I, McNeil HP. Mast cell responses in rheumatoid synovium—association of the MC_{TC} subset with matrix turnover and clinical progression. Arthritis Rheum 1997; 40: 479–489.
217. Cairns JA, Walls AF. Mast cell tryptase stimulates the synthesis of type I collagen in human lung fibroblasts. J Clin Invest 1997; 99:1313–1321.
218. Gruber BL, Kew RR, Jelaska A, Marchese MJ, Garlick J, Ren SL, Schwartz LB, Korn JH.

Human mast cells activate fibroblasts—tryptase is a fibrogenic factor stimulating collagen messenger ribonucleic acid synthesis and fibroblast chemotaxis. J Immunol 1997; 158:2310–2317.

219. Kiener HP, Baghestanian M, Dominkus M, Walchshofer S, Ghannadan M, Willheim M, Sillaber C, Graninger WB, Smolen JS, Valent P. Expression of the C5a receptor (CD88) on synovial mast cells in patients with rheumatoid arthritis. Arthritis Rheum 1998; 41:233–245.
220. Bousquet J, Chanez P, Godard P, Michel FB. Is asthma a disease that remodels the airways? ACI News 1993; 5:5–8.
221. Kawanami O, Ferrans V, Fulmer JD, Crystal RG. Ultrastructure of pulmonary mast cells in patients with fibrotic lung disorders. Lab Invest 1979; 40:717–734.
222. Broide DH, Smith CM, Wasserman SI. Mast cells and pulmonary fibrosis. Identification of a histamine releasing factor in bronchoalveolar lavage fluid. J Immunol 1990; 145:1838–1844.
223. Pesci A, Bertorelli G, Gabrielli M, Olivieri D. Mast cells in fibrotic lung disorders. Chest 1993; 103:989–996.
224. Pesci A, Majori M, Piccoli ML, Casalini A, Curti A, Franchini D, Gabrielli M. Mast cells in bronchiolitis obliterans organizing pneumonia—mast cell hyperplasia and evidence for extracellular release of tryptase. Chest 1996; 110:383–391.
225. Giorno R, Claman HN. Mast cells and neurofibromatosis. Neurofibromatosis 1989; 1:100–104.
226. Nürnberger M, Moll I. Semiquantitative aspects of mast cells in normal skin and in neurofibromas of neurofibromatosis types 1 and 5. Dermatology 1994; 188:296–299.
227. Smith CJ, Smith JC, Finn MC. The possible role of mast cells (allergy) in the production of keloid and hypertrophic scarring. J Burn Care Rehabil 1987; 8:126–130.
228. Chanez P, Lacoste J–Y, Guillot B, Giron J, Barnéon G, Enander I, Godard P, Michel F–B, Bousquet J. Mast cells' contribution to the fibrosing alveolitis of the scleroderma lung. Am Rev Respir Dis 1993; 147:1497–1502.
229. Irani A–MA, Gruber BL, Kaufman LD, Kahaleh MB, Schwartz LB. Mast cell changes in scleroderma: presence of MC_T cells in the skin and evidence of mast cell activation. Arthritis Rheum 1992; 35:933–939.
230. Ryan JJ, Klein KA, Neuberger TJ, Leftwich JA, Westin EH, Kauma S, Fletcher JA, DeVries GH, Huff TF. Role for the stem cell factor/KIT complex in Schwann cell neoplasia and mast cell proliferation associated with neurofibromatosis. J Neurosci Res 1994; 37:415–432.
231. Algermissen B, Hermes B, Feldmann–Boeddeker I, Bauer F, Henz BM. Mast cell chymase and tryptase during tissue turnover: analysis on in vitro mitogenesis of fibroblasts and keratinocytes and alterations in cutaneous scars. Exp Dermatol 1999; 8:193–198.
232. Gruber BL, Marchese MJ, Suzuki K, Schwartz LB, Okada Y, Nagase H, Ramamurthy NS. Synovial procollagenase activation by human mast cell tryptase dependence upon matrix metalloproteinase 3 activation. J Clin Invest 1989; 84:1657–1662.
233. Gordon JR, Galli SJ. Promotion of mouse fibroblast collagen gene expression by mast cells stimulated via the FcεRI. Role for mast cell-derived transforming growth factor-β and tumor necrosis factor-α. J Exp Med 1994; 180:2027–2037.
234. Boesiger J, Tsai M, Maurer M, Yamaguchi M, Brown LF, Claffey KP, Dvorak HF, Galli SJ. Mast cells can secrete vascular permeability factor vascular endothelial cell growth factor and exhibit enhanced release after immunoglobulin E-dependent upregulation of Fc_ε receptor I expression. J Exp Med 1998; 188:1135–1145.
235. Qu ZH, Kayton RJ, Ahmadi P, Liebler JM, Powers MR, Planck SR, Rosenbaum JT. Ultrastructural immunolocalization of basic fibroblast growth factor in mast cell secretory granules: morphological evidence for bFGF release through degranulation. J Histochem Cytochem 1998; 46:1119–1128.

3

Eosinophils

DOUGLAS S. ROBINSON and A. BARRY KAY

Imperial College School of Medicine, National Heart & Lung Institute, London, England

ANDREW J. WARDLAW

University of Leicester, Leicester, England

1 INTRODUCTION

The term ''eosinophile'' was coined by Ehrlich in 1879 to describe granule-containing myelocytes that stained intensely with the acidic dye, eosin (1). These cells were noted to be associated with asthma and allergic disease very soon after their description (2,3). The eosin staining was due to the highly basic eosinophil granule proteins which, in turn, have been implicated in tissue damage in allergic disease (4). In particular, the demonstration that eosinophils are a potent source of bronchoconstrictor lipid mediators, as well as the granule proteins that can damage airway epithelium led to the ''eosinophil hypothesis'' of asthma, which emerged in the late 1970s (5). This suggests that eosinophil mediators contribute to airway narrowing and hyperresponsiveness in asthma, and replaced the earlier idea that eosinophils might serve to ''mop up'' mast cell mediators and thus act to limit tissue damage in allergic disease (6). Although there is much circumstantial evidence to incriminate eosinophils in the pathogenesis of asthma, the tools to specifically target this enigmatic cell in humans are only just emerging. In the next few years these should give important information on this cell's physiological and pathological role.

2 STRUCTURE AND DISTRIBUTION OF EOSINOPHILS

Eosinophils form less than 4% of circulating leukocytes in health. They are principally tissue-dwelling cells, and a bone marrow reserve may allow rapid mobilization to sites

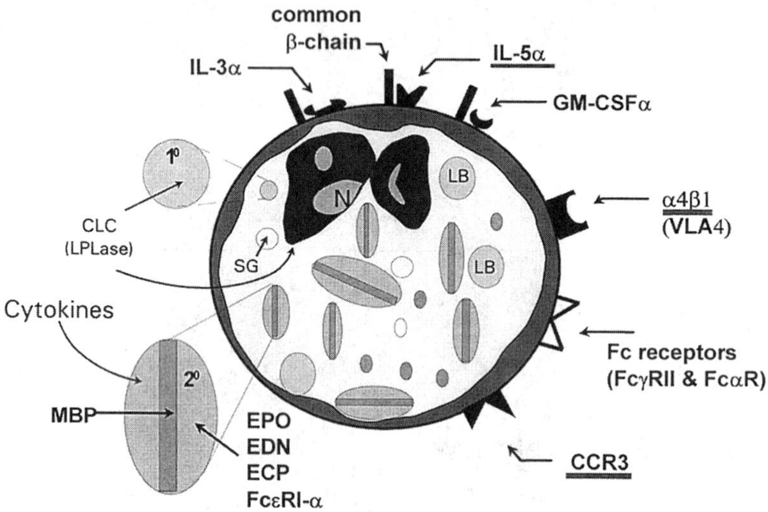

Figure 1 Eosinophil granules and receptors: Eosinophils have characteristic secondary granules containing basic granule proteins (MBP core with EPO, EDN, and ECP in the granule matrix), and primary granules containing Charcot–Leiden crystal lipid (galectin 10). Important surface receptors are $Fc_{\gamma}RII$ and $Fc_{\alpha}R$, which trigger degranulation (whereas $Fc_{\varepsilon}RI$ is intracellular), cytokine receptors for IL-3, IL-5, and GM-CSF, chemokine receptor CCR3, and adhesion receptors including $\alpha_4\beta_1$ integrin: N, nucleus; LB, lipid body (the site of synthesis of lipid mediators, including leuxotrine C_4).

of inflammation. Their life span is estimated at 13 days from development to death, with 6 days storage in bone marrow, and 2 in the circulation (7). Human eosinophils are roughly 8 μm in diameter (although this varies with activation status). The nucleus is characteristically bilobed, although in more mature cells it may be multilobed. Electron microscopists define primary granules that contain Charcot–Leiden crystal protein, and the characteristic secondary granules that contain a crystalline core of major basic protein (MBP) and a matrix including the other basic proteins, eosinophil cationic protein (ECP), eosinophil-derived neurotoxin (EDN), and eosinophil peroxidase (EPO) (8–10). In addition, lipid bodies are recognized. These are a site for synthesis of lipid mediators, and for a number of smaller granule compartments, including phagocytic vesicles. The activity and release of the granule constituents and lipid mediators is considered later. Eosinophil surface receptors and granules are shown in Figure 1.

3 EOSINOPHIL DEVELOPMENT

3.1 Lineage and Maturation

In common with other leukocytes, eosinophils develop from a $CD34^+$ precursor. Eosinophil development and maturation occurs largely in the bone marrow, and on release cells traffic rapidly to tissue, where their half life is close to 13 days (7,11). Eosinophil maturation is T-lymphocyte–dependent in experimental animals, and separate from that of the neutrophil and monocyte–macrophage lineages (12). Although eosinophilic leukemias in humans are relatively uncommon, an association with lymphomas, particularly Hodgkin's disease, supported T-cell–dependence in humans (13). Eosinophil development from CD34$^+$ stem cells is characterized by early expression of mRNA for the granule proteins, which can be detected as early as day 3 in in vitro culture systems (14). Interestingly, common eosinophil–basophil colonies are reported in culture systems, and these cells share a number of granule proteins and surface receptors (15). Much of the defining work on eosinophil–basophil development was performed with conditioned media, and the signals that specifically select for basophil expansion over eosinophils remain to be fully elucidated, although cytokine sensitivity may differ (16).

3.2 Eosinophil Development Factors: The Critical Role of Interleukin-5

The isolation and cloning of cytokines and growth factors in the 1980s and early 1990s established a role for interleukin (IL)-3 and granulocyte–macrophage colony-stimulating factor (GM-CSF) in eosinophil development from bone marrow precursors in both mouse and human (17,18). In 1986 the specific eosinophil differentiation factor IL-5 was cloned and characterized. Early studies suggested that IL-3 and GM-CSF acted early in cell development, and that IL-5 was a lineage-specific factor expanding eosinophil–basophil numbers (18,19). However, more recent work has clarified the interrelation of these factors at the cellular and molecular level and suggests a key role for IL-5 in eosinophil development. Interleukin-5 transgenic mice expressing IL-5 under the CD2 promoter (thus, with constitutive T-cell production of IL-5) showed marked tissue and blood eosinophilia (but no tissue damage), suggesting that IL-5 alone could expand the eosinophil lineage (20). However, it is of note that IL-5 gene-knockout mice, and those lacking the ability to respond to IL-5, IL-3, or GM-CSF still do generate low numbers of eosinophils, suggesting that these factors are not absolutely required for eosinophil development (21,22).

The receptors for IL-3, IL-5, and GM-CSF were cloned in 1991 and form a family with a shared, signaling β-chain, which associates with a cytokine-specific α-chain to form a high-affinity receptor (23,24). The generation of transgenic and gene-deleted mice for these cytokines and their receptors supported the concept that responsiveness of a cell to the members of the IL-3/IL-5/GM-CSF family is determined by cytokine receptor α-chain expression, because cell signaling is through the shared β-chain (through JAK1 and 2 and STAT 5; see Chapter 11) (25–27). Interleukin-5Rα expression is largely limited to eosinophils and basophils in humans, although IL-5 effects are described on B cells (28) and, more recently, smooth-muscle cells (29). Different isoforms of IL-5Rα can be generated by differential gene splicing (30). Responsiveness to IL-5 may be determined by the relative balance of expression of the membrane-anchored signaling (TM) and soluble inhibitor (SOL) isoforms.

We have recently examined factors determining the IL-5 responsiveness of developing eosinophils. Generation of IL-5Rα minigenes had suggested that IL-5 itself could switch on expression of the TM–IL-5Rα isoform on the cell surface, but this effect was not shared by IL-3 and GM-CSF. In cultures of human CD34$^+$ stem cells from umbilical cord blood, IL-5 with IL-3 supported eosinophil development, with concomitant switching to TM–IL-5Rα mRNA expression, detectable surface IL-5Rα, and IL-5 responsiveness (31). However, and in agreement with earlier reports, this was also seen with IL-3 and GM-CSF. Examination of mRNA expression showed that CD34$^+$ cells could produce their own IL-5 early in cultures and, indeed, eosinophil development could be blocked with antibodies to IL-5 in these systems. Thus, IL-5 may be critical to early stages of eosinophil

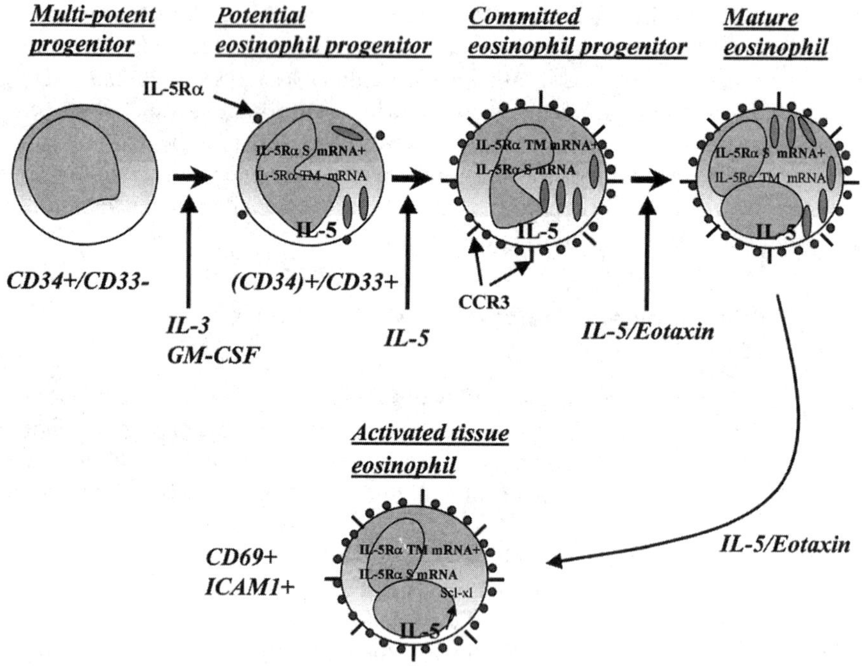

Figure 2 Eosinophil development from CD34$^+$ progenitors: In common with other myeloid cells, eosinophils develop from CD34$^+$ stem cells. A critical step in eosinophil lineage expansion seems to be up-regulation of IL-5 responsiveness (through the IL-5Rα chain), and this may depend on IL-5 itself. In addition CCR3 expression allows response to eotaxin: both eotaxin and IL-5 act in mobilization of eosinophils from the bone marrow. In addition CD69 and ICAM-1 are up-regulation on eosinophil activation.

development, and this may partly explain the IL-5 dependence of eosinophilic responses in animal models of allergic disease (21,32). A proposed model of eosinophil development is shown in Figure 2.

Data from human bone marrow studies (reviewed in the following) also suggests that IL-5Rα expression may be an important step in eosinophil maturation. Thus CD34$^+$/IL-5Rα$^+$ cells have been suggested to represent eosinophil progenitors (33).

4 EOSINOPHIL ACCUMULATION AT SITES OF ALLERGIC INFLAMMATION

Eosinophil accumulation is likely to result from a balance between increased supply from bone marrow precursors, efflux of cells stored in a bone marrow pool, trafficking to sites of inflammation, adhesion to blood vessel endothelium, and egress into the tissue matrix, and finally increased survival owing to growth factor inhibition of apoptosis. Many of these processes are reviewed in detail in other chapters.

4.1 Increased Eosinophil Production

Animal models of atopic airway inflammation and human asthma suggest that there is an increase in eosinophil colony-forming activity in allergic disease. Indeed, increased bone marrow and blood $CD34^+$ cell numbers have been reported in atopic, compared with nonatopic, subjects at baseline and after allergen inhalation challenge (34–36). Furthermore, IL-5Rα expression by bone marrow (BM) $CD34^+$ cells was increased 24 hr after allergen inhalation challenge (33). Eosinophil colony-forming (ECF) cells were detected in the blood during asthma exacerbation (37), and recent evidence supports the notion that eosinophils may mature from progenitors outside the bone marrow, with $CD34^+$/IL-5Rα $mRNA^+$ cells detected in airway mucosal biopsies from atopic asthmatics, and evidence for eosinophil maturation in tissue explants from nasal polyps and bronchial biopsies (38,39). This increase in eosinophil supply may be largely driven by IL-5 acting on a background of allergic inflammation. Although IL-5 transgenic mice have widespread blood and tissue eosinophilia, directed expression suggested that systemic as well as airway expression of IL-5 might be required for eosinophil infiltration, at least in one animal model (40). However, human volunteer studies showed that inhalation of IL-5 was itself sufficient to induce airway eosinophilia and increased bronchial responsiveness in subjects with asthma (41,42).

4.2 Eosinophil Mobilization from the Bone Marrow

Elegant animal studies, involving cannulation of the blood vessels of the guinea pig femur, suggest that there is a bone marrow pool of immature and mature eosinophils that can be mobilized into the circulation by both IL-5 and the C-C chemokine eotaxin (43,44). In particular IL-5 and eotaxin acted cooperatively to greatly increase eosinophil release, which was associated with an increase in β_2-integrin expression and loss of L-selectin (45). Antibodies blocking β_2-integrins inhibited release of eosinophils from the bone marrow, whereas blocking α_4-integrins increased release, suggesting that α_4-integrins may be involved in adhesion to the bone marrow stroma, whereas β_2-integrins may interact with the vascular endothelium of the sinusoids. Recent studies of human bone marrow confirm an increased number of mature and immature eosinophils in the bone marrow of asthmatic subjects compared with both nonatopic and atopic controls. These cells expressed the eotaxin receptor CCR3 in addition to IL-5Rα; thus, they may also be mobilzed by eotaxin and IL-5 (34). The relative contribution from bone marrow sources and eosinophil maturation outside the bone marrow remain to be established.

4.3 Eosinophil Adhesion

Eosinophil recruitment to the tissues requires adhesion to the vessel endothelium followed by extravasation (46). This process is dependent on initial rolling through L-, P-, and E-selectins (CD62L, CD62P, and CD62E). In vitro studies of adhesion of eosinophils to nasal polyp tissue suggested that P-selectin interactions with PSGL may be particularly important for eosinophil adhesion (47). Firm adhesion of eosinophils can occur via LFA-1 (CD11a/CD18) interaction with ICAM-1 (CD54) or 2 (CD102), or via VLA-4 ($\alpha_4\beta_1$-integrin; CD49d/CD29) interaction with endothelial VCAM-1 (CD106) (48–50). This latter pathway may partly account for selective accumulation of eosinophils, rather than neutrophils, at sites of allergic inflammation, because neutrophils do not express VLA-4, and VCAM-1 is up-regulated by IL-4 and IL-13, cytokines prominent in allergic disease (51–53). The $\alpha_5\beta_1$ (CD49e/CD29) and $\alpha_6\beta_1$ (CD49f/CD29) integrins may also play a role in interactions with fibronectin and laminin, respectively (54). Additional adhesion pathways such as $\alpha 4\beta 7$ interaction with the mucosal adressin, MAdCAM may play a role in eosinophil adhesion (55). Although the adhesion molecule CD44 has been detected on human eosinophils, especially those from the airway or sites of allergen exposure, evidence is lacking that it acts in eosinophil adhesion (56). One report suggests the CD44 may have a role in eosinophil development (57).

Adhesion is a two-way process, and both the eosinophil and the endothelial cell may be primed or activated by cytokines produced at the site of inflammation, or by themselves, as described later (58). Thus, IL-1, TNF-α, IL-4, and IL-13 as well as histamine, leukotriene-B4 (LTB_4) and platelet activating factor (PAF), all will up-regulate endothelial expression or avidity of adhesion molecules (51,52,59,60), whereas IL-3, IL-5, GM-CSF, TNF-α, IFN-γ, and C5a act to increase eosinophil adhesion molecules (61). Adhesion itself, for example, can prime the eosinophil for production of superoxide (62), or its own growth factors, such as GM-CSF (63).

4.4 Eosinophil Interaction with Tissue Matrix and Chemotaxis

Eosinophil emigration from the blood vessel into the tissue matrix is a tightly regulated process, involving deadhesion from integrins, with chemoattractant guiding the cell into the tissue, and interaction with tissue matrix proteins, such as fibronectin, laminin, and collagen. As described in the foregoing eosinophil α_4-, α_5-, and α_6/β_1-integrins are likely to be involved in adhesion to tissue matrix. Progress through the tissue depends on a directional release of enzymes capable of degrading matrix (termed matrix metalloproteases or MMPs), followed by neutralization of their activity by tissue inhibitors of metalloproteases (TIMPs). Eosinophils have been reported to be potential sources of MMPs 1, 3, and 9 (64,65).

Migration of eosinophils into sites of allergic inflammation may be in response to specific chemoattractants, providing a gradient or directional signal, in addition to factors such as IL-3, IL-5, GM-CSF, and IL-2 that increase mobility, generally in a chemokinetic manner (66,67). Several potent eosinophil chemoattractants have been defined, including PAF (68), C5a complement fragment (69), LTB_4, 8,15-dihyroxyeicosatetraenoic acid (diHETE) (70), and the bacterial toxin fMLP. More recently, a large family of chemoattractant cytokines, or chemokines, has been described (71). In particular eotaxin, acting on the 7-transmembrane-spanning receptor CCR3, seems relatively specific for eosinophils (as well as basophils and certain T-cell subsets) (72–75). In addition other CC chemokines, including RANTES and monocyte chemotactic proteins (MCP) 3–5, act on CCR3 (76). A subpopulation of individuals also have CCR1 on their eosinophils and are thus responsive to MIP-1α (77). In addition to their role in chemotaxis (and bone marrow egress of eosinophils), many of these agents either activate the cells, for example, in terms of calcium flux or rearrangement of the cytokskeleton to alter cell shape, or prime them to respond to other cytokines or mediators by degranulation or other effector functions (78). CCR3, similar to other chemokine receptors, such as CCR5 and CXCR4, can function as a cofactor for human immunodeficiency virus (HIV) infection, and may do so in brain microglia (79). This may also be relevant to HIV infection of eosinophils, which also express CD4 (80,81). The specificity of CCR3 for eosinophil recruitment makes this an attractive target for therapeutic blockade, and blocking antibodies abrogate eosinophilic responses in animal models of allergen challenge (82).

In addition to chemokines and other eosinophil chemoattractants, significant chemotactic responses of eosinophils to neuropeptides are described. In particular substance P, vasoactive intestinal peptide (VIP), calcitonin gene-related peptide (CGRP), and secretoneurin chemotaxis was blocked by wortmannin, suggesting PI3 kinase dependence (83).

4.5 Eosinophil Survival

Isolated eosinophils undergo spontaneous apoptosis within about 24 hr in culture. *Apoptosis* is programmed cell death, whereby cells show nuclear condensation and DNA fragmentation and are cleared by macrophage uptake without release of toxic granule proteins. This eosinophil apoptosis is prevented by IL-5, IL-3, and GM-CSF (84,85). This survival effect appears to be an important determinant of tissue eosinophilia in allergic disease, in which increased local production of all three cytokines is well documented (86–88). In addition, eosinophils express at least one functional death receptor, the Fas receptor (CD95) (89). Interestingly, nitric oxide (NO), but not the IL-5 family of cytokines, will antagonize Fas-induced eosinophil apoptosis in vitro (90). Because exhaled breath measurements suggest increased NO production in asthma, this mechanism may also contribute to eosinophilic airway inflammation (91).

Corticosteroids block the effects of IL-5 and GM-CSF on eosinophil survival in vitro, and can induce eosinophil apoptosis by raising intracellular calcium levels (92). Steroids also increase macrophage uptake of apoptotic cells.

The signaling pathways and transcription factors involved in eosinophil apoptosis have been studied in some detail (93,94). Apoptosis is an active cell process, blocked by inhibitors of protein synthesis. Furthermore, the rate of apoptosis was greatly increased by inhibitors of the transcription factor NFκB, suggesting that transcription of an NFκB-dependent protein may protect from cell death. A family of proteins of the Bcl-2 family regulate apoptosis in various cell types. Eosinophils constitutively express Bcl_{XL} and Bax, and IL-5 up-regulates the protective factor Bcl_{XL}. A subgroup of patients with hypereosinophilic syndrome have eosinophils that express Bcl-2, and induced expression of Bcl-2 in vitro will prevent eosinophil cell death.

5 ACTIVATION, DEGRANULATION, AND FUNCTION OF EOSINOPHILS

5.1 Eosinophil Effector Mechanisms

5.1.1 Eosinophil Granule Proteins

A major effector limb of eosinophils is the release of the highly basic proteins major basic protein (MBP), eosinophil cationic protein (ECP), eosinophil peroxidase (EPO), and eosinophil-derived neurotoxin, or eosinophil protein X (EDN or EPX). MBP makes up 50% of the granule protein, and is found in the core of the granule where it accounts for virtually all the protein in the core (95). EPO, ECP, and EDN/EPX are found in the granule matrix (96,97).

Major basic protein is a single polypeptide chain of 117 amino acids, with a molecular weight of 13,801 and a pI of 10.9. It contains 17 arginine residues, which accounts for its basicity, and 9 cysteine residues which explains its tendency to form disulfide bonds. MBP (and other granule proteins) is detectable at the mRNA level as early as day 3 of eosinophil development in vitro and by immunocytochemistry at day 6 from $CD34^+$ progenitor cells (98). A study of the MBP promoter suggested that the transcription factors GATA1 and c/EBP-β act synergistically to activate MBP expression (99). Recently, an MBP homologue with a much less basic pI (8.7 rather than 11.4) has been described (100), which interestingly retains many of the functions of the parent molecule. The reduced form of MBP is as toxic for parasites as the native form, but is less potent at activating leukocytes (101). As well as the mature MBP peptide, the cDNA for MBP encodes for a preprosequence which includes a putative signal peptide and a 90-amino acid acidic proprotein that may neutralize MBP's toxicity, as it is processed through the Golgi and is transported to the granule where the prosequence is cleaved (102,103). MBP can also be detected in basophil granules, although basophils contain considerably less MBP than eosinophils (104). Plasma concentrations of MBP are elevated in the sera of pregnant women, with a peak 2–3 weeks before parturition. Placental eosinophils are few and MBP has been shown by immunofluoresence to be in placental X and giant cells (105). The function of MBP in pregnancy is obscure. The gene for mouse MBP maps to chromosome 2, and a gene-knockout animal has been generated, although full publication of the phenotype is awaited.

Eosinophil cationic protein (ECP) is a single-chain polypeptide with a pI in the region of 10.8. On molecular sizing ECP displays marked heterogeneity, probably as a result of differental glycosylation, with molecular weight bands ranging between 16,000 and 21,400. Two isoforms, ECP-1 and ECP-2, can be identified using heparin–Sepharose. The ECP cDNA encodes for a leader sequence of 27 amino acids and a mature protein of 133 amino acids, with a calculated molecular weight of 15,600 (106,107). The amino acid sequence is 66% homologous with EDN and 31% homologous with human pancreatic ribonuclease. ECP does have ribonuclease activity, but it is 100 times less potent than EDN (108). The genes for both EDN and ECP are on chromosome 14q (109). Monoclonal antibodies were described that could distinguish between a form of ECP found in the granules of resting eosinophils (MAb EG1) and a secreted or extracted form of ECP (both MAbs EG1 and EG2) (110). However, recent studies suggest that both MAbs recognize most ECP, although this depends on the fixative used to prepare cells or tissues for immunohistochemistry (111). EG2 also recognizes EDN. There is approximately 5 pg of ECP 9 pg of MBP, 3 pg of EDN, and 12 pg of EPO (111a) per eosinophil. ECP exerts its cytotoxic effect through the formation of membrane pores (112). EDN, also called EPX (113), is a single-chain peptide with a molecular weight on gel electrophoresis of 18.6 kDa and a calculated molecular weight from the cDNA of 15.5 kDa. Similar to ECP, it is a member of a RNase multigene family and has marked ribonuclease activity (113,114). Recently, immunocytochemical studies have suggested that neutrophil granules (but not basophils) also contain both ECP and EDN, although staining is much weaker than for eosinophils (115).

Eosinophil peroxidase (EPO) is a heme-containing protein composed of an approximately 14 kDa (light)- and a 58 kDa (heavy)-subunit derived from the same strand of mRNA and subsequently cleaved. The cDNA encodes for a 381-leader sequence as well as the light and heavy chains (116). EPO shares a 68% amino acid identity with human neutrophil myeloperoxidase and other peroxidase enzymes and is antigenically similar. The human EPO gene is located on chromosome 17 (117). There is approximately 15 pg of EPO per eosinophil.

5.1.2 Eicosanoids

Eicosanoids are oxidation products of arachidonic acid derived from phospholipids by the action of activated phospholipase-A_2 (PLA_2). Eosinophils are rich in the 14-kDa isoform of $sPLA_2$: the functional significance of this compared with other cell types is unknown. Eisosanoid formation occurs at the cell membranes and in lipid bodies (118). The principal pathways for the metabolism of arachidonic acid in eosinophils are through the actions of cyclooxygenase, which produce the prostaglandins and thromboxanes, and 5- and 15-lipoxygenase (LO) that lead to the generation of leukotrienes and the HETEs and di-HETEs, respectively. Recent definition of functionally significant polymorphisms in the 5-LO promoter may have relevance to leukotriene production (119,120).

Eosinophils can generate picogram quantities of prostaglandin-E_2, PGD_2, and PGF_2 (121) although the predominant cyclooxygenase product was thromboxane-B_2 (TXB_2). After stimulation with calcium ionophore human peripheral blood eosinophils produced over 2 ng of TXB_2 per 10^6 cells (122), which is far less than the amounts of 5-LO products produced by these cells (see following).

5-Lipoxygenase (123) catalyzes the oxidation of arachadonic acid at the 5 position to 5-*S*-hydroperoxyeicosatetraenoic acid (5-HPETE) to produce the unstable epoxide leukotriene (LT)-A_4. The activity of 5-lipoxygenase is dependent on an 18-kDa protein called 5-lipoxygenase-activating protein (FLAP) which binds to arachidonic acid (124). Neutrophils contain an epoxide hydrolase (LTA hydrolase), which converts LTA_4 to LTB_4; whereas eosinophils have a specific glutathione-*S*-transferase that links glutathione to LTA_4 to produce the stable sulfidopeptide leukotriene LTC_4 (125). LTC_4 is converted to LTD_4 by the action of γ-glutamyl-transpeptidase, and to LTE_4 by a dipeptidase. LTE_4 is the stable metabolite. Eosinophils generate relatively large amounts (up to 70 ng/10^6 cells) of the sulfidopeptide leukotriene LTC_4 after stimulation with the calcium ionophore, but only negligible amounts of LTB_4 (126,127). Conversely, neutrophils produce large amounts of LTB_4, but little, if any, LTC_4. Interestingly, guinea pig eosinophils resemble human neutrophils in being able to synthesize LTB_4 but not LTC_4 (128). LTC_4, LTD_4, and LTE_4 contain the activity originally known as *slow-reacting substance of anaphylaxis* (SRS-A). Sulfidopeptide leukotrienes have several properties relevant to asthma, including smooth-muscle contraction, mucous hypersecretion, and increased vascular permeability. In addition to calcium ionophore, human eosinophils can also generate LTC_4 following stimulation by IgG-coated Sepharose beads (129), opsonized zymosan (130), or IgG–*Apergillus fumigatus* immune complexes (131). Generation of LTC_4 from eosinophils is inhibited by corticosteroids, such as fluticasone propionate (132).

In general, eosinophils from asthmatics generated more LTC_4 than eosinophils from normal donors (133–135), although there were exceptions. Eosinophils, unlike neutrophils, contain large quantities of 15-lipoxygenase, a 70-kDA cytosolic enzyme homologous with 5-lipoxygenase (136), which catalyzes the insertion of an oxygen at position 15 on arachidonic acid to form 15-hydroperoxyeicosatetraenoic acid (15-HPETE) and, subsequently, 15-HETE (137). Eosinophils can generate microgram quantities of 15-HETE (138). This may be of importance in asthma because 15-HETE stimulated mucus production by cultured human airway (139).

The dual actions of two lipoxygenase enzymes on a molecule of arachidonic acid gives rise to a further set of compounds, termed the lipoxins. Eosinophils can generate lipoxin A_4 (5*S*,6*R*,15*S*-trihydroxy-7,9,13-*trans*-11-*cis*-eicosatetraenoic acid) through the dual actions of 5- and 15-lipoxygenase (140). The activities of lipoxins in relation to eosinophilic inflammation are not entirely clear, but they seem to have a general down-regulatory role, for example, inhibiting neutrophil chemotactic responses to LTB_4 and formyl-methionyl-leucyl-phenylalanine (f-MLP) (141). In a mouse model of airway allergen challenge, inhibitors of 5-LO or FLAP blocked airway production of mucus and eosinophil infiltration, but interestingly, not airway hyperresponsiveness (AHR) (142). This dissociation of eosinophilia from AHR has been observed in other animal models, and is discussed in the following.

Platelet-activating factor (1-*O*-alkyl-2-acetyl-*sn*-glycero-3-phosphocholine; PAF) is a phospholipid formed by the acetylation of its inactive precursor, *lyso*-PAF, through the actions of a specific acetyltransferase. *lyso*-PAF is believed to be generated by the cleavage of an acyl group from the C2 position of 1-*O*-alkyl-2-acyl-glycerophospholipids by phospholipase-A_2. In some situations the acyl group is arachidonic acid, so that eicoanoids and PAF may be generated together. Biodegradation occurs as a result of the actions of an acetyl hydrolase that cleaves the acetyl group to generate *lyso*-PAF (143). Both of these enzymes are present in eosinophils (144,145). PAF has a number of proinflammatory activities and, in particular, acts as a leukocyte chemoattractant and activating agent. Most evidence suggests that PAF can act as an endogenous priming agent and mediator for the effects of cytokines and other agents in eosinophil effector functions, such as degranulation and superoxide generation (146). Inhalation of PAF causes bronchoconstriction in humans and variable increases in bronchial hyperresponsiveness (147). Eosinophils can generate substantial quantities of PAF after stimulation with calcium ionophore, zymosan and IgG-coated Sepharose beads (148,149). Much of the PAF remained cell-associated.

5.1.3 Reactive Oxygen Species

Eosinophil NADPH oxidase and eosinophil peroxidase can generate superoxide, hydroxyl radicals, and peroxynitrites, all of which can contribute to eosinophil cytotoxicity and cell damage (150). Production of these species may be activated or primed by cytokines (such as IL-3, IL-5, and GM-CSF) (151), or other mediators, such as PAF and LTC, or by adhesion, particularly through β_2-integrins (152,153). Activation of NADPH oxidase in eosinophils does not seem dependent on intracellular calcium or protein kinase C (PKC), but is blocked by inhibitors of PI_3 kinase such as wortmannin (154).

5.1.4 Eosinophil Cytokines

In 1993, it was demonstrated that eosinophils could transcribe and translate mRNA for IL-3 and GM-CSF, and further evidence suggested that these cytokines were indeed produced by eosinophils in vivo and that they might act as autocrine growth factors (155–157). Subsequently, it has been shown that eosinophils can produce a large array of cytokines and growth factors. Capron and colleagues have suggested that, as with $CD4^+$ T cells, it may be that eosinophils produce type 1 (IL-2, IFN-γ) or type 2 (IL-4, IL-5, or IL-10) cytokines in response to different stimuli (anti-CD28 triggering type 1 cytokine release, whereas FcαR signaling induced type 2 cytokines), although this remains to be confirmed (158). The subcellular localization of several cytokines to eosinophil granule matrix, together with immunohistochemical staining of cytokines within eosinophils in tissues, raises the possibility that, as for mast cells, eosinophils may store preformed cytokines that can then be released rapidly on activation to alter subsequent cellular responses (159). Eosinophil cytokines may thus amplify or down-regulate allergic inflammation (160). In addition, the release of growth factors, such as insulin-like growth factor, TGF-β, and nerve growth factor, raises the potential of the eosinophil in tissue repair and remodeling (discussed later).

5.1.5 Other Eosinophil-Derived Mediators

A major constituent of the human eosinophil primary granule is Charcot–Leyden crystal (CLC) protein. Cloning revealed a 16.5-kDa polypeptide of 142 amino acids, with similarities to the superfamily of S-type lactose-binding and IgE-binding animal lectins. X-ray crystallography suggested that this is a galectin-like molecule, and it has been designated as galectin-10 (161). Its biological function is unknown. This refutes previous suggestions that CLC-P was a lysophospholipase (162), but LPL activity was detected in galectin-10 preparation, and an LPL that associates with galectin-10, if found, would reconcile these observations.

In addition the eosinophil contains several other granule-stored enzymes the role of which in eosinophil function has not been defined (164). They include acid phosphatase (large amounts of which have been isolated from eosinophils), collagenase, arylsulfatase B, histaminase, phospholipase D, catalase, nonspecific esterases, vitamin B_{12}-binding proteins, and glycosaminoglycans.

6 POTENTIAL ADDITIONAL PROPERTIES OF EOSINOPHILS

Surface expression of various molecules involved in antigen presentation to T cells has been described, including CD4, HLA-DR, CD80, and CD86. Indeed, in vitro presentation of antigen by eosinophils has been described, although whether they are antigen-presenting cells in vivo is uncertain (165–167). In addition, eosinophils express CD40 and IL-4 which together can switch B cells to IgE production (168). However, although switching could be achieved by basophils and mast cells in vitro similar results could not be demonstrated for eosinophils.

6.1 Eosinophil Activation

Release of granule proteins is a major effector limb of eosinophil function. This can be achieved in three broad ways: *exocytosis*, with fusion of the granule and cell membranes and complete release of the granule contents; *piecemeal degranulation* (PMD), with extrusion of small parts of granule contents; or *cytolysis*, with disruption of the whole cell, leading to dispersal of its contents. Eosinophil exocytosis can be induced in vitro and has been studied in detail in elegant patch-clamp experiments in which step increases in capacitance of individual cells occurred with exposure to agonists such as GTPγ-S (169). It is feasible that this process might not be complete and could allow piecemeal degraulation, as is seen in ultrastructural studies in tissue biopsies from sites of allergic inflammation (170). It has been suggested that PMDs allows selective release of one granule constituent over another. However, examination of biopsy material also suggests that eosinophil cytolysis may be an important mechanism for release of granule proteins (171). A family of proteins regulating fusion between granule and cell membranes, termed soluble *N*-ethylmaleimide-sensitive-factor attachment protein (SNAPS) and SNAREs (SNAP receptors) such as the nonneuronal forms of SNAREs (synaptobrevin-2 and syntaxin-4), are expressed by eosinophils and may regulate degranulation (172).

Numerous stimuli have been implicated in eosinophil degranulation, including cytokines, adhesion molecules, and immunoglobulins, and different findings in different reports have confused this area of eosinophil biology. These differences probably reflect different in vitro conditions and donors of eosinophils; a consensus is beginning to emerge. As with many other immunological processes, it is a highly regulated, multistep system. Eosinophil activation in vitro is often best achieved by stimuli that are immobilized on solid surfaces, such as coated to plates or beads, and this may reflect a requirement for surface attachment, such as to helminths or other parasites in vivo. Adhesion through β_2-integrins appears to be an essential step in eosinophil degranulation (173). Thereafter a variety of stimuli including cytokines (IL-5, GM-CSF), lipid mediators such as PAF, small molecules such as C5a, or immunologlobulins such as IgG and secretory IgA, can trigger degranulation (174–176). Charge interactions may also be important, as mucins could inhibit degranulation and neutralizing their negative charge with agents such as polybrene reversed this. Thus, heparin, mucins and sialic acid may decrease eosinophil activation, whereas positively charged molecules, such as the basic granule proteins, may further activate release. In addition endogenous PAF production may provide positive feedback for eosinophil degranulation.

These signals may be integrated to alter subsequent responses to another stimulus, in a process termed priming. Thus IL-5, GM-CSF, and TNF-α prime eosinophils and reduce the threshold for activation (such as degranulation and mediator release) to other stimuli such as PAF or C5a, and vice versa (177). The same is true for adhesion by either intercellular adhesion molecules (ICAM)–β_2-integrins, vascular cell adhesion molecules (VCAM) and β_1-integrins, or matrix proteins such as fibronectin. Priming may also reveal responsiveness to agents (such as IL-8) that show little activity on resting eosinophils. Cell-signaling pathways controlling the processes remain to be fully elucidated. However, inhibitor experiments suggest that p38 kinase and the MEK-ERK pathways may be involved in degranulation in response to IL-5 (178). As described earlier CD28 signaling may induce differential cytokine production by eosinophils. Whether this is through signaling pathways similar to those used in T cells remains to be seen.

Although many of the mediators involved in eosinophil priming and activation (such as IL-5, PAF, and LTC_4) are present at sites of allergic inflammations, the specific triggers for eosinophil activation in allergic disease remain to be well defined. In particular, links between IgE and eosinophil function are uncertain. Although high-affinity receptors for IgE (FcεRI) were detected on eosinophils from donors with the hypereosinophilic syndrome or parasite infections, and these could release EPO (179), evidence for a functional effect of FcεRI in allergic disease is lacking (180). Recent data suggest that eosinophils from allergic donors encode mRNA for the α-, β-, and γ-chains of FcεRI and have intracellular FcεRI, but express very little surface receptor and cannot be triggered by IgE (Fig. 3) (181).

6.2 Eosinophils and Tissue Repair

In addition to airway inflammation in asthma, changes relating to the structure of the airway walls have been reported, including increased airway smooth-muscle mass, epithelial desquamation, elastolysis, hypersecretion of mucus plugging of small airways, and subepithelial fibrosis (''thickening of the epithelial basement membrane''). The term ''airway remodeling'' is often used to describe these structural changes (182). The remodeling process has been attributed to a combination of persistent airway inflammation in response to repetitive insults of antigen-induced injury, on the one hand, and ensuing repair processes, as noted by the increased amounts of structural tissue components, on the other. It is unknown how each of these components contribute to altered airway function in asthma, but it is likely that they are involved in airway narrowing. Over the past few years there have been several reports suggesting that eosinophils may also play a critical role in the *repair* processes associated with allergic tissue injury. Much interest has focused on TGF-β_1 because it is one of the most fibrogenic factors known, and its actions include promoting growth and repair at sites of wound healing and tissue remodeling. In a recent study, Minshall et al. demonstrated that asthmatic individuals exhibited a greater expression of TGF-β_1 mRNA and immunoreactivity in the bronchial submucosa than did normal

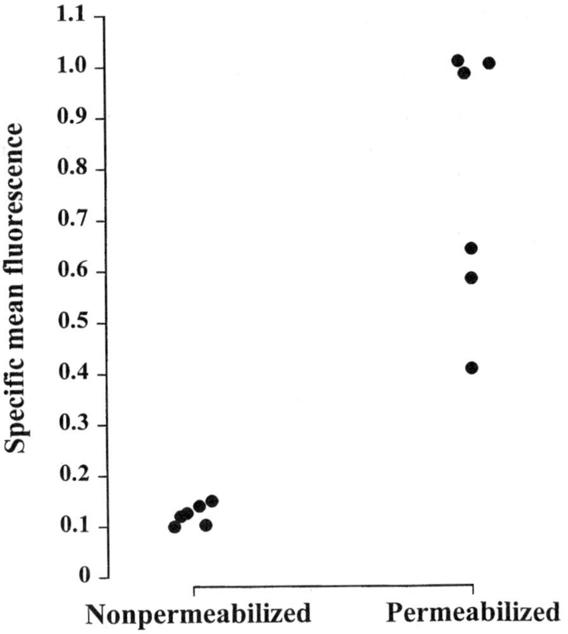

(a)

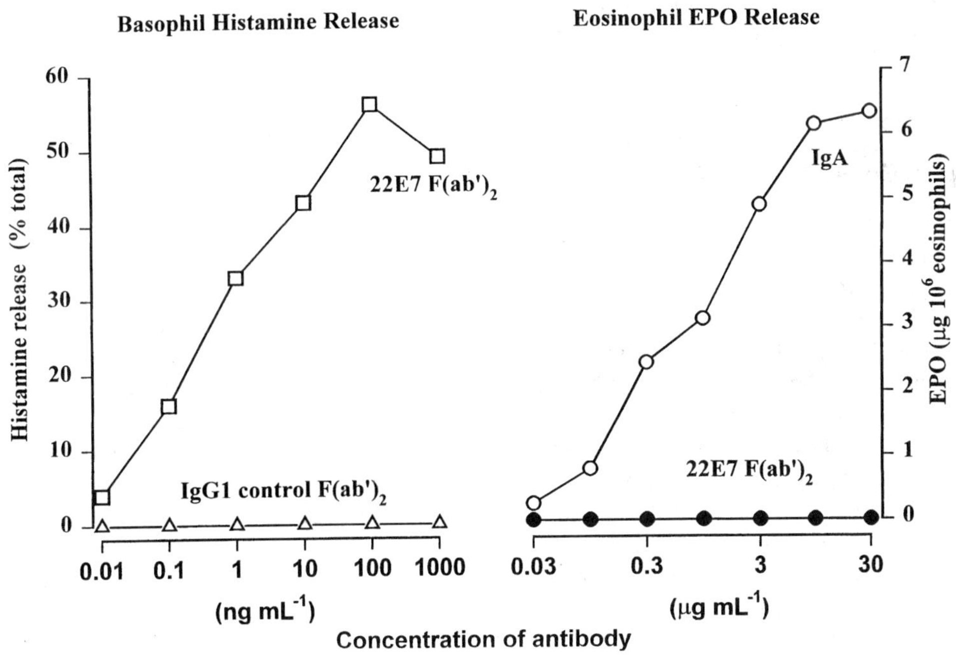

(b)

Figure 3 Eosinophils have intracellular high-affinity IgE receptor α-chain (FcεRIα), but this is not significantly present on the cell surface, nor does it trigger degranulation: (a) Eosinophils were analyzed by flow cytometry with monoclonal antibody 22E7 to FcεRIα before and after cell membrane permeabilization with saponin; (b) Histamine release from basophils compared with eosinophil peroxidase release from eosinophils. Cells were triggered with anti-FcεRIα or with human IgA. (From Ref. 181.)

control subjects (183). Moreover, within the airways of asthmatic individuals, EG2+ve eosinophils represented the major source of TGF-β_1 mRNA and immunoreactivity. Similarly, Ohno et al. investigated the localization of mRNA and protein of PDGF-B chain in nasal polyps and bronchial tissues from mild and severe asthmatics; the vast majority of cells expressing the gene and gene product were eosinophils (184). Eosinophils are a source of various other key molecules implicated in tissue-remodeling processes. These include TGF-α (185), MMP-9 (186), NGF (187), TIMP-1, IL-6 (189), TNF-α (190) and vascular endothelial growth factors (VEGF). However, a number of these studies were performed in vitro using blood eosinophils and, as yet, these GFs, and other agents have not been colocalized to eosinophils infiltrating the site of allergen challenge.

In addition, GF immunoreactivity must be interpreted with caution because it is not necessarily a reflection of biological activity for the following reasons: (1) many GFs are synthesized as an inactive precursor or secreted in the form of an inactive complex with a binding protein; for example, TGF-β_1 associated with latency associated peptide (LAP) is without fibrogenic activity; (2) GF receptors shed into the extracellular milieu may retain a functional binding domain and, therefore, act as specific binding proteins; (3) GFs sequestered to matrix proteins maybe neutralized (e.g., TGF-β_1 bound to decorin). These interactions between GFs and cytokine-binding proteins appear to have a diversity of functions; serving as cytokine reservoirs, protective shields against proteolytic degradation, modifiers of biological activity, or as clearance avenues; accordingly, they represent important control mechanisms that regulate the multifactorial activities of these factors. Therefore, functional studies will be required before any conclusion can be reached on the in vivo importance of any individual mediator.

7 EOSINOPHILS IN ALLERGIC DISEASE

7.1 Eosinophils in Asthma

Blood and sputum eosinophilia have long been recognized as features of asthma. Postmortem studies of patients dying of asthma showed a dense eosinophilic infiltrate in the airway mucosa and lumen, and immunofluorescence studies showed widespread deposition of granule proteins, such as MBP. Eosinophilic inflammation was also observed in the airway submucosa of asthmatics dying from other causes (191,192). The application of fiberoptic bronchoscopy to obtain biopsy and bronchoalveolar lavage specimens from asthmatic and control volunteers confirmed eosinophil infiltration in the airway in asthma, with evidence for release of granule proteins. Furthermore, the numbers of eosinophils seen in biopsies or lavage and the concentrations of their granule proteins have been related to asthma severity, as measured by airflow obstruction (forced expiratory volumn in 1 sec; FEV_1), symptom scores, and airway hyperresponsiveness (193). In addition to MBP and ECP, leukotrienes can be detected in bronchoalveolar lavage (BAL) fluid from asthmatic subjects (193–196). Interleukin-5 mRNA and protein are detected in increased numbers of cells or in higher concentrations in lavage fluid, biopsies, BAL cells, serum, and sputum from asthmatic subjects. Interleukin-5 has also been related to measures of asthma severity, supporting its potential role in eosinophil infiltration (197). Airway eosinophil infiltration is a feature common to atopic and nonatopic (intrinsic) asthma, and is also present in occupational asthma (198,199).

Allergen challenge studies demonstrate eosinophil influx into the airway and degranulation at 6 hr after allergen challenge, and this is sustained through to 24 and 48 hr after inhalation in subjects with a late asthmatic response, and again can be related to the fall in FEV_1 during the late response, and to evidence of IL-5 production (200–203). Studies of the bone marrow from asthmatic and control subjects also confirm a bone marrow pool of mature and immature eosinophils in subjects with asthma, and an increase in $CD34^+$ progenitors in those who are atopic, regardless of asthmatic status. Allergen inhalation challenge resulting in a late asthmatic response is associated with increased bone marrow $CD34^+$/IL-5Rα^+ double-positive cells and eosinophil colony-forming activity in both bone marrow and peripheral blood. Eotaxin expression and CCR3 expressing eosinophils were present in increased numbers in the airway of patients with asthma. The $CD34^+$/IL-5R_α $mRNA^+$ cells are present in increased numbers in the bronchial mucosa of asthmatics at baseline, suggesting that there may be local development of eosinophils, in addition to recruitment from the bone marrow.

Animal models also support a role for eosinophils in asthma, or at least antigen-induced airways hyperresponsiveness (AHR). Inhalation challenge with MBP can, by itself, cause airways hyperresponsiveness in mice and monkeys (204,205). These models allow dissection of the factors contributing to AHR and the role of eosinophils, as discussed in the following.

Several treatments for asthma are associated with changes in airway eosinophil numbers. In particular eosinophil numbers are very sensitive to corticosteroids, indeed eosinophilia is a feature of Addision's disease. Oral and inhaled corticosteroids have been demonstrated to reduce airway eosinophil infiltration and granule protein release, and these effects have been related to improvements in AHR and symptoms. Much of this effect may be indirect through inhibition of T-cell IL-5 production (206–211), but direct effects of corticosteroids are also reported; for example, inhibition of LTC_4 synthesis. In addition other drugs used in treatment of asthma reduce airway mucosal eosinophil infiltrations in biopsy or induced sputum in double-blind studies, including theophyllines, leukotriene receptor antagonists, and anti-IgE (212–214). Successful allergen injection immunotherapy for seasonal birch pollen-induced asthma reduces seasonal airway infiltration with eosinophils (215).

7.2 Eosinophils in Rhinitis

Eosinophil infiltration is also seen in the nasal mucosa in atopic rhinitis, with further increases after either experimental or seasonal allergen challenge (216,217). This process is also thought to be regulated by Th2-type cytokines and CC chemokines, such as eotaxin, and is inhibited by topical corticosteroids (218). Eosinophils are prominent in nasal polyp tissue, which is also rich in cells producing cytokines such as GM-CSF (219). The antigen-driving eosinophil infiltration in most cases of nasal polyposis is uncertain, though eosinophilia is also seen in patients with aspirin-sensitive asthma and nasal polyps. Local instillation of IL-5 into the nose of atopic volunteers will induce eosinophil infiltration (220), and inhalation of IL-5 will cause airway eosinophilia.

7.3 Eosinophils in Allergic Skin Disease

There is a prominent eosinophil infiltration with evidence of degranulation in the dermis in atopic eczema (221), and eosinophils are also seen in the lesional skin of subjects with urticaria (222). The contribution of eosinophils to disease pathology in both conditions is unclear, although granule protein may damage the integrity of the skin in atopic dermatitis. The allergen-induced cutaneous late-phase response has become a useful model for studying the mechanisms and time course of allergen-induced eosinophil infiltration in humans (223). In a recent detailed study we documented an increase in eosinophil numbers in the skin up to 72 hr after challenge, accompanied by variable expression of the chemokines, eotaxin 1, eotaxin 2, MCP-3 and 4, and MIP-1α, and cytokines IL-4 and IL-5 (Fig. 4) (224). In addition IL-13 was prominent in the late-phase skin reaction and this correlated with up-regulation of VCAM–1-bearing cells in the skin (225). The skin late-phase reaction allowed monitoring of resolution of the allergic inflammatory response, with TUNEL

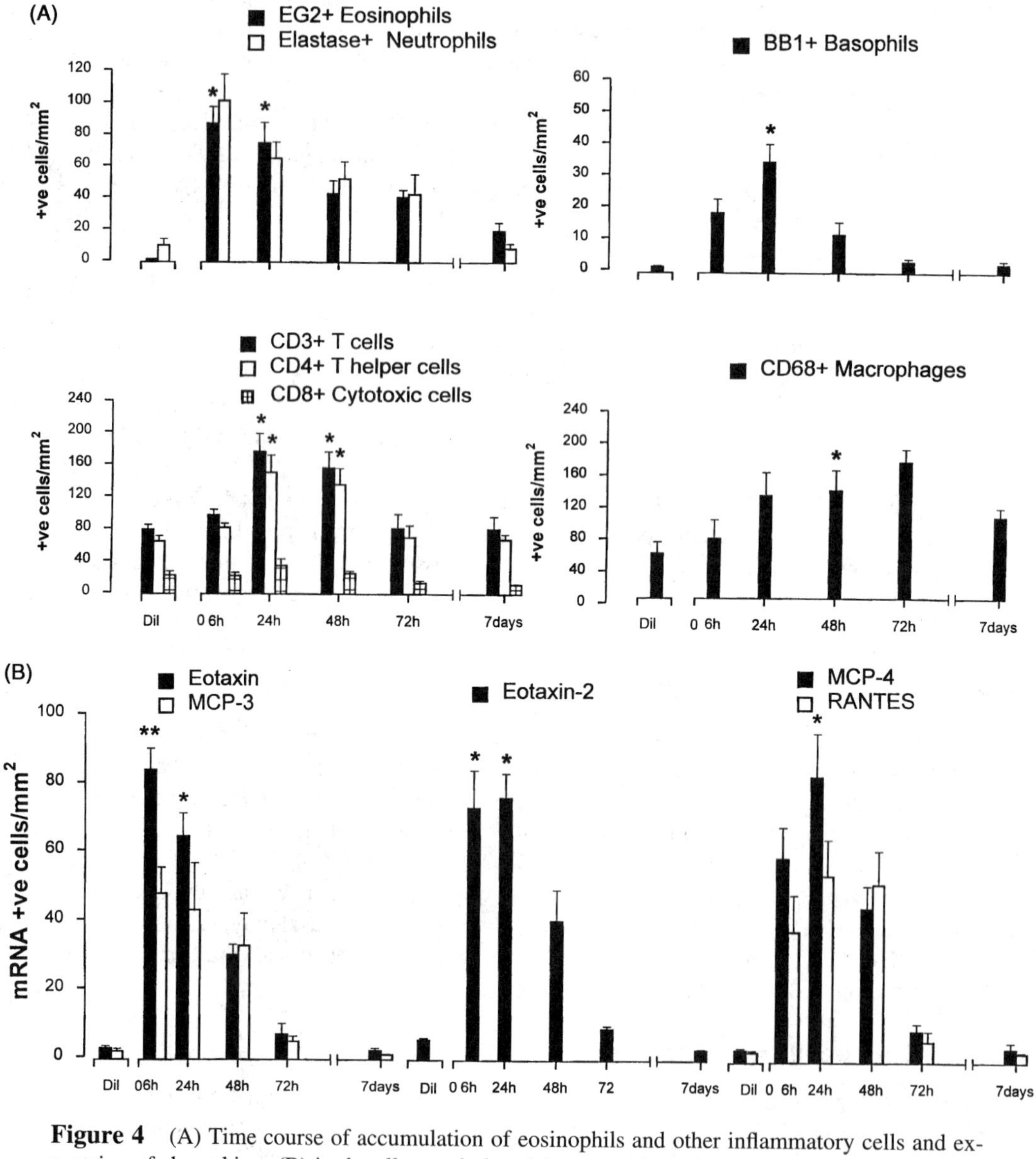

Figure 4 (A) Time course of accumulation of eosinophils and other inflammatory cells and expression of chemokines (B) in the allergen-induced cutaneous late-phase reaction. Cells were enumerated by immunohistochemistry and chemokine expression by in situ hybridization for mRNA. (From Ref. 224.)

evidence of eosinophil apoptosis at 48–72 hr. However, ultrastructural analysis of airway biopsy samples from asthmatic subjects suggest eosinophil cytolysis, rather than apoptosis as a clearance mechanism.

7.4 Other Eosinophilic Diseases

Eosinophilia is a feature of a wide spectrum of diseases, including parasitic infections; some fibrotic diseases, such as systemic sclerosis; dermatological diseases; pulmonary eosinophilias; and the idiopathic hypereosinophilic syndrome. Detailed consideration of all of these syndromes is outside the scope of this chapter, but skin disease, pulmonary eosinophilia, and the idiopathic hypereosinophilic syndrome will be reviewed briefly. There is an eosinophilic infiltrate around some solid tumors, and it is possible that eosinophils have a role in cytotoxicity against cancer cells, and in promoting a fibrotic response that ''walls off'' solid tumors (226). Whether this is a concern for treatments that aim to reduce eosinophil production remains to be seen.

7.4.1 Eosinophilic Skin Disease

In addition to atopic and contact dermatitis and chronic urticaria, eosinophil infiltration has been described in cases of other skin diseases, including psoriasis (227), bullous pemphigoid (228), systemic sclerosis (229), dermatitis herpetiformis (230), and erythema anulare (231). Also described are rarer syndromes involving eosinophilic skin disease. Eosinophilic lymphofolliculosis is a condition of men, involving facial, axillary, and inguinal eosinophilic furunculosis and granulomatous hyperplasia of draining lymph nodes (232). In 1990 a new syndrome of eosinophilic myalgia (EM) was described. Centers for Disease Control and Prevention (CDC) criteria defined this as circulating eosinophil counts of 1×10^9/L or more, with unexplained myalgias (233,234). Some patients had associated eosinophilic skin infiltration or eosinophilic fasciitis, although there is debate about whether the two syndromes are the same. In the EM patients, the disease could affect other systems, and some had life-threatening progressive disease (234). The syndrome was thought to result from ingestion of L-tryptophan or a contaminant in these preparations.

7.4.2 Eosinophil Lung Disease

Pulmonary eosinophilia is seen in a variety of rare syndromes in addition to asthma and tropical diseases (especially, tropical pulmonary eosinophilia, resulting from filarial infection) (235). Most eosinophilic pneumonias are idiopathic and resolve with corticosteroid treatments. Some result from drug reactions or are associated with multisystem granulomatous diseases, such as Churg–Strauss syndrome (236). A possible (rare) association between cysteinyl leukotriene receptor antagonists and Churg–Strauss syndrome has been described, although this may result from a steroid-sparing effect of these drugs, leading to unmasking of disease previously suppressed by corticosteroids (237). More recently, Brightling and colleagues have described the syndrome of eosinophilic bronchitis, which pathologically resembles asthma, but patients lack airflow obstruction and bronchial hyperresponsiveness (238). This may be an important differential diagnosis in unexplained cough, and appears to respond well to inhaled corticosteroids. Sputum induction or even bronchial biopsy may help with diagnosis.

Eosinophils are also prominent in some cases of pulmonary fibrosis, especially that associated with systemic sclerosis, but also some cases of idiopathic pulmonary fibrosis.

The observation that these cells are capable of synthesizing growth factors such as TGF-β suggests that they may contribute to the fibrotic process (239).

7.4.3 The Idiopathic Hypereosinophilic Syndrome

Idiopathic hypereosinophilic syndrome (HES) is an idiopathic leukoproliferative disease of overproduction of eosinophils and a characteristic pattern of organ damage. There are three defining features:

1. Sustained blood eosinophilia of more cells than 1.5×10^9/L for longer than 6 months.
2. All other causes of eosinophilia must have been excluded.
3. There should be signs of organ damage (240).

It occurs predominantly in men (9:1 men/women) aged 20–50. The presenting features are variable, and in some cases the eosinophilia is detected by chance (240–243). Cardiac manifestations are common (50–70% of reported series), with necrosis, thrombosis and, later, endomyocardial fibrosis (244,245). These lead to progressive cardiac failure, and may be recognized on echocardiography as an intracardiac thrombus or a restrictive cardiomyopathy (although dilated cardiomyopathy can also occur). Endomyocardial biopsy may be necessary for diagnosis (246). Neurological disease, which also occurs in 50–70% of cases, may be thromboembolic in some cases. In other cases direct encephalopathy occurs with ataxia, behavioral changes, confusion, memory loss, and upper motor neuron signs (247). Peripheral neuropathies are another manifestation of HES. Cutaneous involvement occurs in about 50% of HES patients, and includes angioedema and urticaria, pruritic nodules, or papules. Although chronic cough is seen in about 40% of patients, asthma is uncommon, and only 15–20% of patients have pulmonary infiltrates caused by eosinophilia. Other organs involved can include the eyes (thromboembolic disease, retinal arteritis), joints (rheumatological disease, large joint involvement with effusions, Raynaud's syndrome, and digital necrosis), and gastrointestinal tract (gastritis, colitis, pancreatitis, or rarely, sclerosing cholangitis). Nearly 40% of patients have a raised total serum IgE, and this may mark a favorable prognosis, with corticosteroid responsiveness (248).

The etiology of HES remains obscure. It is distinct from eosinophilic leukemias, although a few patients demonstrate chromosomal abnormalities, and there is an association with myelodysplasia and myelofibrosis. There may be overproduction of IL-5, but IL-5 transgenic mice show no organ damage despite massive hypereosinophilia, so some activating stimulus must also be present. A T-cell abnormality would be supported by the observation that IL-2 therapy (for solid tumors) is associated with an IL-5-driven eosinophilia (249). The differential diagnosis includes other idiopathic eosinophilic syndromes, outlined in the foregoing, including vasculitides, such as Churg–Strauss syndrome (250). The main distinguishing features are multiorgan and cardiac involvement. A biopsy showing vasculitis and granulomas would favor Churg–Strauss syndrome, as would the presence of asthma. Clinically, treatment is similar. The most important differential to make in the clinic is of parasitic infection: serology may be useful, in some circumstances combined with stool examination for *Strongyloides*. It is important to exclude these infections if high-dose steroids are to be given.

Treatment of Idiopathic Hypereosinophilic Syndrome

If there is no evidence of organ damage, eosinophilia per se is not an indication for treatment, although careful monitoring with echocardiography every 6 months may be required to detect asymptomatic cardiac disease. About 70% of HES patients show a partial or complete response to oral corticosteroids, usually initiated at a dose of 60 mg/day or 1 mg/kg per day of prednisolone, which is then tapered. Other agents that have been used for treatment include hydroxyurea and vincristine, with case reports of etoposide, and cyclosporin also being useful (240). Interferon-alfa was effective even in cases resistant to corticosteroids and cytotoxic agents (250a). Surgical treatment of cardiac disease may be required, and some patients with severe refractory disease have been treated with bone marrow transplantation. Although anticoagulation is logical, it may not prevent thromboembolism. On the whole, the prognosis for HES patients is for control of disease over a long period with 80% 5 to 10-year survival.

8 ANIMAL MODELS OF ALLERGIC DISEASE: WHAT DO THEY TELL US ABOUT EOSINOPHIL INVOLVEMENT?

Animal models of allergen challenge can reproduce the eosinophil infiltrate and airway hyperresponsiveness seen after airway challenge in asthmatic humans. These models allow the application of gene-knockout technology and blocking antibodies to dissect the role of the eosinophil in the changes seen. Studies with blocking antibodies and gene disruption of IL-5, CCR3, and eotaxin, all support a role for eosinophils in AHR in murine allergen challenge (251). These studies were extended to show prolonged diminution of AHR by a single dose of anti-IL-5 monoclonal antibody in a monkey model (252). However, not all models show such eosinophil dependence, and AHR can be observed independently of eosinophils and IgE in animal models. In particular Hogan et al. showed residual $CD4^+$ T-cell–dependent AHR in IL-4 gene-deleted BALB/c mice treated with anti-IL-5 antibodies (253), and Wills-Karp et al. and Grunig et al. showed that blockade of IL-13 could reduce AHR, without affecting airway eosinophilia or IgE (254,255).

9 CONCLUSION: HOW STRONG IS THE EVIDENCE THAT EOSINOPHILS CONTRIBUTE TO AIRWAY HYPERRESPONSIVENESS IN ASTHMA?

There is considerable circumstantial evidence linking eosinophils with asthma, and the current hypothesis is that they contribute to airway hyperresponsiveness through epithelial damage from granule protein release and through lipid mediators. However, there is no direct evidence that this is so. The most direct data will come with the application of strategies to specifically target eosinophils in human asthma. Initial reports are of a dose-finding–tolerance study of anti-IL-5 monoclonal antibody in an allergen challenge protocol. Two doses of anti-IL-5 or a placebo were given to three groups of eight subjects. The antibody significantly reduced blood and sputum eosinophils, but did not alter airway hyperresponsiveness before or 24 hr after allergen challenge, nor did it affect allergen PC_{20} (256). This data is clearly of interest, but more definitive larger studies in day-to-day asthma are in progress, and the results are eagerly awaited. Although airway eosinophilia is seen in almost all asthmatics studied, and the degree of eosinophil infiltration correlates with disease severity, on an individual basis, there are patients with relatively few eosinophils, but marked AHR and symptoms (193,196). In addition a subgroup of patients dying of asthma and some patients with severe chronic asthma appear to have neutrophil-predominant airway inflammation (257,258). These findings could represent the early neutrophilia seen after allergen challenge or the effects of corticosteroid treatment, but equally may suggest that some asthmatics do not have eosinophil-driven disease. Eosinophils are a potent source of fibrogenic cytokines and growth factors and may be involved in repair processes as well as inflammation. The relative role of the eosinophil in airway inflammation and airway remodeling should become clear in the next few years.

REFERENCES

1. Ehrlich P. Uber die specifischen granulationen des Blutes. Arch Anat Physiol Lpz 1879; 3. Physiol Abt 571.
2. Ehrlich P, Lazarus A. Histology of the Blood: Normal and Pathological. W Meyers, ed, trans. London: Cambridge University Press, 1900.
3. Ellis AG. The pathological anatomy of bronchial asthma. Am J Med Sci 1908; 136:407.
4. Gleich GJ, Adolphson CR. The eosinophil leukocyte: structure and function. Adv Immunol 1986; 39:177–253.
5. Gleich GJ. The eosinophil and bronchial asthma: current understanding. J Allergy Clin Immunol 1990; 85:422.
6. Goetzl EJ, Wasserman SI, Austen KF. Eosinophil polymorphonuclear leukocyte function in immediate hypersensitivity. Arch Pathol 1975; 99:4.
7. Steinbach KH, Shick P, Trepel F, Raffler H, Dohrmann J, Heilgeist G, Heltzel W, Li K, Past W, van der Woerd de Lange J, Theml H, Fliedner TM, Begeman H. Estimation of kinetic parameters of neutrophilic, eosinophilic, and basophilic granulocytes in human blood. Blut 1979; 39:27–38.
8. Dvorak AM, Ishizaka T. Human eosinophils in vitro. An ultrastructural morphology primer. Histol Histopathol 1994; 9:339–374.
9. Dvorak AM, Letourneau L, Login GR, Weller PF, Ackerman SJ. Ultrastructural localization of the Charcot–Leyden crystal protein (lysophospholipase) to a distinct crystalloid-free granule population in mature human eosinophils. Blood 1988; 72:150–158.
10. Dvorak AM, Furitsu T, Estrella P, Letourneau L, Ishizaka T, Ackerman J. Ultrastructural localization of major basic protein in the eosinophil lineage in vitro. J Histochem Cytochem 1994; 42:1443–1451.
11. Ogawa M. Hematopoesis. J Allergy Clin Immunol 1994; 94:645–650.
12. Basten A, Beeson PB. Mechanism of eosinophlia. II. The role of the lymphocyte. J Exp Med 1970; 131:1288–1305.
13. Desenne JJ, Acquatella G, Stern R, Muller A, Sanchez M, Somoza R. Blood eosinophilia in Hodgkin's disease: a follow up of 25 cases in Venezuela. Cancer 1992; 69:1248.
14. Shalit M, Sekhsaria S, Mauhorter S, Mahanti S, Malech HL. Early commitment to the eosinophil lineage by cultured human peripheral blood $CD34^+$ cells: messenger RNA analysis. J Allergy Clin Immunol 1996; 98:344–354.
15. Denburg JA, Telizyn S, Messner H, Lim B, Jamal N, Ackerman SJ, Gleich GJ, Bienenstock J. Heterogeneity of human peripheral blood eosinophil-type colonies: evidence for a common basophil–eosinophil progenitor. Blood 1985; 66:312–318.
16. Yamada T, Sun Q, Zeibecoglou K, Bungre J, North J, Kay AB, Lopez AF, Robinson DS. Interleukin-3, interleukin-5, granulocyte-macrophage colony stimulating factor receptor α subunit and common β subunit expression by peripheral leukocytes and blood dendritic cells. J Allergy Clin Immunol 1998; 101:677–682.
17. Clutterbuck EJ, Hirst EM, Sanderson CJ. Human interleukin 5 (IL-5) regulates the production of eosinophils in human bone marrow cultures: comparison and interaction with IL-1, IL-3, IL-6, and GM-CSF. Blood 1989; 73:1504–1512.
18. Yamaguchi Y, Suda T, Suda J, Eguchi M, Miura Y, Harad N, Taminaga A, Takatsu K. Purified interleukin 5 supports the terminal differentiation and proliferation of murine eosinophilic precursors. J Exp Med 1988; 167:43.

19. Sanderson CJ. Interleukin 5, eosinophils and disease. Blood 1992; 79:3101.
20. Dent LA, Strath M, Mellor AL, Sanderson CJ. Eosinophilia in transgenic mice expressing interleukin 5. J Exp Med 1990; 172:1425–1431.
21. Foster PS, Hogan SP, Ramsay AJ, Matthaei KI, Young IG. IL-5 deficiency abolishes eosinophilia, airways hyperreactivity, and lung damage in a mouse asthma model. J Exp Med 1995; 183:195–201.
22. Nishinakamura R, Miyajima A, Mee PJ, Tybulewicz VL, Murray R. Hematopoiesis in mice lacking the entire granulocyte–macrophage colony-stimulating factor/interleukin-3/interleukin-5 functions. Blood 1996; 88:2458–2464.
23. Tavernier J, Devos R, Cornelis S, Tuypens T, van der Heyden J, Fiers W, Plaetinck G. A human high affinity interleukin 5 receptor (IL5R) is composed of an IL-5 specific α chain and a β chain shared with the receptor for GM-CSF. Cell 1991; 66:1175–1184.
24. Kitamura T, Sato N, Arai K, Miyajima A. Expression cloning of the human IL-3 receptor cDNA reveals a shared β subunit for the human IL-3 and GM-CSF receptors. Cell 1991; 66:1165–1174.
25. Burdach S, Nishinakamura R, Dirksen U, Murray R. The physiologic role of interleukin-3, interleukin-5, granulocyte–macrophage colony-stimulating factor, and the beta c receptor system. Curr Opin Hematol 1998; 5:177–180.
26. Takagi M, Hara T, Ichihara M, Takatsu K, Miyajima A. Multi-colony stimulating activity of interleukin-5 (IL-5) on hematopoietic progenitors from transgenic mice that express IL-5 receptor α subunit constitutively. J Exp Med 1995; 181:889–899.
27. Pazdrak K, Stafford S, Alam R. The activation of Jak–STAT1 signalling pathway by IL-5 in eosinophils. J Immunol 1995; 155:397.
28. Huston MM, Moore JP, Mettes HJ, Tavana G, Huston DP. Human B cells express IL-5 receptor messenger ribonucleic acid and respond to IL-5 with enhanced IgM production after mitogenic stimulation with *Moraxella catarrhalis*. J Immunol 1996; 156:1392–1401.
29. Hakonarson H, Maskeri N, Carter C, Chuang S, Grunstein MM. Autocrine interaction between IL-5 and IL-1 beta mediates altered responsiveness of atopic asthmatic sensitized airway smooth muscle. J Clin Invest 1999; 104:657–667.
30. Tavernier J, Tuypens T, Plaetinck G, Verhee A, Fiers W, Devos R. Molecular basis of the membrane-anchored and two soluble isoforms of the human interleukin 5 receptor α subunit. Proc Natl Acad Sci USA 1992; 89:7041–7045.
31. Tavernier J, Van der Heyden J, Verhee A, Brusselle G, Van Ostade X, Vandekerckhove J, North J, Rankin SM, Kay AB, Robinson DS. Interleukin 5 regulates the isoform expression of its own receptor α-subunit. Blood 2000; 95:1600–1607.
32. Mauser PJ, Pitman AM, Fernandez X, et al. Effects of an antibody to interleukin-5 in a monkey model of asthma. Am J Respir Crit Care Med 1995; 52:467–472.
33. Sehmi R, Wood LJ, Watson R, Foley R, Hamid Q, O'Byrne PM, Denburg JA. Allergen-induced increases in IL-5Rα subunit expression on bone-marrow derived $CD34^+$ cells from asthmatic subjects. J Clin Invest 1997; 100:2466–2475.
34. Zeibecoglou K, Ying S, Yamada T, North J, Burman J, Bungre J, Meng Q, Kay AB, Robinson DS. Increased mature and immature CCR3 messenger RNA^+ eosinophils in bone marrow from atopic asthmatics compared to atopic and non-atopic control subjects. J Allergy Clin Immunol 1999; 103:99–106.
35. Sehmi R, Howie K, Sutherland DR, Schragge W, O'Byrne PM, Denburg JA. Increased levels of $CD34^+$ hemopoietic progenitor cells in atopic subjects. Am J Respir Cell Mol Biol 1996; 15:645–655.
36. Wood LJ, Inman MD, Denburg JA, O'Byrne PM. Allergen challenge increases cell traffic between bone marrow and lung. Am J Respir Cell Mol Biol 1998; 18:759–767.
37. Gibson PG, Dolovich J, Girgis–Gabado A, Morris MM, Anderson M, Hargreave FE, Denburg JA. The inflammatory response in asthma exacerbation: changes in circulating eosinophils, basophils, and their progenitors. Clin Exp Allergy 1990; 20:661–668.

38. Robinson DS, Damia R, Zeibecoglou K, Molet S, North J, Yamada T, Kay AB, Hamid Q. CD34$^+$/IL-5Rα mRNA$^+$ cells in the bronchial mucosa in asthma: evidence for airway eosinophil progenitors. Am J Respir Cell Mol Biol 1999; 20:9.
39. Eidelman DH, Minshall E, Dandurand RJ, Schotman E, Song YL, Yasruel Z, Moqbel R, Hamid Q. Evidence for major basic protein immunoreactivity and interleukin 5 gene activation during the late phase response in explanted airways. Am J Respir Cell Mol Biol 1996; 15:582–589.
40. Wang J, Palmer K, Lotvall J, Milan S, Lei XF, Matthaei KI, Gauldie J, Inman MD, Jordana M, Xing Z. Circulating, but not local lung, IL-5 is required for the development of antigen-induced airways eosinophilia. J Clin Invest 1998; 102:1132–1141.
41. Shi H, Qin S, Huang G, Chen Y, Xiao C, Xu H, Liang G, Xie Z, Qin X, Wu J, Li G, Zhang C. Infiltration of eosinophils into the asthmatic airways caused by interleukin-5. Am J Respir Cell Mol Biol 1997; 16:220–224.
42. Shi HZ, Xiao CQ, Zhong D, Qin SM, Liu Y, Liang GR, Xu H, Chen YQ, Long XM, Xie ZF. Effect of inhaled interleukin-5 on airway hyperreactivity and eosinophilia in asthmatics. Am J Respir Crit Care Med 1998; 157:204–209.
43. Collins PD, Marleau S, Griffiths JD, Jose PJ, Williams TJ. Cooperation between interleukin-5 and the chemokine eotaxin to induce eosinophil accumulation in vivo. J Exp Med 1995; 182:1169–1174.
44. Palframan RT, Collins PD, Williams TJ, Rankin SM. Eotaxin induces a rapid release of eosinophils and their precursors from the bone marrow. Blood 1998; 91:2240–2248.
45. Palframan RT, Collins PD, Severs NJ, Rothery S, Williams TJ, Rankin SJ. Mechanisms of acute eosinophil mobilization from the bone marrow stimulated by interleukin 5: the role of specific adhesion molecules and phosphatidylinositol 3-kinase. J Exp Med 1998; 188:1621.
46. Wardlaw AJ, Symon FS, Walsh GM. Eosinophil adhesion in allergic inflammation. J Allergy Clin Immunol 1994; 94:1163–1171.
47. Symon FA, Walsh GM, Watson SR, Wardlaw AJ. Eosinophil adhesion to nasal polyp endothelium is P-selectin-dependent. J Exp Med 1994; 180:371–376.
48. Walsh GM, Hartnell A, Wardlaw AJ, Kurihara K, Sanderson CJ, Kay AB. IL-5 enhances the in vitro adhesion of human eosinophils, but not neutrophils in a leukocyte integrin (CD11/CD18)-dependent manner. Immunology 1990; 71:258–265.
49. Walsh GM, Mermod JJ, Hartnell A, Kay AB, Wardlaw AJ. Human eosinophil, but not neutrophil, adherence to IL-1-stimulated human umbilical vascular endothelial cells is alpha 4 beta 1 (very late antigen-4) dependent. J Immunol 1991; 146:3419–3423.
50. Bochner BS, Schleimer RP. The role of adhesion molecules in human eosinophil and basophil recruitment. J Allergy Clin Immunol 1994; 94:427–438.
51. Thornhill MH, Haskard DO. IL-4 regulates endothelial cell activation by IL-1, tumor necrosis factor, or IFN-gamma. J Immunol 1990; 145:865–872.
52. Bochner BS, Klunk DA, Sterbinsky SA, Coffman RL, Schleimer RP. IL-13 selectively induces vascular cell adhesion molecule-1 expression in human endothelial cells. J Immunol 1995; 154:799–803.
53. Ying S, Meng Q, Barata LT, Robinson DS, Durham SR, Kay AB. Associations between IL-13 and IL-14 (mRNA and protein), vascular cell adhesion molecule-1 expression, and the infiltration of eosinophils, macrophages,and T cells in allergen-induced late-phase cutaneous reactions in atopic subjects. J Immunol 1997; 158:5050–5057.
54. Georas SN, McIntyre BW, Ebisawa M, Bednarczyk JL, Sterbinsky SA, Schleimer RP, Bochner BS. Expression of a functional laminin receptor (alpha 6 beta 1, very late activation antigen-6) on human eosinophils. Blood 1993; 82:2872–2879.
55. Walsh GM, Symon FA, Lazarovils AL, Wardlaw AJ. Integrin alpha 4 beta 7 mediates human eosinophil interaction with MAdCAM-1, VCAM-1, and fibronectin. Immunology 1996; 89: 112–119.
56. Peroni DG, Djukanovic R, Bradding P, Feather IH, Montefort S, Howarth PH, Jones DB,

Holgate ST. Expression of CD44 and integrins in bronchial mucosa of normal and mildly asthmatic subjects. Eur Respir J 1996; 9:2236–2242.
57. Hamann KJ, Dowling TL, Neeley SP, Grant JA, Leff AR. Hyaluronic acid enhances cell proliferation during eosinophilopoiesis through CD44 surface antigen. J Immunol 1995; 154: 4073–4080.
58. Springer TA. Adhesion receptors of the immune system. Nature 1990; 346:425–434.
59. Davies D, Larbi K, Allen A, Sanz M, Weg VB, Haskard DO, Lobb RR, Nourshargh S. VCAM-1 contributes to rapid eosinophil accumulation induced by the chemoattractants PAF and LTB4: evidence for basal expression of functional VCAM-1 in rat skin. Immunology 1999; 97:150–158.
60. Kimani G, Tonnesen MG, Henson PM. Stimulation of eosinophil adherence to human vascular endothelial cells in vitro by platelet-activating factor. J Immunol 1988; 140:3161–3166.
61. Teixeira MM, Rossi AG, Hellewell PG. Adhesion mechanisms involved in C5a-induced eosinophil homotypic aggregation. J Leukoc Biol 1996; 59:389–396.
62. Nagata M, Sedgwick JB, Vrtis R, Busse WW. Endothelial cells upregulate eosinophil superoxide generation via VCAM-1 expression. Clin Exp Allergy 1999; 29:550–561.
63. Anwar AR, Moqbel R, Walsh GM, Kay AB, Wardlaw AJ. Adhesion to fibronectin prolongs eosinophil survival. J Exp Med 1993; 177:839–843.
64. Ohmiya N, Saga S, Ohbayashi M, Kozaki K, Miyaishi O, Kobayashi M, Kasuya S, Arisawa T, Goto H, Hayakawa T. Kinetics and collagenolytic role of eosinophils in chronic gastric ulcer in the rat. Histochem Cell Biol 1997; 108:27–34.
65. Dahlen B, Shute J, Howarth P. Immunohistochemical localisation of the matrix metalloproteinases MMP-3 and MMP-9 within the airways in asthma. Thorax 1999; 54:590–596.
66. Warringa RAJ, Koenderman L, Kok PTM, Krekniet J, Bruijnzeel PLB. Modulation and induction of eosinophil chemotaxis by granulocyte macrophage colony stimulating factor and interleukin-3. Blood 1991; 77:2694–2700.
67. Sehmi R, Wardlaw AJ, Cromwell O, Waltman P, Kurihara K, Kay AB. Interleukin 5 (IL-5) selectively enhances the chemotactic response of eosinophils obtained from normal but not eosinophilic donors. Blood 1992; 79:2952–2959.
68. Wardlaw AJ, Moqbel R, Cromwell O, Kay AB. Platelet activating factor is a potent chemotactic and chemokinetic factor for human eosinophils. J Clin Invest 1986; 78:1701–1706.
69. Gerard NP, Gerard C. The chemotactic receptor for human C5a and anaphylotoxin. Nature 1991; 349:614.
70. Sehmi R, Cromwell O, Taylor GW, Kay AB. The identification of leukotriene B_4 and 18(s)15(s)-diHETE as the principal eosinophil chemotactic factors released during anaphylaxis of the guinea pig lung. J Immunol 1991; 147:2276–2283.
71. Baggiolini M. Chemokines and leukocyte traffic. Nature 1998; 392:565–568.
72. Jose PJ, Griffiths Johnson DA, Collins PD, Walsh DT, Moqbel R, Totty NF, Truong O, Hsuan JJ, Williams TJ. Eotaxin: a potent eosinophil chemoattractant cytokine detected in a guinea pig model of allergic airways inflammation. J Exp Med 1994; 179:881–887.
73. Garcia Zepeda EA, Rothenberg ME, Ownbey RT, Celestin J, Leder P, Luster AD. Human eotaxin is a specific chemoattractant for eosinophil cells and provides a new mechanism to explain tissue eosinophilia. Nat Med 1996; 2:449–456.
74. Daugherty BL, Siciliano SJ, DeMartino JA, Malkowitz L, Sirotina A, Springer MS. Cloning, expression, and characterization of the human eosinophil eotaxin receptor. J Exp Med 1996; 183:2349–2354.
75. Uguccioni M, Mackay CR, Ochensberger B, Loetscher P, Rhis S, LaRosa GJ, Rao P, Ponath PD, Baggiolini M, Dahinden CA. High expression of the chemokine receptor CCR3 in human blood basophils. Role in activation by eotaxin, MCP-4, and other chemokines. J Clin Invest 1997; 100:1137–1143.
76. Ying S, Taborda Barata L, Meng Q, Humbert M, Kay AB. The kinetics of allergen-induced transcription of messenger RNA for monocyte chemotactic protein-3 and RANTES in the

skin of human atopic subjects: relationship to eosinophil, T cell, and macrophage recruitment. J Exp Med 1995; 181:2153–2159.

77. Sabroe I, Hartnell A, Jopling AL, Bel S, Ponath PD, Pease JE, Collins PD, Williams TJ. Differential regulation of eosinophil chemokine signalling via CCR3 and non-CCR3 pathways. J Immunol 1999; 162:2946.
78. Tenscher K, Metzner B, Schopf E, Norgauer J, Czech W. Recombinant human eotaxin induces oxygen radical production, Ca^{2+} mobilzation, actin reorganisation and CD11b upregulation via a pertussis toxin-sensitive heterotrimeric guanine nucleotide binding protein. Blood 1996; 88:3195–3199.
79. He J, Chen Y, Farzan M, Choe H, Ohagen A, Gartner S, Busciglio J, Yang X, Hofmann W, Newman W, Mackay CR, Sodroski J, Gabuzda D. CCR3 and CCR5 are co-receptors for HIV-1 infection of microglia. Nature 1997; 385:645–649.
80. Fox CH, Kotler D, Tierney A, Wilson CS, Fauci AS. Detection of HIV-1 RNA in the lamina propria of patients with AIDS and gastrointestinal disease. J Infect Dis 1989; 159:467–471.
81. Lucey DR, Dorsky DI, Nicolson Weller A, Weller PF. Human eosinophils express CD4 protein and bind human immunodeficiency virus 1 gp120. J Exp Med 1989; 169:327.
82. Grimaldi JC, Yu NX, Grunig G, Seymour BW, Cottrez F, Robinson DS, Hosken N, Ferlin WG, Wu X, Soto H, O'Garra A, Howard MC, Coffman RL. Depletion of eosinophils in mice through the use of antibodies specific for C-C chemokine receptor 3 (CCR3). J Leukoc Biol 1999; 65:846–853.
83. Dunzendorfer S, Meierhofer C, Wiedermann CJ. Signalling in neuropeptide-induced migration of human eosinophils. J Leukoc Biol 1998; 64:828–834.
84. Stern M, Meagher L, Savill J, Haslett C. Apoptosis in human eosinophils: programmed cell death in the eosinophil leads to phagocytosis by macrophages and is modulated by IL-5. J Immunol 1992; 148:3543.
85. Her E, Frazer J, Austen KF, Owen WF Jr. Eosinophil hematopoietins anatagonize the programmed cell death of eosinophils. J Clin Invest 1991; 88:1982–1987.
86. Hamid Q, Azzawi M, Sun Ying, Moqbel R, Wardlaw AJ, Corrigan CJ, Bradley B, Durham SR, Collins JV, Jeffery PK, Quint DJ, Kay AB. Expression of mRNA for interleukin-5 in mucosal bronchial biopsies from asthma. J Clin Invest 1991; 87:1541–1546.
87. Robinson DS, Hamid Q, Sun Ying, Tsicopoulos A, Barkans J, Bentley AM, Corrigan CJ, Durham SR, Kay AB. Predominant T_h2-like bronchoalveolar T lymphocyte population in atopic asthma. N Engl J Med 1992; 326:298–304.
88. Walker C, Bode E, Boer L, Hansel TT, Blaser K, Virchow J–C Jr. Allergic and non-allergic asthmatics have distinct patterns of T cell activation and cytokine production in peripheral blood and bronchoalveolar lavage. Am Rev Respir Dis 1992; 146:109–115.
89. Simon HU, Yousefi S, Dibbert B, Hebestreit H, Weber M, Branch DR, Blaser K, Levi–Schafer F, Anderson GP. Role for tyrosine phosphorylation and *lyn* tyrosine kinase in *fas* receptor mediated apoptosis in eosinophils. Blood 1998; 92:547–557.
90. Hebestreit H, Dibbert B, Balatti I, Braun D, Schapowal A, Blaser K, Simon HU. Disruption of *fas* receptor signaling by nitric oxide in eosinophils. J Exp Med 1998; 187:415–425.
91. Kharitonov SA, Yates D, Robbins RA, Logan–Sinclair R, Shinebourne EA, Barnes PJ. Increased nitric oxide in exhaled air of asthmatic patients. Lancet 1994; 343:133–135.
92. Meagher LC, Cousin JM, Seckl JR, Haslett C. Opposing effects of glucocorticoids on the rate of apoptosis in neutrophilic and eosinophilic granulocytes. J Immunol 1996; 156:4422–4428.
93. Dibbert B, Daigle I, Braun D, Schranz C, Weber M, Blaser K, Zangemeister–Wittke U, Akbar AN, Simon HU. Role for Bcl-xL in delayed eosinophil apoptosis mediated by granulocyte–macrophage colony-stimulating factor and interleukin-5. Blood 1998; 92:778–783.
94. Plotz SG, Dibbert B, Abeck D, Ring J, Simon HU. Bcl-2 expression by eosinophils in a patient with hypereosinophilia. J Allergy Clin Immunol 1998; 102:1037–1040.

95. Lewis DM, Lewis JC, Loegering DA, Gleich GJ. Localization of the guinea pig eosinophil major basic protein to the core of the granule. J Cell Biol 1978; 77:702–713.
96. Egesten A, Alumets J, von Mecklenburg C, Plamegren M, Olssen I. Localization of eosinophil cationic protein, major basic protein and eosinophil peroxidase in human eosinophils by immunoelectron microscopic technique. J Histochem Cytochem 1986; 34:1399–1403.
97. Peters MS, Rodriguez M, Gleich GJ. Localization of human eosinophil granule major basic protein, eosinophil cationic protein and eosinophil-derived neurotoxin by immunoelectron microscopy. Lab Invest 1986; 54:656–662.
98. Popken–Harris P, Checkel J, Loegering D, Madden B, Springett M, Kephart G, Gleich GJ. Regulation and processing of a precursor form of eosinophil granule major basic protein (ProMBP) in differentiating eosinophils. Blood 1998; 92:623–631.
99. Yamaguchi Y, Nishio H, Kishi K, Ackerman SJ, Suda T. C/EBPbeta and GATA-1 synergistically regulate activity of the eosinophil granule major basic protein promoter: implication for C/EBPbeta activity in eosinophil gene expression. Blood 1999; 94:1429–1439.
100. Plager DA, Loegering DA, Weiler DA, Checkel JL, Wagner JM, Clarke NJ, Naylor S, Page SM, Thomas LL, Akerblom I, Cocks B, Stuart S, Gleich GJ. A novel and highly divergent homolog of human eosinophil granule major basic protein. J Biol Chem 1999; 274:14464–14473.
101. O'Donnell MC, Ackerman SJ, Gleich GJ, Thomas LL. Activation of basophil and mast cell histamine release by eosinophil granule major basic protein. J Exp Med 1983; 157:1981.
102. McGrogan M, Simonsen C, Scott R, Griffith J, Ellis N, Kennedy J, Campanelli D, Nathan C, Gabay J. Isolation of a complementary DNA clone encoding a precursor to human eosinophil major basic protein. J Exp Med 1988; 168:2295.
103. Barker RL, Gleich GJ, Pease LR. Acidic precursor revealed in human eosinophil granule major basic protein cDNA. J Exp Med 1988; 168:1493.
104. Ackerman SJ. Characterization and functions of eosinophil granule proteins. In: Makino S, Fukuda, T, eds. Eosinophils. Biological and Clinical Aspects; Boca Raton: CRC Press, 1993: 33–74.
105. Maddox DE, Kephart GM, Coulam CB, Butterfield JH, Benirschke K, Gleich GJ. Localization of a molecule immunochemically similar to eosinophil major basic protein in human placenta. J Exp Med 1984; 160:29–41.
106. Rosenberg HF, Ackerman SJ, Tenen DG. Human eosinophil cationic protein: molecular cloning of a cytotoxin and helminthotoxin with ribonuclease activity. J Exp Med 1989; 67:498.
107. Barker RL, Loegering DA, Ten RM, Hamann KJ, Pease LR, Gleich GJ. Eosinophil cationic protein cDNA. Comparison with other toxic cationic proteins and ribonucleases. J Immunol 1989; 143:952.
108. Slifman NR, Loegering DA, McKean DJ, Gleich GJ. Ribonuclease activity associated with human eosinophil derived neurotoxin and eosinophil cationic protein. J Immunol 1986; 137: 2913.
109. Hamann KJ, Gleich GJ, Checkel JL, Loegring DA, McCall JW, Barker RL. In vitro killing of microfilariae of *Brugia pahangi* and *Brugia malayi* by eosinophil granule proteins. J Immunol 1990; 144:3166–3173.
110. Tai P–C, Spry CJ, Peterson C, Venge P, Olsson I. Monoclonal antibodies distinguish between storage and secreted forms of eosinophil cationic protein. Nature 1984; 309:182–184.
111. Nakajima H, Loegering DA, Kita H, Kephart GM, Gleich GJ. Reactivity of monoclonal antibodies EG1 and EG2 with eosinophils and their granule proteins. J Leukoc Biol 1999; 66:447–454.
111a. Abu–Ghazleh RI, Dunnette SL, Loegering DA, Checkel JL, Kita H, Thomas LL, Gleich GJ. Eosinophil granule proteins in peripheral blood granulocytes. J Leukoc Biol 1992; 52:611–618.
112. Young JDE, Peterson CGB, Venge P, Cohn ZA. Mechanism of membrane damage mediated by human eosinophil cationic protein. Nature 1986; 321:613.

113. Slifman NR, Peterson CGB, Gleich GJ, Dunette SL, Venge P. Human eosinophil-derived neurotoxin and eosinophil protein-X are likely the same protein. J Immunol 1989; 143:2317–2322.
114. Rosenburg HF, Tenen DG, Ackerman SJ. Molecular cloning of the human eosinophil-derived neurotoxin: a member of the ribonuclease gene family. Proc Natl Acad Sci USA 1989; 86: 4460.
115. Sur S, Glitz DG, Kita H, Kujawa SM, Peterson EA, Weiler DA, Kephart GM, Wagner JM, George TJ, Gleich GJ, Leiferman KM. Localisation of eosinophil-derived neurotoxin and eosinophil cationic protein in neutrophilic leukocytes. J Leukoc Biol 1998; 63:715–722.
116. Ten RM, Pease LR, McKean DJ, Bel MP, Gleich GJ. Molecular cloning of the human eosinophil peroxidase. J Exp Med 1989; 169:1757.
117. Sakamaki K, Tomonaga M, Tsukui K, Nagata S. Molecular cloning and characterization of a chromosomal gene for human eosinophil peroxidase. J Biol Chem 1989; 264:16828.
118. Weller PF, Dvorak AM. Arachidonic acid incorporation by cytoplasmic lipid bodies of human eosinophils. Blood 1985; 65:1269.
119. Silverman E, In KH, Yandava C, Drazen JM. Pharmacogenetics of the 5-lipoxygenase pathway in asthma. Clin Exp Allergy 1998; 28(suppl 5):164–170.
120. Drazen JM, Yandava CN, Dube L, Szczerback N, Hippensteel R, Pillari A, Israel E, Schork N, Silverman ES, Katz DA, Drajesk J. Pharmacogenetic association between ALOX5 promoter genotype and the response to anti-asthma treatment. Nat Genet 1999; 22:168–170.
121. Hubscher T. Role of the eosinophil in allergic reactions. II. Release of prostaglandins from human eosinophilic leukocytes. J Immunol 1975; 114:1389.
122. Foegh ML, Maddox YT, Ramwell PW. Human peritoneal eosinophils and formation of arachidonate cyclo-oxygenase products. Scand J Immunol 1986; 23:599.
123. Matsumoto T, Funk CD, Radmark O, Hoog JO, Jornvall H, Samuelsson B. Molecular cloning and amino acid sequence of human 5-lipoxygenase. Proc Natl Acad Sci USA 1988; 85:26.
124. Miller DK, Gillard JW, Vickers PJ, Sadowski S, Leveille C, Mancini JA, Charleson P, Dixon RAF, Ford–Hutchinson AW, Fortin R, Gauthier JY, Rodkey J, Rosen R, Rouzer C, Sigal IS, Strader CD, Evans JF. Identification and isolation of a membrane protein necessary for leukotriene production. Nature 1990; 343:278–281.
125. Samuelsson B. Leukotrienes: mediators of hypersensitivity reactions and inflammation. Science 1983; 220:568–575.
126. Weller PF. Eicosanoids, cytokines and other mediators elaborated by eosinophils. In: Makino S, Fukuda T, eds. Eosinophils, Biological and Clinical Aspects. Boca Raton: CRC Press, 1993; 125–154.
127. Jorg A, Henderson WR, Murphy RC, Klebanoff SJ. Leukotriene generation by eosinophils. J Exp Med 1982; 155:390.
128. Sun FF, Czuk CI, Taylor BM. Arachidonic acid metabolism in guinea pig eosionophils: synthesis of thromboxane B_2 and leukotriene B_4 in response to soluble or particulate activators. J Leukoc Biol 1989; 46:152.
129. Shaw RJ, Walsh GM, Cromwell O, Moqbel R, Spry CJF, Kay AB. Activated human eosinophils generate SRS-A leukotrienes following physiological (IgG-dependent) stimulation. Nature 1985; 316:150–152.
130. Bruijnzeel PL, Kok PT, Hameling ML, Kijne AM, Verhagen J. Exclusive leukotriene C_4 synthesis by purified human eosinophils induced by opsonized zymosan. FEBS Lett 1985; 316:350–354.
131. Cromwell O, Moqbel R, Fitzharris P, Kurlak L, Harvey C, Walsh GM, Shaw RJ, Kay AB. Leukotriene C_4 generation from human eosinophils stimulated with IgG–*Aspergillus fumigatus* antigen immune complexes. J Allergy Clin Immunol 1988; 82:535–544.
132. Sano A, Munoz N, Sano H, Choi J, Zhu X, Jacobs B, Leff AR. Inhibition of cPLA2 translocation and leucotriene C4 secretion by fluticasone propionate in exogenously activated human eosinophils. Am J Respir Crit Care Med 1999; 159:1903–1909.

133. Aizawa T, Tamura G, Ohtsu H, Takashima T. Eosinophil and neutrophil production of leukotriene C_4 and B_4: comparison of cells from asthmatic subjects and healthy donors. Ann Allergy 1990; 64:287–292.
134. Kohi F, Miyagawa H, Agrawal DK, Bewtra AK, Townley RG. Generation of leukotriene B_4 and C_4 from granulocytes of normal controls, allergic rhinitis and healthy donors. Ann Allergy 1990; 65:228–232.
135. Taniguchi N, Mita H, Saito H, Yui Y, Kajita T, Shida T. Increased generation of leukotriene C_4 from eosinophils in asthmatic patients. Allergy 1985; 40:571–573.
136. Sigal E, Craik CS, Highland E, Grunberger D, Costello LL, Dixon RAF, Nade JA. Molecular cloning and primary structure of human 15-lipoxygenase. Biochem Biophys Res Commun 1988; 157:457.
137. Sigal E, Grunberger D, Cashman JR, Craik CS, Caughey GH, Nadel JA. Arachidonate 15-lipoxygenase from human eosinophil enriched leukocytes: partial purification and properties. Biochem Biophys Res Commun 1988; 150:376.
138. Turk J, Maas RL, Brash AR, Roberts L, Oates JA. Arachidonic acid and 15-lipoxygenase products from human eosinophils. J Biol Chem 1982; 257:7068.
139. Marom Z, Shelhamer JH, Sun F, Kaliner M. Human airway monohydroxyeicosatetraenoic acid generation and mucus release. J Clin Invest 1983; 72:122.
140. Serhan CN, Hirsch U, Palmblad J, Samuelsson B. Formation of lipoxin A by granulocytes from eosinophilic donors. FEBS Lett 1987; 217:242.
141. Lee TH, Horton CE, Kyan Aung, Haskaard D, Crea AE, Spur BW. Lipoxin A_4 and lipoxin B_4 inhibit chemotactic responses of human neutrophils stimulated by leukotriene B_4 and *N*-formylmethionine-leucine-phenylalanine. Clin Sci 1989; 77:195.
142. Henderson WR Jr, Lewis DB, Albert RK, Zhang Y, Lamm WJ, Chiang GK, Jones F, Eriksen P, Tien YT, Jonas M, Chi EY. The importance of leukotrienes in airway inflammation in a mouse model of asthma. J Exp Med 1996; 184:483–494.
143. Snyder F. Chemical and biochemical aspects of platelet activating factor: a novel class of acetylated ether linked choline-phosphlipids. Med Res Rev 1985; 5:107–140.
144. Lee T–C, Malone B, Wasserman SI, Fitzgerald V, Snyder F. Activities of enzymes that metabolize platelet-activating factor (1-alkyl-2-acetyl-*sn*-glycero-3-phosphocholine) in neutrophils and eosinophils from human and the effect of a calcium ionophore. Biochem Biophys Res Commun 1982; 105:1303.
145. Lee T–C, Lenihan DJ, Malone B, Roddy LL, Wasserman SI. Increased biosynthesis of platelet activating factor in activated human eosinophils. J Biol Chem 1984; 259:5526.
146. Bartemes KR, McKinney S, Gleich GJ, Kita H. Endogenous platelet-activating factor is critically involved in effector functions of eosinophils stimulated with IL-5 or IgG. J Immunol 1999; 162:2982–2989.
147. Henson PM. PAF—a perspective. Am J Respir Cell Mol Biol 1989; 1:263.
148. Cromwell O, Wardlaw AJ, Osei D, Champion A, Moqbel R, Kay AB. IgG-dependent generation of platelet activating factor by normal and low density human eosinophils. J Immunol 1990; 145:3862–3868.
149. Burke LA, Crea REG, Wilkinson JRW, Arm JP, Spur BW, Lee TH. Comparison of the generation of platelet activating factor and leukotriene C_4 in human eosinophils stimulated by unopsonized zymosan and the calcium inophore A23187: the effects of nedocromil sodium. J Allergy Clin Immunol 1990; 85:26–35.
150. Butterworth AE, Thorne KJI. Eosinophils and parasitic diseases. In: Smith H, Cook RM, eds. Immunopharmocology of Eosinophils. London: Academic Press 1993; 119–150.
151. Horie S, Gleich GJ, Kita H. Cytokines directly induce degranulation and superoxide production from human eosinophils. J Allergy Clin Immunol 1996; 98:371–381.
152. Tool AT, Koenderman L, Kok PT, Blom M, Roos D, Verhoeven AJ. Release of platelet activating factor is important for the respiratory burst induced in human eosinophils by opsonised particles. Blood 1992; 79:2729–2732.

153. Nagata M, Sedgwick JB, Busse WW. Differential effects of granulocyte–macrophage colony-stimulating factor on eosinophil and neutrophil superoxide anion generation. J Immunol 1995; 155:4948–4954.
154. Dent G, Munoz NM, Ruhlmann E, Zhu X, Leff AR, Magnussen H, Rabe KF. Protein kinase C inhibition enhances platelet-activating factor-induced eicosanoid production in human eosinophils. Am J Respir Cell Mol Biol 1998; 18:136–144.
155. Kita H, Ohnishi T, Okubo Y, Weiler D, Abrams JS, Gleich GJ. Granulocyte/macrophage colony-stimulating factor and interleukin 3 release from human peripheral blood eosinophils and neutrophils. J Exp Med 1991; 174:745–748.
156. Moqbel R, Hamid Q, Ying S, Barkans J, Hartnell A, Tsicopoulos A, Wardlaw AJ, Kay AB. Expression of mRNA and immunoreactivity for the granulocyte/macrophage colony-stimulating factor in activated human eosinophils. J Exp Med 1991; 174:749–752.
157. Sun Ying, Humbert M, Barkans J, Corrigan CJ, Pfister R, Menz G, Larche M, Robinson DS, Durham SR, Kay AB. Expression of IL-4 and IL-5 mRNA and protein product by $CD4^+$ and $CD8^+$ T cells, eosinophils, and mast cells in bronchial biopsies obtained from atopic and nonatopic (intrinsic) asthmatics. J Immunol 1997; 158:3539–3544.
158. Woerly G, Roger N, Loiseau S, Capron M. Expression of Th1 and Th2 immunoregulatory cytokines by human eosinophils. Int Arch Allergy Immunol 1999; 118:95–97.
159. Levi–Schaffer F, Lacy P, Severs NJ, Newman TM, North J, Gomperts B, Kay AB, Moqbel R. Association of granulocyte–macrophage colony-stimulating factor with the crystalloid granules of human eosinophils. Blood 1995; 85:2579–2586.
160. Moqbel R, Levi–Schaffer F, Kay AB. Cytokine generation by eosinophils. J Allergy Clin Immunol. 1994; 94:1183–1188.
161. Ackerman SJ, Corrette SE, Rosenberg HF, Bennett JC, Mastrianni DM, Nicholson–Weller A, Weller PF, Chin DT, Tenen DG. Molecular cloning and characterization of human eosinophil Charcot–Leyden crystal protein (lysophospholipase). Similarities to IgE binding proteins and the S-type animal lectin superfamily. J Immunol 1993; 150:456–468.
162. Leonidas DD, Elbert BL, Zhou Z, Leffler H, Ackerman SJ, Acharya KR. Crystal structure of human Charcot–Leyden crystal protein, an eosinophil lysophospholipase, identifies it as a new member of the carbohydrate-binding family of galectins. Structure 1995; 3:1379–1393.
163. Weller PF, Goetzl EJ, Austen KF. Identification of human eosinophils lysophospholipase as the constituent of Charcot–Leyden crystals. Proc Natl Acad Sci USA 1980; 77:7440.
164. Spry CJF. Eosinophils. A Comprehensive Review and Guide to the Medical Literature. London: Oxford University Press, 1988.
165. Lucey DR, Nicolson–Weller A, Weller PF. Mature human eosinophils have the capacity to express HLA-DR. Proc Natl Acad Sci USA 1989; 86:1348.
166. Woerly G, Roger N, Loiseau S, Dombrowicz D, Capron A, Capron M. Expression of CD28 and CD86 by human eosinophils and role in the secretion of type 1 cytokines (interleukin 2 and interferon gamma): inhibition by immunoglobulin A complexes. J Exp Med 1999; 190:487–495.
167. Del–Pozo V, De–Andres B, Martin E, Cardaba B, Fernandez JC, Gallardo S, Tramon P, Leyva–Cobian F, Palomino P, Lahoz C. Eosinophil as antigen-presenting cell: activation of T cell clones and T cell hybridoma by eosinophils after antigen processing. Eur J Immunol 1992; 22:1919–1925.
168. Gauchat JF, Henchoz S, Fattah D, et al. CD40 ligand is functionally expressed on human eosinophils. Eur J Immunol 1995; 25:863–865.
169. Nusse O, Lindau M, Cromwell O, Kay AB, Gomperts BD. J Exp Med 1990; 171:775–786.
170. Erjefalt JS, Anderson M, Gizycki MJ, Greiff L, Korsgren M, Jeffery PK, Persson CGA. Cytolysis and piecemeal degranulation as distinct modes of activation of airway mucosal eosinophils. J Allergy Clin Immunol 1998; 102:286–294.
171. Erjefalt JS, Greiff L, Pettersson H, Mattson E, Linden M, Rogers A, Jeffery PK, Persson

CGA. Eosinophil cytolysis is a primary mechanism for granule protein release in human upper airways. Am J Respir Crit Care Med 1999; 160:304–312.
172. Moqbel R, Lacy P. Exocytotic events in eosinophils and mast cells. Clin Exp Allergy 2000; 30:1667–1671.
173. Horie S, Kita H. CD11b/CD18 (Mac-1) is required for degranulation of human eosinophils induced by human recombinant granulocyte–macrophage colony-stimulating factor and platelet-activating factor. J Immunol 1994; 152:5457–5467.
174. Fujisawa T, Abu–Ghazeleh R, Kita H, Sanderson CJ, Gleich GJ. Regulatory effect of cytokines on eosinophil degranulation. J Immunol 1990; 144:642–646.
175. Kita H, Horie S, Gleich GJ. Extracellular matrix proteins attenuate activation and degranulation of stimulated eosinophils. J Immunol 1996; 156:1174–1181.
176. Kita H, Kato M, Gleich GJ, Abraham RT. Tyrosine phosphorylation and inositol phosphate production: are early events in human eosinophil activation stimulated by immobilized secretory IgA and IgG? J Allergy Clin Immunol 1994; 94:1272–1281.
177. van-der-Bruggen T, Kanters D, Tool AT, Raaijmakers JA, Lammers JW, Verhoeven AJ, Koenderman L. Cytokine-induced protein tyrosine phosphorylation is essential for cytokine priming of human eosinophils. J Allergy Clin Immunol 1998; 101:103–109.
178. Pazdrak K, Olszewska–Pazdrak B, Stafford S, Garofalo RP, Alam R. Lyn, Jak2, and Raf-1 kinases are critical for the antiapoptotic effect of interleukin 5, whereas only Raf-1 kinase is essential for eosinophil activation and degranulation. J Exp Med 1998; 188:421–429.
179. Gounni AS, Lamkhioued B, Ochiai K, Tanaka Y, Delaporte E, Capron A, Kinet J–P, Capron M. High-affinity IgE receptor on eosinophils is involved in defence against parasites. Nature 1994; 367:183.
180. Seminario MC, Saini SS, MacGlashan DW, Bochner BS. Intracellular expression and release of FcεRI-α by human eosinophils. J Immunol 1999; 162:6893–6900.
181. Smith SJ, Ying S, Meng Q, Sullivan MHF, Barkans J, Kon OM, Sihra B, Larche M, Levi–Schafer F, Kay AB. Blood eosinophils from atopic donors express messenger RNA for the α, β and γ subunits of the high affinity IgE receptor (FcεRI) and intracellular, but not cell surface, α subunit protein. J Allergy Clin Immunol 2000; 105:309–317.
182. Redington AE, Howarth PH. Airway wall remodelling in asthma. Thorax 1997; 52:310–312.
183. Minshall EM, Leung DYM, Martin RJ, Song YL, Cameron L, Ernst P, Hamid Q. Eosinophil-associated TGF-β1 mRNA expression and airways fibrosis in bronchial asthma. Am J Respir Cell Mol Biol 1997; 17:326–333.
184. Ohno IY, Yamauchi K, Hoshi H, Honma M, Woolley K, O'Byrne P, Dolovich J, Jordana M, Tamura G, Tanno Y, Shirato K. Eosinophils as a potential source of platelet-derived growth factor β-chain (PDGF-β) in nasal polyposis and bronchial asthma. Am J Respir Cell Mol Biol 1995; 13:639–647.
185. Egesten A, Calafat J, Knol EF, Janssen H, Walz TM. Subcellular localization of transforming growth factor-alpha in human eosinophil granulocytes. Blood 1996; 87:3910–3918.
186. Okada S, Kita H, George TJ, Gleich GJ, Leiferman KM. Migration of eosinophils through basement membrane components in vitro: role of matrix metalloproteinase-9 Am J Respir Cell Mol Biol 1997; 17:519–528.
187. Soloman A, Aloe L, Pe'er J, Frucht–Pery J, Bonini Stefano, Bonini Sergio, Levi–Schaffer F. Nerve growth factor is performed in and activates human peripheral blood eosinophils. J Allergy Clin Immunol 1998; 102:454–460.
188. Levi–Schaffer F, Garbuzenko E, Rubin A, Reich R, Pickholz D, Gillery P, Emonard H, Nagler A, Xavier Maquart FA. Human eosinophils regulate human lung and skin derived fibroblast properties in vitro: a role for transforming growth factor-β. Proc Natl Acad Sci 1999; 96:9660–9665.
189. Hamid Q, Barkans J, Meng Q, Ying S, Abrams JS, Kay AB, Moqbel R. Human eosinophils synthesize and secrete interleukin-6, in vitro. Blood 1992; 80:1496–1501.

190. Costa JJ, Matossian K, Resnick MB, Beil WJ, Wong DT, Gordon JR, Dvorak AM, Weller PF, Galli SJ. Human eosinophils can express the cytokines tumor necrosis factor-alpha and macrophage inflammatory protein-1 alpha. J Clin Invest 1993; 91:2673–2684.
191. Dunnill MS. The pathology of asthma. In: Middleton E Jr, Reed CE, Ellis EF, eds. Allergy: Principles and Practice. St Louis: CV Mosby, 1978:678.
192. Filley WV, Holley KE, Kephart GM, Gleich GJ. Identification by immunofluorescence of eosinophil under granule major basic protein in lung tissue of patients with bronchial asthma. Lancet 1982; 2:11.
193. Bousquet J, Chanez P, Lacoste JY, Barneon G, Ghavanian N, Enander I, Venge P, Ahlstedt S, Simony–Lafontaine J, Godard P, Michel FB. Eosinophilic inflammation in asthma. N Engl J Med 1990; 323:1033–1039.
194. Robinson DS, Assoufi B, Durham SR, Kay AB. Eosinophil cationic protein (ECP) and eosinophil protein X (EPX) concentrations in serum and bronchial lavage fluid in asthma. Effect of prednisolone treatment. Clin Exp Allergy 1995; 25:1118–1127.
195. Bradley BL, Azzawi M, Jacobson M, Assoufi B, Collins JV, Irani A–MA, Schwartz LB, Durham SR, Jeffery PK, Kay AB. Eosinophils, T-lymphocytes, mast cells, neutrophils and macrophages in bronchial biopsy specimens from atopic subjects with asthma: comparison with biopsy specimens from atopic subjects without asthma and normal control subjects and relationship to bronchial hyperresponsiveness. J Allergy Clin Immunol 1990; 88:661–674.
196. Wardlaw AJ, Dunnette S, Gleich GJ, Collins JV, Kay AB. Eosinophils and mast cells in bronchoalveolar lavage in mild asthma: relationship to bronchial reactivity. Am Rev Respir Dis 1988; 137:62–69.
197. Robinson DS, Sun Ying, Bentley AM, Qiu Meng, North J, Durham SR, Kay AB, Hamid Q. Relationships among numbers of bronchoalveolar lavage cells expressing messenger ribonucleic acid for cytokines, asthma symptoms, and airway methacholine responsiveness in atopic asthma. J Allergy Clin Immunol 1993; 92:397–403.
198. Bentley AM, Maestrelli P, Saetta M, Fabbri LM, Robinson DS, Bradley BL, Jeffery PK, Durham SR, Kay AB. Activated T-lymphocytes and eosinophils in the bronchial mucosa in isocyanate-induced asthma. J Allergy Clin Immunol 1992; 89:821–829.
199. Bentley AM, Menz G, Storz CHR, Robinson DS, Bradley BL, Jeffery PK, Durham SR, Kay AB. Identification of T lymphocytes, macrophages and activated eosinophils in the bronchial mucosa in intrinsic asthma. Am Rev Respir Dis 1992; 146:500–506.
200. De–Monchy JG, Kauffman HF, Venge P, Koeter GH, Jansen HM, Sluiter HJ, De–Vries K. Bronchoalveolar eosinophilia during allergen-induced late asthmatic reactions. Am Rev Respir Dis 1985; 131:373–376.
201. Bentley AM, Qiu Meng, Robinson DS, Hamid Q, Kay AB, Durham SR. Increases in activated T lymphocytes, eosinophils, and cytokine messenger RNA expression of IL-5 and GM-CSF in bronchial biopsies after allergen inhalation challenge in atopic asthmatics. Am J Repir Cell Mol Biol 1993; 8:35–42.
202. Robinson DS, Hamid Q, Bentley AM, Sun Ying, Kay AB, Durham SR. $CD4^+$ T cell activation, eosinophil recruitment and interleukin 4 (IL-4), IL-5 and GM-CSF messenger RNA expression in bronchoalveolar lavage after allergen inhalation challenge of atopic asthmatics. J Allergy. Clin Immunol 1993; 92:313–324.
203. Metzger WJ, Richerson HB, Worden K, Monick M, Hunninghake GW. Bronchoalveolar lavage of allergic asthmatic patients following allergen bronchoprovocation. Chest 1986; 89: 477–483.
204. Coyle AJ, Ackerman SJ, Irvin CG. Cationic proteins induce airways hyperresponsiveness dependent on charger interactions. Am Rev Respir Dis 1993; 147:896–900.
205. Gundel RH, Letts LG, Gleich GJ. Human eosinophil major basic protein induces airway constriction and airway hyperresponsiveness in primates. J Clin Invest 1991; 87:1470–1473.
206. Robinson DS, Hamid Q, Sun Ying, Bentley AM, Assoufi B, North J, Qui Meng, Durham SR, Kay AB. Prednisolone treatment in asthma is associated with modulation of bronchoal-

veolar lavage cell interleukin-4, interleukin-5 and interferon-gamma cytokine gene expression. Am Rev Respir Dis 1993; 148:401–406.
207. Bentley AM, Hamid Q, Robinson DS, Schotman E, Meng Q, Assoufi B, Kay AB, Durham SR. Prednisolone treatment in asthma. Reduction in the numbers of eosinophils, T cells, tryptase-only positive mast cells, and modulation of IL-4, IL-5, and interferon-gamma cytokine gene expression within the bronchial mucosa. Am J Respir Crit Care Med 1996; 153: 551–556.
208. Wilson JW, Djukanovic R, Howarth PH, Holgate ST. Inhaled beclomethasone dipropionate downregulates airway lymphocyte activation in atopic asthma. Am J Respir Crit Care Med 1994; 149:86–90.
209. Adelroth E, Rosenhall L, Johansson SA, Linden M, Venge P. Inflammatory cells and eosinophilic activity in asthmatics investigated by bronchoalveolar lavage. The effects of antiasthmatic treatment with budesonide or terbutaline. Am Rev Respir Dis 1990; 142:91.
210. Trigg CJ, Manolitsas ND, Wang J, et al. Placebo-controlled immunopathologic study of four months of inhaled corticosteroids in asthma. Am J Respir Crit Care Med 1994; 150:17–22.
211. Leung DY, Martin RJ, Szefler SJ, Sher ER, Ying S, Kay AB, Hamid Q. Dysregulation of interleukin 4, interleukin 5, and interferon gamma gene expression in steroid-resistant asthma. J Exp Med 1995; 181:33–44.
212. Sullivan P, Bekir S, Jaffar Z, Page C, Jeffery P, Costello J. Anti-inflammatory effects of low-dose oral theophylline in atopic asthma. Lancet 1994; 343:1006–1008.
213. Macfarlane AJ, Dworski R, Sheller JR, Pavord ID, Kay AB, Barnes NC. Sputum cysteinyl leukotrienes increase 24 hours after allergen inhalation challenge in atopic asthmatics. Am J Respir Crit Care 2000; 161:1553–1558.
214. Fahy JV, Fleming HE, Wong HH, Liu JT, Su JQ, Reimann J, Fick RB Jr, Boushey HA. The effect of an anti-IgE monoclonal antibody on the early- and late-phase responses to allergen inhalation in asthmatic subjects. Am J Respir Crit Care Med 1997; 155:1828–1834.
215. Rak S. Effects of immunotherapy on the inflammation in pollen asthma. Allergy. 1993; 48(17 suppl):125–128.
216. Varney VA, Jacobson MR, Sudderick RM, Robinson DS, Irani AM, Schwartz LB, Mackay IS, Kay AB, Durham SR. Immunohistology of the nasal mucosa following allergen-induced rhinitis. Identification of activated T lymphocytes, eosinophils, and neutrophils. Am Rev Respir Dis 1992; 146:170–176.
217. Bentley AM, Jacobson MR, Cumberworth V, Barkans J, Moqbel R, Schwartz LB, Irani, A–M, Kay AB, Durham SR. Immunohistology of the nasal mucosa in seasonal allergic rhinitis: increase in activated eosinophils and epithelial mast cells. J Allergy Clin Immunol 1992; 89: 877–883.
218. Masuyama K, Till SJ, Jacobson MR, Kamil A, Cameron L, Juliusson S, Lowhagen O, Kay AB, Hamid QA, Durham SR. Nasal eosinophilia and IL-5 mRNA expression in seasonal allergic rhinitis induced by natural allergen exposure: effect of topical corticosteroids. J Allergy Clin Immunol 1998; 102:610–617.
219. Ohno I, Lea R, Finotto S, Marshall J, Denburg J, Dolovich J, Gauldie J, Jordana M. Granulocyte/macrophage colony-stimulating factor (GM-CSF) gene expression by eosinophils in nasal polyposis. Am J Respir Cell Mol Biol 1991; 5:505–510.
220. Terada N, Konno A, Tada H, Shirotori K, Ishikawa K, Togawa K. The effect of recombinant human interleukin-5 on eosinophil accumulation and degranulation in human nasal mucosa. J Allergy Clin Immunol 1992; 90:160–168.
221. Leiferman K, Ackerman SJ, Sampson H, Haugen H, Venencie P, Gleich GJ. Dermal deposition of eosinophil granule protein in atopic dermatitis. N Engl J Med 1985; 313:282–285.
222. Peters MS, Schroeter AL, Kephart GM, Gleich GJ. Localization of eosinophil granule major basic protein in chronic urticaria. J Invest Dermatol 1983; 81:39–43.
223. Frew AJ, Kay AB. The relationship between infiltrating $CD4^+$ lymphocytes, activated eosino-

phils and the magnitude of the allergen induced late-phase response in man. J Immunol 1988; 141:4158.
224. Ying S, Robinson DS, Meng Q, Barata LT, McEuen AR, Buckley MG, Walls AF, Askenase PW, Kay AB. C-C chemokines in allergen-induced late-phase cutaneous responses in atopic subjects: association of eotaxin with early 6-hour eosinophils, and of eotaxin-2 and monocyte chemoattractant protein-4 with the later 24-hour tissue eosinophilia, and relationship to basophils and other C-C chemokines (monocyte chemoattractant protein-3 and RANTES). J Immunol 1999; 163:3976–3984.
225. Ying S, Meng Q, Barata LT, Robinson DS, Durham SR, Kay AB. Associations between IL-13 and IL-4 (mRNA and protein), vascular cell adhesion molecule-1 expression, and the infiltration of eosinophils, macrophages, and T cells in allergen-induced late-phase cutaneous reactions in atopic subjects. J Immunol. 1997; 158:5050–5057.
226. Samoszuk M. Eosinophils and human cancer. Histol Histopathol 1997; 12:807–812.
227. Steigleder GK, Inderwisch R. Eosinophilic granulocytes in the skin lesions of psoriasis and neurodermatitis. Arch Dermatol Res 1975; 254:253–256.
228. Sams WM, Gammon WR. Mechanism of lesion production in pemphigus and pemphigoid. J Am Acad Dermatol 1982; 6:431–452.
229. Falanga V, Medsger TA, Reichlin M, Rodnan GP. Linear scleroderma: clinical spectrum, prognosis, and laboratory abnormalities. Ann Intern Med 1986; 104:849–857.
230. Blenkinsopp WK, Haffenden GP, Fry L, Leonard JN. Histology of linear IgA disease, dermatitis herpetiformis and bullous pemphigoid. Am J Dermatol 1983; 5:547–554.
231. Silverman RA, Rabinowitz AD. Eosinophils in the cellular infiltrate of granuloma annulare. J Cutan Pathol 1985; 12:13–17.
232. Wells GC, Whimster IW. Subcutaneous angio-lymphoid hyperplasia with eosinophilia. Br J Dermatol 1969; 81:1–15.
233. Silver RM, Heyes MP, Maize JC, Quearry B, Vionnet–Fuasset M, Sternberg EM. Scleroderma, fasciitis, and eosinophilia associated with the ingestion of tryptophan. N Engl J Med 1990; 322:874–881.
234. Varga J, Kahari VM. Eosinophilia myalgia syndrome, eosinophilic fascitis and related fibrosing disorders. Curr Opin Rheumatol 1997; 9:562–570.
235. Gibbs AR, Anderson G. Pulmonary vasculitis and eosinophilic pneumonia. In: Brewis RAL, Gibsin GJ, Geddes DM, eds. Respiratory Medicine, London: Balliere Tindall, 1990:1164–1182.
236. Churg J, Straus L. Allergic granulomatosis, allergic angiitis and polyarteritis nodosa. Am J Pathol 1951; 27:277.
237. Stirling RG, Chung KF. Leukotriene antagonists and Churg–Strauss syndrome: the smoking gun. Thorax 1999; 54:865–866.
238. Brightling CE, Ward R, Goh KL, Wardlaw AJ, Pavord ID. Eosinophilic bronchitis is an important cause of chronic cough. Am J Respir Crit Care Med 1999; 160:406–410.
239. Levi–Schaffer F, Garbuzenko E, Rubin A, Reich R, Pickholz D, Gillery P, Emonard H, Nagler A, Maquart FA. Human eosinophils regulate human lung- and skin-derived fibroblast properties in vitro: a role for transforming growth factor beta (TGF-beta). Proc Natl Acad Sci USA 1999; 96:9660–9665.
240. Weller PF, Bubley GJ. The hypereosinophlic syndrome. Blood 1994; 83:2759–2779.
241. Fauci AS, Harley JB, Roberts WC, Ferrans VJ, Gralnick HR, Bjornson BH. The idiopathic hypereosonphilic syndrome. Clinical, pathophysiologic, and therapeutic considerations. Ann Intern Med 1982; 97:78.
242. Lefebvre C, Bletry O, Degoulet P, Guillevin L, Bentata–Pesayre M, Le Thi HD, Godeau P. Facteurs pronostiques du syndrome hypereosinophilique. Ann Med Interne 1989; 140:253.
243. Spry CJ, Davies J, Tai PC, Olsen EG, Oakley CM, Goodwin JF. Clinical features of fifteen patients with the hypereosinophilic syndrome. QJ Med 1983; 52:1.
244. Parillo JE, Borer JS, Henry WL, Wolff SM, Fauci AS. The cardiovascular manifestations

of the hypereosinophilic syndrome. Prospective study of 26 patients with review of the literature. Am J Med 1979; 67:572.
245. Davies J, Spry CJ, Sapsford R, Olsen EG, De PG, Oakley CM, Goowin JF. Cardiovascular featues of 11 patients with eosinophilic endomyocardial disease. QJ Med 1983; 52:23.
246. Spry CJ, Take M, Tai PC. Eosinophilic disorders affecting the myocardium and endocardium: a review. Heart Vessels Suppl 1985; 1:240.
247. Moore PM, Harley JB, Fauci AS. Neurologic dysfunction in the idiopathic hypereosinophilic syndrome. Ann Intern Med 1985; 102:109.
248. Parillo JE, Lawley TJ, Frank MM, Kaplan AP, Fauci AS. Immunologic reactivity in the hypereosinophilic syndrome. J Allergy Clin Immunol 1979; 64:113.
249. Van Haelst Pisani C, Kovach JS, Kita H, Leiferman KM, Gleich GJ, Silver JE, Dennin R, Abrams JS. Administration of interleukin-2 (IL-2) results in increased plasma concentrations of IL-5 and eosinophilia in patients with cancer. Blood 1991; 78:1538.
250. Varon D, Watzler M, Berrebi A. Hypereosinophilic syndrome associated with polycythaemia vera. Arch Intern Med 1986; 146:1440.
250a. Butterfield JH, Gleich GJ. Interferon-α treatment of six patients with idiopathic hypereosinophilic syndrome. Ann Intern Med 1994; 121:648–653.
251. Chand N, Harrison JE, Rooney S, Pillar J, Jkubicki R, Nolan K, Diamantis W. Sofia D. Anti-IL-5 monoclonal antibody inhibits allergic late phase bronchial eosinophila in guinea pigs: a therapeutic approach. Eur J Pharmacol 1992; 211:121–123.
252. Mauser PJ, Pitman AM, Fernandez X, Foran SK, Adams GK 3rd, Kreutner W, Egan RW, Chapman RW. Effects of an antibody to interleukin-5 in a monkey model of asthma. Am J Respir Crit Care Med 1995; 152:467.
253. Hogan SP, Matthaei KI, Young JM, Koskinen A, Young IG, Foster PS. A novel T cell-regulated mechanism modulating allergen-induced airways hyperactivity in BALB/c mice independently of IL-4 and IL-5. J Immunol 1998; 161:1501–1509.
254. Wills–Karp M, Luyimbazi J, Xu X, Schofield B, Neben TY, Karp CL, Donaldson DD. Interleukin-13: central mediator of allergic asthma. Science 1998; 282:2258–2261.
255. Gruing G, Warnock M, Wakil AE, Venkayya R, Brombacher F, Rennick DM, Sheppard D, Mohrs M, Donaldson DD, Locksley RM, Corry DB. Requirement for IL-13 independently of IL-4 in experimental asthma. Science 1998; 282:2261–2263.
256. Leckie MJ, ten Brinke A, Lordan J, Khan J, Diamant Z, Walls CM, Cowley H, Hansel TT, Djukanovic R, Sterk PJ, Holgate ST, Barnes PJ. A humanised anti-IL-5 monoclonal antibody: initial single dose safety and activity in patients with asthma [abstr.]. Am J Respir Crit Care Med 1999; 159:A624.
257. Sur S, Crotty TB, Kephart GM, Hyman BA, Colby TV, Reed CE, Hunt LW, Gleich GJ. Sudden-onset fatal asthma. A distinct entity with few eosinophils and relatively more neutrophils in the airway submucosa? Am Rev Respir Dis 1993; 148:713–719.
258. Wenzel SE, Schwartz LB, Langmack EL, Halliday JL, Trudeau JB, Gibbs RL, Chu HW. Evidence that severe asthma can be divided pathologically into two inflammatory subtypes with distinct physiologic and clinical characteristics. Am J Respir Crit Care Med 1999; 160: 1001–1008.

4

Neutrophils

BURTON ZWEIMAN

University of Pennsylvania School of Medicine, Philadelphia, Pennsylvania

1 NEUTROPHIL STRUCTURE AND FUNCTION

1.1 Origin, Maturation, and Circulation of Neutrophils

Polymorphoneutrophils (PMN), which constitute 50–80% of the circulating blood leukocytes, are derived from phagocytic stem cells in the bone marrow (1). Over about 7–10 days, these stem cells mature first into nongranulated myeloblasts, then into promyelocytes containing primary granules that arise from the Golgi apparatus. In the next maturation stage, myelocytes, primary granule synthesis ceases, but cells continue to divide, diluting the number of primary granules per cell. Myelocytes also synthesize secondary (specific) granules.

Following this stage, these cells do not divide, but undergo progressive segmentation and condensation of the nucleus. This proceeds from indentation of the round nucleus (metamyelocytes), to a bilobed nucleus (band form), and then a polysegmented nucleus of mature cells. In the latter, three or four lobes containing much of the genomes are joined by thin DNA-containing filaments (2). It is possible that such segmented nuclei enhance the capacity of PMN to crawl through small spaces as they emigrate from the blood and migrate within the tissues.

About 50% of the 5×10^{10} PMN in the adult vascular compartment are carried in the axial stream and are those sampled by venipuncture. The other 50% (the marginal pool) migrate along the vascular endothelium, particularly in the vascular bed of certain organs. The average PMN circulates in the blood for less than 12 hr, then emigrates into the tissues, at a rate of about 1×10^{11} PMN per day for the average adult. A rapid replacement of new PMN from the bone marrow is necessary to maintain steady-state levels in the blood. Presumably, PMN do not return to the bloodstream once they have emigrated into the tissues.

It was often assumed that PMN died naturally by disintegration or necrosis, with the potential for surrounding tissue damage caused by released PMN contents (3). However, more recent studies have shown that PMN undergo apoptosis, with subsequent macrophage recognition and phagocytosis of the dying PMN, without triggering the release of macrophage mediators (4,5). Several PMN functions such as phagocytosis and granule release are down-regulated during apoptosis, which may also limit the chance of tissue injury by the dying PMN (5,6). Leukotriene-B_4 (LTB_4), a potent attractant and activator of PMN, can inhibit PMN apoptosis through G protein and tyrosine kinase activation, raising the possibility that the viability of PMN may be extended in inflammatory sites containing LTB_4 (7).

1.2 Emigration of PMN from the Vascular Compartment into Tissue Sites

The subject of leukocyte emigration from the circulation is discussed in detail in Chapter 6 of this text. In brief, three continuous events are important in such emigration (8,9). In the initial, *rolling stage*, the circulation of PMN in the postcapillary venules is slowed in sites of inflammation owing to interactions of members of the selectin family on the surface of activated endothelial cells with their ligands on PMN. P-selectin (CD62P) on endothelial cells interacts with platelet and endothelial selectin glycoprotein ligands (PSGL-1, ESGL-1). E-selectin (CD62E) on endothelial cells binds to sialyl Lewis^x on PMN, whereas L-selectin (CD62L) binds to unidentified structure on endothelium (8). In combination with the shear forces of blood flow, this reversible binding results in the PMN rolling along the endothelium without activation of either cell type (9). PMN adhering to endothelium can act as *nucleation* sites for a second layer of rolling PMN (10).

In inflammatory sites, rolling is followed by adhesion due to *activation of the* β_2-*integrin* CD11/CD18 family of adhesion molecules on the PMN surface, stimulated by local activating substances, such as platelet activating factor (PAF) and interleukin-8 (IL-8). These integrins bind to the intracellular adhesion molecules 1 and 2 (ICAM-1, CD54; ICAM-2, CD102) in a firmer interaction than seen in the E-selectin–ligand interaction which may also occur in this stage. These adherent PMN are more responsive to stimuli for chemotaxis. At this point in their activation, PMN begin to shed some of their surface adhesion molecules. This, in turn, may decrease recruitment of additional PMN and thus down-regulate continued inflammatory responses (11). In the third stage called *diapedesis*, the PMN migrates between endothelial cells through junctions (mainly where three endothelial cells meet) into the extracellular matrix (ECM). This activity occurs through the integrins–ICAM interaction as previously noted (12). This is a complex process involving a spatially coordinated sequence of adhesion–deadhesion, locomotion, reversible localized proteolysis of vascular basement membranes, and subsequent adhesion of the PMN to the ECM (13). GPI-anchored proteins on the PMN surface, and phosphoinositide-3 kinase appear to be important in regulating PMN extravasation and migration (14). Such transmigration involves PMN activation and also appears to delay apoptosis (15). Exposure to IL-8 may decrease PMN responses to other chemotactic stimuli (16).

Once in the extracellular tissue milieu, PMN appear to migrate by an integrin-dependent interaction with ECM proteins such as fibronectin and laminin (8). Such integrin-mediated adhesion is accompanied by PMN activation with cytoskeletal changes and release of intracellular products, including reactive oxidant species (8,17–19).

1.3 Neutrophil Motility and Chemotaxis

Neutrophils are inherently motile cells as a reflection of their cytoskeletal apparatus. This motility is increased when PMN become activated by various stimuli, including agents that may be released in allergic inflammatory reactions. PMN exhibit two types of motion: *random* and *directed.* The latter, important in inflammatory responses, involves ameboid movement along a chemical gradient (chemotaxis) triggered by a variety of chemoattractants (20). Some of these agents are listed in Table 1. They include (1) cleaved components of complement C3 and C5; (2) *N*-formylated peptides (e.g., fMLP) that may mimic bacterial- or mitochondrial-encoded proteins; (3) PAF, released from a variety of cell types; (4) LTB-4, formed by the activation of the lipooxygenase on arachidonic acid; and (5) chemotactic cytokines (chemokines).

The latter, 8- to 10-kDa proteins, are discussed in detail in Chapter 11 of this text. Of particular relevance to the PMN are the CXC chemokines IL-8, melanoma growth stimulating activity (MGSA), and neutrophil-activating peptide-2 (NAP-2), which generally act on PMN but not on other leukocytes (20). Two receptors for IL-8 (IL8-RA; CXCR-1, and IL8-RB; CXCR-2) have different functional activities, that are partly dependent on the degree of receptor phosphorylation (21).

Following engagement of PMN receptors by chemoattractants, several unrelated classes of signals are generated: (1) production and then enzymatic catabolism of the phosphatidylinositol 3,4,5-triphosphate (PIP_3), a membrane phospholipid; by phospholipase C, generating diacylglycerol (DAG); and inositol triphosphate (IP_3); (2) 2 types of cytosolic G protein exchanges; guanosine diphosphate (GDP) for guanosine triphosphate (GTP), and then GTP binding to and activation of phospholipase C. Other cellular factors can accelerate or inhibit the the G protein-dependent hydrolytic activity; (3) phospholipase C can also be activated when it becomes phosphorylated following binding of its receptor by a chemoattractant.

The breakdown products IP_3 and DAG play important roles in PMN activation: (1) DAG activates protein kinase C to phosphorylate key intracellular proteins and serves as a substrate for DAG lipase, generating arachidonic acid; (2) IP_3 stimulates release of Ca^{2+} from cytoplasmic vesicles into the cytosol, with resultant enhancement of phospholipase C activity and activation of several intracellular reactions, including the contractile activity

Table 1 Some Chemoattractants[a] for Neutrophils

Chemokines: IL-8, MGSA, NAP-2
Arachidonic acid metabolites: LTB_4, LXB_4[b]
Platelet-activating factor
Complement components: C3a, C5a
N-Formyl peptides

[a] IL-8, interleukin-8; MGSA, melanoma growth-stimulating activity; NAP-2, neutrophil-activating peptide-2; LTB_4, leukotriene-B_4; LXB_4, lipoxin B_4.
[b] Inhibits leukocyte–endothelial interaction.

of myosin. Once activated, PMN appear to crawl toward the chemotactic stimulus, in the tissues in a tank-tread fashion. Up-regulated integrins expressed on their surface adhere to ECM fibers, providing the functional face for interaction with the chemoattractant gradient. As they move, these adherent membrane sites are moved progressively to the rear of the cell where they detach from the ECM through the formation or polymerization and subsequent destruction of a system of actin fibers. Meanwhile, newly expressed integrin molecules at the leading edge of the PMN adhere to the ECM, continuing the directed movement. Once the PMN is no longer exposed to a chemotactic gradient, as in the center of an inflammatory reaction, directed movement ceases and the PMN becomes relatively sessile. It should be emphasized that a number of other PMN activities are increased during a prominent chemotactic response, to be discussed later (21,22).

1.4 Neutrophil Granules

The PMN cytoplasm contains a variety of granules that can be classified in several ways, including that of azurophilic and specific granules, referred to earlier (23). Some of the contents of these granules are shown in Table 2. These granules should be considered as a continuum from those containing myeloperoxidase to granules rich in metalloprotease (23). Discussions of PMN granules have traditionally focused on their important microbicidal, enzymatic, and proinflammatory activities. However, some granules also store membrane proteins that become incorporated into the plasma membrane during fusion of granules to plasma membranes during exocytosis (24). Also, secretory vesicles, specialized endocytic structures in the PMN cytoplasm, have plasma proteins in their lumen and large amounts of receptors such as CR1, CR3 (Mac-2), and Fcγ (receptor for IgG) on the vesicle membrane (23,25).

The profiles of diverse proteins in the different PMN granules appears to be related to the timing of synthesis of different granule proteins during PMN development (23). Also, some proteins cannot exist together in the same granule or secretory vesicle. Effective PMN function appears to depend on the mobilization of different granule or vesicle contents in a differential fashion.

Inflammatory stimuli generally first cause exocytosis of vesicle contents, then release of the contents of specific granules and, finally, stimulation of the azurophilic granule proteins. The proteins of the latter are released predominantly into adjacent phagocytic vesicles during phagocytosis; they are less readily and more slowly secreted into the extracellular environment (23,24).

Table 2 Some Neutrophil Granule Components Relevant to Inflammatory Reactions

Predominantly in azurophilic granules
Serine esterases: elastase, cathepsin G, protease 3
Heme protein: myeloperoxidase
Cationic peptides: defensins
Cationic enzyme: lysozyme[a]
Predominantly in specific granules
Matrix metalloproteases: collagenase (MMP-8), gelatinase A and B (MMP-2, MMP-9)
Iron-binding protein: lactoferrin

[a] Present in both azurophilic and specific granules.

The results of this differential exocytosis of PMN proteins include (1) increased PMN surface CD11b expression, converting a rolling PMN to a cell more adherent to endothelial surface ICAM (as described earlier); (2) degradation of type IV collagen in vascular basement membrane by released gelatinase, permitting transmigration of PMN into the tissues. The signal transduction pathways that control this differential mobilization of granule subpopulations have not been defined clearly. However, smaller granules and those controlled by VAMP-2, a fusion protein, may be more readily mobilized (26,27).

1.5 Reactive Oxygen Species

Activated PMN frequently generate by-products of O_2 that can be damaging to microbes and tissue proteins. Current concepts of the reactions involved have been reviewed in detail (28,29) and will be discussed only briefly here. The enzyme NADPH oxidase becomes activated by assembly at the cytosolic face of the plasma membrane leading to a series of transfers of single electrons from NADPH to O_2, leading to superoxide (O_2^-) formation. H_2O_2 can be produced and then further reduced to the highly reactive hydroxyl (OH^-) radical in the presence of unstable iron (Fe^{2+}) (Fig. 1a). Myeloperoxidase (MPO), found in rich supply in the azurophilic granules of PMN, can convert H_2O_2 in the presence of halides, such as chloride, to hypochlorous acid, another potent oxidant.

In most instances, these reactive oxygen species (ROSs) of PMN are secreted mainly across invagination of the plasma membrane into phagocytic vesicles during phagocytosis, with resultant damage to many ingested microbes. However, in greatly or persistently stimulated PMN, ROSs are liberated into the nearby extracellular spaces with the potential for damaging nearby cells by oxidative degradation of essential cellular components (30). Also, certain ROS can up-regulate the transcription factor, nuclear factor kappa B (NF-κB), which regulates the expression of genes for several adhesion molecules and proinflammatory cytokines (30). The extracellular toxic effects of the ROS may be countered, to a degree, by antioxidants, such as vitamins C and E, which scavenge free radicals and inhibit activation of NF-κB.

A second major oxidant-generating pathway relevant to inflammation involves inducible nitric oxide synthetase (iNOS) which appears in activated PMN (see Fig. 1b). This enzyme reacts with L-arginine to generate nitric oxide (NO), which is mildly reactive with tyrosine-containing amino acids, sometimes impairing protein function while being converted to the more toxic peroxynitrates. The latter, in turn, can be converted to the OH^- radical. Peroxynitrites bind to glutathione, which may inhibit some of their activity.

1.6 Arachidonic Acid Metabolites

This subject is reviewed in detail in Chapter 10 of this text and will be discussed here only briefly as they relate to PMN function. In activated PMN, arachidonic acid (AA) is removed from membrane phospholipids by phospholipase-A_2 and is metabolized mainly by the 5-lipoxygenase (5-LO) pathway in the presence of the 5-lipoxygenase-activating protein (FLAP) into leukotriene-A_4(LTA_4). In turn, this is catabolized by the ample amounts of LTA_4 hydrolase to LTB_4 (31), which is a potent attractant for leukocytes, particularly PMN. It also stimulates production of proinflammatory cytokines and mediators that can act in an autocrine–paracrine manner to induce and augment tissue inflammation. However, LTB_4 is rapidly metabolized to relatively inactive 20-OH LTB_4, with possible down-regulatory effects on inflammation (31). PMN do not secrete LTC_4 themselves because they lack the LTC_4 synthase (32); however, activated PMN may export LTA_4 to

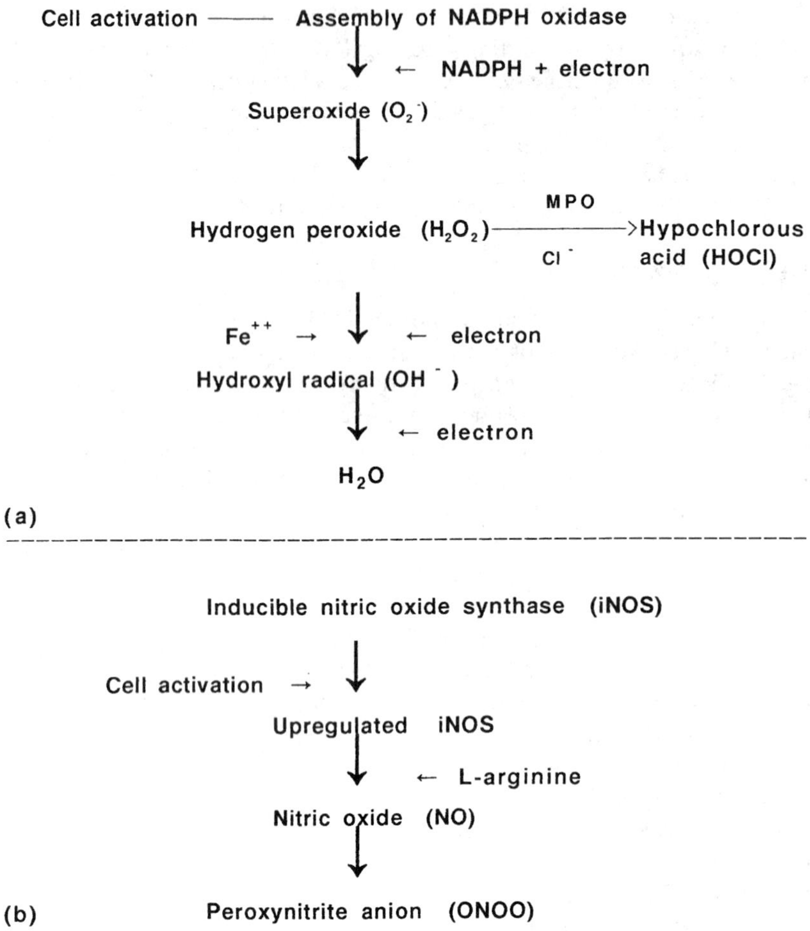

Figure 1 Biochemical pathways for formation of (a) reactive oxygen species; (b) nitric oxide and its derivatives. NADPH, reduced nicotinamide-adenine dinucleotide phosphate.

nearby cells, which then can convert this into LTC_4 (32). LTC_4 has several proinflammatory effects, including an increase in microvascular permeability, contraction of airway smooth muscle, and stimulation of mucous secretion (33). Some products of 5-LO enzymatic activity within PMN may down-regulate inflammatory responses. Lipoxins A_4 and B_4 are eicosanoids, formed through transcellular biosynthetic pathways, that inhibit PMN–endothelial interactions and the subsequent PMN emigration into inflammatory sites (34,35).

1.7 Cytokines

The role of these agents in inflammation is discussed in detail in Chapter 11 of this text and will be mentioned only briefly as related to the possible role of PMN in allergic inflammation. Several general principles apply to such a discussion: (1) PMN may secrete both proinflammatory and anti-inflammatory cytokines under different conditions (36); (2) PMN contain much less mRNA and synthetic capacity for cytokines per cell than do monocytes and lymphocytes; (3) nevertheless, the large number of PMN in some inflammatory responses may serve as a major source of cytokines; (4) the type and magnitude of cytokine synthesis by PMN may depend on the nature of the stimulus; (5) some cytokines made by PMN will also stimulate these cells in an autocrine–paracrine manner (e.g., IL-8, TNF-α) (36).

1.8 Neutrophil Granule Components

Before discussing the actions of some PMN granule components, several general characteristics of inflammatory tissue sites bear mention: 1) Diapedesis and migration of inflammatory cells, such as PMN, likely requires interaction of the emigrating cell with laminin and fibronectin in the vascular basement membrane and extracellular matrix (ECM); 2) ECM (discussed in detail in Chap. 7) is not just a scaffold that maintains tissue architecture, but is also an interactive substratum that regulates the shape, migration, growth, and differentiation of local cells (37); the ECM also plays a role in the orderly repair of damaged tissues; 3) the inflammatory process is generally associated with exudation of plasma components that may be processed by PMN or, conversely, may modulate selected PMN activities; 4) the discharge of PMN granule components is frequently associated with the generation of ROS. Thus, there is potential for ROS and enzymatic activities to interact in a paracrine manner; 5) ROS are short-lived, react stochiometrically and but once, and act rather nonspecifically on protein targets (37). However, the PMN granules contain over 20 proteins, some of which can remain active for relatively long periods after being released, permitting prolonged action on specific protein targets (37) (see Table 2).

1.8.1 Azurophilic Granule Enzymes

Most of these enzymes are secreted into phagocytic vacuoles during phagocytosis (38). However, with vigorous stimulation, proteolytic enzymes can be discharged into the surrounding extracellular milieu. Some investigators have described ''frustrated phagocytosis'' in which the PMN cannot ingest a large particle to which it adheres; lysosomal enzymes are secreted into empty phagocytic vacuoles, the membranes of which are in continuity with the plasma membrane, resulting in extracellular discharge of vacuole contents (37,39).

Serine Proteases

ELASTASE. Present in large amounts in the PMN (1.5 $\mu g/10^6$ cells), elastase is a potent omnivorous enzyme that attacks small hydrophobic residues in proteins, degrading almost all components of the ECM, including elastin and glycoproteins (37,39). Furthermore, it can cleave a variety of plasma proteins, such as immunoglobulins, complement proteins, and coagulation factors, and can even attract inflammatory cells (37,40). Elastase may actually inhibit some PMN functions, such as phagocytosis and associated lysosomal enzyme release (39). Thus, elastase might exert some anti-inflammatory as well as proinflammatory activities.

However, the potent proinflammatory effects of elastase are countered by the rapid binding of plasma protein α_1-antiprotease and the slower inhibition by plasma α_2-macroglobulin (called by some the ''antiprotease shield'') that exude into the inflammatory sites (37,39). α_1-Antiprotease can also be synthetized and secreted by activated PMN. In addition, a secretory leukocyte protease inhibitor is secreted by respiratory epithelial cells (41). Yet, this antiprotease shield can be broken. Chlorinated ROS, formed in the PMN, can oxidize and inactivate these antiproteases (37). Also, some metalloproteases released from activated PMN can inactivate these antiproteases (39). Once elastase binds to its targets, it cannot readily be inhibited by antiproteases. Thus, there appears to be a race between the binding of the surrounding antiprotease inhibitors to elastase released from stimulated PMN and the damage to these inhibitors by chlorinated oxidants and enzymes released from the same PMN. There may be a gradient effect, with the greatest elastolytic activity immediately around the PMN where the ratio of released elastase to inhibitor is greatest (39).

CATHEPSIN G. Expressed in a pattern similar to elastase in azurophilic granules; it predominantly attacks the sites adjacent to aromatic amino acids in proteins (39). Cathepsin G can attack basal lamina of blood vessels and certain other membranes (42). Similar to elastase, it can damage elastin, fibronectin, and proteoglycan, and it may enhance the activity of elastase, including inactivation of TNF-α (43,44). Cathepsin G is also a chemoattractant for monocytes, possibly explaining the sequential accumulation of PMN, then monocytes in some inflammatory sites (45). It is also a potent platelet activator (46).

PROTEASE-3. PR3 has a high degree of structural homology with elastase and cathepsin G. It can bind to PMN and endothelial cells and stimulate IL-8 production by the latter (47). In this way, PR3 could perpetuate inflammatory reactions by the IL-8-induced attraction of more PMN to the site. PR3 also has proteolytic activity, binding to small hydrophobic residues. It also participates, with cathepsin G, in platelet aggregation. PR3 is the major target for the serum antineutrophil cytoplasmic antibody found in Wegener's granulomatosis (47).

Myeloperoxidase (MPO)

The role of the heme protein MPO in the formation of chlorinated reactive oxygen species (HOCl) in the PMN is been described in the foregoing. HOCl oxidizes and inactivates antiproteases; also, it oxidizes the inactive form of metalloproteases leading to their activation (48). This is another example of the intimate interactions of ROS and proteases, leading to the pro-inflammatory activities of PMN. MPO-catalyzed H_2O_2 activity can also inhibit certain lymphocyte functions (49). Yet, individuals with a hereditary deficiency of MPO appear to have normal host defenses against infection and inflammatory responses (50). MPO is the target for antineutrophil cytoplasmic antibodies found in many individuals with small-vessel vasculitis and certain forms of glomerulonephritis (51).

Defensins

Defensins are small, cationic peptides, without enzymatic activities, that constitute 30–50% of the protein in azurophilic granules (52). In addition to their antimicrobial actions, defensins induce IL-8 synthesis and are cytotoxic to airway epithelial and endothelial cells. Thus, defensins could mediate some of the pathogenic effects of PMN in the airways. However, defensins also inhibit the toxic effects of elastase, whereas, elastase can inactivate defensins (52).

Lysozyme

Lysozyme is a cationic enzyme present in both azurophilic and specific granules of PMN as well as in salivary secretions (53). It has bacteriolytic properties caused by both enzymatic and nonenzymatic mechanisms (54). This can occur both within and outside the PMN (53). Lysozyme is not proinflammatory and may actually suppress PMN chemotaxis and ROS formation (55).

1.8.2 Specific Granule Components

These proteins are readily transferred to the plasma membrane or secreted into the surrounding extracellular milieu (38). The major components relevant to inflammation follow:

Collagenase

This matrix metalloprotease (MMP-8) is one of a family of Zn^{2+} containing endoproteases that share structural domains, but differ in substrate specificity (48). Collagenase exists in a latent form that can be oxidized to an activated form by HOCl released during PMN activation (37). This could explain the greater release of active collagenase from PMN, which is stimulated by ingestion of opsonized particles, than by soluble stimulants such as PAF (37,56). The collagenase released from PMN preferentially degrades type I collagen at a triple-helical locus (57). Types II and III collagen are affected to lesser degrees. The resultant alteration of collagen structure likely contributes to enhanced passage of inflammatory cells through interstitial tissue and subsequent tissue remodeling. Collagenase can also degrade α_1-antiprotease, possibly leading to prolonged activity of the PMN serine protease activity described earlier (58).

Gelatinases A and B

These metalloproteases (MMP-2 and MMP-9, respectively), are thought to reside in specific granules and in a third, less dense, type of granule (59). Along with elastase and collagenase, gelatinase can degrade all the major components of the ECM (59). These gelatinases may be activated by the OH^- radical and elastase. Gelatinase may play an important role in the diapedesis of PMN into inflammatory sites by its effect on collagen type IV in the vascular basement membrane (59).

Lactoferrin

Lactoferrin, which is liberated readily from activated PMN, inhibits the iron-catalyzed formation of OH^- from O_2^- and H_2O_2 by avid binding of iron into a noncatalytic form (60). Therefore, lactoferrin could be one of the control mechanisms down-modulating pathogenic activities of PMN. However, lactoferrin may also enhance some toxic effects of ROS by presenting iron more efficiently within PMN (61).

1.9 Surface Receptors

Surface receptors for the Fc region of IgG (FcγR) play an important role in the phagocytosis of IgG-coated particles by PMN (62). When FcγR type III (CD16)—the major FcγR on PMN—is cross-linked, actin polymenzation and granule protein exocytosis occur in addition to phagocytosis. Binding of IgG to FcγR type II (CD32) leads to both granule protein extrusion and reactive oxidant formation (63,64). Stimulated PMN express FcγR type I (CD64) and receptors for C3b (CR1) and C3bi (CR3), also playing roles in enhanced phagocytosis (65). Although resting PMN generally do not express the high-affinity IgE receptor or the lower-affinity CD23 receptor for IgE, activated PMN do express an IgE-binding protein called galectin-3 (Mac-2/εBP), one of the β-galactoside-binding lectins (66,67). Also, PMN stimulated by GM-CSF can express CD23 (67). These expressions of receptors for IgE could play a role in allergic inflammation as PMN entry sites of IgE-mediated reactions and become activated when local allergen interacts with IgE on their surface.

2 THE POSSIBLE ROLE OF PMN IN ALLERGIC REACTIONS

Pathological mechanisms in different allergic reactions and diseases are discussed in detail in other chapters in this text. Here, evidence for possible roles of PMN in such reactions will be considered.

2.1 Late-Phase Reactions

In the skin, an indurated late-phase reaction (LPR) follows the immediate-whealing reactions to intradermal allergen injection in about 50% of sensitive subjects. As reviewed (68), sequential biopsies of such sites have shown that PMN are the first inflammatory cells entering these sites, starting within 20 min after the allergen challenge, and somewhat before prominent eosinophil accumulation. Skin chamber studies have shown that such PMN are activated, with ROS formation and granule protein release (68). The pathogenic role of PMN in such sites is still unclear. The accumulation of PMN may be decreased, although not as impressively as eosinophil reduction, following corticosteroid administration, which inhibits the gross LPR (69–71). Of note, antihistamine treatment or cyclooxygenase inhibition does not alter LPR expression or PMN accumulation (72,73).

2.2 Asthma

Neutrophils are generally considered to be infrequent and play little role in the asthmatic inflammatory reaction, unlike the situation in chronic bronchitis and chronic obstructive pulmonary disease (COPD) (74,75). However, more recent studies have found a correlation between the frequency of PMN and MPO levels in induced sputum and the clinical severity of asthma (76). PMN are particularly prominent in the airways in certain asthmatic situations (Table 3).

2.2.1 Fatal Asthma

Several studies have found that PMN are much more prominent than eosinophils in the airways of some individuals who die within several hours of the onset of a severe asthma exacerbation (77,78). The pathogenic effects of PMN in such cases are not defined. The frequency of lymphocytes and airway thickness were not significantly different between the patients in whom PMN predominated or in those in whom eosinophils were the predominant inflammatory cell (78). PMN components, such as elastase, are prominent in the extracellular tissues of the patients whose asthma progressed rapidly to a fatal outcome (77). PMN may be prominent in some individuals with acute, severe, but nonfatal, asthma episodes requiring intensive care unit (ICU) treatment whether or not an infectious trigger is identified (79,80). Wenzel et al. have found increased PMN accumulation in the airways

Table 3 Presentations of Asthma with Prominent Neutrophil Accumulation in Airways

1. Fatal and near-fatal asthma
2. Some acute, severe asthma exacerbations
3. Chronic, steroid-dependent asthma
4. Some steroid-insensitive asthma
5. Occupational asthma

of those with chronic, severe, steroid-dependent asthma whether or not there was prominent eosinophila accumulation in these airways (81).

2.2.2 Steroid Unresponsive Asthma

Although several factors may be responsible for corticosteroid insensitivity in asthma (82), some groups have found that the minority of chronic asthmatics who have PMN, but few eosinophils, in the airway secretions are less clinically responsive to corticosteroid therapy (83,84).

2.2.3 Occupational Asthma

A higher frequency of PMN accumulation and lower degree of eosinophilic inflammation has been reported in occupational asthma caused by low molecular weight compounds than in nonoccupational asthma (85,86). Jung and Park also found prominent PMN as well as eosinophils in occupational asthma caused by grain dust or TDI (85).

Thus, it appears that PMN can accumulate prominently in sites of some cases of asthma. What is the stimulus for this PMN response? Several studies have found that PMN, as well as eosinophils, of asthmatic patients are activated with increased respiratory burst and granule protein secretion (87,88). Stimuli for this could include IL-8, TNF-α, and IL-1, which are secreted by cells in the respiratory mucosa during allergic reactions (89). Also, IL-8 and LTB_4 released locally by activated PMN could attract additional PMN to the site.

2.3 Allergic Rhinitis

A late-phase reaction to inhaled allergens is thought to play a major role in chronic allergic rhinitis (AR) (90). Eosinophil exudation has been considered to be the major inflammatory cell response during AR in response to environmental exposures or nasal challenge (91,92). However, increased numbers of PMN and increase MPO levels are found in nasal lavages 6–24 hr after local allergen challenge (92,93). Levels of MPO, as a marker of PMN accumulation or activation, but not ECP levels, correlated well with IL-8 levels in the same lavage material (93). PMN as well as eosinophil responses are increased during allergen rechallenge 3 days after the initial allergen nasal challenge, possibly because of a local priming effect (94). PMN are found in the nasal secretions of uninfected children with perennial AR in some, but not other studies (95,96). Their accumulation increased markedly during superinfection (94). PMN are not prominent in the nasal mucosa or in polyps from aspirin-reactive individuals, in contrast with the prominent PMN accumulation in polyps seen in cystic fibrosis patients (96,97). The local stimulus for any PMN accumulation in AR is undefined. Gosset et al. have found increased neutrophil chemotactic activity in the nasal secretions of such patients, inhibited only weakly by prior incubation with an anti–IL-8 antibody (98).

2.4 Urticaria

The usual histological patterns in chronic idiopathic urticaria (CIU) is described in detail in Chapter 17. Neutrophils are usually not prominent in the lesional areas (99). However, there appears to be a small subset of CIU cases in which PMN accumulation is prominent; this has been called ‘‘neutrophilic urticaria’’ by some investigators (Table 4) (100,101). Such neutrophil-prominent CIU cases are frequently characterized by an increased sedimentation rate, leukocytosis, more lesional vasodilation, and expression of TNF-α and

Table 4 Characteristics of Neutrophilic Urticaria

1. Neutrophils are predominant inflammatory cells in lesions.
2. Increased expression of TNF-α, IL-3, but not IL-8, in lesions.
3. Prominent vasodilation in lesions.
4. Associated blood leukocytosis and increased sedimentation rate.
5. Poor clinical response to H_1 antihistamines; may respond to dapsone or colchicine.

Source: Refs. 100 and 101.

IL-3, but not IL-8 (100). Treatment with antihistamines is often ineffective, although this type of urticaria may be controlled by dapsone or colchicine, which affect PMN function (101).

2.5 Atopic Dermatitis

The inflammatory responses in atopic dermatitis (AD) are discussed in Chapter 16. PMN and their granule proteins are not prominent in AD (102), although increased levels of LTB_4 in AD skin have been reported (103). As noted earlier, LTB_4 is a potent PMN chemoattractant.

3 MODULATION OF PMN ACTIVITY

3.1 Cytokines

Of the various cytokines synthesized by PMN, IL-8 is released in the greatest abundance (104). Such IL-8 can act in an autocrine or paracrine manner to activate and attract PMN through binding to one or both IL-8 receptors (CXCR-1 and CXCR-2) (105). Other inflammatory reactants that stimulate IL-8 production include TNF-α, IL-1β, IL-15, and IL-17, through binding to specific surface receptors that may be partially shed during PMN recruitment and activation (106–108). TNF-α also stimulates PMN apoptosis, associated with caspase activation, an effect countered by effects of GM-CSF and G-CSF (109). G-CSF also exerts proinflammatory (ROS production) and anti-inflammatory (decreased granule protein release) effects (110). Chemokines, such as RANTES and eotaxin, are generally chemotactic for eosinophils, but not for PMN; however, IFN-γ-treated PMN may be attracted by these agents because the CCR1 and CCR3 receptors are up-regulated on these PMN (111).

3.2 Granulocyte Proteins

Eosinophil major basic protein (EMBP)—but not other eosinophil granule proteins—stimulates both IL-8 production and PMN apoptosis (104). Elastase released from PMN can actually inhibit some PMN functions (39). Lactoferrin may also have anti-inflammatory effects in different organs (60). Prostaglandin E_2 (PGE_2) may inhibit PMN activation, possibly related to induction of intracellular cyclic-AMP. Cyclooxygenase (COX) inhibition can markedly reduce prostaglandin synthesis in allergen-challenged sites, but has variable effects on allergic inflammation (73,113). *Salicylates* may reduce PMN diapedesis by inhibiting adhesion molecule expression on endothelial cells and PMN, not related to cyclooxygenase inhibition (114). *Substance P* appears to induce the PMN accumulation seen in neurogenic inflammation by up-regulating vascular E-selectin expression (115). Some H_1-antihistamines can inhibit several PMN activities in vitro, as well as inhibiting the binding of histamine to the H_1-receptor (116). However, as noted, treatment with antihistamine generally does not affect PMN accumulation or activation in allergen-challenged sites. *Corticosteroids (CS)*—among the extensive anti-inflammatory effects of corticosteroids (discussed in Chap. 22) are the actions of these agents on PMN activities. CS can inhibit chemotaxis, adhesion, diapedesis, oxidative bursts, and possibly the induction of annexin-1 (lipocortin-1) activity (117). They also inhibit PMN synthesis and secretion of several proinflammatory cytokines (118). However, these CS effects on PMN may not be as prominent as on eosinophils, possibly explaining the less impressive improvement after CS treatment of asthma in which PMN accumulation is prominent (described earlier). This could be because corticosteroids promote apoptosis of eosinophils, but inhibit PMN apoptosis (119). *β_2-Adrenergic agonists*—although the major clinical effect of these agents is bronchodilation, some β_2-agonists do inhibit certain PMN activities; however, there appears to be little in vivo anti-inflammatory effects of these agents (120).

4 CONCLUDING COMMENTS

Neutrophils are short-lived, but very active, granulocytes with many pro-inflammatory activities, reviewed here. PMNs appear to play a much less prominent role than eosinophils or basophils in allergic inflammation. However, in a minority of cases of asthma, perennial rhinitis, and urticaria, PMN participation is more prominent. There are both similarities and differences in the modulation of PMN and eosinophil activities by endogenous and therapeutic agents. Therefore, the role of PMN in allergic diseases merits continued investigation.

REFERENCES

1. Babior BM, Stossel T. Phagocytes and non neoplastic phagocyte disease. In: Pathophysiologic Approach. London: Churchill-Livingstone, 1994.
2. Sanchez JA, Wangh IJ. New insights into the mechanisms of nuclear segmentation in human neutrophils. J Biochem 1999; 73:1–10.
3. Hurley JV. Termination of inflammation. In: Hurley JV, ed. Acute Inflammation. London: Churchill Livingston, 1983.
4. Savill JS, Wyllie AH, Henson JE, Walport MJ, Henson PM, Haslett C. Macrophage phagocytosis of aging neutrophils in inflammation—programmed cell death in the neutrophil leads to its recognition by the macrophages. J Clin Invest 1989; 83:865–875.
5. Meagher LC, Savill JS, Baker A, Fuller RW, Haslett C. Phagocytosis of apoptotic neutrophils does not induce macrophage release of thromboxane B_2. J Leukoc Biol 1992; 52:269–273.
6. Haslett C, Savill JS, Whyte MK, Stern M, Dransfield I, Meagher LC. Granulocyte apoptosis and the control of inflammation. Trans R Soc Lond B Biol Sci 1994; 345:3327–3333.
7. Hébert M–J, Takano T, Holthöfer H, Brady HR. Sequential morphologic events during apoptosis of human neutrophils. Modulation by lipoxygenase-derived eicosanoids. J Immunol 1996; 157:3105–3115.
8. Bochner B. Cellular adhesion and its antagonism. J Allergy Clin Immunol 1997; 100:581–590.

9. Parent C, Eichacker PQ. Neutrophil and endothelial cell interactions in sepsis. Infect Dis Clin North Am 1999; 13:427–447.
10. Hamann A, Hogg N. Adhesion molecules and chemokines. Immunologist 1995; 3:204–205.
11. Strausbaugh HJ, Green PG, Lo E, Tangemann K, Reichling DB, Rosen SD, Levine JD. Painful stimulation suppresses joint inflammation by inducing shedding of L-selectin from neutrophils. Nat Med 1999; 5:1057–1060.
12. Burns AR, Walker DC, Brown ES, Thurmon LT, Bowden RA, Keese CR, Simon SJ, Entman ML, Smith CW. Neutrophil transendothelial migration is independent of tight junctions and occurs preferentially at tricellular corners. J Immunol 1997; 159:2893–2903.
13. Sendo F, Araki Y. Regulation of leukocyte adherence and migration by GPI-anchored proteins. J Leukoc Biol 1999; 369–374.
14. Ebisawa M, Toshimitsu T, Bickel C, Klunk D, Schleimer RP. Eosinophil transmigration induced by cytokines. J Immunol 1994; 153:2153–2160.
15. Watson RWG, Rotstein OD, Nathens AB, Parodo J, Marshall JC. Neutrophil apoptosis is modulated by endothelial transmigration and adhesion molecule engagement. J Immunol 1997; 158:945–953.
16. Kitayama J, Carr MW, Roth SJ, Buccola J, Springer TA. Contrasting responses to multiple chemotactic stimuli in transendothelial migration. Heterologous desensitization in neutrophils and augmentation of migration in eosinophils. J Immunol 1997; 158:2340–2349.
17. Lowell CA, Berton G. Integrin signal transduction in myeloid leukocytes. J Leukoc Biol 1999; 65:313–320.
18. Zweiman B, von Allmen C. Comparative effects of anti-lactoferrin antibodies and tumor necrosis factor on neutrophil adherence to matrix proteins. Clin Diagn Lab Immunol 1999; 6:364–368.
19. Cox EA, Huttenlacher A. Regulation of integrin-mediated adhesion during cell migration. Microvasc Res Technol 1998; 43:412–419.
20. Rothenberg ME, Zimmermann N, Mishra A, Brandt E, Birkenberger LA, Hogan SP, Foster PS. Chemokines and chemokine receptors: their role in allergic airway disease. J Clin Immunol 1999; 19:250–264.
21. Boulay F, Naik N, Giannini E, Tardif M, Brouchon L. Phagocyte chemoattractant receptor. Ann NY Acad Sci 1997; 832:69–81.
22. Yasui K, Yamazaki M, Miyabayashi M, Tsuno T, Komiyama A. Signal transduction pathway in human polymorphonuclear leukocytes for chemotaxis induced by a chemotactic factor. J Immunol 1994; 152:5922.
23. Borregaard N. Development of neutrophi granule diversity. Ann NY Acad Sci 1997; 832: 62–68.
24. Borregaard N. Current opinion about neutrophil granule physiology. Curr Opin Hematol 1996; 3:11–20.
25. Sengelov HL, Kjeldsen L, Diamond MS, Springer TA, Borregaard N. Sub-cellular localization and dynamics of Mac-1 ($\alpha_m\beta_2$) in human neutrophils. J Clin Invest 1993; 92:1467–1476.
26. Lollike K, Borregaard N, Lindall M. The exocytotic fusion pore of small granules has a conductance similar to an ion channel. J Cell Biol 1995; 129:99–104.
27. Brumell JH, Volchuck A, Sengelov HL, Borregaard N, Cieutat AM, Bainton DF, Grinstein S, Klip A. Subcellular distribution of docking/fusion proteins in neutrophils, secretory cells with multiple exocytic compartments. J Immunol 1995; 155:5750–5759.
28. Ward P, Lertsch AB. The acute inflammatory response and its regulation. Arch Surg 1999; 134:666–669.
29. Clark RA. Activation of the neutrophil respiratory burst oxidase. J Infect Dis 1999; 179(suppl 2):309–317.
30. Jourd'heuil D, Morise Z, Conner EM, Grisham MB. Oxidants, transcription factors and intestinal inflammation. J Clin Gastroenterol 1997; 24(suppl 1):61–72.

31. Crooks SW, Stockley RA. Leukotriene B_4. Int J Biochem Cell Biol 1998; 30:173–178.
32. Sala A, Zarini S, Folco G, Murphy RC, Henson PM. Differential metabolism of exogenous and endogenous arachidonic acid in human neutrophils. J Biol Chem 1999; 274:28264–28269.
33. Busse WW. Leukotrienes and inflammation. Am J Respir Crit Care Med 1998; 157(suppl): 210–213.
34. Papayianni A. Serhan CN, Brady HR. Lipoxin A_4 and B_4 inhibit leukotriene-stimulated interactions of human neutrophils and endothelial cells. J Immunol 1996; 156:2264–2272.
35. Diamond P, McGinty A, Sugrue D, Brady HR, Godson C. Regulation of leukocyte trafficking by lipoxins. Clin Chem Lab Med 1999; 37:293–297.
36. Cassatella MA. Neutrophil-derived proteins: selling cytokines by the pound. Adv Immunol 1999; 73:369–509.
37. Weiss SJ. Tissue destruction by neutrophils. N Engl J Med 1989; 320:365–376.
38. Lehrer RI, Ganz T, Selsted ME, Babior BM, Curnutte JT. Neutrophils and host defense. Ann Intern Med 1998; 109:127–142.
39. Doring A. The role of neutrophil elastase in chronic inflammation. Am J Respir Crit Care Med 1994; 150:114–17.
40. Janoff A. Elastase in tissue injury. Am Rev Med 1985; 36:206–216.
41. Sallenave J–M, Si-Tahar M, Cox G, Chignard M, Gauldie J. Secretory leukocyte proteinase inhibitor is a major leukocyte elastase inhibitor in human neutrophils. J Leukoc Biol 1997; 61:695–702.
42. Glinski W, Kuligowski M, Pierozynska–Dubowska M, Glinska–Ferenz M, Jablonska S. Ultrastructural changes of the skin induced by human leukocyte elastase and cathepsin G. Acta Derm Venereol 1991; 71:277–282.
43. Kubes P, Smith R, Grisham MD, Granger DN. Neutrophil-mediated proteolysis. Differential roles for cathepsin G and elastase. Inflammation 1993; 17:321–332.
44. Scuderi P, Nez PA, Duerr ML, Wong BJ, Valdez CM. Cathepsin-G and leukocyte elastase inactivate human tumor necrosis factor and lymphotoxin. Cell Immunol 1991; 135:299–313.
45. Chertov O, Ueda H, Xu LL, Tani K, Murphy WJ, Wang JM, Howard OM, Sayers TJ, Oppenheim JJ. Identification of human neutrophil-derived cathepsin G and azurocidin CAP37 as chemoattractants for mononuclear cells and neutrophils. J Exp Med 186:739–747.
46. LaRosa CA, Rohrer MJ, Benoit SE, Rodino LJ, Barnard MR, Michelson AD. Human neutrophil cathepsin G is a potent platelet activator. J Vasc Surg 1994; 19:306–318.
47. Berger S, Seelen MAJ, Gerritsman JSJ, Heemskerk E, van der Woude FJ. Proteinase 3, the major autoantigen of Wegener's granulomatosis, enhances IL-8 production by endothelial cells in vitro. J Am Soc Nephrol 1996; 7:694–701.
48. Goetzl EJ, Bondo MJ, Leppert D. Matrix metalloproteinases in immunity. J Immunol 1996; 156:4–7.
49. El-Hag A, Lipsky PE, Bennett M, Clark RA. Immunomodulation by neutrophil myeloperoxidase and hydrogen peroxide: differential susceptibility of human lymphocyte functions. J Immunol 1986; 136:3420–3426.
50. Lanza F. Clinical manifestation of myeloperoxidase deficiency. J Mol Med 1998; 76:676–681.
51. Savige J, Gillie D, Benson E, Davies D, Esnault V, Falk RJ, Hagen EC, Jayne D, Jennette JC, Paspaliaris B, Pollock W, Pusey C, Savage CO, Silvestrini R, van der Woude F, Wieslander J, Wiik A. International Consensus Statement on Testing and Reporting of Antineutrophil Cytoplasmic Antibodies (ANCA). Am J Clin Pathol 1999; 111:507–513.
52. Van Wetering S, Mannesse–Lazeroms SP, Dijkman JH, Hiemstra PS. Effect of neutrophil serine proteinases and defensins on lung epithelial cells: modulation of cytotoxicity and IL-8 production. J Leukoc Biol 1997; 62:217–226.
53. Taylor DC, Cripps AW, Clancy RL. A possible role for lysozyme in determining acute exacerbation in chronic bronchitis. Clin Exp Immunol 1995; 102:406–416.

54. Levy O. Antibiotic proteins of polymorphonuclear leukocytes. Eur J Haemotol 1996; 56: 263–277.
55. Gordon LI, Douglas SD, Kay NE, Yamada O, Osserman EF, Jacob HS. Modulation of neutrophil function by lysozyme. Potential negative feedback system of inflammation. J Clin Invest 1979; 64:225–232.
56. Chathan WW, Heck LW, Balckburn WD Jr. Ligand-dependent release of active neutrophil collagenase. Arthritis Rheum 1990; 33:228–235.
57. Hasty A, Stricklin GP, Hibbs MS, Mainardi CL, Kang WH. Immunologic relationship of human neutrophil and collagenases. Arthritis Rheum 1987; 30:695–705.
58. Sorsa T, Konttinen YT, Lindy O, Suomalainen K, Ingman T, Saari H, Halinen S. Doxycycline protects serum alpha-1-antitrypsin from human neutrophil collagenase. Agents Action 1993; 39(suppl):225–259.
59. Hibbs MS, Bainton DF. Human neutrophil gelatinase is a component of specific granules. J Clin Invest 1989; 84:1395–1402.
60. Britigan BE, Serody J, Cohen MS. The role of lactoferrin as an anti-inflammatory molecule. Adv Exp Med Biol 1994; 357:143–56.
61. Vercellotti GM, van Asbeck BS, Jacob HS. Oxygen radical-induced erythrocyte hemolysis by neutrophils. J Clin Invest 1985; 76:956–962.
62. McKenzie SE, Schreiber AD. Fc gamma receptors in phagocytes. Curr Opin Hematol 1998; 5:16–21.
63. Huizinga TW, Roos D, von dem Borne AE. Neutrophil Fc-gamma receptors: a two-way bridge in the immune system. Blood 1990; 75:1211–1214.
64. Salmon JE, Brogle NL, Edberg JC, Kimberly RP. Fcγ receptor III induces actin polymerization in human neutrophils and primes phagocytosis mediated by Fcγ receptor II. J Immunol 1991; 146:997–1004.
65. Zhou MJ, Poo H, Todd RF III, Petty HR. Surface-bound immune complexes trigger transmembrane proximity between complement receptor type 3 and the neutrophil's cortical microfilaments. J Immunol 1992; 148:3550–3553.
66. Truong MJ, Gruart V, Kusnierz JP, Papin JP, Loiseau S, Capron A, Capron M. Human neutrophils express immunoglobulin E (IgE)-binding proteins (Mac-2/epsilon BP) of the S-type lectin family: role in IgE-dependent activation. J Exp Med 1993; 177:243–248.
67. Yamaoka KA, Arock M, Issaly F, Dugas N, Le Goff L, Kolb JP. Granulocyte macrophage colony stimulating factor induces Fc epsilon RII/CD23 expression on normal human polymorphonuclear neutrophils. Int Immunol 1996; 8:479–490.
68. Zweiman B. Inflammatory responses in late-phase allergic reactions in the skin. Can J Allergy Clin Immunol 1999; 4:336–344.
69. Slott RI, Zweiman B. Histologic studies of human skin test responses to ragweed and compound 48/80. II. Effect of corticosteroid therapy. J Allergy Clin Immunol 1975; 55:232–238.
70. Talbot S, Atkins PC, Bedard PM, Zweiman B. In vivo effects of corticosteroids on human allergic responses. I. Effects of systemic administration of steroids. Ann Allergy 1987; 58: 363–365.
71. Charlesworth EN, Kagey–Sobotka A, Schleimer RP, Norman PS, Lichtenstein LM. Prednisone inhibits the appearance of inflammatory mediator and the influx of eosinophils and basophils associated with the cutaneous late-phase response to allergen. J Immunol 1991; 146:671–676.
72. Zweiman B, Atkins PC, Moskovitz AR, von Allmen C, Ciliberti M, Grossman S. Cellular inflammatory responses during immediate developing and established late phase allergic cutaneous reactions: effects of cetirizine. J Allergy Clin Immunol 1997; 100:341–347.
73. Atkins PC, Zweiman B, Littman B, Presti C, von Allmen C, Moskovitz A, Eskra JD. Products of arachidonic acid metabolism and the effects of cyclooxygenase inhibition on ongoing cutaneous allergic reactions in human beings. J Allergy Clin Immunol 1995; 95:742–747.

74. Jeffery PK. Differences and similarities between chronic obstructive pulmonary disease and asthma. Clin Exp Allergy 1999; 2(suppl):14–26.
75. Keatings VM, Barnes PJ. Granulocyte activation markers in induced sputum: comparison between chronic obstructive pulmonary disease, asthma, and normal subjects. Am J Respir Crit Care Med 1997; 155:449–453.
76. Jatakanon A, Uasuf C, Maziak W, Lim S, Chung KF, Barnes PJ. Neutrophilic inflammation in severe persistent asthma. Am J Respir Crit Care Med 1999; 160:1532–1539.
77. Sur S, Crotty TB, Kephart GM, Hyma BA, Colby TV, Reed CE, Hunt LW, Gleich GJ. Sudden onset fatal asthma. A distinct entity with few eosinophils and relatively more neutrophils in the airway submucosa? Am Rev Respir Dis 1993; 148:713–719.
78. Carroll N, Carello S, Cooke C, James A. Airway structure and inflammatory cells in fatal attacks of asthma. Eur Respir J 1996; 9:709–715.
79. Fahy JV, Kim KW, Liu J, Boushey HA. Prominent neutrophilic inflammation in sputum from subjects with asthma. J Allergy Clin Immunol 1995; 95:843–852.
80. Lamblin C, Gosset P, Tillie–Leblond I, Saulnier F, Marquette CH, Wallaert B, Tonnel AB. Bronchial neutrophilia in patients with noninfectious status asthmaticus. Am J Respir Crit Care Med 1998; 157:394–402.
81. Wenzel SE, Schwartz LB, Langmack EL, Halliday JL, Trudeau JB, Gibbs RL, Chu HW. Evidence that severe asthma can be divided pathologically into two inflammatory subtypes with distinct physiologic and clinical characteristics. Am J Respir Crit Care Med 1999; 160: 1001–1008.
82. Hamid QA, Wenzel SE, Hauk PJ, Tsicopoulos A, Wallaert B, Lafitte JJ, Chrousos GP, Szefler SJ, Leung DY. Increased glucocorticoid receptor beta in airway cells of glucocorticoid-insensitive asthma. Am J Respir Crit Care Med 1999; 159:1600–1604.
83. Cox G. The role of neutrophils in inflammation. Can Respir J 1998; 5(suppl A):L37–40.
84. Hargreaves FE. Induced sputum for the investigation of airway inflammation: evidence for its clinical application. Can Respir J 1999; 6:169–174.
85. Jung KS, Park HS. Evidence for neutrophil activation in occupational asthma. Respirology 1999; 4:303–306.
86. Leigh R, Hargreave FE. Occupational neutrophilic asthma. Can Respir J 1999; 6:194–196.
87. Carlson M, Hakansson L, Peterson C, Stalenheim G, Venge P. Secretion of granule proteins from eosinophils and neutrophils is increased in asthma. J Allergy Clin Immunol 1991; 87: 27–33.
88. Joseph BZ, Routes JM, Borish L. Activities of superoxide dismutases and NADPH oxidase in neutrophils obtained from asthmatic and normal donors. Inflammation 1993; 17:361–370.
89. Shelhamer JH, Levine SJ, Wu T, Jacoby DB, Kaliner MA, Rennard SI. NIH Conference. Airway Inflammation. Ann Intern Med 1995; 123:288–304.
90. Segura T, Casale TB. Allergic rhinitis: basic pathophysiology and therapeutic strategies. Can J Allergy Clin Immunol 1999; 4:318–330.
91. Wilson SJ, Lau L, Howarth PH. Inflammatory mediators in naturally occurring rhinitis. Clin Exp Allergy 1998; 28:220–227.
92. Miadonna A, Milazzo N, Gibelli S, Salmaso C, Lorini M, Tedeschi A. Nasal response to a single antigen challenge in patients with allergic rhinitis—inflammatory cell recruitment persists up to 48 hours. Clin Exp Allergy 1999; 29:941–949.
93. Jacobi HH, Poulsen LK, Reimert CM, Skov PS, Ulfgren AK, Jones I, Elfman LB, Malling HJ, Mygind N. IL-8 and the activation of eosinophils and neutrophils following nasal allergen challenge. Int Arch Allergy Immunol 1998; 116:53–59.
94. Ciprandi G, Ricca V, Landi M, Passalacqua G, Bagnasco M, Canonica GW. Allergen-specific nasal challenge: response kinetics of clinical and inflammatory events to rechallenge. Int Arch Allergy Immunol 1998; 115:157–161.
95. Shinogi J, Majima Y, Takeuchi K, Harada T, Sakakura Y. Quantitative cytology of nasal

secretions with perennial allergic rhinitis in children: comparison of noninfected and infected conditions. Laryngoscope 1998; 108:703–705.
96. Varga EM, Jacobson MR, Masuyama K, Rak S, Till SJ, Darby Y, Hamid Q, Lund V, Scadding GK, Durham SR. Inflammatory cell populations and cytokine mRNA expression in the nasal mucosa in aspirin-sensitive rhinitis. Eur Respir J 1999; 14:610–615.
97. Rowe–Jones JM, Trendell–Smith N, Shembekar M, Mackay IS. Polypoid rhinosinusitis in patients with host defence deficiencies: cellular infiltration and disease severity. Rhinology 1997; 35:113–117.
98. Gosset P, Tillie–Leblond I, Malaquin F, Durieu J, Wallaert B, Tonnel AB. Interleukin-8 secretion in patients with allergic rhinitis after an allergen challenge: interleukin-8 is not the main chemotactic factor present in nasal lavages. Clin Exp Allergy 1997; 27:379–388.
99. Sabroe RA, Poon E, Orchard GE, Lane D, Francis DM, Barr RM, Black MM, Black AK, Greaves MW. Cutaneous inflammatory cell infiltrate in chronic idiopathic urticaria: comparison of patients with and without anti-Fc epsilon R1 or anti-IgE autoantibodies. J Allergy Clin Immunol 1999; 103:484–493.
100. Toppe E, Haas N, Henz BM. Neutrophilic urticaria: clinical features, histologic changes and possible mechanisms. Br J Dermatol 1998; 13:248–253.
101. Tharp MD. Chronic urticaria: pathophysiology and treatment approaches. J Allergy Clin Immunol 1996; 98(suppl):325–330.
102. Leiferman KM. Eosinophils in atopic dermatitis. J Allergy Clin Immunol 1994; 94:1310–1317.
103. Thorsen S, Fogh K, Broby–Johansen U, Sondergaard J. Leukotriene B_4 in atopic dermatitis: increased skin levels and altered sensitivity of peripheral blood T-cells. Allergy 1990; 45: 457–463.
104. Page SM, Gleich GJ, Roebuck KA, Thomas LL. Stimulation of neutrophil interleukin-8 production by eosinophil granule basic protein. Am J Resper Cell Mol Biol 1999; 21:230–237.
105. Ben–Baruch A, Grimm M, Bengali K, Evans GA, Chertov O, Wang JM, Howard OM, Mukaida N, Matsushima K, Oppenheim JJ. The differential ability of IL-8 and neutrophil-activating peptide-2 to induce attenuation of chemotaxis is mediated by their divergent capabilities to phosphorylate CXCR2 (IL-8 receptor B). J Immunol 1997; 158:5927–5933.
106. Strieter RM, Kasahara K, Allen RM, Standiford TJ, Rolfe MW, Becker FS, Chensue SW, Kunkel SL. Cytokine-induced neutrophil-derived interleukin-8. Am J Pathol 1992; 141:397–407.
107. Laan M, Cui ZH, Hoshino H, Lotvall J, Sjostrand M, Gruenert DC, Skoogh BE, Linden A. Neutrophil recruitment by human IL-17 via C-X-C chemokine release in the airways. J Immunol 1999; 162:2347–2352.
108. Simms H, D'Amico R. Regulation of polymorphonuclear leukocyte cytokine receptor expression. The role of altered oxygen tensions and matrix proteins. J Immunol 1996; 157:3605–3616.
109. Fadeel B, Ahlin A, Henter JI, Orrenius S, Hampton MB. Involvement of caspases in neutrophil apoptosis: regulation by reactive oxygen species. Blood 1998; 92:4808–4818.
110. Heard SO, Fink MP. Counterregulatory control of the acute inflammatory response: granulocyte colony-stimulating factor has anti-inflammatory properties. Crit Care Med 1999; 27: 1019–1021.
111. Bonecchi R, Polentarutti N, Luini W, Borsatti A, Bernasconi S, Locati M, Power C, Proudfoot A, Wells TN, Mackay C, Mantovani A, Sozzani S. Up-regulation of CCR1 and CCR3 and induction of chemotaxis to CC chemokines by IFN-gamma in human neutrophils. J Immunol 1999; 162:474–449.
112. Wenzel SE. Arachidonic acid metabolites: mediators of inflammation in asthma. Pharmacotherapy 1997; 17:3–12.
113. Gronneberg R, Zetterstrom O. Inhibition of the late phase response to anti-IgE in humans by indomethacin. Allergy 1985; 40:36–41.

114. Pierce JW, Read MA, Ding H, Luscinskas FW, Collins T. Salicylate inhibit 1kB-α phosphorylation, endothelial–leukocyte adhesion molecule expression, and neutrophil transmigration. J Immunol 1996; 156:3961–3969.
115. Smith CH, Barker JNWN, Morris RW, MacDonald DM, Lee TH. Neuropeptides induce rapid expression of endothelial cell adhesion molecules and elicit granulocytic infiltration in human skin. J Immunol 1993; 151:3274–3282.
116. Marone G, Granata F, Spadaro G, Onorati AM, Triggiani M. Anti-inflammatory effects of oxatomide. J Invest Allergol Clin Immunol 1999; 9:207–214.
117. Goulding NJ, Euzger HS, Butt SK, Perretti M. Novel pathways for glucocorticoid effects on neutrophils in chronic inflammation. Inflamm Res 1998; 47:158–165.
118. Schwiebert LM, Beck LA, Stellato C, Bickel CA, Bochner BS, Schleimer RP. Glucocorticosteroid inhibition of cytokine production: relevance to anti-allergic actions. J Allergy Clin Immunol 1996; 97:143–152.
119. Meagher LC, Cousin JM, Seckl JR, Haslett C. Opposing effects of glycocorticoids on the rate of apoptosis in neutrophilic and eosinophilic granulocytes. J Immunol 1996; 156:4422–4428.
120. Barnes PJ. Effect of beta-agonists on inflammatory cells. J Allergy Clin Immunol 1999; 104(suppl):10–17.

5

Lymphocytes

SERGIO ROMAGNANI

University of Florence, Florence, Italy

1 INTRODUCTION

The history of discoveries on the pathogenesis of atopic allergy started in 1879, when Ehrlich first described mast cells and eosinophils. Then in 1921, Prausnitz and Kustner discovered that the allergic reactivity could be transferred by soluble factors (reagins), which in 1968 were characterized as antibodies of the IgE class by Ishizaka and Johansson, independently. The allergic reaction emerging at the end of this series of discoveries exhibited the pattern of an inflammatory process, resulting from the interaction between common environmental allergens and allergen-specific IgE antibodies bound to mast cells–basophils, that induced the release of both preformed and neosynthesized mediators, and was characterized by the simultaneous, but unexplained, presence in the blood and in the target tissues of elevated numbers of eosinophil granulocytes.

The demonstration, provided between 1986 and 1988 (1) in mice, and in humans (2,3), that the IgE antibody production by B cells was regulated by T-helper (Th)-cell-derived interleukins (IL) underlined the central role of lymphocytes in the pathogenesis of allergic reactions. Subsequently, in mice (4) and in humans (5) the existence of two different types of $CD4^+$ Th cells were described based on the different cytokine profiles produced, which were defined as type 1 (Th1) and type 2 (Th2), respectively. Of note, the cytokines produced by Th2 cells (IL-4, IL-5, IL-10, and IL-13) allowed us to explain the joint involvement of IgE-producing B cells, mast cells, and eosinophils in allergic inflammation (see later discussion), Thus, because of these discoveries, as well as of many other findings that have not been mentioned here, in the last 10 years the concept of allergic inflammation has dramatically changed. At present, allergic inflammation is considered by the great majority of authors as the final result of a Th2-type T-lymphocyte response to one or more common environmental allergens. The allergen-specific Th2 response indeed represents the triggering event for the recruitment and the involvement not only of IgE-producing B cells, mast cells, and eosinophils, but also of other cell types, as well as a high number of soluble factors and adhesion molecules, thus giving rise to an inflammatory cascade of unequaled complexity (see later discussion). Based on these findings, *atopic allergy* may presently be defined as a Th2-driven hypersensitivity to innocuous antigens (allergens) of complex genetic and environmental origins, which is currently known as the "Th2 hypothesis in allergy" (6).

2 FUNCTIONAL PROPERTIES OF Th1 AND Th2 CELLS

Murine type 1 T-helper (Th1) and type 2 T-helper (Th2) cells represent two polarized forms of the $CD4^+$ Th cell-mediated, specific immune response that develops in response to infections by intracellular bacteria and some viruses, or during infestations by complex parasites, such as gastrointestinal nematodes, respectively. Th1 cells produce interferon (IFN)-γ, IL-2, and tumor necrosis factor (TNF)-β, which affect the production by B cells of IgG2a opsonizing, complement-fixing antibodies and antibodies involved in antibody-dependent cell cytotoxicity (ADCC), activation of macrophages, activation of cytotoxic T lymphocytes (CTL), and induction of cell-mediated immunity (CMI). Therefore, Th1-dominated immune responses predominantly produce a pattern of phagocyte-dependent inflammation (7,8) (Fig. 1). On the other hand, murine Th2 cells provide optimal help not only for humoral immune responses, including IgE and IgG1 isotype switching, but also mucosal immunity, through production of mast cell and eosinophil growth and differentiation factors. Moreover, some Th2-derived cytokines, such as IL-4, IL-10, and IL-13 inhibit several macrophage functions. Therefore, the activation of these cells usually results in a phagocyte-independent inflammation (7,8) (see Fig. 1). Other cytokines, such as IL-3, granulocyte–macrophage colony-stimulating factor (GM-CSF), and TNF-α are produced by both Th1 and Th2 cells. Moreover, Th1 and Th2 are not the only immune response patterns possible, but rather are strongly polarized forms of more heterogeneous T-cell effector response. T cells expressing cytokines of both patterns have been designated type 0 (Th0). T cells producing high amounts of transforming growth factor (TGF)-β have been termed type 3 (Th3), and additional patterns have been described among long-term clones and during immune responses in vivo. Th0 cells probably represent a heterogeneous population of partially differentiated effector cells consisting of multiple discrete subsets, which can secrete both Th1 and Th2 cytokines. The cytokine response at the effector level can remain mixed, or it can be induced to further differentiate into the Th1 or Th2 pathway under the influence of signals received from the microenvironment (see later discussion). Some studies, however, have demonstrated heterogeneity of cytokine synthesis at the single-cell level, even in polarized Th1 and Th2 responses. Moreover, each of the cytokine genes seems to be under unique control, with distinct tendencies for concordant (e.g., IL-4 and IL-5) or discordant (e.g., IL-4 and IFN-γ) development. Thus, a more likely possibility is that cytokine profiles are largely random at the clonal level and that the exogenous signals that appear to direct T cells to differentiate into Th1 or Th2 cells (see following) act by increasing the probability for expression of certain cytokine genes at the population level, rather than by activating the expression of a cassette of transcriptionally linked genes in the individual cell. Thus, Th1 and Th2 cells are certainly not the result of a preexisting functional dichotomy of $CD4^+$ T cells, but rather, they can be considered as polarized forms of the specific immune response that frequently develop

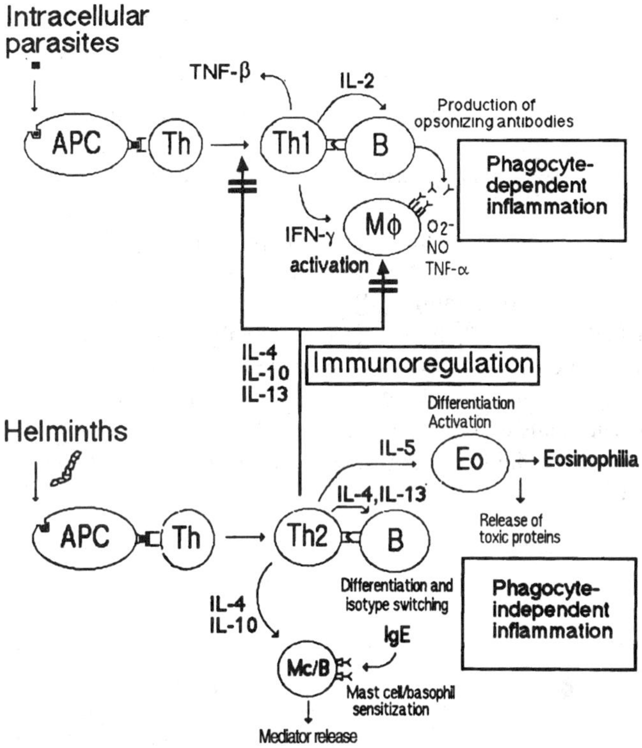

Figure 1 Main properties and functions of Th1- or Th2-polarized responses: APC, antigen-presenting cell; Th, T helper cell; Th1, type 1 Th; B, B lymphocyte; Mϕ, macrophage; Eo, eosinophil; Th2, type 2 Th; Mc/B, mast cell/basophil; IFN, interferon; TNF, tumor necrosis factor; IL, interleukin. See text for explanations. (From Ref. 12.)

under the combined action of genetic and environmental factors (7,8). In general, human Th1 and Th2 cells have a less restricted cytokine profile than murine T cells. Interleukin-2, IL-6, IL-10, and IL-13 tend to segregate less clearly among human $CD4^+$ subsets than in the mouse (8). Therefore, the majority of authors now define as Th2 or Th2-like those $CD4^+$ T cells that have been differentiated to produce IL-4, but not IFN-γ, and as Th1 or Th1-like cells those $CD4^+$ T cells that produce IFN-γ, but not IL-4, without considering the other set of Th1 or Th2 cytokines. It has also been suggested to consider as Th2 cells $CD4^+$ T-effector lymphocytes that maintain the ability to produce IL-4, and as Th1 cells those $CD4^+$ effectors that have lost this ability. If we keep all these points in mind, the Th1–2 paradigm may provide an useful model for understanding the pathogenesis of several pathophysiological conditions and possibly for the development of novel immunotherapeutic strategies (8).

3 METHODS FOR DETECTION OF Th1 AND Th2 CELLS

The possibility of detecting the presence of Th1- or Th2-dominated responses in normal and pathological conditions is limited by serious methodological problems. First, all cytokines are produced by T cells in small amounts, and some of them are not released in the microenvironment, but are directly transmitted from one cell to another during cell-to-cell contact. Therefore, it is virtually impossible to measure or even detect most spontaneously secreted cytokines in biological fluids even in supernatants of T-cell suspensions. Second, some cytokines, such as IL-4, are practically undetectable even in supernatants of T cells activated in short-term cultures, because repeated in vitro stimulation is required to obtain the production of measurable amounts of IL-4. To characterize the cytokine profile of Th–cell-mediated effector responses, different methodological approaches have been proposed. They include (1) cloning procedures, (2) reverse transcriptase–polymerase chain reaction (RT–PCR) assay, (3) in situ hybridization, (4) immunocytochemistry, (5) enzyme-linked immunoassay (ELISPOT) and (6) flow cytometric analysis of intracellular cytokine synthesis. The advantages and disadvantages of the different techniques are summarized in Table 1. At present, the best method for detection of cytokine production in cell suspensions is flow cytometric analysis of intracellular cytokine synthesis (Fig. 2), whereas in situ hybridization is more reliable for the identification of cells producing a given cytokine in tissue specimens (8).

Table 1 Methods Used to Detect Polarized Th1 or Th2 Responses

Method	Advantages	Disadvantages
Cloning	Cytokine profile easily detectable	Labor-intensive and time-consuming Reflects potential, rather than current, cytokine profile
RT–PCR	High sensitivity Possibility to assess tissue specimens	High risk for nonspecific reactions Possibility that a cytokine is transcribed, but not secreted Impossibility to characterize the cell type
In situ hybridization	Identification of the cell type Possibility to examine tissue specimens	More labor-intensive than RT–PCR
Immunocytochemistry	Identification of the cell type Possibility to examine tissue specimens	Not all cytokines detectable (e.g., IL-4)
ELISPOT	Relatively simple	Overcome by the technique of intracellular staining by flow cytometry
Intracellular staining by flow cytometry	Relatively simple and highly sensitive Allows detection of cytokine synthesis at single cell level	Usable only on cell suspensions

Source: Ref. 8.

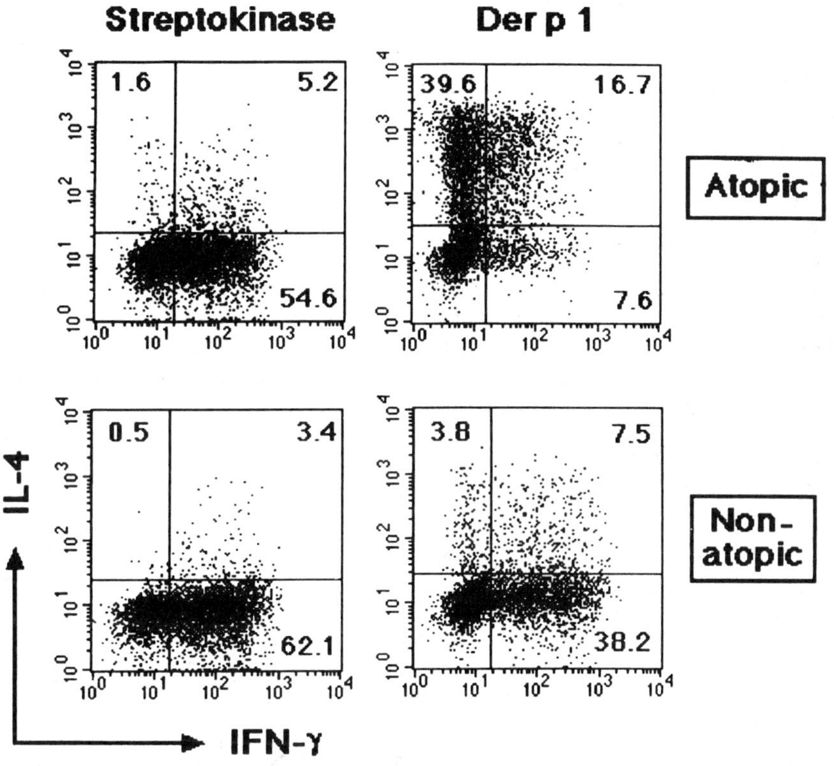

Figure 2 Different production of IL-4 and IFN-γ by streptokinase or *Dermatophagoides pteronyssinus* group 1 (Der p 1)-specific T-cells from one atopic and one nonatopic donor. Streptokinase- and Der p 1-specific T-cells were assessed on day 15 for intracellular cytokine synthesis following 4-hr stimulation with PMA plus ionomycin.

4 SURFACE MOLECULES PREFERENTIALLY ASSOCIATED WITH Th1 OR Th2 CELLS

The possibility that the Th1 or Th2 polarization of the effector response associates with the expression of distinctive molecules on the cell surface has also been investigated. Although specific markers for a given cell type probably do not exist, several molecules showing preferential association with Th1 or Th2 cells have been described (Table 2). This is sometimes because their expression is dependent on, or up-regulated by, the production of a given cytokine. For example, LAG-3 expression is up-regulated by IFN-γ, CD30 is dependent on the production of IL-4, CXCR4 is up-regulated by IL-4 and down-regulated by INF-γ, the IL-12 receptor (R) β-chain is up-regulated by IFN-γ and down-regulated by IL-4. By contrast, the preferential association of CD62L, CCR3, CCR4, CCR8, and CRTH2 with Th2 cells and of CCR5 and CXCR3 with Th1 cells is because these molecules represent chemokine receptors or adhesion molecule ligands involved in the attraction and permanence of Th2 or Th1 cells at the level of inflamed tissues, respectively (8). In our hands, the molecules more selectively associated both in vitro and in vivo with Th1 or Th2 cells are CCR5 for Th1 and CRTH2 for Th2, respectively (Fig. 3).

Table 2 Surface Molecules Preferentially Expressed by Human Th1 or Th2 Cells

Cell	Surface molecule	Ligand(s)
Th1	CD26	ADA, FN
	LAG-3	MHC class II
	IL-12R β-chain	IL-12
	CXCR3	IP-10, MIG, I-TAC
	CCR5	RANTES, MIP-1α, MIP-1
Th2	CD30	CD30L
	CCR3	Eotaxin(s), RANTES, MCP-3, MCP-4
	CCR4	MDC, TARC
	CCR8	I-309
	CXCR4	SDF-1
	CRTH2	PGD_2

ADA, adenosine deaminase; FN, fibronectin; LAG-3, lymphocyte activation gene-3; RANTES, regulated on activation, normal T-cell expressed and secreted; MIP, macrophage inflammatory protein; IP-10, interferon-induced protein 10; MIG, monokine induced by IFN-γ; I-TAC, IFN-inducible T-cell α-chemoattractant; CD30L, CD30 ligand; MCP, monocyte chemoattractant protein; MDC, macrophage-derived chemokine; TARC, thymus and activation-regulated chemokine; SDF-1, stromal-derived factor-1; PGD_2, prostaglandin D_2.
Source: Ref. 12.

5 MECHANISMS RESPONSIBLE FOR Th1 OR Th2 POLARIZATION

Both Th1 and Th2 cells develop from the same Th-cell precursor under the influence of environmental and genetic factors acting at the level of antigen presentation (7,8). The environmental factors that play the most important role in this process are (1) the route of antigen entry, (2) the physical form of immunogen, (3) the type of adjuvant, and (4) the dose of antigen. The genetic mechanisms that concur in controlling the type of Th-cell differentiation still remain unclear. The environmental and genetic factors act together to influence the Th1–Th2 differentiation, mainly by modulating (1) a group of contact-dependent factors and (2) the predominance of a given cytokine in the microenvironment of the responding Th cell. The most important contact-dependent factors are (1) the extent of T-cell receptor (TCR) ligation and (2) the signals delivered by costimulatory molecules, such as B7-C28 and OX40–OX40L. OX40L–OX40 interaction enhances IL-4 expression at priming and promotes the differentiation of naive CD4 T cells into high IL-4-producing effectors. The role of B7-CD28 interactions is more complex and still controversial. However, IL-4 production by naive T cells also appears to be highly dependent on B7 molecules. Naive CD4 T cells seem to be receptive to CD28-dependent IL-4 production only if they receive a weak T-cell receptor (TCR) signal. Thus, naive Th cells themselves are able to produce small amounts of IL-4 from their initial activation, and the concentration of IL-4 that accumulates at the level of the Th cell response increases with increasing lymphocyte activation. The inducing effect of IL-4 dominates over other cytokines, so that if IL-4 levels reach a necessary threshold, differentiation of the Th cell into the Th2 phenotype occurs (Fig. 4). Under certain circumstances another IL-4 source may be a small subset of $CD4^+NK1.1^+$ cells capable of recognizing antigens presented in association with the nonpolymorphic β_2-microglobulin–associated molecule, CD1. Finally, the role of IL-

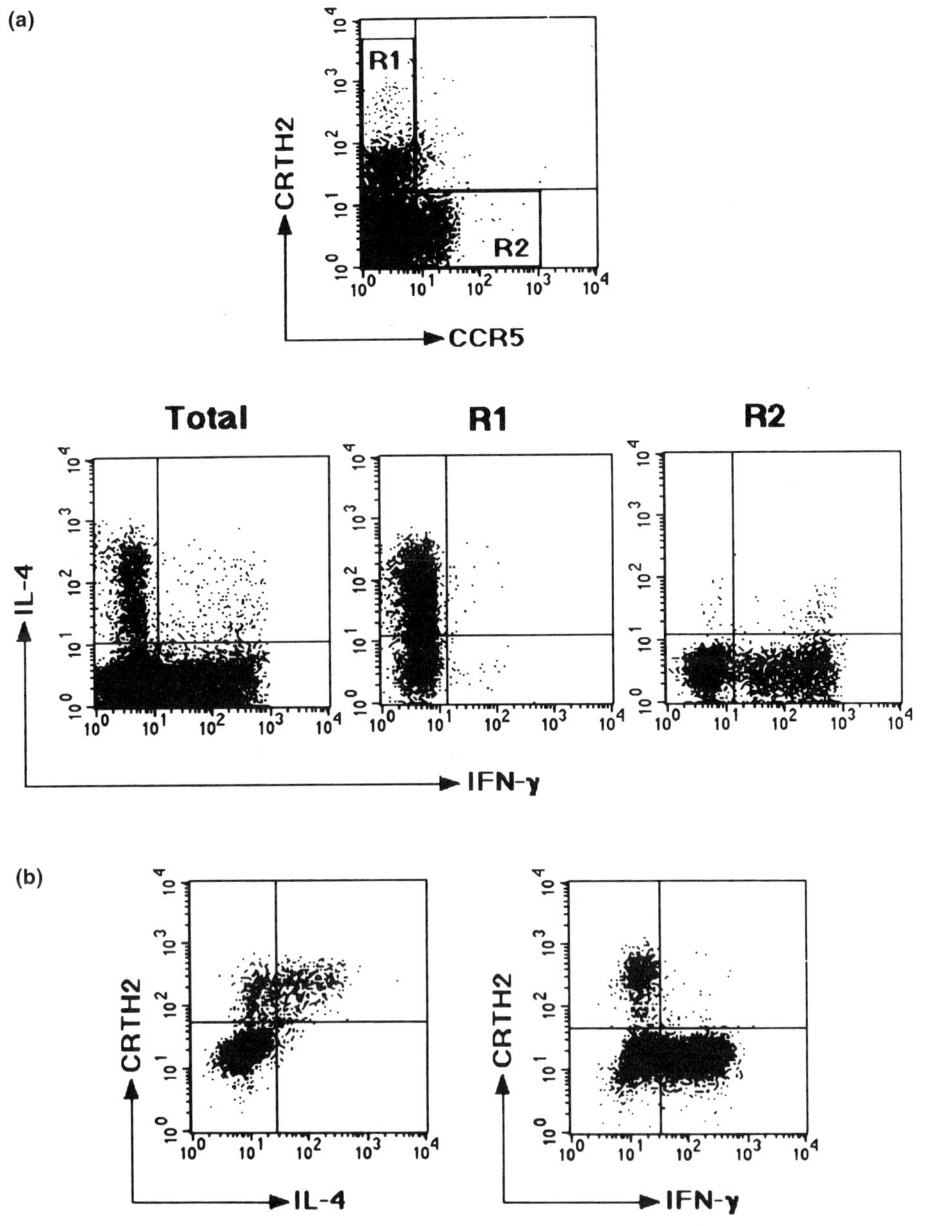

Figure 3 Alternative expression of CCR5 and CRTH2 by human Th1 or Th2 cells, respectively: (a) Detection by flow cytometry of CRTH2 and CCR5 on peripheral blood mononuclear cells (top) and of intracellular production IL-4 and IFN-γ induced by 4-hr stimulation with PMA plus ionomycin of the total, as well as of the CRTH2- or CCR5-enriched, population. (b) Intracellular synthesis of IL-4 (left) and IFN-γ (right) of the circulating CRTH2-expressing population in a subject with severe atopic disorder.

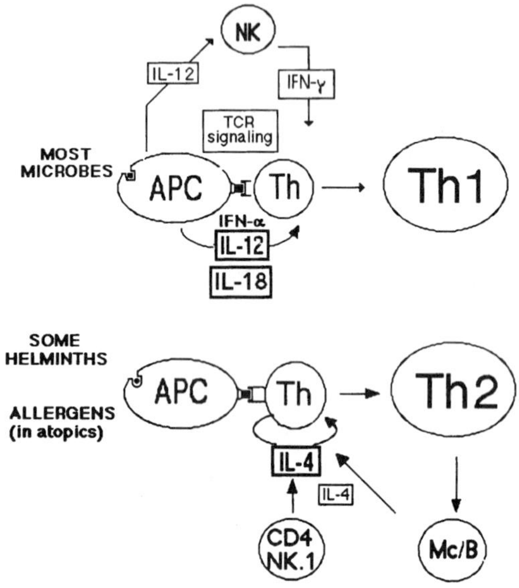

Figure 4 Cytokines responsible for the Th1- or Th2-polarization and their sources: NK, natural killer; TCR, T-cell receptor; for other abbreviations, see legend of Figure 1 and see text for explanations. (From Ref. 12.)

4 released by mast cells or basophils in promoting the differentiation of Th cells into the Th2 pathway has been suggested. However, IL-4 released by mast cells or basophils may amplify established Th2 responses, but its role in promoting the development of Th2 cells in the primary response is unlikely, because obvious mechanisms determining FcεR-independent IL-4 production for the great majority of antigens have not yet been defined.

In contrast to IL-4, the early production of IL-12, IL-18, and IFNs favors Th1 development (see Fig. 4). IL-12, which is the most powerful Th1-inducing agent, is produced mainly by dendritic cells (DC) under the stimulation provided by exogenous signals and is up-regulated by both CD40L–CD40 interaction and the presence of IFN-γ. Of interest, IFN-γ plays an important role in mice, whereas both IFN-γ and IFN-α promote the Th1 differentiation in humans, the latter up-regulating the expression of the IL-12R β-chain. Prostaglandin-E_2 (PGE_2), and IL-10, which can also be produced by DC, inhibit IL-12 production, thus biasing naive Th cells' development toward the Th2 pathway. Thus, different signals by pathogens or other antigens can modulate the type and the amount of cytokines produced by DC, or more likely, may stimulate functionally distinct DC subsets. Hormones also play some role in TH cells' differentiation: glucorticoids, calcitriol, and progesterone favoring Th2, whereas androgen steroids and relaxin favor Th1 cells' development (8). Recently, it has been shown that Th cell fate is regulated not only by differentiative signals delivered by cytokines, T cell receptor (TCR) ligation, and costimulatory molecules, but is also dependent on cell cycle expression (i.e., the number of postactivation cell divisions). These studies suggest that there is an opportunity for a Th cell to initiate cytokine gene expression at each cell division and that the probability of this occurring varies between cytokines. It is of interest that these division relations and probabilities of expression do not appear to be heavily dependent on the genetic background of the T cells, but rather, on epigenetic events that may control cytokine gene accessibility. Thus, both deterministic and probabilistic processes concur to determine the final choice in the cytokine pattern during the specific Th cell's response (9).

6 TRANSCRIPTION FACTORS THAT REGULATE THE DEVELOPMENT OF Th1 AND Th2 CELLS

The demonstration that early IL-4 expression during an immune response is critical for determining the development of Th2 cells has raised interest in the molecular basis of its regulation (10,11). The binding of cytokines to their receptors typically results in rapid tyrosine phosphorylation of signal transducers and activators of transcription (STATs). Of these, STAT6 appears selectively activated by IL-4 and knockout of the *Stat6* gene results in deficient Th2 responses, inasmuch as in these animals T cells are unable to develop into Th2 cells and the production of IgE and IgG1 is virtually abolished. However, there is as yet no direct evidence that STAT6 transactivates the IL-4 promoter in T cells, or that the STAT6 site of the IL-4 promoter is required for promoter activity. Other transcription factors of the nuclear factor of activated T cells (NF-AT) family (NF-ATp, NF-ATc, NF-AT3, NF-AT4) are able to transactivate the IL-4 promoter, but they are expressed in both Th1 and Th2 cells. However, in NF-ATc-deficient chimeric mice, severe T-cell defects in IL-4 production and Th2 differentiation were observed. By contrast, NF-ATp-deficient mice displayed increased Th2 and decreased Th1 responses, suggesting that, unlike NF-ATc, NF-ATp behaves as negative regulator of the Th2 responses. Another molecule that appears to be a repressor of Th2 responses is the proto-oncogene *BCL-6*, which inhibits STAT-6 transcription. *BCL-6* represses IL-4–induced activation of CD23 expression and targeted deletion of the *BCL* gene led to a massive inflammatory response, characterized by eosinophilic infiltration. Moreover, IgE responses were elevated in immunized BCL-6-deficient mice. NIP45 (NF-AT interacting protein) is also a factor expressed in Th2 cells that appears to function as a potent coactivator of IL-4 gene transcription, but its expression in Th1 cells is unclear. Other transcription factors expressed by many cell types are important for Th2 gene expression. Mice genetically deficient in the NF-κB subunit p50 failed to express IL-5 and eotaxin, as well as to develop airway inflammation. The transcription factors C/EBP and AP-1 are important for the expression of Th2 cytokine genes. Finally, the proto-oncogene c-*maf* is selectively expressed in Th2 clones and is induced during Th2, but not during Th1, differentiation. More importantly, its activity appears to be specific to the IL-4 promoter, inasmuch as it is unable to transactivate the promoters of other Th2 cytokine genes, such as IL-5 or IL-10.

A transcription factor that may be more widely involved in the induction and maintenance of the Th2 pattern of cytokine secretion is GATA-3. GATA-3 is expressed in both immature and mature T cells, and is selectively suppressed during Th2, but not during Th1, differentiation. Thus, in contrast to c-*maf*, which appears to be IL-4–specific, GATA-3 may function as a more general regulator of Th2 cytokine expression. Moreover, GATA-3 also inhibits IFN-γ expression, thereby also behaving as an inhibitory factor for Th1 effector development (10,11). However, the hierarchy of transcription factors and their differential control in Th2 gene expression, as well as the precise relation between the different factors, are still unclear.

The molecular mechanisms by which IL-12, IL-18, and IFNs promote the development of naïve T cells into Th1 effectors are even less clear. The interaction of IL-12 with its receptor results in a rapid and selective tyrosine phosphorylation of STAT6, which has been suggested to directly regulate the IFN-γ gene. However, another transcription factor,

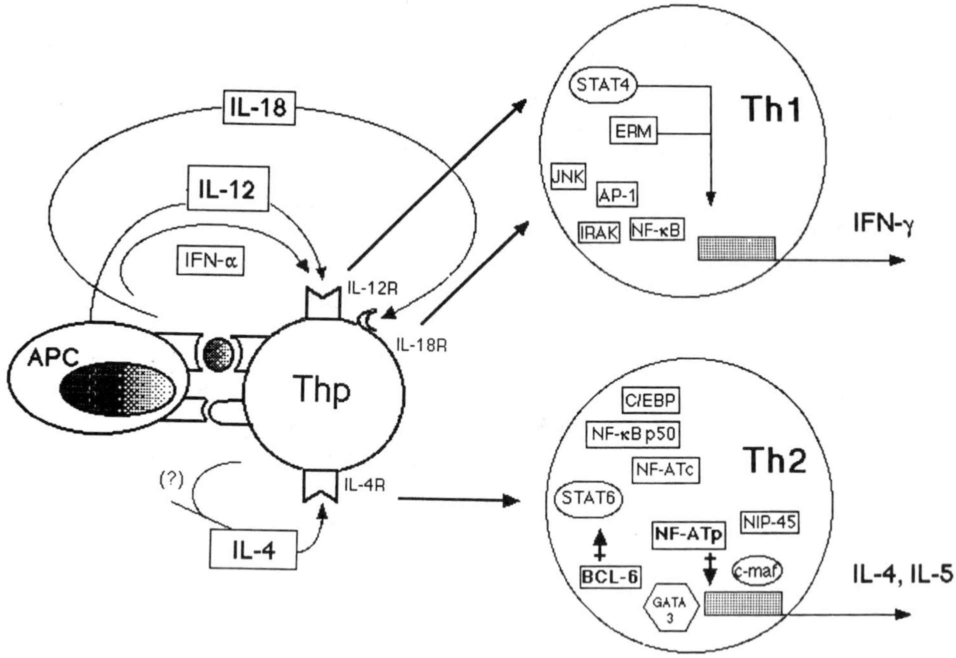

Figure 5 Transcription factors involved in the Th1- or Th2-polarization: Thp, Th cell precursor; IL-12R, IL-12 receptor; IL-18R, IL-18 receptor; IL-4R, IL-4 receptor; STAT, signal transducer and activator of transcription; JNK, c-Jun *N*-terminal kinase; IRAK, IL-1 receptor-associated kinase; AP-1, activator protein-1; NF-κB, nuclear factor-kappa B; C/EBP, CCAAT enhancer-binding proteins; NF-AT, nuclear factor of activated T-cells; NIP-45, NF–AT interacting protein. *BCL-6* and c-*maf* are proto-oncogenes. For other abbreviations see legend of Figure 1 and see text for explanations. Bar in the arrows means inhibitory effect. (From Ref. 12.)

ERM, has recently been identified, which is selectively expressed by Th1 cells after activation in the presence of IL-12 in a STAT4-dependent manner. In addition, STAT4 alone is not sufficient to induce IFN-γ. IL-18 signaling, which involves the activation of JNK, AP-1, NF-κB, and IRAK, also regulates the transcriptional activity of the IFN-γ promoter. Thus, probably, the synergistic expression of IFN-γ induced by IL-12 and IL-18 results from the interplay of multiple transcription factors in differential regulation of IFN-γ promoter activity (12) (Fig. 5).

7 DATA SUPPORTING THE ROLE OF ALLERGEN-SPECIFIC Th2 CELLS IN THE PATHOGENESIS OF ATOPIC ALLERGY

Both conceptual and experimental data support the validity of the Th2 hypothesis in the pathogenesis of atopic allergy. Conceptually, Th2 cells are the only cells that can both directly recognize the allergen peptides by the T-cell receptor (TCR) and account for the joint involvement of IgE-producing B cells (IL-4; IL-13), mast cells (IL-4; IL-10), and eosinophils (IL-5) in the allergic inflammation. The experimental data supporting the Th2 hypothesis originate both from experiments performed in animal models of allergy and asthma, as well as in human allergic diseases.

7.1 Cytokines in Animal Models of Allergy and Asthma

7.1.1 Injection of Cytokines or Anticytokine Antibodies

Antigen challenge to the lungs of sensitized mice produces an intense influx of eosinophils into the BAL fluid and lung tissue. Bronchial hyperreactivity is an important feature of asthmatic airways and can be demonstrated in sensitized mice following repeated exposure to antigen. There is also increased expression of IL-4 and IL-5 mRNA, as well as IL-4 and IL-5 protein levels, but not significant increases in IFN-γ, in the lungs of allergic mice, the main source being from T cells. Administration of anti-IL-4 antibodies or soluble IL-4 receptors inhibits IgE and IgG1 production, as well as airway hyperreactivity (AHR), but not eosinophilia, in sensitized mice, whereas administration of anti-IL-5 antibody at levels that suppressed eosinophils to less than 1% of recruited cells had no effect on the subsequent airway response. The possibility that IL-4 can induce tissue inflammation has been demonstrated by injection of murine Th2 cells into the footpad of naive animals. Th2 cells induced swelling that peaked at 6 hr and lasted about 48 hr and was completely blocked by anti-IL-4 antibody or soluble IL-4 receptors. However, most data suggest that AHR is also IL-5-dependent. First, antibodies to IL-5 inhibit both pulmonary eosinophilia and AHR in allergic mice. More importantly, in IL-5-deficient mice, the eosinophilia, lung damage, and AHR normally resulting from allergen challenge are abolished. The role of Th2-type cytokines in the induction and maintenance of allergic inflammation is supported by the observation that administration of recombinant IFN-γ, induction of endogenous IFN-γ by poly-I:C, or administration of IL-12 (which all down-regulate Th2 responses), inhibit antigen-induced eosinophil infiltration in the murine trachea and AHR. The inhibitory effect of IL-12 on antigen-induced AHR was dependent on IFN-γ activity, whereas depletion of eosinophils was only partially IFN-γ-dependent. Parenteral administration of IFN-γ also failed to decrease IgE production and to normalize airways function, but treatment regimens of sensitized mice with nebulized IFN-γ caused a decrease in cutaneous reactivity and normalization of AHR. The possible role of increased numbers of IFN-γ–producing $CD8^+$ T cells in this process was suggested. Finally, mice that lack the IFN-γ receptor have an impaired ability to resolve lung eosinophilic inflammatory reactions associated with Th2 responses (13).

AHR and eosinophil infiltration into lung tissue and bronchoalveolar lavage (BAL) fluid are also a characteristic feature of antigen challenge to the airways of sensitized guinea pigs. Treatment with antibodies to IL-5, inhibits these pulmonary responses. Furthermore, administration of murine IL-5 to normal guinea pigs lungs induces a small, but significant, increase in bronchoconstrictor reactivity and an increase in the number of inflammatory cells in the BAL fluid. IL-5 is also involved in the development of eosinophilic lung inflammation and AHR in monkeys, because treatment with an anti-IL-5 antibody inhibits both eosinophil influx into the airways and early- and late-phase bronchoconstriction and AHR in antigen-challenged *Ascaris suum*-sensitive cynomolgus monkeys. Interestingly, inhibition of the pulmonary eosinophilia and AHR by the anti-IL-5 antibody was seen to persist for at least 3 months after a single treatment. These results demonstrate the importance of Th2 cytokines, especially of IL-5, in the induction of allergic pulmonary inflammation and AHR in both rodents and nonhuman primates. Finally, tracheal instillation of IL-9, another Th2-derived cytokine, resulted in the increase of eosinophils in the BAL and significantly elevated serum IgE levels. Taken together, these studies suggest that IL-4, IL-5, and IL-9 are involved in the induction of both allergy and asthma induced in animal models (13).

7.1.2 Effect of Transfer of Th1 or Th2 Cells

Transfer of Th2, but not Th1 cells into recipient mice induces airway eosinophilia, hypersecretion of mucus and AHR. However, IL-4 appears to be essential for Th2-cell recruitment to the lung and for migration of eosinophils from lung tissue to the airways, but has no direct role in production of mucus. In the absence of IL-4, IL-13 may be critical for Th2-induced mucus production and eosinophilia. Thus, these studies suggests that signaling through IL-4Rα (shared by IL-4 and IL-13) is critically important in Th2 stimulation of allergic inflammation and mucus production (14). By contrast, Th1 cells induced such production, but not eosinophilic infiltration in IFN-γR gene-deficient mice, but both mucus production and eosinophilia were inhibited by IFN-γ, suggesting an important protective role for IFN-γ. According to the results of other models; however, Th1 cells do not seem to play a protective role on the lung inflammation induced by Th2 cells, and even they are required to promote the eosinophil recruitment to the airways and to increase the allergic inflammation (15). Of great interest was the recent observation that the transfer of Th1-cell lines, which were engineered to secrete TGF-β, strongly down-modulated allergic inflammation and AHR in a mouse model of asthma, based on the transfer of Th2 cells (16). This suggests that T cells secreting TGF-β in the respiratory mucosa can regulate Th2-induced airway inflammation and AHR and may be key regulatory cells in asthma.

7.1.3 Knockout Mice Showing Deficient Th2 Responses

The role of Th2 cells in allergic inflammation is not limited to their ability to induce the production of allergen-specific IgE antibodies by B cells and to promote the eosinophilic infiltration in target tissues. Data obtained in knockout (KO) mice support the concept that Th2 cells are critical for both allergic inflammation and asthma, but they also suggest that at least some pathophysiological consequences of allergic reaction may also occur in the absence of the IgE response (17). Indeed, B-cell, IgE, CD40, and mast cell gene knockout mice can develop asthma, whereas $CD4^+$ T-cell, IL-4, STAT-6, and IL-5 gene knockout mice cannot. Of note, in IL-4 gene knockout mice, only the passive transfer of T, but not of non-T, cells may restore both their ability to develop Th2 cells and to produce IgE antibodies. Thus, based on knockout models, IL-4 produced by T cells seems to be essential for the development of Th2 cells and, therefore, for the production of both IgE antibodies and IL-5; however, IL-5-mediated effects appear to be even more important than IL-4-related activities at effector levels.

7.1.4 Effect of Overexpression of Cytokines in the Airway Epithelium of Transgenic Mice

Data obtained in transgenic mice that exhibit overexpression of Th2 cytokines in the airway epithelium provide additional support for the validity of the Th2 hypothesis in allergy and asthma (18). The overexpression of IL-13 in the lung and airways caused a profound phenotype characterized by eosinophilic and mononuclear inflammation, with mucous metaplasia, subepithelial fibrosis, airway obstruction, AHR, and eotaxin production (see later discussion). Similarly, the overexpression of IL-9 and IL-4 caused a mixed mononuclear and eosinophilic inflammatory response, and IL-5 overexpression caused both subepithelial fibrosis and AHR.

The IL-6-type cytokine family contains IL-6, IL-11, cardiotropic-1, oncostatin-M, and ciliary neurotropic factor. These cytokines have similar structure, all use the promiscuous gp130 molecule in their multimeric receptor complexes, and exhibit overlapping functions. Overexpression of IL-6 in the murine airway caused impressive subepithelial fibrosis, with collagen deposition and the endothelial accumulation of α-smooth–muscle actin-containing stromal cells. By contrast IL-6 overexpression did not cause tissue eosinophilia, mucous metaplasia, or AHR. Overexpression of IL-11 by eosinophils and epithelial cells caused an airway phenotype characterized by (1) subepithelial fibrosis; (2) the enhanced deposition of type III and type I, but not of type IV, collagens; (3) the enhanced accumulation of fibroblasts, myofibroblasts and myocites; and (4) baseline airway obstruction and AHR. Tissue eosinophilia and mucous metaplasia are not features of the lungs of IL-11-overexpressing animals. Moreover, this cytokine was able to inhibit the acute eosinophilic response and Th2 gene expression, suggesting it may represent a healing molecule in the airway (18).

7.2 Cytokines in Allergic Human Diseases

The prevalent expression of Th2 cytokines in allergic disorders has been suggested by an impressive series of observations performed both in vitro and in vivo (13).

7.2.1 Vernal Conjunctivitis

The first description of the cytokine profile of T-cells from tissue in allergic disease was in vernal conjunctivitis, a condition of papillary hyperthrophy of the conjunctiva with eosinophil and lymphocyte infiltration and associated high serum IgE. T-cell clones were made from tissues by initial expansion with phytohemagglutinin (PHA) followed by IL-2. Clones from the conjunctival tissue of three patients were mostly $CD4^+$ and produced IL-4, but little IFN-γ. These clones supported IgE synthesis in vitro. More recently, these data have been confirmed using flow cytometry to assess cytokine production by tear T-cells. Interestingly, an allergic-like blepharitis (inflammation of the eyelid) with a mononuclear cell infiltrate was observed in a cohort of IL-4 transgenic mice that expressed IL-4 at the level of B lymphocytes.

7.2.2 Allergic Rhinitis

In patients with allergic rhinitis, nasal allergen provocation, followed by nasal mucosa biopsy 24 hr after allergen challenge, is associated with a cellular infiltrate in which $CD4^+$ T-cells and eosinophils are prominent. By use of the complementary techniques of immunohistology and in situ hybridization an increase in cytokine mRNA expression for IL-3, IL-4, IL-5, and GM-CSF was found, which correlated with the degree of local eosinophilia. Accordingly, $CD4^+$ T-cell clones generated from the nasal mucosa after allergen challenge, many of which were specific for the allergen used in the challenge test, showed a prevalent Th2 profile. However, in another study performed on patients with perennial allergic rhinitis, there was a complete lack of any cytokine immunoreactivity localized to tissue lymphocytes. Mast cells accounted for more than 90% of IL-4 and IL-6 and more than 50% of IL-5 immunoreactive cells. These findings leave open the question of whether allergic inflammation in the mucosa of patients with allergic rhinitis is initiated by Th2 cells that, however, do not accumulate cytokines in sufficient concentrations to be consistently detected by immunohistochemical methods, or by mast cells that may be able to secrete Th2 cytokines rapidly and in high concentrations (13). However, recent findings based on the measurement of cytokines in nasal lavage fluids of children with seasonal allergic rhinitis support the concept that reactivity to pollen exposure follows the cytokine pattern consistent with Th1–Th2 concept.

7.2.3 Bronchial Asthma

Asthma in humans is a complex disorder characterized by intermittent, reversible airway obstruction, and by airway hyperresponsiveness and inflammation. Although its cause(s) remain unknown, we now recognize that asthma is a syndrome for which the common pathological expression is inflammation of the airways. From clinical and laboratory findings, asthma may be divided into allergic (extrinsic) and nonallergic (intrinsic) forms. Allergic asthma usually starts during childhood and is characterized by allergen-dependent, often seasonal symptoms, with positive skin tests to allergens and elevated total and allergen-specific serum IgE. In contrast, nonallergic asthma usually begins in adulthood, is perennial and more severe, has no elevation in serum IgE, and is often associated with sinusitis and nasal polyposis. Both allergic and intrinsic asthma are characterized by infiltration of the bronchial mucosa with large numbers of activated eosinophils and the presence of elevated concentrations of eosinophil-derived proteins, such as major basic protein (MBP) and the eosinophil cationic protein (ECP). By specific immunostaining of bronchial mucosal biopsies obtained with the fiber-optic bronchoscope, a significant increase in the number of IL-2 receptor-positive (activated T-cells) in the airways of mild, steady-state asthmatics was observed. With in situ hybridization technique, cells showing mRNA for Th2, but not Th1, cytokines were found at the site of late-phase reactions in skin biopsies from atopic patients, and in mucosal bronchial biopsies or BAL of patients with atopic asthma. By use of immunomagnetic separation, most IL-4 and IL-5 mRNA in the BAL cells from asthmatic subjects was associated with $CD2^+$ T cells. Interestingly, glucocorticosteroid (GCS) treatment in asthma resulted in the down-regulation of BAL cells expressing mRNA for IL-4 and IL-5, whereas the number of cells expressing mRNA for IFN-γ was increased. GCS, as well as the immunosuppressants FK506 and cyclosporin A, also suppress IL-5 production by peripheral blood mononuclear cells (PBMC) from mite-sensitive atopic asthmatics. In contrast, no effect on the number of BAL cells expressing mRNA for IL-4 and IL-5 was observed, suggesting that steroid-resistant asthma may be associated with a dysregulation in the expression of the genes encoding for Th2 and Th1 cytokines in airway cells. To assess whether the T-cell response to inhaled allergens induced activation and recruitment of allergen-specific Th2 cells in the airway mucosa of patients with respiratory allergy, T-cell clones were generated from biopsy specimens of bronchial mucosa of patients with grass pollen-induced asthma or rhinitis, taken 48 hr after positive bronchial provocation test with the relevant allergen. Proportions ranging from 14 to 22% of $CD4^+$ T-cell clones derived from the stimulated mucosa of grass-allergic patients were specific for grass allergens and most of them exhibited a definite Th2 profile and induced IgE production by autologous B cells in the presence of the specific allergen (13).

Because many studies addressing abnormalities of T-lymphocyte cytokine secretion in asthma have been performed on subjects who are also atopic, the question has been assessed of whether disordered cytokine synthesis by T lymphocytes in asthmatics simply reflects the existence of atopy or do they imply a role in asthma pathogenesis. In recent studies, peripheral blood mononuclear cells (PBMC) from atopic and nonatopic asthmatic children were stimulated with PHA in vitro, and concentrations of both IL-4 and IFN-γ released into cell supernatants were measured. Although PHA-stimulated PBMC from the atopic asthmatics secreted significantly more IL-4 and significantly less IFN-γ than those from both the nonatopic asthmatics and the normal controls, no significant differences were observed in the secretion of both cytokines by cells from the nonatopic asthmatics or those from the normal controls, suggesting that the imbalance in cytokine secretion relates to the atopic state, rather than specifically to the presence of asthma, and that ''intrinsic'' asthma is a distinct immunopathological entity. Indeed, although increased levels of IL-4 and IL-5 were measured in the BAL of allergic asthmatics, in nonallergic asthmatics IL-2 and IL-5 predominated. Moreover, $CD4^+$ and $CD8^+$ T-cell lines generated from the BAL of patients with asthma secreted significantly higher quantities of IL-5 and GM-CSF than lines from the atopic and nonatopic controls. More recently, however, the comparison in bronchial biopsies from atopic and intrinsic asthmatics of mRNA for IL-4, IL-5, IL-3, IL-13, and GM-CSF, as well as of the CC chemokines eotaxin, eotaxin 2, RANTES, MCP-3, and MCP-4, showed the existence of more similarities than differences (19). Thus, it is highly likely that elevated synthesis of Th2-type cytokines and related chemokines (see following) is a feature shared by both atopic and intrinsic asthmatics.

Of note, both IL-4 and IL-13 act on human lung fibroblasts by inducing upregulation of β_1-integrin and vascular cell adhesion (VCAM)-1 and production of IL-6 and monocyte-chemoattractant protein (MCP)-1, suggesting their possible role in subendothelial fibrosis (20). Mucin production is also a common feature of asthma and an important contributor to airway obstruction. A recent study performed in cultured epithelial cells showed that samples of asthmatic fluid stimulated mucin synthesis severalfold more potently than nonasthmatic fluid. Of note, antibody blockade of ligand–receptor interaction for IL-9 (but not for IL-5 or IL-13) inhibited mucin stimulation by airway fluid. This suggests that IL-9 may account for most of the mucin-stimulating activity of lung fluids in allergic airway disease (21).

7.2.4 Atopic Dermatitis

Atopic dermatitis (AD) is the cutaneous disorder of atopic allergy caused by chronic skin inflammation that results from the exposure to foreign proteins. Most patients with AD (>80%) have positive intracutaneous skin test reactions to one or more environmental allergens and elevated serum IgE levels, which represent antibodies specific to the allergens concerned. The histological appearance of lesional AD skin is characterized by dermal perivascular infiltrates of mononuclear cells, mainly consisting of $CD4^+$ T-cells and eosinophils. However, the relation between allergy and the pathogenesis of the skin lesions in AD is still unclear. By using the RT–PCR technique, spontaneous mRNA IL-4 expression was found in PBMC from AD patients, whereas IL-13, another IgE-switching cytokine, was not produced. IFN-γ mRNA expression was also increased in PBMC from AD patients, but IFN-γ production was reduced, suggesting a posttranscriptional defect of IFN-γ secretion (22). IFN-γ production by PBMC from AD patients was deficient in response to stimulation with toxic shock syndrome toxin-1 (TSST-1) or IL-12, whereas both IL-12 production and IL-12R expression in the same patients were normal. However, neutralization of IL-4, and even more of IL-10, activity caused a great augmentation of IFN-γ production. These data suggest that PBMC from AD patients, despite normal levels of IL-12 production and IL-12R expression, are unable to generate normal IL-12-induced IFN-γ responses, which may be related to the excess production of IL-4 and IL-10. High proportions of Dermatophagoides pteronyssinus (Dp)-specific Th2-like $CD4^+$ T-cell clones were obtained from the skin lesions of patients with AD, indicating accumulation or expansion of these T cells in lesional skin. Interestingly, Dp-specific Th2-like clones were also derived from biopsy specimens of intact skin taken after contact challenge with

Dp, suggesting that percutaneous sensitization to aeroallergens may play a role in the induction of skin lesions in patients with AD. More recent data partially confirm both the Der p-specificity and the Th2-type profile of high proportions of T-cell clones derived from Der p-induced patch test lesions of AD patients. However, the majority of T-cell clones derived from the lesional skin of patients with AD had a mixed (Th0-like) phenotype and only a few of them were specific for Dp. Interestingly, Der p-specific T-cell clones generated from the skin of AD patients usually have a more polarized Th2 cytokine profile than those obtained from the peripheral blood of the same patients, and that consistently produce IL-10 in addition to IL-4 and IL-5. In some patients, most T-cell clones derived from lesional skin exhibited high IFN-γ production, and a few of them appeared to be specific for bacterial antigens. More importantly, the presence of both Dp-specific and Th2-like cells in the skin of AD patients did not correlate with the presence in the serum of Dp-specific IgE antibody or the serum levels of IgE protein. By using the RT–PCR technique, overexpression of IL-10, but not of IL-4, was found in AD lesions in comparison with allergic contact dermatitis lesions and tuberculin reactions. Moreover, by assessing the kinetics of T-cell–derived cytokine production, it was found that in the initiation phase (APT skin site) IL-4 production is predominant over IFN-γ production. This is in line with the recent demonstration that epicutaneous exposure of protein antigens can induce a predominant Th2-like response with high IgE production in mice. In the late and chronic phase (lesional skin), the situation may be reversed and IFN-γ production predominates over IL-4 production. Taken together, these data suggest that Th2-like responses against Dp or other allergens at skin level are involved in the initiation of skin lesions, but there is a subsequent influx of Th1 cells, which may be responsible for the aggravation of the inflammation (21). However, the relation between aeroallergen sensitization and pathogenesis of AD still remains unclear.

7.3 Chemokines in Allergic Diseases

Over the last years, a family of chemotactic cytokines (chemokines) has been identified that appears to have specificity for the type of leukocytes that are recruited to the site of inflammation. Several chemokines have been identified in human allergic reactions, the production of which appears to be related to the severity of the inflammatory response. Several of these chemokines, including IL-8, regulator on activation, normal T-cell expressed and secreted (RANTES), macrophage chemotactic protein (MCP-3), and MCP-4 have been identified that induce eosinophil recruitment. However, the most important chemokine in eosinophil recruitment is eotaxin, which binds to a single receptor; CCR3, that is highly expressed by eosinophils, but also by basophils, mast cells, and even to a smaller extent, by Th2 cells. Eotaxin gene-deficient mice showed significantly less eosinophil accumulation compared with littermate controls. Moreover, in human asthma, eotaxin was produced at high levels and localized to the airway epithelium and smooth-muscle cells. It was also highly expressed, together with CCR3, in lesional skin from atopic dermatitis. Thus, this chemokine may play an important role in the attraction and homing of different cell types involved in allergic inflammation, such as eosinophils, basophils, mast cells, and even Th2 cells, in the target organs of allergic reactions. Of note, eotaxin also potentiates antigen-dependent basophil IL-4 production (23).

Other chemokines that play an important role in the pathogenesis of allergic inflammation are macrophage-derived chemokine (MDC) and thymus and activation-regulated chemokine (TARC). MDC is produced by not only macrophages and DC, but also by Th2 cells and interacts with the CCR4 receptor present on the same cells. Moreover, both IL-4 and IL-13 stimulate the production of MDC by DC, thereby providing an important amplification circuit for allergic inflammation. Accordingly, overproduction of Th2-specific chemokines MDC and TARC, as well as hyperexpression of their receptor CCR4, have recently been described in NC-Nga mice exhibiting atopic dermatitis-like lesions (23).

8 MECHANISMS RESPONSIBLE FOR ALLERGEN-SPECIFIC Th2 RESPONSES IN ATOPIC INDIVIDUALS

It has been well known for many years that the expression of the allergic phenotype is dependent on two major factors: a genetic predisposition and the environmental interactions.

8.1 Genetic Predisposition

It is clear that the pattern of allergic inheritance does not follow mendelian concepts usually associated with single-gene diseases. Rather, the pattern of inheritance is that of a complex poligenic disorder. This is consistent with the fact that the development of a prevalent Th2 response is up- and down-regulated by the activity of a series of cytokines, cytokine receptors, and transcription factors. Therefore, linkages to asthma and allergy have been found at multiple gene levels (Table 3). For example, both allergy and asthma have been linked to polymorphisms associated with the IL-4 gene and IL-4R gene. In addition, the apparent linkage to chromosome 12 includes several genes that may also influence IL-4 production (IFN, SCF, and NF-YB) or function (STAT-6). Additional candidate genes for the development of asthma include those associated with the leukotriene cascade, including 5-lipoxygenase (5-LO), the 5-LO-activating peptide, and leukotriene-C_4 synthase. Finally, abnormalities in β_2-adrenergic responsiveness have long been recognized in asthma, making the β_2-adrenergic receptor an important candidate (24).

Table 3 Linkages to Asthma and Allergy

Chromosome	Candidate genes
1p	IL-12R
2q	CD28
3p24	BCL-6 (STAT6 binding inhibition)
5q23–35	IL-3, IL-4, IL-5, IL-9, IL-13, GM-CSF, LTC_4 synthase, M-CSF-R, β_2-adrenergic-R, GCS-R
6p21–23	MHC, TNF, TAP-1 and TAP-2, LMP
10q	5-lipoxygenase
11q13	FcεR1 β-chain, Clara cell protein, fibroblast growth factor 3
12q14–24	IFN-γ, SCF, NO synthase (constitutive), NF-YB, I-LGF-1, LTA_4 hydrolase, STAT6
13q21–24	No known candidates
14q11–13	TCR (α/δ chains), NF-κB inhibitor
16p11–12	IL-4R

Source: Ref. 24.

8.2 Environmental Factors Acting Before Birth

Environmental factors may influence the differentiation of allergen-specific T-cells into a prevalent Th2 phenotype and, therefore, the development of atopic allergy by acting both before and after birth. Some years ago, we first showed that the immune response to DP begins during fetal life, a finding that has then been confirmed by others. In pregnancy, a Th2-skewed priming probably occurs in all cases, owing to the maternal environment. Successful pregnancy may indeed be characterized by a switch from Th1 to Th2 at the maternofetal interface to reduce the reactivity of the maternal immune system against the fetal allograft. Accordingly, progesterone, at the concentrations present at fetomaternal interface, favors the development of T-cells into IL-4-producing cells. More recently, we found that T-cell clones generated from the decidua of women suffering from unexplained recurrent abortions showed significantly reduced production of IL-4, IL-10, and leukemia inhibitory factor (LIF), which is required for egg implantation, in comparison with T-cell clones generated from the decidua of women with underlying voluntary abortion (normal gestation). Thus, the pregnancy-related environment may favor a weak Th2-skewed priming to transplacental allergens, which is obviously enhanced under the influence of an ''atopic'' genetic background (13).

8.3 Environmental Factors Acting After Birth

Environmental factors acting after birth, however, are certainly more important in influencing the individual outcome in the Th-response to ubiquitous allergens and can account for the increased prevalence of allergy over the last decades in western countries. Indeed, a genetic mechanism with steep changes in gene frequency is highly unlikely in the absence of extraordinary mutation rates or very powerful darwinian selection. More importantly, we know that following the occurrence of random TCR rearrangements and the processes of positive and negative selection in the thymus, the educational process of the immune system continues in the periphery, especially in the first years of life, throughout repeated interactions with infectious agents, ''innocuous antigens,'' and the commensal flora. This process results in both the fine tuning of the TCR repertoire and the progressive shifting of the T-cell effector balance from Th2 to Th1 (23). Given this knowledge, as well as our data showing that cytokines (IL-12 and IFNs) produced by cells of the ''natural immunity,'' such as macrophages, dendritic cells (DC), and natural killer (NK) cells, in response to *Mycobacterium tuberculosis* or its components, were able to shift, at least in vitro, the development of allergen-specific T-cells from the Th2/Th0 to the Th1 profile, six years ago I hypothesized that the increasing prevalence of allergy could be related to changes incurred in the infectious environment of children after the Second World War,

Table 4 Main Epidemiological Studies Supporting the ''Hygiene'' Hypothesis

The number of siblings decreases the risk for allergy, which is higher in the firstborn.
There is an inverse relation between risk for atopy and the occurrence of some infections in childhood.
There is reduced prevalence of allergy or asthma in patients with multiple sclerosis, a Th1-mediated disorder.
Total serum IgE levels decline in subjects infested by parasites after treatment for tuberculosis.
Prevalence of atopy is lower in children from anthroposophic families.

Source: Ref. 23.

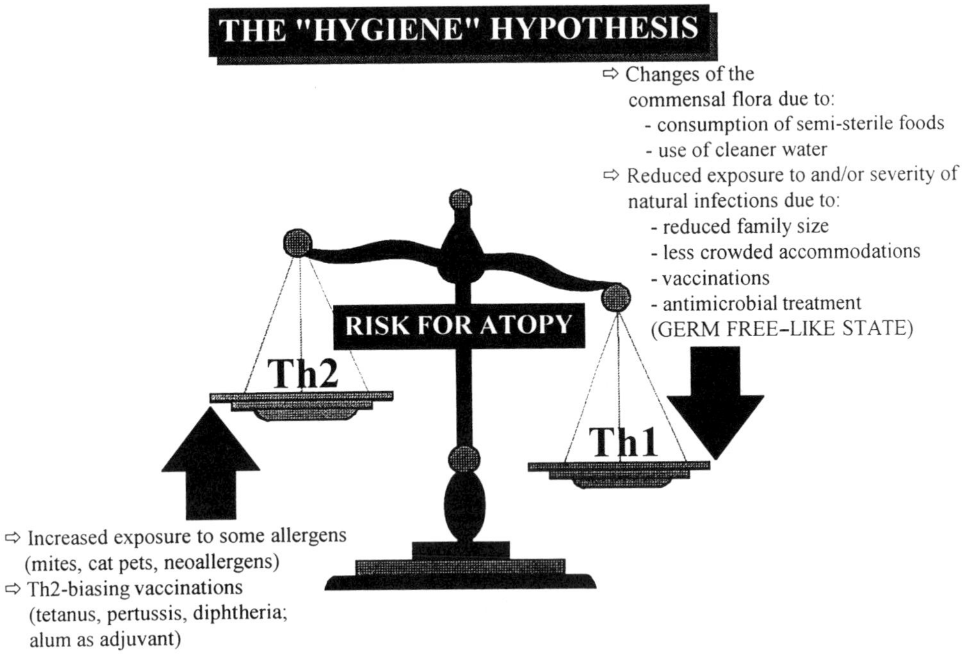

Figure 6 Factors that have contributed to a change in the infectious environment during childhood, thus favoring the alteration of balance between Th1 and Th2 responses to innocuous antigens (allergens) in favor of Th2 responses. (From Ref. 23.)

rather than to pollution (6). This hypothesis has been confirmed by studies performed in mice, showing that IFN-γ produced during the Th1 immune response against bacille calmette-guerin (BCG) suppresses the development of local inflammatory Th2 responses in the lung. More importantly, several epidemiological studies strongly suggest that changes in the infectious environment and in the pattern of microbial exposure of children associated with westernization are an important factor underlying the rising severity and prevalence of atopic disorders over the last decades in developed countries (Table 4). The major causes of changes in microbial environment, which alter the balance between Th1 and Th2 responses in favor of these latter, thus sustaining the validity of the so-called ''hygiene'' hypothesis, are summarized in Figure 6.

9 IMMUNOTHERAPEUTIC STRATEGIES BASED ON THE Th2 HYPOTHESIS IN ALLERGY

The insights in the pathogenesis of allergic disorders are providing exciting opportunities for the development of novel immunomodulatory regimens (25). The new approaches are addressed to target allergen-specific T-cells (allergen-specific immunotherapy) or their effector molecules (nonallergen-specific immunotherapy). The allergen-specific immunotherapy may consist of induction of unresponsiveness in T-cells or prevention or redirection of Th2 responses. Nonallergen-specific immunotherapy may be based on antagonization of Th2 cytokines and on anti-IgE therapies (Table 5).

Table 5 Novel Immunotherapeutic Strategies Based on the Th2 Hypothesis in Allergy

A. Allergen-specific immunotherapy
   1. Induction of anergy in Th2 cells by allergen-derived peptides
   2. Redirection of allergen-specific Th2 responses
      Allergen plus Th1-inducing cytokines
      Altered allergen peptide ligands
      Allergen peptides incorporated in recombinant micro-organisms or appropriate adjutants
      Plasmid DNA (allergen epitope) gene therapy
      CpG dinucleotides

B. Nonallergen-specific immunotherapy
   1. Targeting selective Th2 transcription factors (c-Maf, STAT6)
   2. Targeting IL-4 (soluble IL-4 receptors; IL-4 mutant protein)
   3. Targeting IL-5 (humanized anti-IL-5 antibody; inhibitors of IL-5 transcription
   4. Targeting IgE (''intelligent'' humanized anti-IgE antibody)

Source: Ref. 25.

9.1 Induction of Anergy in Allergen-Specific Th2 Cells

Anergy, or the induction of a state of functional nonresponsiveness, in allergen-specific Th2 cells was achieved, at least in vitro, by incubation of Dp-specific Th2 clones with high doses of the relevant Dp-derived peptides in the absence of antigen-presenting cells (APC). A similar approach had previously been performed on influenza virus-specific human T-cell clones incubated with the relevant virus-specific hemagglutinin peptide. Under these experimental conditions, both influenza- and DP-specific T-cell clones lost the ability to respond to subsequent stimulation with the intact antigen and APC, as well as to provide B-cell help for IgE production even in the presence of exogenous IL-4 and IL-13. However, there is still limited information on the possibility to tolerize allergen-specific Th2 responses in vivo. The activation of allergen-specific T-cells and immunoglobulin synthesis in mice can be inhibited in vivo by intranasal, oral, or subcutaneous administration of Dp or certain Dp peptides. Subcutaneous immunization with a dominant peptide of the major cat allergen *Felix domesticus* group 1 (Fel d 1) resulted in decreased T-cell responses, as measured by reduced IL-2 production to subsequent challenge with this peptide in Fel d 1-primed mice. Furthermore, pretreatment of mice with two Fel d 1-derived immunodominant peptides induced T-cell tolerance to a subsequent challenge with the entire recombinant Fel d 1 chain, suggesting that peptides containing some of the T-cell epitopes in a large polypeptide can tolerize T-cells for subsequent challenge with that larger polypeptide protein. Finally, rush immunotherapy with an equimolar mixture of three phospolipase-A_2 (PLA) peptides appeared to be protective against live bee sting and resulted in the induction of T-cell tolerance toward the entire PLA antigen, which could be reversed by in vitro treatment of cells with IL-2 and IL-15.

Thus, the foregoing studies support the possibility of using peptide-induced T-cell anergy to treat human allergic diseases. The major advantage of this type of specific immunotherapy, in comparison with the classic therapy with crude extracts or purified native allergens, is its major potential safety. Binding of allergen-specific IgE to allergen-derived peptides is strongly reduced with the desired effects on T-cells unaltered. However, some conceptual and practical problems still need to be overcome. First, although peptides containing minimal T-cell epitopes cannot cause anaphylactic reactions, the possibility that high amounts of IL-4 and IL-5 are produced during initiation of peptide vaccination, thus causing initial worsening of the allergic reactions, cannot be excluded. More importantly, most allergens contain multiple T-cell epitopes that are restricted by different MHC class II antigens. Thus, although some studies have shown that total T-cell responses to complex native proteins are limited to a few immunodominant epitopes, the possibility exists that T-cells can escape the induction of tolerance in the presence of other, nonimmunodominant T-cell epitopes, which become available after in vivo processing of native allergen. This problem, however, may be circumvented by administering mixtures of overlapping allergen-derived peptides representing the entire series of T-cell activation-inducing epitopes on the corresponding native allergen, thereby avoiding both mapping of all T-cell activation-inducing epitopes and precise MHC class II typing of patients. A clinical trial, based on vaccinating cat allergic patients with immunodominant peptides derived from the major cat allergen Fel d 1 has already been performed. The results show that the treatment is safe and may result in clinical improvement. Likewise, a trial with bee venom phospholipase-A_2-derived peptides has shown good clinical efficacy with no adverse reactions (25).

9.2 Redirection of Allergen-Specific Th2 Responses

Another strategy for the neutralization of allergen-specific Th2 responses would be to change the cytokine profile of allergen-specific $CD4^+$ T-cells. One possibility to induce a T-cell class switch in the cytokine profile may be to act directly on allergen-specific Th2 cells. This strategy raises the question of the stability of established Th2 effectors. Once established, the Th2 phenotype appears to be more stable than that of the Th1 in both mice and humans. Fully polarized murine Th2 cells are resistant to a reversal in their cytokine production patterns, which may reflect the lack of receptors for Th1 induction on these cells. Likewise, the activation of established Th2-like human T-cell clones in the presence of IL-12 can result in the transient expression of very low amounts of IFN-γ, which is lost if the stimulation is repeated in the absence of IL-12. Strongly polarized allergen-specific human Th2 clones are even unable to respond to IL-12, as shown by the total lack of IL-12-induced phosphorylation of STAT4. Thus, it is reasonably clear that reversibility of polarized Th2 effectors is lost after long-term stimulation.

The possibility to influence the development of memory Th cells seems more likely. Initial studies suggested that once naive T-cells were committed to Th1 or Th2 patterns of cytokine secretion, even their memory populations would secrete identical arrays of cytokine after antigen restimulation. However, more recent findings indicate that, regardless of prior commitment memory, $CD4^+$ T-cells may retain the capacity to be further influenced during effector cell development to become subsets that are at least temporarily polarized to a particular pattern of cytokine secretion. For example, administration of IL-12 to mice reverses detrimental *Leishmania major*-specific Th2 responses, when given with a drug, which reduces the parasite load. These findings support our previous findings on human Th subsets suggesting that memory cells previously committed in vivo to the Th2 pattern of cytokine secretion can be induced to produce cytokines of the opposite phenotype by restimulation in vitro in the presence of IFN-γ and anti-IL-4 antibody, IFN-α, or IL-12. Accordingly, human neonatal T-cells primed to Th2-cell phenotype by IL-4 were not stable and could revert into a population predominantly containing Th0 and Th1 cells, after a single restimulation in the presence of IL-12. In addition, successful specific immunotherapy in vivo is associated with changes in the cytokine profile of allergen-reactive Th2 cells. Thus, a potentially successful approach should be to prime memory allergen-specific Th cells in a manner that selects for prevalent Th1 phenotype. Indeed, predominant secretion of Th1-type cytokines in response to allergen will result not only in development and recruitment of different effector responses (IgG production and macrophage activation instead of IgE production and eosinophil activation), but also will probably inhibit the function of established Th2 responses as a result of cross-regulatory circuits (25).

9.2.1 Th1-Inducing Cytokines

Up-regulation of allergen-specific Th1 responses was achieved in vitro by using cytokines, such as IFN-α and IFN-γ. It was subsequently demonstrated that the Th1-inducing effect of IL-12 was mainly due to its ability to prime T-cells to IFN-γ production. A similar effect was observed by adding into bulk PBMC culture an antibody directed against the signaling lymphocyte activation molecule (SLAM), a novel 70-kDa T-cell surface receptor capable of inducing or enhancing IFN-γ production by human T-cells. Up-regulation of allergen-specific Th1 cell development was also obtained with poly-I:C, that induced high production of both IFN-α and IL-12 by macrophages or DC. Interestingly, IFN-α not only modulated the cytokine profile of allergen-specific T-cells, but also affected their TCR repertoire. The regulatory effects of Th1-inducing cytokines on allergen-specific responses have been demonstrated also in vivo. Mice lacking the IFN-γR have impaired ability to resolve a lung eosinophilic inflammatory response associated with a prolonged capacity of T-cells to exhibit a Th2 cytokine profile. Moreover, nebulized IFN-γ decreases IgE production and normalizes airway function in a murine model of allergen sensitization. IFN-γ inhibits the eosinophil and $CD4^+$ T-cell infiltration induced into the trachea of ovalbumin (OVA)-immunized mice. IL-12 can block the antigen-induced AHR and pulmonary inflammation in vivo by suppressing Th2 cytokine expression. These data suggest that the injection of selected allergen peptides in combination with Th1-inducing cytokines may represent the basis for a novel immunotherapeutic strategy in allergic disorders (25).

9.2.2 Altered Peptide Ligands

Several experimental models suggest that certain epitopes can preferentially induce one of the two subsets of Th cells. Varying either the antigenic peptide or the MHC class II molecules can determine whether Th1-like or Th2-like responses are obtained. High MHC class II peptide density on the APC surface favored Th1-like responses, whereas low ligand densities favored Th2-like responses. Likewise, when using a set of ligands with various class binding affinities, but unchanged T-cell specificity, stimulation with the highest-affinity ligand resulted in IFN-γ production. In contrast, ligands that demonstrated relatively lower MHC class II binding induced only IL-4 secretion. A single MHC polymorphism may dictate Th1–Th2 selection by determining the level of peptide presented to a given TCR on APC. Recently, the p28–40 analogues, with alanine residues at positions 34 and 36 of the dominant T-cell epitope of the group 2 allergen, were able to alter the IFN-γ/IL-4 ratio production in human Th0 cells by selectively enhancing IFN-γ secretion. Likewise, replacement of the 21st residue arginine with lysine of the peptide fragment ^{18}RSLRTVTPIRMQGG^{31}, derived from a *D. farinae* group 1 allergen, resulted in a significant increase in IFN-γ production, with remarkable changes in IL-4 production, by a specific human Th0 clone, which was also associated with an increased production of IL-12. More recently, a Th1-skewing peptide, analogue of a dominant allergen peptide, was able to modulate the Th2 response in vivo and to ameliorate the disease process in a murine model of allergic asthma (25).

9.2.3 Recombinant Microrganisms and Other Adjuvants Incorporating Allergen Peptides

In general, it appears that corpuscolate immunogens more easily promote Th1 responses than soluble antigens. The Th1-inducing activity of corpuscolate immunogens is probably related to their greater ability to induce IL-12 production by macrophages that are responsible for phagocytosis. Recombinant *M. bovis* (BCG) strains have been proposed as optimal adjuvants for the induction of Th1 responses. Orally administered live recombinant *Salmonella* also elicits dominant antigen-specific Th1-type responses in both mucosal and systemic tissues, in the absence of expression of Th2 cytokines I1-4 and IL-5. Thus, allergens may be engineered into recombinant mycobacteria or other appropriate microrganisms. Antigen polymerization also preferentially evokes Th1-type responses in comparison with the unmodified antigen. Following administration of high molecular weight OVA polymers, there was marked inhibition of OVA-specific IgE and a strong increase of IgG2a production. This was due to marked up-regulation of IFN-γ and down-regulation of IL-10 production, whereas the frequency of IL-4-producing cells was unchanged in response to the polymerized form of antigen. The type of adjuvant is also important in determining the profile of cytokine secretion. Complete Freund's adjuvant (CFA) evokes Th1 responses, probably because the components of the mycobacterial cell wall induce high IL-12 production by macrophages, with subsequent up-regulation of IFN-γ production (see later discussion), whereas incomplete Freund's adjuvant, alum, acellular *Bordetella pertussis* toxin, and cholera toxin expand prevalent Th2 responses. Moreover, influenza virus envelop proteins incorporated in immunostimulating complexes stimulate a prevalent Th1 response, whereas the same antigens in a micelle induce a more prominent Th2 response. Of interest is the recent finding indicating that conjugation of recombinant antigens with the polysaccharide mannan (polymannose) under reducing conditions favors predominantly Th2 responses. By contrast, the same antigen coupled with oxidized mannan selectively promotes Th1 responses (25).

9.2.4 Plasmid DNA (Allergen Epitope) Gene Therapy

Another revolutionary approach to the treatment of allergic disorders, originally developed for gene therapy, may be based on vaccination with plasmid vectors. These genetic vaccines are commonly called naked DNA or polynucleotide vaccines. Naked DNA consists of a desired gene inserted into a plasmid that can enter, and remain episomally in, cells close to the injection site, where it is subsequently transcribed and translated, causing expression of the gene product. There are three major advantages with this technique. First, naked DNA vaccines could bypass the numerous problems associated with other vectors, such as immune responses against the delivery vectors and concern about safety related to the use of any viral vector. Second, they could induce the expression of antigens that resemble native epitopes more closely than do standard vaccines for which the process of manufacturing can alter the structure of protein and, thereby, lower the antigenicity of the vaccine. Third, they may be constructed so that genes from several different allergens are included on the same plasmid, thus potentially decreasing the number of vaccinations required. Finally, and most importantly, the gene protein enters the cells' MHC class I pathway because only proteins that originate inside a cell are processed by this pathway. This results in the stimulation of $CD8^+$ CTL and evokes CMI. Accordingly, the results of a recent study suggest that intradermal immunization of BALB/c mice with naked plasmid DNA encoding for *Escherichia coli* β-galactosidase (β-gal) induces a Th1 immune response, as demonstrated by a highly restricted IgG2a antibody response to β-gal together with IFN-γ, but not IL-4 or IL-5, secretion by in vitro β-gal-stimulated splenic $CD4^+$ T-cells, whereas immunization with the corresponding protein, β-gal, in saline or alum induces a Th2 response. Moreover, intramuscular injection in mice of a gene construct containing an important house dust mite allergen gene (*Der p 5*) resulted in the induction of Der p 5-specific IgG antibodies, but not IgE antibody. The suppression of specific IgE response could be adaptively transferred with $CD8^+$ T-cells producing high levels of IFN-γ, suggesting that allergen–gene transfer is indeed effective in modulation of allergen-specific IgE responses (25).

9.2.5 Oligodeoxynucleotides

More recently, it was shown that bacterial DNA contains immunostimulatory motifs consisting of unmethylated CpG dinucleotides, which rapidly trigger an innate immune response characterized by T-cell–independent polyclonal B-cell activation, direct NK-cell stimulation, and production of IL-6, IL-12, IL-18, and IFN-α by macrophages or dendritic cells. Synthetic oligodeoxynucleotides (ODN) that contain unmethylated CpG motifs also bias the specific immune response to a Th1-dominated cytokine pattern. How mouse mac-

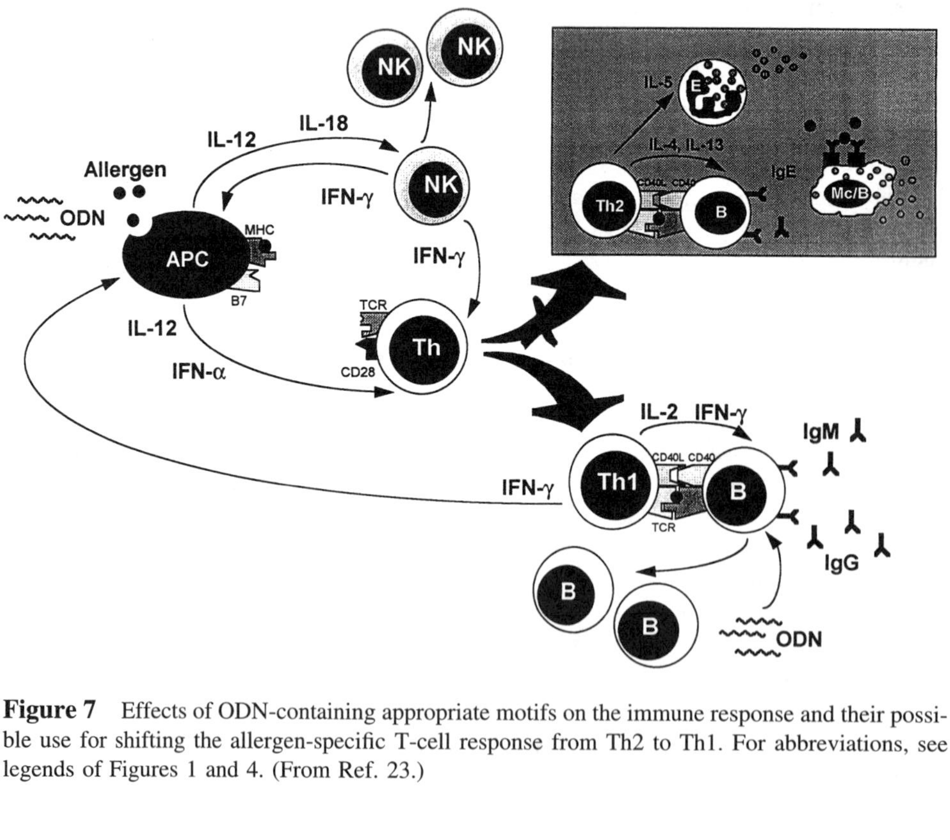

Figure 7 Effects of ODN-containing appropriate motifs on the immune response and their possible use for shifting the allergen-specific T-cell response from Th2 to Th1. For abbreviations, see legends of Figures 1 and 4. (From Ref. 23.)

rophages, B lymphocytes, and NK cells recognize specific DNA sequences in bacterial DNA is still unclear. The immunostimulatory CpG motifs could theoretically bind to complementary sequences in DNA or mRNA, or interact with one or more signal transduction molecules in the cytoplasm, or on the plasma membrane. At least in mice, the Th1-inducing effect of ODN appeared to be related to their ability to induce the production of IL-12 and IFN-α by monocytes or dendritic cells and possibly the production of IFN-γ by NK cells. Similar results were recently obtained in my laboratory by assessing the ability of selected ODN on the development of allergen-specific human T-cells in vitro. The characterization of ODN sequences responsible for the effects on cells of both innate and adaptive immune response in humans is less clear than in mice. In agreement with the results reported in mice, our findings demonstrate that the Th1-shifting effect of ODN requires phosphorothioation, is abolished by cytosine methylation, and is related to the stimulation of Th1-inducing cytokines by cells of the natural immunity (Fig. 7). However, differently from the results obtained in the murine experimental models, several sequences were able to stimulate B-cell proliferation and to modulate the functional profile of allergen-specific T-cells. We found indeed that all the phosphorothioate nonrepetitive sequences were effective, irrespective of the presence or absence of the CpG motifs that had been previously defined in mice. Actually, a CpG motif-lacking ODN exerted the maximal activity. Moreover, CpG dinucleotides per se did not appear to be sufficient, for a PT-repetitive sequence of CpG (poly-CG), of similar length as the other ODN, was completely ineffective. Finally, the active ODN, in which CpG dinucleotides were inverted to GpC retained its immunomodulatory activity, even if to a lower extent. This suggests that CpG dinucleotides may be important to obtain the maximal effect, but they are not necessarily required to induce an immunomodulatory activity in human T-cells (26).

9.3 Targeting Th2 Cells or Th2-Dependent Effector Molecules

Other potentially efficient therapeutic strategies may be based on targeting Th2 cells or the effector molecules produced as a consequence of activation of Th2 cells. This approach has become conceptually acceptable after evidence was accumulated to suggest that probably Th2 responses are not critical for survival and protection. First, IL-4 gene-knockout mice, which do not develop Th2 responses, are better protected than wild animals against the great majority of infections. Th2 cells are indeed more protective than Th1 cells only against gastrointestinal nematodes; Th2 cells do not kill nematodes, but make their life habitat unpleasant through the effects exerted by IL-4 on gastrointestinal function. At present, however, gastrointestinal nematodes do not represent a health problem, at least in developed countries. On the other hand, subjects homozigous for deletions involving the ε gene look perfectly normal, suggesting that at least one of the most important IL-4-dependent effector mechanisms (i.e., production of IgE antibody) is not critical for human life or its quality. Thus, targeting of either Th2 cells or Th2-dependent effector molecules may be a reasonable form of immunotherapy in patients with severe atopic disorders (25).

9.3.1 Targeting Transcription Factors Related to Th2 Cells

The demonstration that some transcription factors are critical for IL-4 production or Th2 cell development (see foregoing), such as the c-*maf* oncogene product and STAT6, suggests that they may be appropriate targets for manipulating Th2 responses. The c-*maf* oncogene is indeed selectively transcribed in Th2 cells and appears to control tissue expression of IL-4. On the other hand, signaling by IL-4 occurs through activation of STAT6, and knockout of *stat 6* gene results in deficient Th2 responses (discussed earlier).

9.3.2 Antagonizing IL-4

The activity of IL-4 may be antagonized by soluble IL-4R, as well as by a human IL-4 mutant protein. Interestingly, this protein also antagonizes the biological activity of IL-13, as well as the IL-4-driven differentiation of Th2 cells in vitro. Recently, soluble IL-4R has been shown to be able to inhibit airway inflammation following allergen challenge in a mouse model of asthma (27).

9.3.3 Antagonizing IL-5

The activity of IL-5 has been antagonized by humanized antibodies to IL-5, which appeared to be capable of inhibiting eosinophil infiltration and normalizing airway hyperreactivity in monkeys challenged with *Ascaris suis*. IL-5 activity has also been antagonized by soluble IL-5R or an IL-5-specific gene transcription inhibitor (25).

9.3.4 Targeting IgE

Intelligent humanized antihuman IgE antibodies have recently been developed. These antibodies bind to IgE residues critical for receptor binding, thereby reacting with both membrane IgE from B cells and soluble IgE, but not with mast cell- or basophil-bound IgE. Interestingly, one form of this antibody not only neutralized serum IgE, but also inhibited the recruitment of eosinophils into the lungs of DP-sensitized mice, as well as the production of IL-4 and IL-5, but not IFN-γ, by inhibiting IgE–CD23-facilitated antigen presentation to T-cells. Thus, IgE targeting not only blocks the IgE-mediated allergic inflammation, but also down-regulates Th2 responses and the subsequent infiltration of eosinophils into the airways. Human preclinical safety of anti-IgE humanized antibody appears to be satisfying, and the clinical studies performed so far have shown that this therapy may have a significant influence on symptoms of patients suffering from allergic rhinitis (28) or asthma (29).

10 CONCLUDING REMARKS

In the last few years, evidence has been accumulated to suggest that allergen-reactive Th2-polarized CD4$^+$ T lymphocytes play a triggering role in the activation or recruitment of IgE antibody-producing B cells (through IL-4 and IL-13), mast cells (through IL-4 and IL-10), and eosinophils (through IL-5), the cellular triad involved in allergic inflammation. More recently it has been shown that Th2 responses can also account for other hallmarks of allergic inflammation and asthma, such as hyperproduction of mucus (by IL-4, IL-9, and IL-13) and subendothelial fibrosis (by IL-4 and IL-13). Chemokines attracting both Th2 cells and cells activated by Th2 cells, such as eotaxin or produced by Th2 cells themselves, such as MDC, also contribute to the amplification of the allergic inflammation.

Th2 cells do represent a polarized arm of the effector-specific response that provides protection against some gastrointestinal nematodes. Th2 cells are generated from precursor naive Th cells when the specific antigen is encountered in an IL-4-containing microenvironment. However, the source of IL-4 required at the initiation of response for the development of naive Th cells into Th2 effectors is still unknown. Both FcεR non-T-cells and a specialized subset of CD1-restricted NK1.1$^+$CD4$^+$ T-cells have been suggested to provide IL-4 quickly to the naive Th cell; however, a more likely possibility is that the maturation into the Th2 pathway depends mainly on the levels and the kinetics of autocrine IL-4 production by naive Th cells themselves at priming.

The question of how these Th2 responses are enhanced in atopic patients is also unclear. Both the nature of the TCR signaling provided by the allergen peptide ligand and a disregulation of IL-4 production likely concur to determine the Th2 profile of allergen-specific Th cells, the genetic disregulation of IL-4 production probably being overwhelming. Some gene products selectively involved in the development of Th2 cells, such as GATA-3, or selectively controlling the expression of IL-4, such as STAT6 and c-*maf*, have been described.

Moreover, cytokines, such as IL-12, IL-18, IFN-γ, and IFN-α, that dampen the production of IL-4, as well as the development or the function of Th2 cells, have been identified. These findings suggest that an inherited disregulation of gene(s) controlling IL-4 expression or alterations of mechanisms that regulate Th2 development and function may favor Th2 responses against common environmental allergens, particularly in patients who develop severe atopic disorders. However, the role of environmental factors influencing the balance between Th1 and Th2 responses in the development of mild or common atopy also has to be considered. For example, the strong decrease occurred in both the prevalence and the severity of childhood infections with consequent reduced production of cytokines antagonistic to Th2 development at early age, may be partly responsible for the rising prevalence of allergy observed in the last decades in developed countries.

The new insights in the pathophysiology of T-cell responses in atopic diseases provide exciting opportunities for the development of novel immunotherapeutic strategies. These include the induction of nonresponsiveness in allergen-specific Th2 cells by allergen peptides or redirection of allergen-specific Th2 responses by Th1-inducing cytokines, altered peptide ligands, allergens incorporated into recombinant microrganisms or bound to appropriate adjuvants, and plasmid DNA vaccination. In patients with severe atopic disorders, the possibility of non-allergen-specific immunotherapeutic regimens, designed to target Th2 cells or Th2-dependent effector molecules, is also being considered.

REFERENCES

1. Coffman RL, Carty J. A T-cell activity that enhances polyclonal IgE production and its inhibition by interferon-gamma. J Immunol 1986; 136:949–954.
2. Del Prete G, Maggi E, Parronchi P, Chretien I, Tiri A, Macchia D, Ricci M, Banchereau J, De Vries J, Romagnani S. IL-4 is an essential factor for the IgE synthesis induced in vitro by human T-cell clones and their supernatants. J Immunol 1988; 140:4193–4198.
3. Pene J, Rousset F, Briere F, Chretien I, Paliard X, Banchereau J, Spits H, De Vries JE. IgE production by normal human B-cells induced by alloreactive T cell clones is mediated by IL-4 and suppressed by IFN-gamma. J Immunol 1988; 141:1218–1224.
4. Mosmann TR, Coffman RL. TH1 and TH2 cells: different patterns of lymphokine secretion lead to different functional properties. Annu Rev Immunol 1989; 7:145–173.
5. Romagnani S. Human T_H1 and T_h2: doubt no more. Immunol Today 1991; 12:256–257.
6. Romagnani S. Regulation of Th2 development in allergy. Curr Opin Immunol 1994; 6:838–846.
7. Abbas AK, Murphy KM, Sher A. Functional diversity of helper T lymphocytes. Nature 1996; 383:787–793.
8. Romagnani S. The Th1/Th2 interleukins. In: Oppenheim JJ, Feldman M, Durum S, Hirano T, Vilcek J, Nicola NA, eds. Cytokine Database. New York: Academic Press, 2000. In press.

9. Fitzpatrick DR, Kelso A. Nature versus nurture in T cell cytokine production. J Leukoc Biol 1999; 66:869–875.
10. Szabo SJ, Glimcher LH, Ho I–C. Genes that regulate interleukin-4 expression in T-cells. Curr Opin Immunol 1997; 9:776–781.
11. Ray A, Cohn L. Th2 cells and GATA-3 in asthma: new insights into the regulation of airway inflammation. J Clin Invest 1999; 104:985–993.
12. Romagnani S. Th cell subsets (Th1 vs. Th2). Ann Allergy Asthma Immunol 2000 (in press).
13. Romagnani S. The Th1/Th2 Paradigm in Disease. Heidelberg: Springer, 1997.
14. Cohn L, Homer RJ, Niu N, Bottomly K. T helper 1 cells and interferon gamma regulate allergic airway inflammation and mucus production. J Exp Med 1999; 190:1309–1318.
15. Randolph DA, Stephens R, Carruthers CJ, Chaplin DD. Cooperation between Th1 and Th2 cells in a murine model of eosinophilic airway inflammation. J Clin Invest 1999; 104:1021–1029.
16. Hansen G, McIntire JJ, Yeung VP, Berry G, Thorbecke GJ, Chen L, DeKruyff RD, Umetsu DT. $CD4^+$ T helper cells engineered to produce latent TGF-1β reverse allergen-induced airway hyperreactivity and inflammation. J Clin Invest 2000; 105:61–70.
17. Ricci M, Matucci A, Rossi O. New advances in the pathogenesis and therapy of bronchial asthma. Ann Ital Med Int 1998; 13:93–110.
18. Elias JA, Zhu Z, Chupp G, Homer RJ. Airway remodeling in asthma. J Clin Invest 1999; 104: 985–999.
19. Humbert M, Menz G, Ying S, Corrigan CJ, Robinson DS, Durham SR, Kay AB. The immunopathology of extrinsic (atopic) and intrinsic (non-atopic) asthma: more similarities than differences. Immunol Today 1999; 20:528–533.
20. Doucet C, Brouty–Boye D, Pottin–Clemenceau C, Canonica GW, Jasmin C, Azzarone B. Interleukin (IL) 4 and IL-13 act on human lung fibroblasts. Implication in asthma. J Clin Invest 1998; 101:2129–2139.
21. Longphre M, Li D, Gallup M, Drori E, Ordonez CL, Redman T, Wenzel S, Bice DE, Fahy JV, Basbaum C. Allergen-induced IL-9 directly stimulates mucin transcription in respiratory epithelial cells. J Clin Invest 1999; 104:1375–1382.
22. Grewe M, Bruijnzeel–Koomen CA, Schopf E, Thepen T, Langeveld–Wildschut AG, Ruzicka T, Krutmann J. A role for Th1 and Th2 cells in the immunopathogenesis of atopic dermatitis. Immunol Today 1998; 19:359–361.
23. Romagnani S. The role of lymphocytes in allergic disease. J Allergy Clin Immunol 1999; 105: 399–408.
24. Borish L. Genetics of allergy and asthma. Ann Allergy Asthma Immunol 1999; 82:413–426.
25. Parronchi P, Maggi E, Romagnani S. Redirecting Th2 responses in allergy. Curr Top Microbiol Immunol 1999; 238:27–56.
26. Parronchi P, Brugnolo F, Annunziato F, Manuelli C, Sampognaro S, Mavilia C, Romagnani S, Maggi E. Phosphorotbioate oligodeoxynucletides promote the in vitro development of human allergen-specific $CD4^+$ T-cells into Th1 effectors. J Immunol 1999; 163:5946–5953.
27. Henderson WR, Chi EY, Maliszewski CR. Soluble IL-4 receptor inhibits airway inflammation following allergen challenge in a mouse model of asthma. J Immunol 2000; 164:1086–1095.
28. Casale TB, Bernstein IL, Busse WW, Tinkelman DG, Stoltz RR, Dockhorn RJ, Reimann J, Su JQ, Fick RB Jr, Adelman DC. Use of an anti-IgE humanized monoclonal antibody in ragweed-induced allergic rhinitis. J Allergy Clin Immunol 1997; 100:110–121.
29. Milgrom H, Fick RB Jr, Su JQ, Reimann JD, Bush RK, Watrous ML, Metzger WJ. Treatment of allergic asthma with monoclonal anti-IgE antibody, rhuMAB-E25 Study Group. N Engl J Med 1999; 341:1966–1973.

6

Leukocyte–Blood Vessel Interactions

KELLY L. DAVENPECK

Thomas Jefferson University, Philadelphia, Pennsylvania

BRUCE S. BOCHNER

Johns Hopkins University School of Medicine, Baltimore, Maryland

1 INTRODUCTION

Eosinophils, basophils, T cells, and other leukocyte subtypes have been implicated in the development of chronic allergic inflammatory responses. Whereas early studies on leukocyte recruitment in allergic disease focused on leukocyte-specific chemoattractants, the more recent identification and characterization of a large group of molecules, referred to collectively as cell adhesion molecules, has led to a plethora of studies examining the role of adhesion molecules in leukocyte recruitment in allergic inflammation. The process of leukocyte recruitment involves multiple steps, including leukocyte–endothelial interactions (rolling and firm adhesion), transendothelial migration (diapedesis), directed movement through tissues (chemotaxis and haptotaxis), and in the airway, transepithelial migration. Each of these steps is mediated by sequential interactions between adhesion molecules and their molecular counterligands. These molecules, which mediate both cell–cell and cell–substratum interactions, have been subdivided into families, such as the selectins and their sialomucin counterligands, the integrins, and immunoglobulin-like structures, based on shared structural characteristics and functions. The overall goal of this chapter is to summarize the cell adhesion molecules that function during leukocyte–blood vessel interactions during cellular recruitment in allergic inflammation. Particular attention will be given to the molecules that mediate eosinophil recruitment, as eosinophil accumulation in allergic disease is one of the best-studied models of selective leukocyte recruitment.

2 ADHESION MOLECULE FAMILIES

2.1 Selectins

There are three known selectin molecules, E-selectin, L-selectin, and P-selectin, which are also referred to as CD62 followed by their respective first letters (CD62E, CD62L, and CD62P) (1). Although the selectins can mediate adhesion under static conditions, it is now felt that the major function of selectins in vivo is to mediate the initial step of leukocyte recruitment—leukocyte–endothelial tethering and rolling—under conditions of flow or shear stress. The structures of the selectins are shown schematically in Figure 1. The most critical portion of the selectin molecule for adhesion is the lectin domain, although the conformation of the adjacent epidermal growth factor (EGF) domain may influence binding. Soluble forms of all three selectins, as well as other adhesion molecules, can be detected in blood and other body fluids, and may possess biological activity.

E-selectin is expressed exclusively on activated endothelium. E-selectin expression is not constitutive, but is inducible within hours after exposure to various stimuli, including interleukin (IL)-1, tumor necrosis factor (TNF), and lipopolysaccharide (LPS). Expression is transient, declining over 24–48 hr toward undetectable levels. E-selectin functions as a ligand for leukocytes, including neutrophils, monocytes, eosinophils, basophils, and subsets of T lymphocytes bearing the cutaneous lymphocyte antigen (CLA; see later discussion) (2).

P-selectin originally received its name because of its stimulus-dependent expression on platelets, but it is also rapidly and transiently expressed on endothelial cells. Unlike E-selectin, P-selectin exists preformed within Weibel–Palade bodies in the endothelial cell

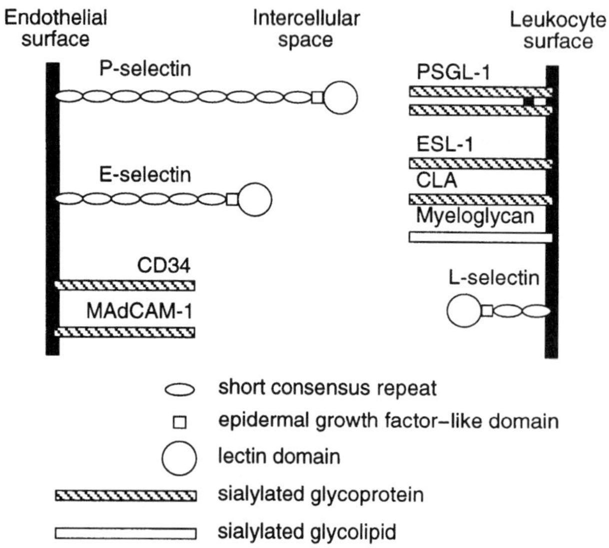

Figure 1 Basic structures of selectins on leukocytes and endothelium. Examples of extensively glycosylated, mucin-like counterligands for each selectin are also displayed. The transmembrane and intracytoplasmic domains for each of these structures are not shown. PSGL-1, P-selectin glycoprotein-1; ESL-1, E-selectin ligand-1; CLA; cutaneous lymphocyte antigen; MAdCAM-1, mucosal addressin cell adhesion molecule-1. (From Ref. 2.)

and is expressed within minutes after stimulation with agents such as histamine, thrombin, phorbol esters, peroxides, leukotriene-C_4, and C5a (2). P-selectin can also be up-regulated by prolonged exposure to cytokines such as IL-3 or IL-4, where changes in expression are gradual and sustained. Once expressed, P-selectin acts as a ligand for many cell types, including neutrophils, eosinophils, basophils, monocytes, and some T lymphocytes. P-selectin-mediated interactions have been demonstrated to alter leukocyte functions, such as integrin-mediated phagocytosis, and production of superoxide, cytokines, and chemokines (3,4). Leukocyte activation can reduce adhesion to P-selectin by altering the topographical location and by shedding of the P-selectin ligand (5,6).

L-selectin is found exclusively on leukocytes. Originally discovered as a peripheral lymph node-homing receptor responsible for lymphocyte attachment to high endothelial venules found in lymph nodes, it also functions as an adhesion molecule for nonlymphoid vascular endothelium under conditions of shear stress (7). Leukocyte stimulation leads to rapid L-selectin shedding from the leukocyte surface through activation of an endogenous protease that releases the molecule at a site close to the cell membrane (8).

2.2 Selectin Ligands

Many of the functional characteristics of E-, L-, and P-selectin–selectin ligand interactions are similar. For example, all are glycosylated, require calcium, and function under conditions of shear stress (1). A variety of carbohydrate-containing mucin-like ligands for selectins have been identified (9) (see Fig. 1). For instance, the tetrasaccharide sialyl Lewis^x (sLe^x or CD15s), which contains α(2,3)-linked terminal sialic acid residues and α(1,3)-linked fucose, appears to be a common factor in selectin binding as it can bind to all three selectins. Biosynthesis of the important selectin–ligand molecule sLe^x results from the sequential activity of sialyl- and fucosyltransferases, in particular, α(1,3)-fucosyltransferases (Fuc-T) on α(2,3)-sialylated lactosamine-type oligosaccharides (10). At least five forms of α(1,3)-fucosyltransferases have been cloned, but one in particular, Fuc-TVII, is especially important for leukocyte synthesis of sLe^x, and thus, functional selectin ligands (11). Cytokine regulation of Fuc-TVII, as well as other transferase enzymes, in both leukocytes and endothelial cells may play a role in regulation of leukocyte recruitment responses. Several studies have demonstrated that naive CD4 T cells do not express Fuc-TVII, leaving these cells unable to support P- or E-selectin–mediated interactions (12,13). However, Th1-type cytokine stimulation (IL-12) of naive CD4 T cells results in rapid up-regulation of Fuc-TVII, permitting selectin-mediated leukocyte–endothelial interactions and subsequent migration into inflammatory sites. Conversely, stimulation with the Th2-type cytokine IL-4, inhibits enzyme up-regulation and selectin-mediated recruitment (14). For endothelial cells, transfection with Fuc-TVII and a newly cloned enzyme GlcNAcβ:6-sulfotransferase up-regulates ligands for L-selectin (15). Support for the critical role of these glycosylation events in leukocyte trafficking in vivo has been provided by generation of a Fuc-TVII knockout mouse, which manifests leukocytosis, impaired leukocyte recruitment in inflammation, and impaired lymphocyte homing (16). In addition, in humans a rare genetic disease termed leukocyte adhesion deficiency disease type II (LAD type II), in which sLe^x synthesis and leukocyte rolling and recruitment responses are impaired owing to abnormal GDP-fucose biosynthesis (17).

Several important differences in selectin–selectin ligand interactions exist. For P-selectin, a specific disulfide-linked homodimer named P-selectin glycoprotein ligand-1 (PSGL-1; CD162), has been identified (18) (see Fig. 1). PSGL-1 is constitutively expressed on most leukocyte subtypes, and is shed after leukocyte activation (6). Although PSGL-1 can bind all three selectins, it binds with the highest affinity to P-selectin, and PSGL-1–blocking antibodies can completely inhibit neutrophil, eosinophil, and basophil interactions with P-selectin (6,18,19).

For E-selectin, possible ligands include carbohydrates displayed on CD65, CD66, L-selectin, ESL-1 (E-selectin ligand-1, a murine molecule with, as yet, no human homologue), as well as glycolipid ligands termed myeloglycans (2,9). For subsets of memory skin-homing lymphocytes, additional sialylated molecules recognized by monoclonal antibodies, such as HECA-452 [the cutaneous lymphocyte antigen (CLA), a modified form of PSGL-1 (20)], appear to mediate binding to E-selectin, but not to P-selectin (21). In addition, B-lymphocyte rolling on E-selectin has recently been attributed to a novel 240-kDa E-selectin ligand that has not yet been fully characterized (22).

For L-selectin, the first identified ligands were sialomucins, such as the fucosylated, sialylated, sulfated molecule CD34, and mucosal addressin cell adhesion molecule-1 (MAdCAM-1) found in the gut and associated with lymphocyte trafficking (23). More recently, podocalyxin-like protein, a transmembrane sialomucin structurally similar to CD34, has been described on high endothelial venules in lymph nodes to support L-selectin-mediated lymphocyte rolling (24). L-selectin ligands are also up-regulated by cytokines on vascular endothelium. Although these structures have yet to be fully elucidated, a CLA-bearing ligand has been implicated as a possible L-selectin ligand (25). In view of the vast array of potential ligands for the selectins, more studies are clearly needed to distinguish among specific and nonspecific selectin ligands on human cells, and to determine the functions of these molecules during leukocyte trafficking in humans.

2.3 Integrins

The integrins are a large family of structurally similar heterodimeric molecules with non–covalently associated α- and β-subunits (26,27). At least 16 α-subunits and 8 β-subunits have been identified that can combine to generate at least 23 different heterodimers (Table 1) (2,28–33). A site on the α-subunit important in integrin binding is the inserted, or ''I'' domain. This domain is a conserved structural characteristic of many integrins including all four of the α-chains that associate with β_2-integrin chains, as well as the α_1- and α_2-chains of β_1-integrins.

Integrins recognize a wide variety of ligands, including other cell-surface adhesion molecules, such as those of the immunoglobulin gene family (see later), extracellular matrix protein, and complement protein fragments (see Table 1). In tissues, their primary function is to mediate adhesion to basement membrane and other matrix proteins, whereas for leukocytes, the integrins mediate the processes of firm adhesion, locomotion, and trans-endothelial migration. Surface expression of integrins is highly variable from one cell type to another. For example, endothelial cells express several β1-integrins (α2β1, α3β1, α5β1, α6β1), as well as αvβ3 (34), whereas respiratory epithelial cells express these β1-integrins as well as α9β1, αvβ1, α6β4, αvβ5, and αvβ6 (35). Integrin expression on leukocytes and mast cells is also quite varied (Table 2) (2,28–30,36). For example, eosinophils express α4β1 and α6β1, basophils express α4β1 and α5β1, and mast cells express α3β1, α4β1, and α5β1. Although β_1- and β_3-integrins are expressed on both leukocytes and tissue-resident cells (endothelium, epithelium), β_2-integrin expression is restricted to leukocytes. Ligands for β_2-integrins include ICAM-1, ICAM-2, and ICAM-3, as well as fibrinogen, the complement fragment C3bi, and other structures (see Table 1).

Table 1 Biochemical and Functional Characteristics of Integrins

Subunit (CD, name)	kDa	Ligands
α1β1 (49a/29, VLA-1)	210/130	Laminin, collagen
α2β1 (49b/29, VLA-2)	160/130	Collagen, laminin, ECHO virus
α3β1 (49c/29, VLA-3)	150/130	Collagen, laminin, others
α4β1 (49d/29, VLA-4)	150/130	VCAM-1, fibronectin CS-1 domain, osteopontin, α4β1, α4β7
α5β1 (49e/29, VLA-5)	160/130	Fibronectin
α6β1 (49f/29, VLA-6)	150/130	Laminin
α7β1 (α7/29)	97/130	Laminin
α8β1 (α8/29)	180/130	Fibronectin, osteopontin
α9β1 (α9/29)	130/130	Fibronectin, tenascin, VCAM-1, osteopontin
αvβ1 (51/29)	135/130	Fibronectin, vitronectin
αLβ2 (11a/18, LFA-1)	180/95	ICAM-1, ICAM-2, ICAM-3
αMβ2 (11b/18, Mac-1)	170/95	ICAM-1 and -2, C3bi, fibrinogen, heparin
αXβ2 (11c/18, p150,95)	150/95	C3bi, fibrinogen
αdβ2 (αd/18)	150/95	ICAM-3, VCAM-1
αIIbβ3 (41/61, gpIIb/IIIa)	120/105	Fibrinogen, other RGD peptides
αvβ3 (51/61)	163/105	Vitronectin, PECAM-1, osteopontin, other RGD-containing proteins
α6β4 (49f/104)	150/205	Laminin
αvβ5 (51/β5)	163/100	Vitronectin
αvβ6 (51/β6)	163/106	Fibronectin, tenascin
α4β7 (49d/β7, ACT-1)	150/105	MAdCAM-1, VCAM-1, fibronectin CS-1 domain
αEβ7 (103/β7, HML-1)	175/105	E-cadherin
α1β8 (49a/β8)	210/95	Laminin, collagen, fibronectin
αvβ8 (51/β8)	150/95	Laminin, collagen, fibronectin

Source: Refs. 2, 28–33.

Defects in β_2-integrin expression, such as in leukocyte adhesion deficiency disease type I (LAD type I) lead to impaired leukocyte recruitment responses, especially in neutrophils (37). A variant of this disorder, in which expression is normal, but function is abnormal, was termed LAD type I variant (38,39). Although many integrin molecules are constitutively expressed on the cell surface, expression of integrins can be altered during processes such as cellular activation and hematopoiesis. For example, certain β_1-integrins are expressed only on lymphocytes after prolonged activation, hence, the name very late activation antigens (VLAs). In contrast, other integrins, such as $\alpha M\beta_2$ and $\alpha d\beta_2$, exist constitutively on the cell surface and also in intracytoplasmic granules, and can be rapidly translocated to the cell surface following cell activation (2).

In addition to the level of adhesion molecule expression, functional changes can occur in integrins, resulting in rapid and reversible changes in binding avidity (26,27,40). Beyond their role as adhesion molecules, integrins also have important functions as signal-transducing molecules, mediating so-called outside-in signaling (41). Cross-talk between G–protein-coupled chemokine receptors and integrins has been identified; for example, involving alterations in nucleotides in the GTP-binding protein RhoA (42). Signaling by integrin clustering does not appear to occur exclusively through the integrins themselves. Integrins, such as α3β1, α4β1, and α6β1, associate with other nonintegrin cell surface molecules, such as CD9 and members of the transmembrane 4 family of proteins that

Table 2 Surface Expression of Integrins and Other Adhesion Molecules on Human Leukocytes and Mast Cells

Integrin (CD, name)	Lymph[a]	Mono	Neut	Eos	Baso	Mast
$\alpha1\beta1$ (49a/29, VLA-1)	+	−	−	−	−	−
$\alpha2\beta1$ (49b/29, VLA-2)	+	+	−	−	−	−
$\alpha3\beta1$ (49c/29, VLA-3)	+	−	−	−	−	+
$\alpha4\beta1$ (49d/29, VLA-4)	+	+	−	+	+	+
$\alpha5\beta1$ (49e/29, VLA-5)	+	+	+	−	+	+
$\alpha6\beta1$ (49f/29, VLA-6)	+	+	+	+	−	−
$\alpha9\beta1$ (49i/29, VLA-9)	−	±	+	−	−	?
$\alpha L\beta2$ (11a/18, LFA-1)	+	+	+	+	+	−
$\alpha M\beta_2$ (11b/18, Mac-1)	−	+	+	+	+	−
$\alpha x\beta2$ (11c/18, p150,95)	+	+	+	+	+	+
$\alpha d\beta2$ (αd/18)	+	+	+	+	+	−
$\alpha v\beta3$ (51/16)	−	+	−	−	−	+
$\alpha4\beta7$ (49d/$\beta7$, ACT-1)	+	+	−	+	+	−
$\alpha E\beta7$ (103/$\beta7$, HML-1)	+	−	−	−	−	−
Other adhesion molecules						
Sialyl Lewis[x] (CD15s)	+	+	+	+	+	−
PECAM-1 (CD31)	+	+	+	+	+	−
CD44	+	+	+	+	+	+
L-VAP-2 (CD73)	+	−	−	−	−	−
PSGL-1 (CD162)	+	+	+	+	+	−
CLA	+	−	−	−	−	−
VAP-1	+	−	−	−	−	−

Abbreviations: Lymph, lymphocytes; Mono, monocytes; Neut, neutrophils; Eos, eosinophils; Baso, basophils; Mast, mast cells; +, present; −, absent; ±, weak; ?, not studied.
[a] Expression may be restricted to subsets of these cells.
Source: Refs. 2, 28–30, 36.

include CD53, CD63, CD81, and CD82 (43); these colocalized structures may be involved in the regulation of integrin function. Outside-in signaling may occur as a result of interactions between integrins and other associated molecules, such as cytoskeletal proteins (44). Integrins possess intracytoplasmic domains, with distinct sites for phosphorylation and for attachment to cytoskeletal elements such as talin, vinculin, α-actinin, filamin, paxillin, and actin. During adhesion, integrins and associated cytoskeletal proteins localize on the cell surface within contact sites called focal adhesions.

Of particular interest in allergic inflammation is the $\alpha4\beta1$ (VLA-4) integrin. Because of its prominent expression on eosinophils, basophils, and T lymphocytes, and its absence on neutrophils, VLA-4 has been targeted as a molecule that may in large part mediate selective cellular recruitment in allergic inflammation (45). VLA-4 binds to regions within the first and fourth domains of VCAM-1 (vascular cell adhesion molecule-1, containing the consensus amino acid sequent IDS), a molecule expressed on activated endothelial cells, to the alternatively spliced CS-1 (connecting segment-1) portion of the IIICS (type III connecting segment) region of fibronectin (containing the related consensus amino acid sequence LDV), and to osteopontin, a matrix protein found in bone and other tissues (2,32). Very recent studies have identified two additional integrin ligands for VCAM-1: $\alpha d\beta2$ (29) and $\alpha9\beta1$ (28). These integrins have patterns of surface expression different from VLA-4, including expression on neutrophils. In addition, VLA-4 and $\alpha d\beta_2$ are unique in that they are the only integrins that, similar to the selectins, can mediate leukocyte rolling under conditions of shear stress (30,46). The α_4 subunit can also pair with another β-subunit, β_7 (α4β7). Similar to VLA-4, α4β7 binds to fibronectin and VCAM-1, but unlike VLA-4, it binds to another cytokine-inducible adhesion molecule, mucosal addressin cell adhesion molecule-1 (MAdCAM-1) (23). The β_7-subunit can also pair with an another subunit, αE, expressed on lymphocytes (but not granulocytes) where it functions as a ligand for E-cadherin, a molecule found on the basolateral surface of intestinal epithelial cells (47).

2.4 Immunoglobulin Gene Superfamily

There are more than a dozen members of the immunoglobulin gene superfamily (IgSF), which consists of molecules that have a series of globular domains, formed by disulfide bonds, resembling those found in immunoglobulins (2). The structures of several important IgSF family members involved in endothelial cell–endothelial cell, endothelial cell–leukocyte, and leukocyte–leukocyte adhesion are shown schematically in Figure 2. Similar

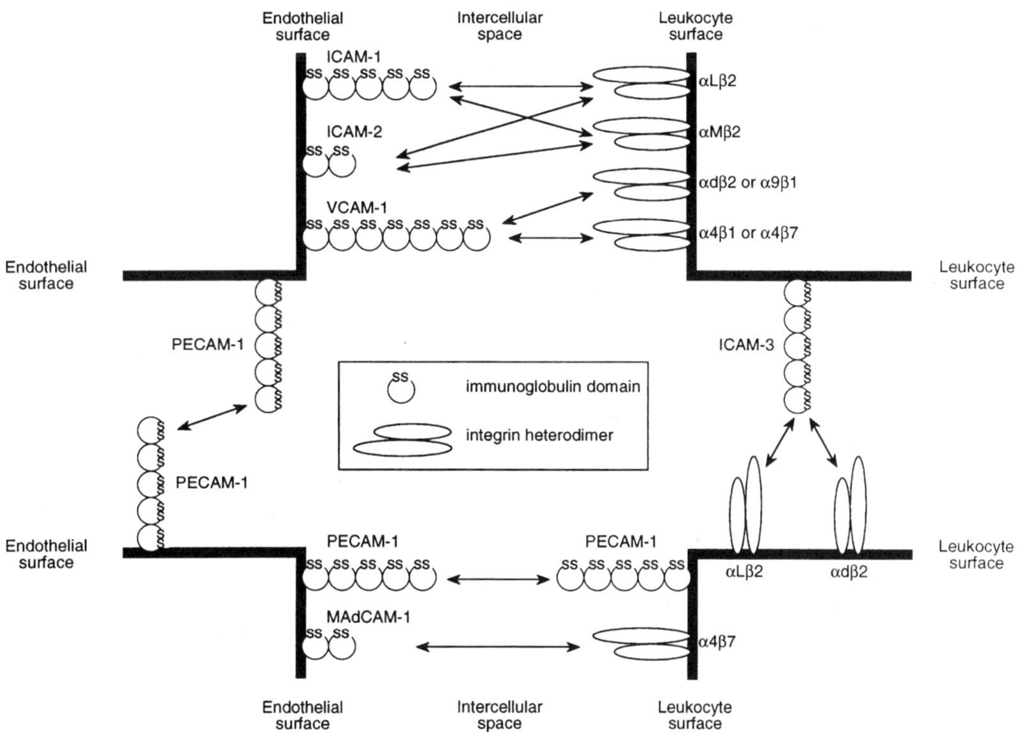

Figure 2 Schematic representation of several immunoglobulin gene superfamily molecules expressed on endothelial cells and leukocytes. Counterligands, most of which are integrins, are also shown. Arrows denote ligand–counterligand interactions, but do not indicate domains used for binding. MAdCAM-1 expression appears to be limited to endothelium in the lamina propria of the gut and to Peyer's patches, whereas others, such as VCAM-1, require specific stimuli to induce expression. (From Refs. 2, 28, 29.)

to integrins, these molecules are responsible for adhesion to other cell-surface ligands and have important signaling functions. Other IgSF family members, which are not directly involved in leukocyte adhesion or recruitment, include CD2, CD3, CD4, CD8, CD58, MHC class I and II, the T-cell receptor, and the sialic acid-binding IgSF subfamily, called siglecs, that include CD22 and CD33 (48).

Two members of the immunoglobulin superfamily, known as the intracellular adhesion molecules (ICAMs), share a similar structure and ligand binding and are implicated in leukocyte–endothelial interactions. The first of these molecules, ICAM-1 (CD54) was originally described as a 90-kDa molecule responsible for heterotypic cell adhesion. Ligands for the first N-terminal domain include LFA-1, fibrinogen, and most serotypes of rhinovirus, whereas the third domain is recognized by Mac-1 (2). ICAM-1 is expressed on a wide variety of cells types, including endothelial cells, respiratory epithelial cells, and leukocytes. ICAM-1 is constitutively expressed on endothelial cells, and various stimuli, including IL-1, TNF, LPS, and IFN-γ are capable of inducing or enhancing its expression.

The second molecule, ICAM-2 (CD102), was originally detected as an LFA-1-dependent, ICAM-1-independent endothelial adhesion molecule. ICAM-2 has only two immunoglobulin-like extracellular domains that possess 34% homology with the first two domains of ICAM-1 (49). Similar to ICAM-1, the ligand-binding site for LFA-1 is located in the first N-terminal domain. In addition to its expression on endothelial cells, ICAM-2 is also constitutively expressed on mononuclear cells, basophils, mast cells, and platelets. Studies with ICAM-2-deficient mice revealed few abnormalities except for an unexpected alteration in eosinophil airways recruitment and prolonged airways hyperactivity in an allergen challenge model (50).

Another member of the immunoglobulin family potentially involved in leukocyte recruitment is platelet–endothelial cell adhesion molecule-1 (PECAM-1; CD31) (51). Although the name implies limited expression, PECAM-1 is not only constitutively expressed on endothelial cells and platelets, but is also expressed on most leukocytes. PECAM-1 is found at particularly high concentrations at interendothelial cell interfaces, and PECAM-1 can mediate endothelial cell–endothelial cell interactions by homotypic interactions (51,52). Heterotypic adhesion by PECAM-1 has also been reported, as is the case for PECAM-1 interactions with the integrin $\alpha v\beta 3$ (see Fig. 2). PECAM-1 appears to play a critical role in transendothelial migration in vitro and in vivo because blocking antibodies prevent leukocyte migration between endothelial cells (53). However, with the appreciation that the intracellular portion of PECAM-1 contains immunoreceptor tyrosine-based inhibitory motifs (ITIMs), it has been proposed that its primary function after engagement may, in fact, be more relevant to inhibition of tyrosine kinase-mediated signaling rather than as an adhesion molecule (54).

One additional immunoglobulin superfamily molecule implicated in leukocyte–endothelial cell adhesion that may play a significant role in allergic inflammation because of its interaction with VLA-4, as mentioned earlier, is vascular cell adhesion molecule-1 (VCAM-1; CD106) (2). This molecule can be expressed on endothelium in two alternatively spliced versions, existing in a seven-domain form (with two VLA-4–binding sites) and infrequently in a six-domain form (lacking one of the two VLA-4–binding sites). In the more prevalent seven-domain form, there is extensive homology between the three N-terminal domains and the fourth through sixth domains. VCAM-1 expression has also been detected on cell types other than endothelium, including macrophages, dendritic cells, epithelial cells, and bone marrow stromal cells (35,55). It can be induced de novo within several hours after exposure to IL-1, TNF, or LPS, and expression is maximal by 24–48 hr. These treatment conditions lead to increased expression of other endothelial adhesion molecules including ICAM-1 and E-selectin. However, VCAM-1 can be selectively upregulated by treatment of endothelial cells with IL-4 or IL-13 (56,57). The combination of IL-4 or IL-13 with TNF or IL-1 is synergistic (58).

2.5 Other Adhesion Molecules

Several other adhesion molecules that may function during leukocyte recruitment responses, have also been identified on endothelial cells or leukocytes. For example, vascular adhesion protein-1 (VAP-1) is a 90-kDa sialylated lymphocyte ligand that has been identified in synovial, mucosal, peripheral lymph node endothelium, and at sites of inflammatory disorders including the liver (not on unstimulated or activated umbilical vein endothelium) (59). Recent cloning of murine VAP-1 revealed a molecule with both adhesive and enzymatic functions (monoamine oxidase activity) (60). A similar molecule is L-VAP-2 (lymphocyte–vascular adhesion protein-2; CD73), a 70-kDa structure constitutively expressed on endothelial cells and some lymphocytes. Antibody-blocking studies suggest that this molecule also functions as a lymphocyte ligand (61). Another molecule, CD44 (formerly Hermes antigen, H-CAM or pgp-1), is found at high levels on most leukocytes, endothelial cells, epithelial cells, and other cell types (62), and many spliced variant forms of differing molecular weights have been identified (85–160 kDa; 90 kDa being most predominant). These molecules have been implicated as adhesion molecules for peripheral lymph nodes, hyaluronic acid, and T-cell signaling. Cytokines, such as IL-3, IL-5, and GM-CSF increase CD44 levels on eosinophils, but the significance of this is uncertain because eosinophils do not bind hyaluronate in vitro (63,64).

3 ADHESION MOLECULE PHYSIOLOGY: ROLLING, TETHERING, FIRM ADHESION, AND TRANSENDOTHELIAL MIGRATION

It is generally accepted that leukocyte emigration from the intravascular compartment into tissue sites is a multistep process, involving numerous adhesion molecules (40). Under the shear forces of blood flow, cells undergo the first step of leukocyte emigration, which is the reversible process of rolling. Leukocyte rolling is mediated primarily by the three selectins and their carbohydrate counterligands (1), although the integrins VLA-4 and $\alpha d\beta 2$, interacting with their counterligand VCAM-1, can also participate in cell rolling (30,46,65).

The next step of leukocyte emigration is firm adhesion of the leukocyte to the endothelial surface. This step is felt to require leukocyte activation, which may result from exposure of leukocytes to activating factors produced by, or displayed on, the surface of endothelial cells, such as chemokines (40). It is hypothesized that in association with leukocyte activation are increases in both avidity and expression of integrins on the leukocyte surface, leading to enhanced binding to immunoglobulin family molecules such as ICAM-1, ICAM-2, and VCAM-1, although recent studies suggest that this may differ between β_1-and β_2-integrins in that decreased adhesion by β_1-integrins, presumably to permit deadhesion associated with cell migration, also occurs (66). Subsequently, transendothelial migration, during which time the leukocytes emigrate between endothelial cells and penetrate the basement membrane to enter the extravascular space, is mediated in part by PECAM-1 (52), although integrins, selectins, and selectin ligands may also participate in this process (67). In addition to adhesion molecules, cytokines, chemokines, and other chemotactic factors act to direct the migration response and bring about preferential leukocyte recruitment (40,68).

4 SELECTIVE EOSINOPHIL, BASOPHIL, AND T-CELL RECRUITMENT IN ALLERGIC INFLAMMATION: ROLE OF ENDOTHELIAL ADHESION MOLECULES

Tissue accumulation of subsets of leukocytes, especially eosinophils, basophils, and Th2 lymphocytes, is a hallmark of chronic allergic inflammation. Extensive studies over the last several years, reviewed elsewhere (2,68–71), have utilized in vitro and in vivo systems to characterize the adhesion molecule phenotype of these cells (see Table 2); to examine the effects of cytokines and chemokines on the adhesion molecule phenotype and function; to determine the result of altered adhesion molecule function on leukocyte recruitment; and to examine endothelial expression of adhesion molecules in response to allergen challenge and allergic inflammation.

Most studies examining adhesion molecule phenotype have identified relatively subtle differences in adhesion molecule expression among these cell types. This is particularly true for eosinophils and neutrophils. For example, for selectins, both eosinophils and neutrophils express L-selectin and bind to cytokine-activated endothelium under rotational conditions in an L-selectin–dependent manner, but neutrophil adhesion is greater, and one L-selectin antibody, LAM 1-11, selectively inhibited eosinophil, but not neutrophil, adhesion under these conditions (72). Eosinophils express about twice as much PSGL-1 as neutrophils. As a result, eosinophils attach as well as or better than neutrophils to P-selectin that is immobilized on plastic surfaces (73). Eosinophil PSGL-1 is 10-kDa larger than neutrophil PSGL-1, the difference being primarily due to altered glycosylation (6,74). Eosinophils, similar to neutrophils, bind to E-selectin, but eosinophil binding to E-selectin is lower than neutrophil binding, because there is tenfold lower amounts of the sialyl Lewis^x and sialyl-dimeric Lewis^x ligand on the eosinophil surface (75). Other leukocyte types, including basophils and mast cells, are implicated in the development of the allergic inflammatory response. Basophils, similar to other granulocytes, express L-selectin and shed it after activation, but the shedding is less complete (76); its function on basophils has not been studied. Basophils and mouse mast cells are also known to express PSGL-1 and have interactions with P-selectin similar to other leukocytes (19,77), but normal human mast cells appear to lack PSGL-1 expression. Levels of the selectin ligands sialyl Lewis^x and sialyl-dimeric Lewis^x, as well as binding to E-selectin, is similar for basophils and neutrophils (78).

In some situations, expression of adhesion molecules among leukocytes is vastly different. One important difference between lymphocytes, or at least subsets of lymphocytes, and all other leukocytes, is their expression of CLA, CD73, and certain β_1- and β_7-integrins (21) (see Table 2). Another major difference among leukocytes is the absence of α_4-integrins on neutrophils, suggesting that VCAM-1 might play a role in inflammatory conditions in which neutrophils do not predominate, such as chronic allergic diseases. This is consistent with studies showing that cytokines such as IL-4 and IL-13, which are associated with allergic inflammation, selectively induce VCAM-1 expression on endothelial cells, enhancing eosinophil and basophil, but not neutrophil, adhesion in vitro (56,57,78). Under conditions of flow, IL-4 induced up-regulation of VCAM-1-mediated (together with P-selectin) eosinophil rolling and subsequent firm adhesion (79). Other in vitro studies have begun to analyze the mechanisms regulating eosinophil transendothelial migration. Differences between eosinophils and neutrophils have been noted for these functions and most involve the VCAM-1–VLA-4 adhesion pathway (67,80). For instance, treatment of endothelial monolayers with IL-1 or TNF increased eosinophil transendothelial migration in a CD18-dependent manner. However, unlike neutrophils, a combination of VCAM-1, ICAM-1, and E-selectin antibodies was more effective at inhibiting eosinophil migration than ICAM-1 antibody alone. Furthermore, incubation of eosinophils with antibodies that activate β_1-integrins stimulates adhesion, but inhibits eosinophil transendothelial migration, presumably by preventing deadhesion needed for migration (81).

The current paradigm of leukocyte recruitment contends that adhesion molecules work in concert with cytokines, chemokines, and other chemotactic factors, to direct selective leukocyte migration (40). For example, exposure to CCR3-active chemokines causes eosinophil and basophil chemotaxis and transendothelial migration (67,68). These effects on eosinophils are synergistic with IL-5 in promoting CD18- and VLA-4–dependent transmigration across IL-1-activated endothelium. Furthermore, in vitro adhesion of eosinophils from asthmatics to VCAM-1 and ICAM-1 is enhanced compared with normals (82). These and other studies suggest that cytokines and chemokines can activate certain adhesion pathways while inactivating or not affecting others, and suggest that cytokines and chemokines with selective chemotactic activity may work in concert with adhesion molecules to mediated preferential leukocyte recruitment.

5 ROLE OF ENDOTHELIAL ADHESION MOLECULES IN ALLERGIC INFLAMMATION: IN VIVO STUDIES

A variety of studies in both animals and humans have implicated adhesion molecules in allergic inflammation. For example, knockout mouse technology and antibody-blocking studies in vivo indicate that VCAM-1–VLA-4 interactions, along with ICAM-1 and P-selectin, work cooperatively to mediate selective eosinophil and T-cell migration, whereas E- and L-selectins have little or no contribution (45,83–90). The effectiveness of antagonists directed at the VCAM-1–VLA-4 adhesion pathway and the selective nature of these antagonists has made them targets for clinical trials in allergic disease (45,91,92). However, there are situations in vivo in which acute or chronic eosinophil accumulation occurs without detectable endothelial VCAM-1 expression (93,94). Similarly, there are conditions under which VCAM-1 is expressed at relatively high levels, but little or no eosinophil accumulation is seen (95). This, combined with the aforementioned discovery of other VCAM-1 ligands, besides α4-integrins, on eosinophils, neutrophils, and other cells suggests alternative adhesive pathways may be operational in vivo.

The role of adhesion molecules in allergic diseases in vivo has been also been studied by correlating endothelial adhesion molecule expression with cell influx at sites of allergic inflammation. Immunohistochemistry has been utilized to detect adhesion molecule expression in the skin, nose, and lower airways following experimental allergen challenge, as well as in allergic and other eosinophilic diseases (94,96,97). In challenge studies, intradermal injection of allergic subjects with allergen results in endothelial expression of E-selectin and VCAM-1, and increased expression of ICAM-1 (97). Intranasal allergen challenge also resulted in increased VCAM-1 expression, with numbers of infiltrating eosinophils modestly correlating with the extent and intensity of VCAM-1 staining, and in nasal polyps, increased VCAM-1 is seen (96). Similarly, endobronchial allergen challenge resulted in increased endothelial VCAM-1 staining and epithelial ICAM-1 staining, and a significant correlation was seen between these parameters and eosinophil influx (94).

There is additional indirect evidence that endothelial activation occurs within the human airway following intrabronchial allergen challenge, because increased levels of soluble forms of E-selectin, ICAM-1, and VCAM-1 are observed in BAL fluids (94). Studies in the airways demonstrated a correlation with soluble VCAM-1, or VCAM-1 in biopsies, with eosinophil influx and levels of both IL-4 and IL-5 (98–100), whereas another study, in the skin, found a correlation between IL-13 (not IL-4) and eosinophil influx and VCAM-1 expression (101).

6 CONCLUSION

Inflammation is a complex process involving interactions between tissue resident cells and recruited leukoytes. The vascular endothelium is situated in a key location, and plays a crucial role in initiating, perpetuating, and terminating this response. In allergic diseases, the endothelial contribution to the relatively unique pattern of inflammation is a result of its expression of specific adhesion molecules, many of which are regulated by Th2 cytokines. The local generation and display of chemokines and other chemoattractants, together with the unique phenotypic pattern of expression of adhesion molecules and chemokine receptors on leukocyte subsets, combine to facilitate the selective emigration and accumulation of eosinophils, basophils, and Th2 lymphocytes at sites of chronic allergic inflammation. Novel therapies currently under development that target adhesion molecules may soon provide the pharmacological verification of their importance in allergic diseases.

REFERENCES

1. Tedder TF, Steeber DA, Chen A, Engel P. The selectins: vascular adhesion molecules. FASEB J 1995; 9:866–873.
2. Bochner BS. Cellular adhesion in inflammation. In: Middleton J, Reed C, Ellis E, Adkinson J, Yunginger J, Busse W, eds. Allergy Principles and Practice. 5th ed. St. Louis: Mosby, 1998:94–107.
3. Hidari KIP, Weyrich AS, Zimmerman GA, McEver RP. Engagement of P-selectin glycoprotein ligand-1 enhances tyrosine phosphorylation and activates mitogen-activated protein kinases in human neutrophils. J Biol Chem 1997; 272:28750–28756.
4. Weyrich AS, McIntyre TM, McEver RP, Prescott SM, Zimmerman GA. Monocyte tethering by P-selectin regulates monocyte chemotactic protein-1 and tumor necrosis factor-α secretion. J Clin Invest 1995; 95:2297–2303.
5. Lorant DE, McEver RP, McIntyre TM, Moore KL, Prescott SM, Zimmerman GA. Activation of polymorphonuclear leukocytes reduces their adhesion to P-selectin and causes redistribution of ligands for P-selectin on their surfaces. J Clin Invest 1995; 96:171–182.
6. Davenpeck KL, Brummet ME, Sterbinsky SA, Mayer RJ, Bochner BS. Activation of human leukocytes reduces surface P-selectin glycoprotein ligand-1 (PSGL-1, CD162) and adhesion to P-selectin in vitro. J Immunol 2000; 165:2764–2772.
7. Butcher EC, Picker LJ. Lymphocyte homing and homeostasis. Science 1996; 272:60–66.
8. Feehan C, Darlak K, Kahn J, Walcheck B, Spatola AF, Kishimoto TK. Shedding of the lymphocyte L-selectin adhesion molecule is inhibited by a hydroxamic acid-based protease inhibitor. J Biol Chem 1996; 271:7019–7024.
9. Varki A. Selectin ligands: will the real ones please stand up? J Clin Invest 1997; 99:158–162.
10. Lowe JB. Specificity and expression of carbohydrate ligands. In: Wegner CD, ed. Adhesion Molecules. London: Academic Press, 1994:113–140.
11. Knibbs RN, Craig RA, Natsuka S, Chang A, Cameron M, Lowe JB, Stoolman LM. The

fucosyltransferase FucT-VII regulates E-selectin ligand synthesis in human T cells. J Cell Biol 1996; 133:911–920.

12. Lim YC, Henault L, Wagers AJ, Kansas GS, Luscinskas FW, Lichtman AH. Expression of functional selectin ligands on Th cells is differentially regulated by IL-12 and IL-4. J Immunol 1999; 162:3193–201.
13. Blander JM, Visintin I, Janeway CA Jr, Medzhitov R. alpha(1,3)-Fucosyltransferase VII and alpha(2,3)-sialytransferase IV are up-regulated in activated CD4 T cells and maintained after their differentiation into Th1 and migration into inflammatory sites. J Immunol 1999; 163: 3746–3752.
14. Wagers AJ, Waters CM, Stoolman LM, Kansas GS. Interleukin 12 and interleukin 4 control T cell adhesion to endothelial selectins through opposite effects on α1,3-fucosyltransferase VII gene expression. J Exp Med 1998; 188:2225–2231.
15. Kimura N, Mitsuoka C, Kanamori A, Hiraiwa N, Uchimura K, Muramatsu T, Tamatani T, Kansas GS, Kannagi R. Reconstitution of functional L-selectin ligands on a cultured human endothelial cell line by cotransfection of $\alpha 1 \rightarrow 3$ fucosyltransferase VII and newly cloned GlcNAcbeta:6-sulfotransferase cDNA. Proc Natl Acad Sci USA 1999; 96:4530–4535.
16. Maly P, Thall AD, Petryniak B, Rogers GE, Smith PL, Marks RM, Kelly RJ, Gersten KM, Cheng GY, Saunders TL, Camper SA, Camphausen RT, Sullivan FX, Isogai Y, Hindsgaul O, von Andrian UH, Lowe JB. The α(1,3) fucosyltransferase Fuc-TVII controls leukocyte trafficking through an essential role in L-, E-, and P-selectin ligand biosynthesis. Cell 1996; 86:643–653.
17. Karsan A, Cornejo CJ, Winn RK, Schwartz BR, Way W, Lannir N, Gershoni–Baruch R, Etzioni A, Ochs HD, Harlan JM. Leukocyte adhesion deficiency type II is a generalized defect of de novo GDP-fucose biosynthesis—endothelial cell fucosylation is not required for neutrophil rolling on human nonlymphoid endothelium. J Clin Invest 1998; 101:2438–2445.
18. Yang J, Furie BC, Furie B. The biology of P-selectin glycoprotein ligand-1: its role as a selectin counterreceptor in leukocyte–endothelial and leukocyte–platelet interaction. Thromb Haemost 1999; 81:1–7.
19. Taylor ML, Brummet M, Hudson SA, Miura K, Bochner BS. Expression and function of P-selectin glycoprotein ligand-1 (PSGL-1, CD162) on human basophils. J Allergy Clin Immunol 2000; 106:918–924.
20. Fuhlbrigge RC, Kieffer JD, Armerding D, Kupper TS. Cutaneous lymphocyte antigen is a specialized form of PSGL-1 expressed on skin-homing T cells. Nature 1997; 389:978–981.
21. Leung DYM, Picker LJ. Adhesion pathways controlling recruitment responses of lymphocytes during allergic inflammatory reactions in vivo. In: Bochner BS, ed. Adhesion Molecules in Allergic Diseases. New York: Marcel Dekker, 1997:297–314.
22. Montoya MC, Holtmann K, Snapp KR, Borges E, Sanchez–Madrid F, Luscinskas FW, Kansas G, Vestweber D, de Landazuri MO. Memory B lymphocytes from secondary lymphoid organs interact with E-selectin through a novel glycoprotein ligand. J Clin Invest 1999; 103: 1317–1327.
23. Briskin M. Pathways of cell recruitment to mucosal surfaces. In: Bochner BS, ed. Adhesion Molecules in Allergic Diseases. New York: Marcel Dekker, 1997:105–128.
24. Sassetti C, Tangemann K, Singer MS, Kershaw DB, Rosen SD. Identification of podocalyxin-like protein as a high endothelial venule ligand for L-selectin: parallels to CD34. J Exp Med 1998; 187:1965–75.
25. Tu L, Delahunty MD, Ding H, Luscinskas FW, Tedder TF. The cutaneous lymphocyte antigen is an essential component of the L-selectin ligand induced on human vascular endothelial cells. J Exp Med 1999; 189:241–252.
26. Hunt SW III, Kellermann S–A, Shimizu Y. Integrins, integrin regulators and the extracellular matrix: the role of signal transduction and leukocyte migration. In: Bochner BS, ed. Cell Adhesion Molecules in Allergic Disease. New York: Marcel Dekker, 1997:73–104.

27. Loftus JC, Liddington RC. New insights into integrin-ligand interaction. J Clin Invest 1997; 99:2302–2306.
28. Taooka Y, Chen J, Yednock T, Sheppard D. The integrin $\alpha9\beta1$ mediates adhesion to activated endothelial cells and transendothelial neutrophil migration through interaction with vascular cell adhesion molecule-1. J Cell Biol 1999; 145:413–420.
29. Grayson MH, Van der Vieren M, Sterbinsky SA, Gallatin WM, Hoffman PA, Staunton DE, Bochner BS. $\alpha_d\beta_2$ Integrin is expressed on human eosinophils and functions as an alternative ligand for VCAM-1. J Exp Med 1998; 188:2187–2191.
30. Van der Vieren M, Crowe DT, Hoekstra D, Adams L, Vazeux R, Grayson MH, Bochner BS, Staunton DE. The leukocyte integrin $\alpha d\beta2$ binds VCAM-1: evidence for a binding interface between I domain and VCAM-1. J Immunol 1999; 163:1984–1990.
31. Yokosaki Y, Matsuura N, Sasaki T, Murakami I, Schneider H, Higashiyama S, Saitoh Y, Yamakido M, Taooka Y, Sheppard D. The integrin $\alpha9\beta1$ binds to a novel recognition sequence (SVVYGLR) in the thrombin-cleaved amino-terminal fragment of osteopontin. J Biol Chem 1999; 274:36328–36334.
32. Bayless KJ, Meininger GA, Scholtz JM, Davis GE. Osteopontin is a ligand for the alpha4 beta1 integrin. J Cell Sci 1998; 111:1165–1174.
33. Denda S, Reichardt LF, Muller U. Identification of osteopontin as a novel ligand for the integrin alpha8 beta1 and potential roles for this integrin-ligand interaction in kidney morphogenesis. Mol Biol Cell 1998; 9:1425–1435.
34. Ebisawa M, Schleimer RP, Bickel C, Bochner BS. Phenotyping of purified human peripheral blood eosinophils using the blind panel mAb. In: Schlossman S, Boumsell L, Gilks W, Harlan J, Kishimoto T, Morimoto C, Ritz J, Shaw S, Silverstein R, Springer T, Tedder T, Todd R, eds. Leukocyte Typing V: White Cell Differentiation Antigens. New York: Oxford University Press, 1995:1036–1038.
35. Polito AJ, Proud D. Epithelial cells: phenotype, substratum and mediator production. In: Bochner BS, ed. Cell Adhesion Molecules in Allergic Disease. New York: Marcel Dekker, 1997:43–72.
36. Kishimoto T, Goyert S, Kikutani H, Mason D, Miyasaka M, Moretta L, Ohno T, Okumura K, Shaw S, Springer TA, Sugamura K, Sugawara H, von dem Borne AEGK, Zola H. Leucocyte Typing VI. White Cell Differentiation Antigens. New York: Garland Publishing, 1997: 1221–1244.
37. Harlan JM. Leukocyte adhesion deficiency syndrome—insights into the molecular basis of leukocyte emigration. Clin Immunol Immunopathol 1993; 67:S16–S24.
38. Kuijpers TW, van Lier RAW, Hamann D, de Boer M, Thung LY, Weening RS, Verhoeven AJ, Roos D. Leukocyte adhesion deficiency type 1 (LAD-1)/variant—a novel immunodeficiency syndrome characterized by dysfunctional β_2 integrins. J Clin Invest 1997; 100:1725–1733.
39. Hogg N, Stewart MP, Scarth SL, Newton R, Shaw JM, Law SK, Klein N. A novel leukocyte adhesion deficiency caused by expressed but nonfunctional β_2 integrins Mac-1 and LFA-1. J Clin Invest 1999; 103:97–106.
40. Springer TA. Traffic signals on endothelium for lymphocyte recirculation and leukocyte emigration. Annu Rev Physiol 1995; 57:827–872.
41. Wahl SM, Feldman GM, McCarthy JB. Regulation of leukocyte adhesion and signaling in inflammation and disease. J Leukoc Biol 1996; 59:789–796.
42. Laudanna C, Campbell JJ, Butcher EC. Role of Rho in chemoattractant-activated leukocyte adhesion through integrins. Science 1996; 271:981–983.
43. Hemler ME. Integrin associated proteins. Curr Opin Cell Biol 1998; 10:578–585.
44. Schoenwaelder SM, Burridge K. Bidirectional signaling between the cytoskeleton and integrins. Curr Opin Cell Biol 1999; 11:274–286.
45. Bochner BS. Targeting VLA-4 integrin function: potential therapeutic implications. In:

Mousa SA, ed. Cell Adhesion Molecules and Matrix Proteins in Health and Disease. Georgetown, TX: Springer-Verlag, Landes Bioscience, 1998:113–131.

46. Sriramarao P, von Andrian UH, Butcher EC, Bourdon MA, Broide DH. L-selectin and very late antigen-4 integrin promote eosinophil rolling at physiological shear rates in vivo. J Immunol 1994; 153:4238–4246.
47. Cepek KL, Shaw SK, Parker CM, Russell GJ, Morrow JS, Rimm DL, Brenner MB. Adhesion between epithelial cells and T lymphocytes mediated by E-cadherin and the $\alpha_E\beta_7$ integrin. Nature 1994; 372:190–193.
48. Munday J, Floyd H, Crocker PR. Sialic acid binding receptors (siglecs) expressed by macrophages. J Leukoc Biol 1999; 66:705–711.
49. Staunton DE, Dustin ML, Springer TA. Functional cloning of ICAM-2, a cell adhesion ligand for LFA-1 homologous to ICAM-1. Nature 1989; 339:61–64.
50. Gerwin N, Gonzalo JA, Lloyd C, Coyle AJ, Reiss Y, Banu N, Wang BP, Xu H, Avraham H, Engelhardt B, Springer TA, Gutierrez–Ramos JC. Prolonged eosinophil accumulation in allergic lung interstitium of ICAM-2-deficient mice results in extended hyperresponsiveness. Immunity 1999; 10:9–19.
51. Newman PJ. The biology of PECAM-1. J Clin Invest 1997; 99:3–7.
52. Muller WA. The role of PECAM-1 (CD31) in leukocyte emigration: studies in vitro and in vivo. J Leukoc Biol 1995; 57:523–528.
53. Vaporciyan AA, DeLisser HM, Yan H–C, Mendiguren II, Thom SR, Jones ML, Ward PA, Albelda SM. Involvement of platelet-endothelial cell adhesion molecule-1 in neutrophil recruitment in vivo. Science 1993; 262:1580–1582.
54. Newman PJ. Switched at birth: a new family for PECAM-1. J Clin Invest 1999; 103:5–9.
55. Rice GE, Munro JM, Corless C, Bevilacqua MP. Vascular and nonvascular expression of INCAM-110. Am J Pathol 1991; 138:385–393.
56. Schleimer RP, Sterbinsky SA, Kaiser J, Bickel CA, Klunk DA, Tomioka K, Newman W, Luscinskas FW, Gimbrone MA Jr, McIntyre BW, Bochner BS. Interleukin-4 induces adherence of human eosinophils and basophils but not neutrophils to endothelium: association with expression of VCAM-1. J Immunol 1992; 148:1086–1092.
57. Bochner BS, Klunk DA, Sterbinsky SA, Coffman RL, Schleimer RP. Interleukin-13 selectively induces vascular cell adhesion molecule-1 (VCAM-1) expression in human endothelial cells. J Immunol 1995; 154:799–803.
58. Thornhill MH, Haskard DO. IL-4 regulates endothelial cell activation by IL-1, tumor necrosis factor, or IFN-γ. J Immunol 1990; 145:865–872.
59. Salmi M, Tohka S, Berg EL, Butcher EC, Jalkanen S. Vascular adhesion protein 1 (VAP-1) mediates lymphocyte subtype-specific, selectin-independent recognition of vascular endothelium in human lymph nodes. J Exp Med 1997; 186:589–600.
60. Bono P, Salmi M, Smith DJ, Jalkanen S. Cloning and characterization of mouse vascular adhesion protein-1 reveals a novel molecule with enzymatic activity. J Immunol 1998; 160: 5563–5571.
61. Airas L, Niemela J, Salmi M, Puurunen T, Smith DJ, Jalkanen S. Differential regulation and function of CD73, a glycosyl-phosphatidylinositol-linked 70-kD adhesion molecule, on lymphocytes and endothelial cells. J Cell Biol 1997; 136:421–431.
62. Lesley JR, Hyman R, Kincade PW. CD44 and its interaction with extracellular matrix. Adv Immunol 1993; 54:271–298.
63. Matsumoto K, Appiah–Pippim J, Bickel C, Schleimer RP, Bochner BS. The cell surface antigens CD44 and CD69 are activation markers for human eosinophils (EOS). J Allergy Clin Immunol 1996; 97:274.
64. Matsumoto K, Appiah–Pippim J, Schleimer RP, Bickel CA, Beck LA, Bochner BS. CD44 and CD69 represent different types of cell surface activation markers for human eosinophils. Am J Respir Cell Mol Biol 1998; 18:860–866.

65. Kubes P, Jutila M, Payne D. Therapeutic potential of inhibiting leukocyte rolling in ischemia/reperfusion. J Clin Invest 1995; 95:2510–2519.
66. Tachimoto H, Burdick M, Hudson SA, Kikuchi M, Konstantopoulos K, Bochner BS. CCR3-active chemokines promote rapid detachment of eosinophils from VCAM-1 in vitro. J Immunol 2000; 165:2748–2754.
67. Ebisawa M, Bochner BS, Schleimer RP. Eosinophil-endothelial interactions and transendothelial migration. In: Bochner BS, ed. Adhesion Molecules in Allergic Diseases. New York: Marcel Dekker, 1997:173–186.
68. Nickel R, Beck LA, Stellato C, Schleimer RP. Chemokines and allergic disease. J Allergy Clin Immunol 1999; 104:723–742.
69. Wardlaw AJ. Molecular basis for selective eosinophil trafficking in asthma: a multistep paradigm. J Allergy Clin Immunol 1999; 104:917–926.
70. Bochner BS. Cellular adhesion and its antagonism. J Allergy Clin Immunol 1997; 100:581–585.
71. Schleimer RP, Bochner BS. The role of adhesion molecules in allergic inflammation and their suitability as targets of antiallergic therapy. Clin Exp Allergy 1998; 28:15–23.
72. Knol EF, Tackey F, Tedder TF, Klunk DA, Bickel CA, Bochner BS. Comparison of human eosinophil and neutrophil adhesion to endothelial cells under non-static conditions: the role of L-selectin. J Immunol 1994; 153:2161–2167.
73. Wein M, Sterbinsky SA, Bickel CA, Schleimer RP, Bochner BS. Comparison of eosinophil and neutrophil ligands for P-selectin: ligands for P-selectin differ from those for E-selectin. Am J Respir Cell Mol Biol 1995; 12:315–319.
74. Symon FA, Lawrence MB, Williamson ML, Walsh GM, Watson SR, Wardlaw AJ. Functional and structural characterization of the eosinophil P-selectin ligand. J Immunol 1996; 157:1711–1719.
75. Bochner BS, Sterbinsky SA, Bickel CA, Werfel S, Wein M, Newman W. Differences between human eosinophils and neutrophils in the function and expression of sialic acid-containing counterligands for E-selectin. J Immunol 1994; 152:774–782.
76. Bochner BS, Sterbinsky SA. Altered surface expression of CD11 and Leu-8 during human basophil degranulation. J Immunol 1991; 146:2367–2373.
77. Sriramarao P, Anderson W, Wolitzky BA, Broide DH. Mouse bone marrow-derived mast cells roll on P-selectin under conditions of flow in vivo. Lab Invest 1996; 74:634–643.
78. Bochner BS, Sterbinsky SA, Saini SS, Briskin M, MacGlashan DW Jr. Counter-receptors on human basophils for endothelial cell adhesion molecules. J Immunol 1996; 157:844–850.
79. Patel KD. Eosinophil tethering to interleukin-4-activated endothelial cells requires both P-selectin and vascular cell adhesion molecule-1. Blood 1998; 92:3904–3911.
80. Yamamoto H, Sedgwick JB, Busse WW. Differential regulation of eosinophil adhesion and transmigration by pulmonary microvascular endothelial cells. J Immunol 1998; 161:971–977.
81. Kuijpers TW, Mul EPJ, Blom M, Kovach NL, Gaeta FCA, Tollefson V, Elices MJ, Harlan JM. Freezing adhesion molecules in a state of high-avidity binding blocks eosinophil migration. J Exp Med 1993; 178:279–284.
82. Hakansson L, Bjornsson E, Janson C, Schmekel B. Increased adhesion to vascular cell adhesion molecule-1 and intercellular adhesion molecule-1 of eosinophils from patients with asthma. J Allergy Clin Immunol 1995; 96:941–950.
83. Abraham WM, Sielczak MW, Ahmed A, Cortes A, Lauredo IT, Kim J, Pepinsky B, Benjamin CD, Leone DR, Lobb RR, Weller PF. α_4-Integrins mediate antigen-induced late bronchial responses and prolonged airway hyperresponsiveness in sheep. J Clin Invest 1994; 93:776–787.
84. Wegner CD, Gundel RH, Reilly P, Haynes N, Letts LG, Rothlein R. Intercellular adhesion molecule-1 (ICAM-1) in the pathogenesis of asthma. Science 1990; 247:456–459.
85. Gonzalo JA, Lloyd CM, Kremer L, Finger E, Martinez C, Siegelman MH, Cybulsky M,

Gutierrez–Ramos JC. Eosinophil recruitment to the lung in a murine model of allergic inflammation—the role of T cells, chemokines, and adhesion receptors. J Clin Invest 1996; 98:2332–2345.

86. Broide DH, Sullivan S, Gifford T, Sriramarao P. Inhibition of pulmonary eosinophilia in P-selectin– and ICAM-1–deficient mice. Am J Respir Cell Mol Biol 1998; 18:218–225.
87. Wolyniec WW, De Sanctis GT, Nabozny G, Torcellini C, Haynes N, Joetham A, Gelfand EW, Drazen JM, Noonan TC. Reduction of antigen-induced airway hyperreactivity and eosinophilia in ICAM-1-deficient mice. Am J Respir Cell Mol Biol 1998; 18:777–785.
88. Fryer AD, Costello RW, Yost BL, Lobb RR, Tedder TF, Steeber DA, Bochner BS. Antibody to VLA-4, but not to L-selectin, protects neuronal M_2 muscarinic receptors in antigen-challenged guinea pig airways. J Clin Invest 1997; 99:2036–2044.
89. Sanz MJ, Marinova–Mutafchieva L, Green P, Lobb RR, Feldmann M, Nourshargh S. IL-4-induced eosinophil accumulation in rat skin is dependent on endogenous TNF-α and α_4 integrin/VCAM-1 adhesion pathways. J Immunol 1998; 160:5637–5645.
90. Sanz MJ, Ponath PD, Mackay CR, Newman W, Miyasaka M, Tamatani T, Flanagan BF, Lobb RR, Williams TJ, Nourshargh S, Jose PJ. Human eotaxin induces α_4 and β_2 integrin-dependent eosinophil accumulation in rat skin in vivo: delayed generation of eotaxin in response to IL-4. J Immunol 1998; 160:3569–3576.
91. Metzger WJ. Therapeutic approaches to asthma based on VLA-4 integrin and its counter receptors. Springer Semin Immunopathol 1995; 16:467–478.
92. Abraham WM, Ahmed A, Sielczak MW, Narita M, Arrhenius T, Elices MJ. Blockade of late-phase airway responses and airway hyperresponsiveness in allergic sheep with a small-molecule peptide inhibitor of VLA-4. Am J Respir Crit Care Med 1997; 156:696–703.
93. Beck LA, Dalke S, Leiferman KM, Bickel CA, Hamilton R, Rosen H, Bochner BS, Schleimer RP. Cutaneous injection of RANTES causes eosinophil recruitment: comparison of nonallergic and allergic human subjects. J Immunol 1997; 159:2962–2972.
94. Montefort S, Holgate ST. Expression of cell adhesion molecules in asthma. In: Bochner BS, ed. Adhesion Molecules in Allergic Diseases. New York: Marcel Dekker, 1997:315–338.
95. Briscoe D, Cotran R, Pober J. Effects of TNF, LPS, and IL-4 on the expression of VCAM-1 in vivo: correlation with $CD3^+$ T cell infiltration. J Immunol 1992; 149:2954–2960.
96. Beck LA, Georas SN. Expression of cell adhesion molecules in eosinophilic disorders of the skin and nose. In: Bochner BS, ed. Adhesion Molecules in Allergic Diseases. New York: Marcel Dekker, 1997:339–366.
97. Bochner BS, Beck LA. Adhesion molecules and their role in allergic skin diseases. In: Leung DYM, Greaves M, eds. Allergic Skin Diseases: A Multidisciplinary Approach. New York: Marcel Dekker, 1999:87–112.
98. Zangrilli JG, Shaver JR, Cirelli RA, Cho SK, Garlis CG, Falcone A, Cuss FM, Fish JE, Peters SP. sVCAM-1 levels after segmental challenge correlate with eosinophil influx, IL-4 and IL-5 production, and the late phase response. Am J Respir Crit Care Med 1995; 151: 1346–1353.
99. Ohkawara Y, Yamauchi K, Maruyama N, Hoshi H, Ohno I, Honma M, Tanno Y, Tamura G, Shirato K, Ohtani H. In situ expression of the cell adhesion molecules in bronchial tissues from asthmatics with air flow limitation: in vivo evidence of VCAM-1/VLA-4 interaction in selective eosinophil infiltration. Am J Respir Cell Mol Biol 1995; 12:4–12.
100. Fukuda T, Fukushima Y, Numao T, Ando N, Arima M, Nakajima H, Sagara H, Adachi T, Motojima S, Makino S. Role of interleukin-4 and vascular cell adhesion molecule-1 in selective eosinophil migration into the airways in allergic asthma. Am J Respir Cell Mol Biol 1996; 14:84–94.
101. Ying S, Meng Q, Barata LT, Robinson DS, Durham SR, Kay AB. Associations between IL-13 and IL-4 (mRNA and protein), vascular cell adhesion molecule-1 expression, and the infiltration of eosinophils, macrophages, and T cells in allergen-induced late-phase cutaneous reactions in atopic subjects. J Immunol 1997; 158:5050–5057.

7

Extracellular Matrix

CLIVE R. ROBERTS, DAVID C. WALKER, and R. ROBERT SCHELLENBERG

The University of British Columbia, Vancouver, British Columbia, Canada

1 INTRODUCTION: EXTRACELLULAR MATRIX STRUCTURE AND FUNCTION IN HEALTH AND DISEASE

The extracellular matrix can be classified into basal lamina, which underlies epithelial and endothelial cells, and the interstitial matrix, which is maintained by tissue fibroblasts. The components of the matrix may be classified as predominantly structural or predominantly adhesive. The fibrillar collagens I, II, and III contribute to the tensile modulus of tissues, elastin gives tissue elasticity, and aggregating proteoglycans contribute to compressive and hysteretic properties of tissue. Several glycoproteins bind both structural elements and cell surface receptors, performing important adhesive functions that may have profound effects on cell biology. For example, the basal lamina protein laminin binds type IV collagen and the proteoglycan perlecan and, through cell surface integrin receptors for laminin, mediates a signaling process that contributes to the basal lamina's powerful effects on maintenance of differentiated functions in epithelial cells. Homeostatic effects of the extracellular matrix have been described in numerous systems, over many years. Perhaps the best-studied system is the influence of the extracellular matrix on mammary gland epithelial cell gene expression, delineated in the concept of "dynamic reciprocity," coined by Bissell and co-workers in the late 1970s and early 1980s. A body of evidence showed that epithelial cells both synthesize and maintain their underlying matrix, and respond to it in the expression of tissue-specific genes. Interestingly, in the mammary gland system, normal gene expression was responsive to both the composition of the matrix and mechanical stresses in it. (Bissell et al., 1982; Lee et al., 1984).

It has long been known that the inflammatory process leads to changes in the matrix, including altered synthesis and local extracellular matrix degradation. Serine proteases, such as elastase and cathepsin G, are released by granulocytes early in inflammation, and macrophages and connective tissue cells release various powerful matrix metalloproteases, including MMP-1 MMP-3, and MMP-7 (macrophages), and MMP-2, MMP-3, and MMP-9 (connective tissue cells) in inflammation and remodeling conditions that have been studied. This combination of enzymes has the capacity to degrade fibrillar collagens (MMP-1), elastin (elastase, cathepsin G, and MMP-7), gelatinized collagen (MMP-2, -9, and -7) and matrix glycoproteins and proteoglycan core proteins (MMP2, -3, -7, -9, elastase, and cathepsin G). Matrix degradation is considered an unwanted side effect of a limited proteolytic process that is required for immune and phagocytic cells to be able to enter inflammatory sites, or as the unwanted side effect of release of enzymes for which the primary function is degradation of microorganisms. In addition to simple damage to the matrix, a body of work suggests that, in chronic inflammation, such degradation exposes new epitopes in extracellular matrix molecules to which the immune system becomes sensitized, thereby initiating autoimmune disease. Examples may include collagen type II in arthritis (Champion and Poole, 1981), the proteoglycan aggrecan in relapsing polychondritis and ankylosing spondylitis (Glant et al., 1987), and proteoglycan aggregate components late in the process of osteoarthritis (Guerassimov et al., 1999). Inflammation leads to increased synthesis of matrix glycoproteins, under the control of several growth factors. Indeed, the extracellular matrix of chronic inflammatory and healing sites, at which mesenchymal cell proliferation occurs, is distinct from normal matrix. This ''provisional'' or ''transitional'' matrix has been well studied in the remodeling lung in a variety of allergic and nonallergic conditions and will be discussed at some length. Just as cells respond to the normal matrix in the maintenance of their differentiated phenotype, connective tissue cells in inflammatory sites both synthesize and respond to the altered ''provisional matrix'' in ways that are currently being elucidated. The focus of this chapter is lung extracellular matrix, and our interest is in remodeling inflammatory processes associated with interstitial fibrosis and the airway disease asthma.

2 EXTRACELLULAR MATRIX IN NORMAL TISSUE STRUCTURE

The epithelium is our largest interface with the environment and, consequently, has important barrier functions. In the airways, barrier functions are balanced against the need for cellular trafficking into the airway, and the epithelial basal lamina is adapted to allow regulated passage of inflammatory cells. The airways from the trachea to the alveoli are dynamic structures, always in motion, some areas in particular undergoing large changes in distention and deformation. Elastic fibers and smooth-muscle cells maintain tissue mechanics over a range of architectures and levels of distension. An upper limit must be set for the range of motion to preserve the integrity of the organ system. Fibrillar collagen, composed primarily of types I and III collagen, although capable of rearrangement within the connective tissue, provides the ultimate high-tensile modulus to the tissue when fully extended.

2.1 Basal Lamina

The basal lamina provides a foundation on which is attached the continuous epithelium of the nose, airways, and alveoli. The principal constituents of the basal lamina are type IV collagen (Scott, 1983), laminin (Sage, 1982; Scott, 1983) and the proteoglycan perlecan (Murdoch et al., 1992) that are contained in the lamina densa, the electron-dense middle layer of basal lamina as detected by electron microscopy. These structural elements are apparently produced by the respiratory epithelium (Laurie and Leblond, 1983). Perlecan has its globular protein core in the lamina densa and its heparan sulfate side chains extending to the lamina rara externa (Laurie et al., 1993), the electron translucent layer between the lamina densa and the plasma membrane of the epithelial cells. Below the lamina densa, hoops of type VII collagen-anchoring fibrils link the basal lamina to fibrillar elements of the interstitium (Kawanami et al., 1979; Olsen and Ninomiya, 1993). Wasano and Yamamoto (1985) have suggested that the link between basal lamina and underlying fibrillar extracellular matrix elements is rather a reticulum of ''microthread'' filaments.

The basal lamina is not a continuous sheet; rather, there are fixed holes in it through which a variety of contacts and processes occur in both the conducting airways (MacDonell et al., 1998) and alveoli (Walker et al., 1995; Behzad et al., 1996). Clearly, there must be fixed apertures through which nerves penetrate into the epithelium of the conducting airways (Fig. 1A), and apertures must exist for migratory cells to accumulate in the conducting airway epithelium (see Fig. 1B). Fixed apertures in the basal lamina below type II pneumonocytes permit contacts between myofibroblasts and type II pneumonocytes (Vaccaro and Brody, 1981; Adamson et al., 1990, 1991; Behzad et al., 1996), and they may serve as passages through which leukocytes migrate into the alveoli (Damiano et al., 1980; Walker et al., 1995; Behzad et al., 1996). Similar holes have been demonstrated in the basal lamina of conducting airways of guinea pigs, rabbits, and humans (MacDonell et al., 1998). It is possible that these fixed apertures become the sites of fixed tunnels through the thickened basement membrane of the bronchioles of patients with asthma, through which inflammatory cells migrate to the airway lumen (Fig. 2A, B). The epithelium of both the skin (Fine, 1991) and the gut (Komuro and Hashimoto, 1990) is also subtended by a continuous basal lamina that is perforated by numerous apertures. The apertures in the basal lamina of the gut epithelium also permit epithelial–fibroblast contacts (Parker et al., 1974). Immediately below the basal lamina of the conducting airways, a population of squamous fibroblasts have been described that may ensheath up to 70% of the airway in rats (Evans et al., 1993).

The basal lamina can be considered a mat of adhesive glycoproteins, including laminin and heparan sulfate proteoglycans, associated with a structural network of type IV collagen (Yurchenco and Ruben, 1987; van der Rest and Garrone, 1991). The basal lamina appears to impart fundamental positional information to the cells of the lung, which may be mediated by integrins and promotes cell growth through the presentation of basal lamina proteoglycan-bound growth factors to cell surface receptors, as for basic fibroblast growth factor (Yayon et al., 1991). The importance of intact basal lamina for tissue repair is shown by the studies of Vracko (1972), who demonstrated that even after epithelial and endothelial desquamation, regeneration and function were completely restored if basal laminae remained intact (see Sec. IV).

2.2 Elastic Fibers

Elastic fibers have been subdivided into three types: elastic, elaunan, and oxytalin (Montes, 1992) that can be distinguished both histochemically (Gawlik, 1965) and ultrastructurally (Böck and Stockinger, 1994). The oxytalin fibers consist of characteristic 10-nm microfibrils that run approximately parallel in bundles of various sizes (Fig. 3A, B). Elaunin fibers consist of the same bundles of microfibrils with the addition of small amounts of amorphous elastin among the fibrils (see Fig. 3A, B). Elastic fibers consist almost entirely of elastin, with microfibrils usually visible only around the perimeter of the fiber when

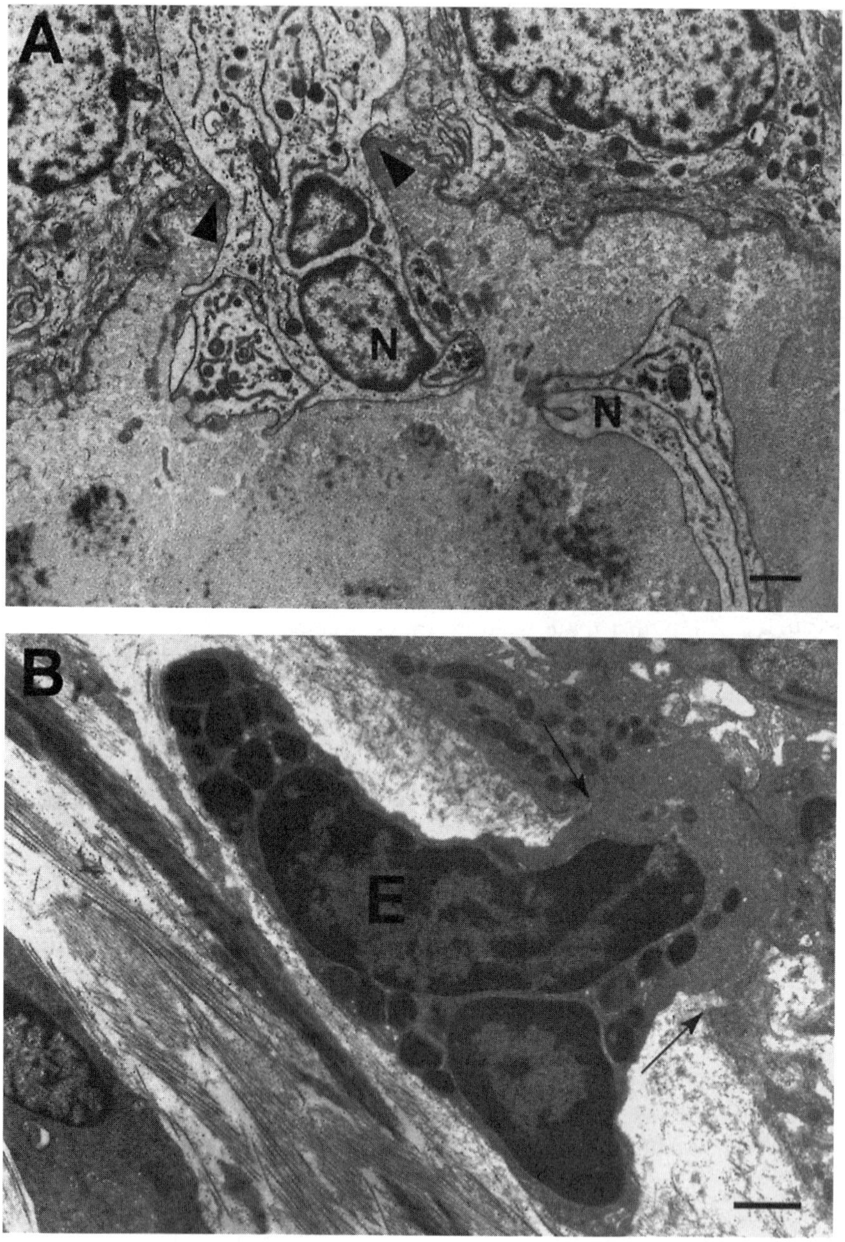

Figure 1 Fixed apertures in the basal laminae of conducting airway epithelia: (A) Basal region of a human bronchiolar epithelium; the edges of the aperture (arrowheads) in the basal lamina are in contact with the nerve (N) which extends from below in the basement membrane through the aperture into the epithelium. (B) lamina propria and basal region of guinea pig trachea; an eosinophil (E) extends from the lamina propria, through an aperture in the basal lamina (arrows) into the epithelium. Scale bars = 1 μm.

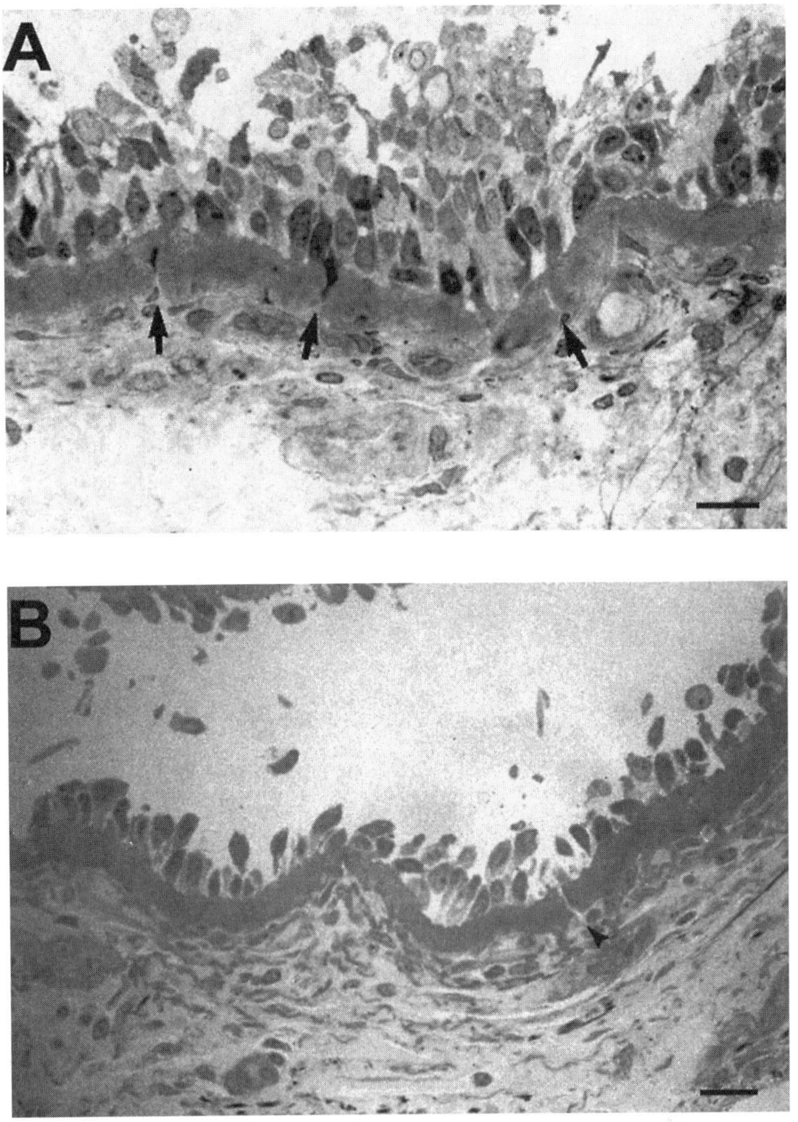

Figure 2 Fixed basement membrane tunnels and basal lamina apertures in the airways of asthmatics: (A) A region of human asthmatic bronchiole in which three tunnels through the basement membrane (arrows) are observed to contain parts of migrating cells. (B) A region of human asthmatic bronchiole in which a tunnel penetrates the thickened basement membrane (arrowhead) and is not occupied by a migrating cell. Scale bars = 20 μm.

viewed in cross section (see Fig. 3A). Elastic fiber development begins with the deposition of the microfibrils that contain fibrillins (Sakai et al., 1986; Hollister et al, 1990); a scaffold on which elastin is deposited and cross-linked (Fahrenbach et al., 1966; Greenlee et al., 1966). It has been suggested that the three different types of fibers actually represent interrupted elastogenesis when they occur in mature tissue (Cotta–Pereira et al., 1977), and in support of this, all three fibers are actually continuous (Cotta–Pereira et al., 1976).

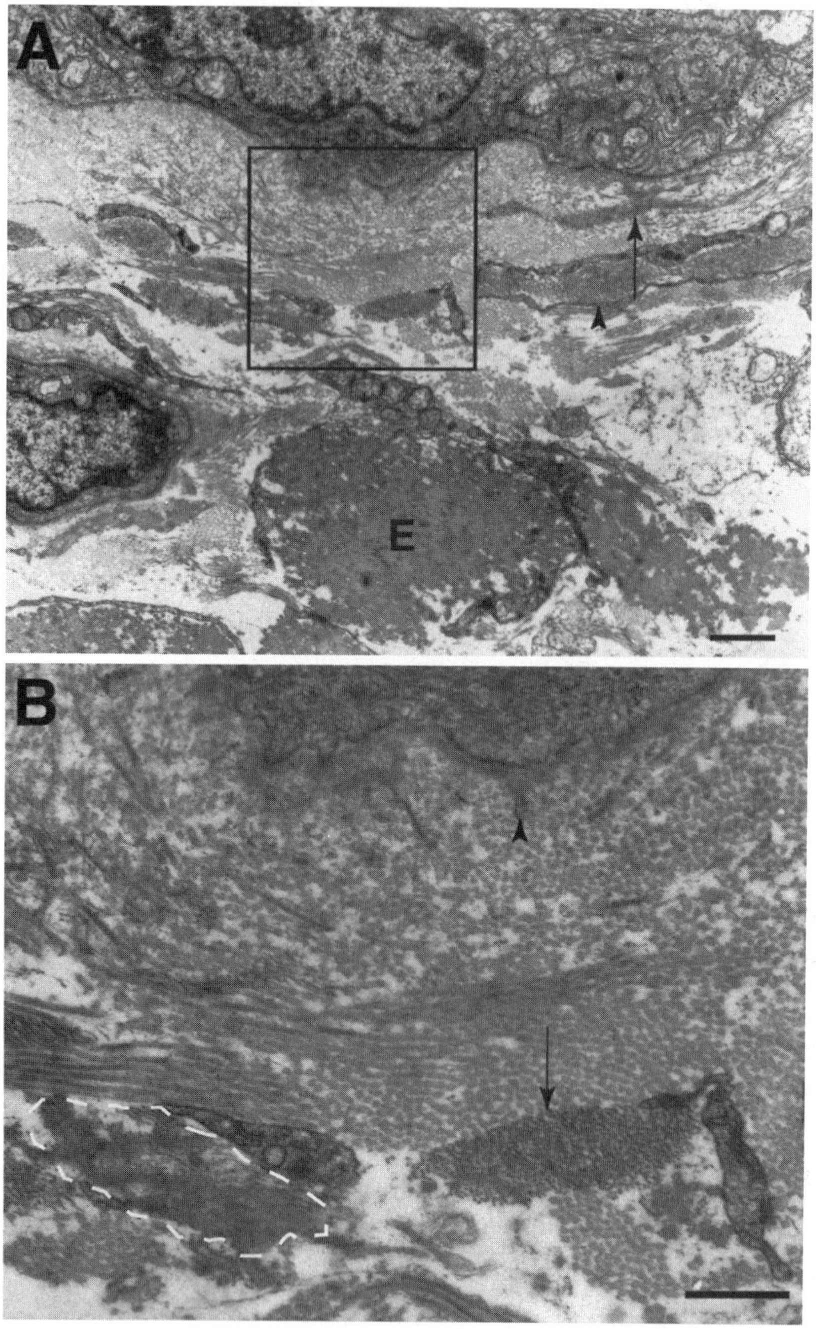

Figure 3 Elastic fibers of human bronchioles: (A) Lamina propria of a human bronchiole; large elastic fibers (E) are made of amorphous elastin with microfibrils visible only at the perimeter. Oxytalan fibers (arrowhead) contact the basal lamina (arrow). Elaunin fibers are observed among the oxytalan fibers in the lamina propria (within the box, enlarged in panel B). (B) Elaunin fibers (within dashed line) are distinguished from oxytalan fibers (arrow) by the presence of some elastin among the microfibrils. Anchoring fibrils are observed at the internal surface of the lamina densa of the basal lamina (arrowhead). Scale bars = 1 μm.

The elastic fiber system in the connective tissues of the respiratory system extends from the larynx, down airways, and through the lung parenchyma to the pleura, where there is more elastin (Macklin, 1922; Wright, 1961). From very early studies (Miller, 1937), the connective tissues of the lung were described as being supported by a myoelastic system of smooth muscle and elastic fibers. The intimate association between smooth-muscle cells and elastic fibers is shown in Figure 4. The organization of the elastic elements of this system in the conducting airways may be appreciated in Figure 5A–C. The most prominent elastic fibers run longitudinally and are grouped in a layer, an elastic lamina, that separates the lamina propria from the submucosa of the conducting airways (see Fig. 5B, C) (Rhodin, 1974). Smaller oxytalan and elaunin fibers are observed in the lamina propria, and oxytalan fibers often end at the epithelial basal lamina (Leick–Maldonado and Lemos, 1997) as shown in Figure 3A and B. Elastic fibers are also present throughout the submucosal dense irregular tissue in fewer numbers (Figs. 5B and C); however, these encircle bundles of smooth muscle and penetrate between the smooth-muscle cells (see Figs. 4, 5B, C). Ultrastructurally, oxytalan and elaunin fibers are present among the smooth-muscle cells (see Fig. 4). Whereas oxytalan fibers may terminate at smooth-muscle basal lamina (see Fig. 4), elastic fibers may terminate at smooth-muscle cell plasma membranes. Leick–Maldonado and Lemos (1997) have shown that elastic fibers penetrate from the lamina propria between the smooth-muscle bundles into the deeper submucosa and adventitia and suggest that they play a role in epithelial folding during bronchoconstriction. A very similar arrangement of the elastic fibers of the dermis of the skin has been described (Cotta–Pereira et al., 1976). Cotta–Pereira et al. (1976) also demonstrated that the elastic, elaunin, and

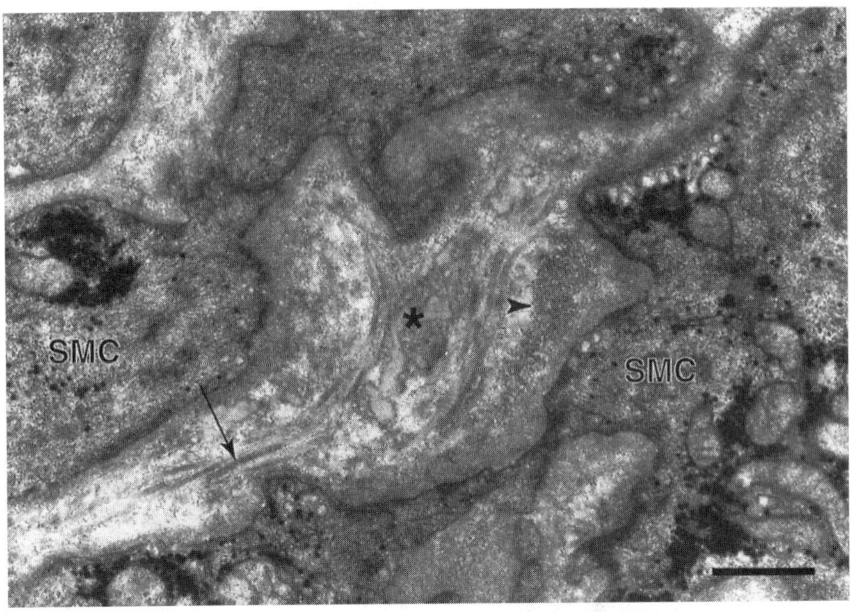

Figure 4 Submucosal smooth muscle cells of a human bronchiole: Small elastic (*) and oxytalan (arrowhead) fibers are observed in the intercellular spaces along with type III collagen (arrow). Oxytalan fibrils contact the basal lamina (between the oxytalan microfibril bundle and the smooth-muscle cell (SMC) plasma membrane). Scale bar = 0.5 μm.

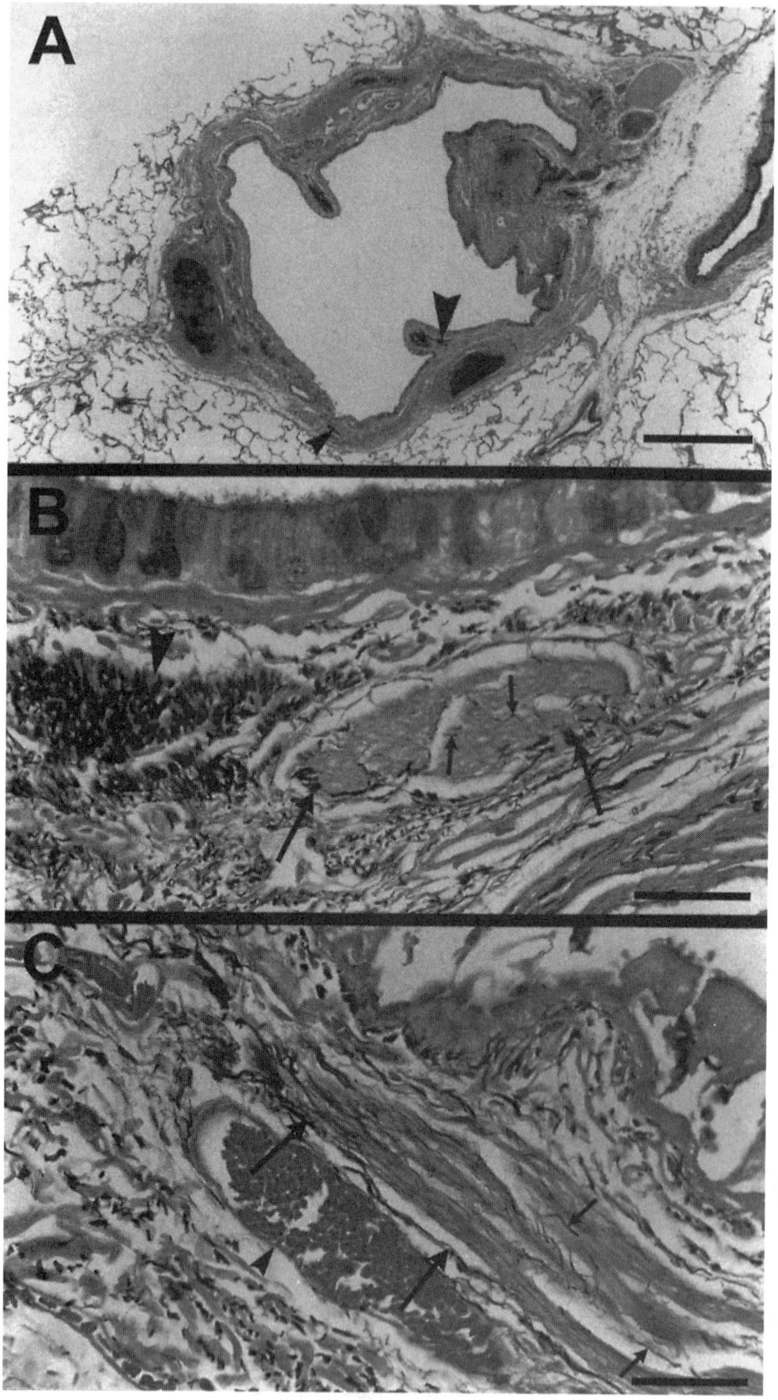
A
B
C

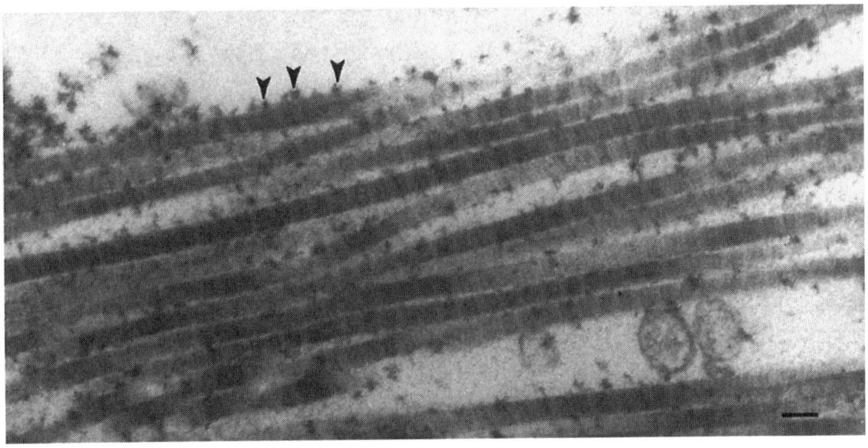

Figure 6 Long section of type I fibrillar collagen in which the banding pattern is clear and associated proteoglycans are labeled with lanthanum chloride (arrowheads). Scale bar = 0.1 μm.

oxytalan fibers were confluent, all part of a single reticulum, moving from the elastic lamina up into the papilli, where oxytalan fibers terminated at the epithelial basal lamina. In lung parenchyma most of the elastic fibers are located in the openings of alveoli along the alveolar ducts where they occur as hoops at the mouth of each alveolus (Mercer and Crapo, 1990; Wright, 1961; Jones and Barson, 1971; Peirce and Ebert, 1965).

2.3 Collagen

Collagens are the most abundant proteins in the body. The best understood collagens are the fibril-forming collagens types I, II, III, V, and XI (Olsen and Ninomiya, 1993), and these form the major matrix element that resists tensile stresses. A classification of collagens is found in van der Rest and Garrone (1991). The collagens are a group of molecules united by the fact that they contain a characteristic left-handed triple helix, formed from the tight association of three polypeptide α-chains. The collagenous regions of the α-chains are composed of repeats of triplet Gly-x-y sequences, of which the glycine residues occupy the core of the triple helix, so that the molecule takes the form of a braided three-strand rope that resists tensile forces. In addition to the fibril-forming collagens, the collagen triple helix forms a structural element in various other modular proteins, including

---

Figure 5 Acid fuchsin trichrome stain of a human airway illustrating the myoelastic system: (A) Low-magnification image; the region illustrated in B is indicated by the large arrowhead, and that indicated by the smaller arrowhead is illustrated in C. Scale bar equals 1 mm. (B) Elastic lamina and smooth muscle in the submucosa; elements of the elastic lamina may aggregate (arrowhead). Smooth-muscle cell clusters are surrounded by large elastic fibers (larger arrows) and penetrated by smaller fibers (smaller arrows) that attach to basal laminae. Scale bar equals 50 μm. (C) Longitudinal section of a smooth-muscle bundle; surrounding larger elastic fibers (large arrows) and penetrating smaller fibers (small arrows) connect the smooth-muscle bundles to the elastic system. Postcapillary venule (arrowhead) contains RBCs. Scale bar = 50 μm.

the so-called minor collagens and nonmatrix molecules, such as complement component C1q. Types I, III, and V are abundant in the interstitium of the lung; types II and XI collagen are usually observed in hyaline cartilage and vitreous humor of the eye (Olsen and Ninomiya, 1993). Fibers containing principally type I collagen constitute the major fibrous elements of dense connective tissue, whereas fibers in the lamina propria (Junqueira et al., 1983) and surrounding smooth-muscle cells (see Fig. 4) and neurons (Montes et al., 1984) contain more type III. These type III collagen fibrils constitute the extracellular matrix element reticulin, as defined by histochemical and ultrastructural observations (Montes et al., 1980), and are smaller in diameter than type I fibrils (Montes et al., 1984) and less closely packed, a phenomenon attributed to the greater abundance of fibril-associated proteoglycans (Montes et al., 1980) (see Fig. 6).

In summary, the epithelium is attached to a basal lamina that it synthesizes, composed mainly of type IV collagen, laminin, fibronectin, and the proteoglycan perlecan. The basal lamina provides important positional information to epithelial cells that are fundamental for homeostasis and tissue repair after minor injury. Apertures permit contact between epithelial cells and fibroblasts, the migration of cells, and the innervation of the epithelium. Type VII collagen and oxytalin fibers anchor the interstitial surface of the basal laminae to deeper connective tissue elements. Oxytalin fibers arise from elaunin fibers that have aborized from elastic fibers from below. In the airways there is an elastic lamina or membrane that lies at the border between the lamina propria and the submucosa. Elements of this layer extend into the smooth-muscle bundles and end at smooth muscle cell basal laminae. At some points, elastic fibers contact smooth-muscle cell plasma membranes. The arrangement of collagen and elastic fibers in the airway wall and parenchyma reflects and is adapted to resist the dynamic forces experienced by each tissue.

3 INTERACTION OF INFLAMMATORY CELLS, CONNECTIVE TISSUE CELLS, AND EPITHELIUM WITH ECM

Cells interact with the matrix through the actions of several classes of receptors. Anchorage, migration, growth, and differentiation, all are highly responsive to matrix composition. Matrix receptors form a link between the structural and adhesive components of the extracellular matrix and the cytoskeleton, transmitting biochemical and biomechanical information into cells, and transducing forces that contract, organize,or assemble the matrix around cells. By far the most important matrix receptors are the integrins, a large family of membrane glycoproteins, each of which is a heterodimer composed of an α- and a β-subunit (see Ruoslahti, 1996 for a review). The α-subunits contain cation-binding sites; the β-subunits a cysteine-rich knot close to the transmembrane region. The α- and β-subunits can combine noncovalently to form numerous integrins; this generates great diversity in the abilities of cells to recognize matrix substrates, and to transduce intracellular signals on ligation of receptors (see Giancotti and Ruoslahti, 1999 for a review). Integrins form a diversity of receptors including the collagen receptors (α1,2,3-β1), fibronectin receptors (α2,3,4,5,V-β1), laminin receptors ($\alpha_6\beta_1$) and vitronectin receptors ($\alpha V\beta_5$, $\alpha V\beta_3$, αIIbβ3), tenascin receptors (α_9) (Yokosaki et al., 1994) and ligands for adhesion molecules, such as ICAM-1 (LFA-1/CD11/CD18, or αLβ2), influencing cell–cell adhesion. Normal cells, particularly mesenchymal cells such as fibroblasts, proliferate at a low rate when attached to their normal matrix. There is evidence that β_2-integrins down-regulate cell proliferation in this context. If removed from this regulatory influence (e.g., in tissue culture) many of the cells undergo apoptosis or anoikis (Frisch and Ruoslahti,

1997), but can be rescued in the presence of ligands, such as fibronectin or vitronectin, that are also found in the provisional matrix of inflammatory sites or healing wounds. The potent effects of fibronectin on cell proliferation are particularly well studied (Bourdoulous et al., 1998). Modification of matrix composition in inflammatory sites, together with changes in integrin expression as a result of growth factor activities, or feedback from altered matrix composition, could give rise to a seemingly endless diversity of cell–matrix and matrix–cell effects. In this context, it has recently been shown that subtle changes in integrin–ligand-binding properties influence cell migration speed (Palacek et al., 1997). The provisional matrix, the matrix that surrounds cells at remodeling sites, is associated with various specific integrins; integrins for fibronectin, vitronectin, and tenascin, all are expressed by mesenchymal and epithelial cells at these sites. There is evidence that ligation of these integrins influences protease production and, hence, pericellular matrix turnover, an effect that is likely to be important at remodeling sites in chronic inflammation. Many cells possess cell surface receptors for the abundant extracellular matrix glycosaminoglycan hyaluronan. Hyaluronan is synthesized early in inflammatory sites; its synthesis is responsive to interleukin (IL)-1, prostaglandin $(PGE)_2$ and PDGF; and it is believed that interactions between hyaluronan receptors and hyaluronan may be important for migration of inflammatory cells in inflammatory sites. Hyaluronan receptors include CD44, a pleiomorphic receptor, the variants of which derive from alternative mRNA splicing (Lesley et al., 1993), and intercellular cell adhesion molecule-1 (ICAM-1) (McCourt et al., 1994). The function of RHAMM, a hyaluronan-binding protein and putative hyaluronan receptor (Turley, 1989; Yang et al., 1994) is now uncertain (Hoffmann et al., 1998; Assmann et al., 1998).

4 REGULATION OF MATRIX SYNTHESIS IN RESOLUTION OF INFLAMMATION, CHRONIC INFLAMMATION, AND SCARRING

The process of matrix synthesis and deposition in the lung, associated with acute and chronic inflammation is best studied in pulmonary fibrosis, a disease process that can be initiated by either allergic or nonallergic stimuli; at least 150 causes or associations are known. Pulmonary fibrosis is a dynamic process, driven by chronic inflammation, that involves matrix degradation, cell migration, and proliferation, an ordered sequence of matrix changes, and ultimately, the accumulation of collagenous matrix, that replaces and distorts lung architecture (Fig. 7). The process may be initiated by inhaled particles, such as asbestos or silica; by inhaled gases, such as nitrogen dioxide; by xenobiotics, such as the chemotherapeutic agent bleomycin; by systemic autoimmune disease, such as scleroderma; by the reaction to aeroallergens, such as fungal spores or to infectious agents such as mycobacteria; or by as yet, undefined predisposing genetic factors. In most individual patients the cause is impossible to determine and the disease is termed idiopathic and classified based on histological appearance (see Fraser et al., 1991 for review). The most prevalent ILDs are idiopathic pulmonary fibrosis (IPF), occupationally induced fibrosis caused by particle inhalation, and sarcoidosis, a multisystem idiopathic granulomatous disease. The early stages of ILD involve inflammation and fluid exudation onto the surface of the lung, recruitment and activation of polymorphonuclear (PMN) leukocytes and mononuclear phagocytes, and damage to, and regeneration of, epithelial cells. If the exudate persists, the next step of the process occurs: Fibroblasts colonize the exudate, and synthesize a fibronectin–versican proteoglycan–hyaluronan- and tenascin-rich provisional matrix in which they proliferate. In the final, irreversible step in the progression to fibrosis,

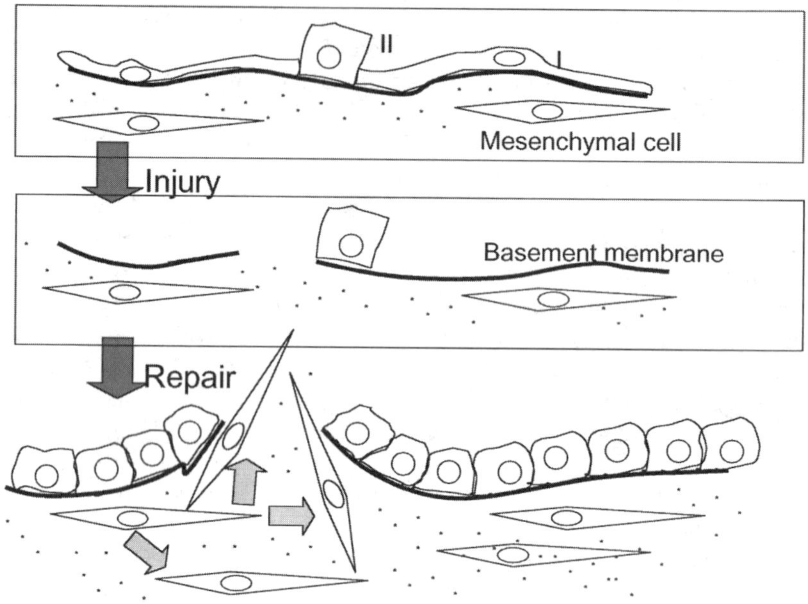

Figure 7 Cell biology of remodeling in inflammation and fibrosis: Epithelial injury leads to epithelial regrowth and subepithelial fibroblast proliferation. Pathological features of epithelial hyperplasia, increased subepithelial fibroblast proliferation, and subepthelial provisional matrix deposition is observed in early IPF in a few cases, and shows similarities with changes in asthma. (From Roberts, 1995; Roberts and Burke, 2000.)

provisional matrix is replaced by collagenous matrix. The fibroblasts are contractile, and their contractility, together with the local replacement of the normal architecture of the lung with collagenous matrix causes changes in tissue mechanics and function. The progressive replacement of normal lung architecture with fibrosis is responsible for the insidiously progressive nature of the disease. Current anti-inflammatory therapy, with corticosteroids or cytotoxic agents, slows the rate of deterioration in lung function in only 10–30% of ILD patients, but does not reverse fibrotic changes that have already occurred.

A paradigm for the disease process leading to fibrosis is established, based on studies of human biopsies and animal models (Crystal et al, 1981; Kuhn and McDonald, 1991).

4.1 Epithelial Injury, Inflammation, and Exudate

Infectious agents or inhaled toxins damage the epithelium, leading to the release from alveolar macrophages of cytokines that recruit granulocytes into the lung and activate them (Rochester and Elias, 1993). Alternatively, epithelial injury may result from allergic inflammation (e.g., in allergic alveolitis). Injury may be mediated by oxidants (Cantin et al., 1987) or proteases released from granulocytes or macrophages in the inflammatory process. The basal lamina is damaged ultrastructurally in IPF, consistent with proteolysis (Raghu et al., 1985). Inflammation may become chronic, because of repeated or persistent insult, or because epithelial regeneration is prevented (Hatschek and Witschi, 1979). A fibrinous exudate, containing inflammatory cells, fibrin, and fibronectin covers, the alveolar surface (McDonald, 1990). Fibroblasts migrate through holes in the basal lamina into this alveolar clot. Hyaluronan is found in these early lesions (Bensadoun et al., 1996). Fibroblasts isolated from individuals with adult respiratory distress syndrome (ARDS) use the hyaluronan receptor CD44 to invade fibronectin- and hyaluronan-containing matrices in vitro (Svee et al., 1996), suggesting that hyaluronan receptors may be important as fibroblasts invade exudates in vivo.

Prostaglandin E_2 (Karlinsky and Goldstein, 1989), tumor necrosis factor (TNF), and interleukin-1 (Sampson et al., 1992), all increase hyaluronan synthesis by fibroblasts in vitro, and could be responsible for increased hyaluronan synthesis early in lung inflammation. Migrating fibroblasts in IPF are surrounded by a pericellular matrix containing the hyaluronan-binding proteoglycan versican (Roberts and Burke, 2000), which may influence cell adhesion.

4.2 Structural and Biological Functions of Provisional Matrix

The characteristic early lesions of fibrosis that had been interpreted as thickened interstitium (''subepithelial fibroblast foci'') were shown by Kuhn et al., (1989) and Kuhn and Macdonald (1991) to result from the colonization of former airspaces by fibroblasts (Zhang et al., 1994) that synthesize type I collagen and express α-smooth muscle actin. These lesions consist of a matrix (provisional matrix) that contains fibronectin, a macromolecular aggregate of hyaluronan and the 1-million–Da proteoglycan, versican (Bensadoun et al., 1996; Roberts and Burke, 2000), together with several glycoproteins that are considered antiadhesive, including tenascin and thrombospondin (Kuhn and Mason, 1995) (Fig. 8). Each major component of this system binds at least two other components (see Yamada, 1991; Yamagata et al., 1986; Apsberg, 1995; Yokosaki et al., 1994, for discussions of the

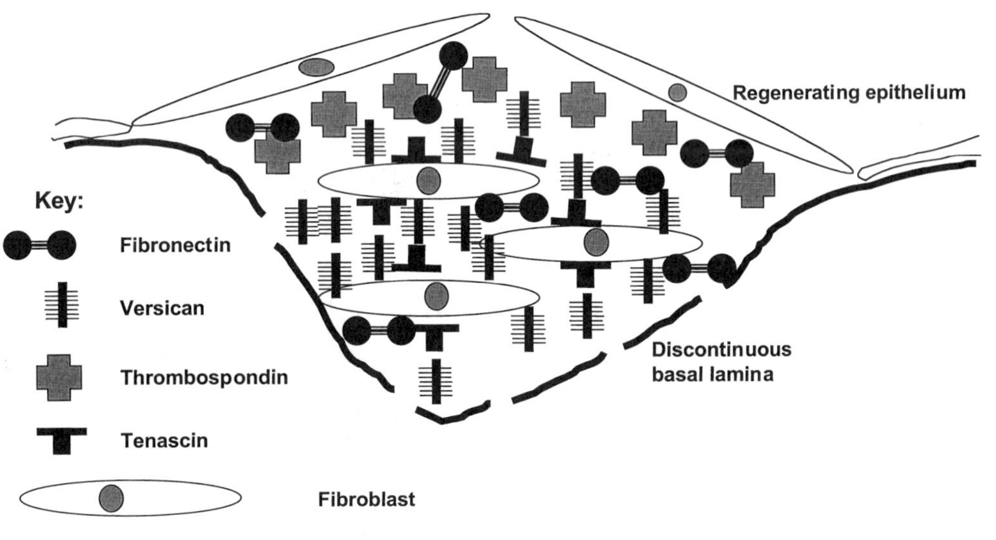

Figure 8 Structure and biological functions of provisional matrix in the remodeling lung: Inflammation leads to exudation of fibrin- and cell-containing fluid into airspace. The exuidate is colonized by fibroblasts, through holes in the basal lamina. Fibroblasts in the former exudate synthesize a versican–hyaluronan matrix to which is bound fibronectin (dumbbell shape) tenascin (T) and thrombospondin (+). Epithelial cells overgrow the provisional matrix. New collagen is synthesized by ''myo'' fibroblasts in these lesions, which evolve to become collagenous scar tissue.

binding properties of fibronectin, versican, and tenascin), so the provisional matrix can be considered a gel with multiple cell growth factor- and protein-binding activities). Provisional matrix appears to facilitate migration and proliferation of myofibroblasts, and it is in this matrix that they begin to synthesize and assemble collagen fibers. As cells isolated from their normal matrix usually undergo apoptosis or anoikis, the provisional matrix in chronic inflammatory sites must contain factors that support cell survival and proliferation (Fig. 9). Such signals may include integrins that bind tenascin, or fibronectin, or both, or growth factors that specifically localize to the provisional matrix. Myofibroblasts express the fibronectin receptor integrin α5b1 (Fukuda et al., 1995), which may be a major permissive factor for cell proliferation (Bourdoulous et al., 1998). Our recent data show that several growth factors and cytokines with the ability to bind heparin also bind the chondroitin sulfate that is part of versican, suggesting that provisional matrix may concentrate these signals and modulate their biological activities, which may also contribute to the ability of provisional matrix to support mesenchymal cell proliferation (Roberts, McQuibban, and Overall, manuscript in preparation). Tenascin C colocalizes with versican in development (Shinomura et al., 1990), in healing wounds, and the matrix of malignant tumors (Erickson and Bourdon, 1989; Yeo et al., 1991, Isogai et al., 1996). Tenascin–fibronectin complexes (but not either alone) stimulate secretion of matrix-degrading metalloproteases by fibroblasts (Tremble et al., 1994). Proteases so induced might contribute to the removal of this versican–tenascin–fibronectin provisional matrix, a process that must occur in the evolution of the lesions to form areas of collagen-rich and proteoglycan-poor fibrosis (Bensadoun et al., 1996, 1997; Roberts and Burke, 2000). Concomitantly the myofibroblasts disappear, presumably by apoptosis. This sequence of events is common to the remodeling process driven by chronic inflammation, whether the cause is acute severe injury as in ARDS

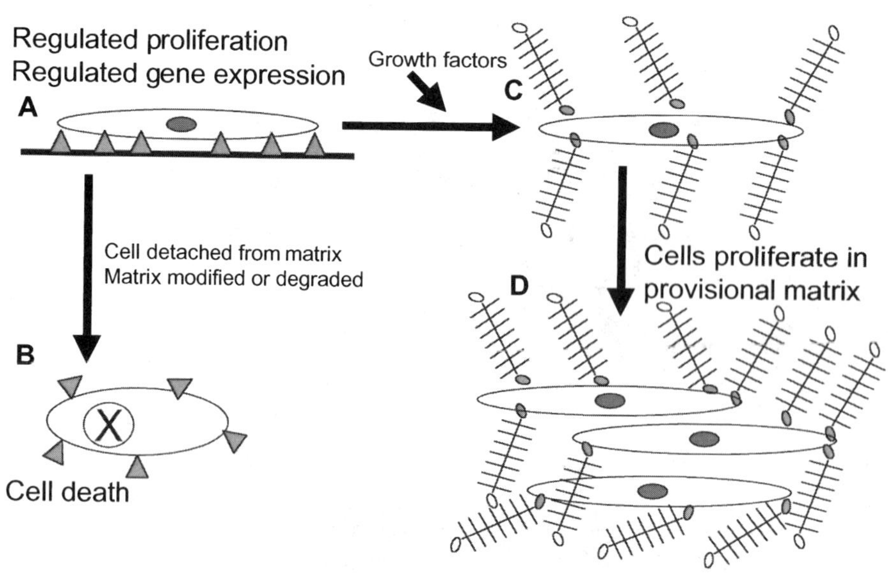

Figure 9 Provisional matrix supports cell migration and proliferation: Normal cell–matrix interactions are altered in inflammatory sites. Provisional matrix in presence of growth factors supports cell migration and proliferation.

(Bensadoun et al., 1996), idiopathic bronchitis obliterans and organizing pneumonia (BOOP) or IPF (Bensadoun et al., 1996), allergic injury in extrinsic allergic alveolitis (Bensadoun et al., 1997), and encapsulation of a chronic inflammatory stimulus such as *Mycobacterium tuberculosis* (Bensadoun et al., 1997). We have also shown that increased deposition of versican in airway walls is a feature of severe asthma (Roberts, 1995).

4.3 Platelet-Derived Growth Factor and Transforming Growth Factor-β Localize to Sites of Fibroblast Proliferation and Matrix Deposition

Expression of platelet-derived growth factor (PDGF) is increased in IPF (Martinet et al., 1987), and is localized to the fibroblast foci (Limper et al., 1991) and to sites of injury in experimental asbestos-induced fibrosis (Liu et al., 1997). PDGF is a stimulator of smooth-muscle cell proliferation (Ross et al., 1986), hyaluronan synthesis (Papakonstantinou et al., 1995), and versican synthesis (Schonherr et al., 1991). Transforming growth factor-β, (TGF-β) is also found in the fibroblast foci (Khalil et al., 1991; Broekelmann et al., 1991), and is synthesized by regenerating epithelial cells in IPF (Khalil et al., 1991). Indeed, thrombospondin, a component of the provisional matrix (Kuhn and Mason, 1995) appears to be able to activate TGF-β (Schultz–Cherry et al., 1995), as can integrin $\alpha v\beta 6$ (Munger et al., 1999), which may release TGF-β from its latent complex at remodeling sites. TGF-β_1 induces expression of genes for α-smooth-muscle actin (Hautmann et al., 1997) and various matrix proteins, including hyaluronan (Westergren-Thorsson et al., 1990), versican (Schonherr et al., 1991), and collagen. Mononuclear phagocytes overproduce PDGF (Martinet et al., 1987), and TGF-β in human pulmonary fibrosis (Khalil et al., 1991), and are able to activate TGF-β_1 in a process that involves endogenous plasmin (Khalil et al., 1996). Thus PDGF and TGF-β, released by macrophages locally, could induce cell proliferation, expression of α-smooth-muscle actin, and synthesis of hyaluronan and versican in target mesenchymal cells (Fig. 10). Both TGF-β and PDGF are strongly linked to cell proliferation and accumulation of ECM in wound healing and fibrosis in many organs, and modulation of their biological activities is a key therapeutic goal in the treatment of many diseases that involve aberrant matrix synthesis.

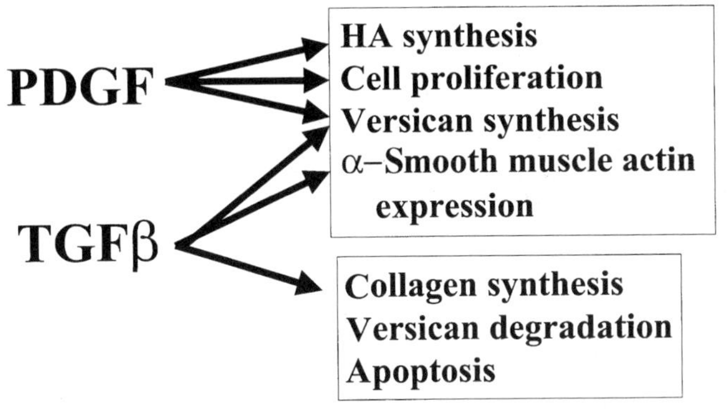

Figure 10 Matrix changes in evolving fibrotic lesions: Many of the changes that occur associated with myofibroblasts in evolving fibrotic lesions can be reproduced by the action of platelet-derived growth factor and transforming growth factor-β in vitro.

4.4 Cell Biology of Pulmonary Fibrosis: Parallels with Wound Healing

In wound healing, a well-established sequence of events occurs (Fig. 11). Cellular injury and vascular leak is followed by platelet activation, blood clotting, and release of mediators of acute inflammation. Polymorphonuclear leukocytes (PMN) and macrophages enter the exudate; PMN endocytose and kill microorganisms, and macrophages remove erythrocytes, fibrin, and cellular debris. The macrophages' release of plasmin, from plasminogen activator, is important in this process. Fibroblasts proliferate and migrate into the area of the exudate and lay down a new extracellular matrix; these cells have a distinct phenotype and are known as myofibroblasts. Myofibroblasts express α-(smooth-muscle) actin, resemble smooth-muscle cells ultrastructurally, and contract in response to agonists that cause smooth-muscle contraction (Gabbiani et al., 1972; Ryan et al., 1974). These cells not only synthesize and assemble structural elements of the matrix, but also contract the granulation tissue, a phenomenon important in closing the wound. The origin of the myofibroblasts that are central to wound healing is controversial. They may be derived from tissue fibroblasts, from expansion of a preexistent pool of α-actin-positive connective tissue cells such as pericytes, in the microvasculature as occurs in the skin (Sundberg et al., 1996) and liver (Bedossa et al., 1994), or ''myofibroblasts'' in the sub-epithelial matrix of the airways of the lung (Brewster et al., 1990), or even, more controversially, from a circulating pool of mesenchymal cells originating in the bone marrow (Prockop et al., 1997). Although macrophages are still generally considered to direct the remodeling process, older studies have shown that wounds in animals depleted of macrophages heal adequately, although leaving a repair cluttered with debris (Ross, 1969). This indicates that myofibroblast proliferation, migration, and new matrix synthesis can occur, at least in the skin, independently of macrophage-derived factors. The signals that stimulate the proliferation of connective tissue cells and the generation of myofibroblasts are incompletely understood. However, a relatively simple mechanism exists that could be central in inducing the generation of myofibroblasts adjacent to the exudate, their proliferation, and synthesis of new matrix. Thrombin, produced from its zymogen in the coagulation cascade, is a strong inducer of fibroblast and smooth-muscle cell proliferation (through its actions on protease-activated receptors (PAR 1 and PAR 2) (Bretschneider et al., 1999). Thrombin also releases the smooth-muscle cell mitogen PDGF from matrix stores by proteolyis

•Inflammation
•Fibroblast proliferation
•Fibroblast migration
•Provisional matrix synthesis
•Wound contraction
•Collagen synthesis
•Matrix degradation
•Apoptosis

Figure 11 Cell biology of wound healing.

(Soyombo and Di Corleto, 1994), and it also induces synthesis of TGF-β by smooth-muscle cells (Bachhuber et al., 1997). Although other schemes are possible, this relatively simple mechanism links coagulation and inflammation to the production of the mitogen PDGF, and the production of TGF-β, a potent inducer of both the expression of α-smooth-muscle actin and matrix accumulation. Such a mechanism depends on competent mesenchymal cells in vivo responding to thrombin as cultured smooth-muscle cells do in vitro. After the granulation tissue has been replaced by collagen-rich scar tissue, the myofibroblasts disappear, and this appears to involve apoptosis (Desmouliere et al., 1995), rather than a change to the fibroblast phenotype, for there is a decrease in cellularity at this stage. The cellular signals that control this process are as yet unknown, but they are of great interest in seeking to control tissue repair and fibrosis.

4.5 Why Pulmonary Fibrosis, Rather Than Wound Healing in the Lung?

Lung architecture can return to normal after inflammation and fluid exudation; most cases of pneumonia resolve successfully. Pulmonary fibrosis is considered by many to be an example of wound repair that is aberrant because of some combination of the magnitude, kind, repetitive nature of the injury, or defective removal of the initial clot (McDonald, 1991). What is abnormal about the healing process in pulmonary fibrosis?

4.5.1 Persistence of Initial Injury?

The initiating stimulus clearly is likely to be persistent in forms of lung fibrosis that have a major autoimmune component, such as scleroderma, or if exposure to antigen is not discontinued, as in allergic alveolitis. The pneumoconioses are initiated by toxic particles that cannot be effectively neutralized by phagocytes or other cells (Morris et al., 1996), and animal studies convincingly demonstrate that rapid generation of growth factors, including PDGF, at the site of injury is linked to fibrotic changes (Liu et al., 1997; Brass et al., 1999). Such stimulation likely persists as long as the particulate remains in the lung (i.e., indefinitely).

4.5.2 Slower Than Normal Clot Dissolution?

The dissolution of the fibronectin–fibrin clot is believed to be important in promoting resolution (McDonald, 1990). Alveolar fibrinolytic activity is diminished in human IPF (Chapman et al., 1986); and there is evidence from animal studies that increased susceptibility to fibrosis is associated with a decreased propensity to synthesize plasminogen activator. The implication of this is that the longer a fibrin-rich clot covers the original epithelium, the more likely it is that this will be colonized by fibroblasts and, ultimately, be coopted as part of the collagenous matrix of the lung, as opposed to being cleared and architecture returned to normal.

4.5.3 Magnitude of Inital Injury?

The studies of Vracko (1972), using a model in which lung inflammation in dogs was elicited by increasing doses of oleic acid, showed that a greater degree of damage to the subepithelial basal lamina correlated with the likelihood that complete restoration of lung architecture could not occur. He suggested that the basal lamina provides information to epithelium and mesenchymal cells that defines the original architecture of the lung, and that loss of this information (implicitly, owing to matrix degradation in inflammation) results in ineffective repair. In support of the hypothesis that fibrosis may result from excessive proteolysis in inflammation, fibrosis is a frequent consequence of the adult respiratory distress syndrome (ARDS), in which PMN arrest in large numbers in the lung and release large amounts of proteolytic enzymes. Consistent with the hypothesis that basal lamina proteolysis is an important determinant of progression to fibrosis, holes appear in the alveolar basal lamina early in IPF (Raghu et al., 1985). This mechanism may be most relevant to ARDS-initiated fibrosis, when initial injury is widespread and severe and leads to significant fibrosis in 50% of survivors.

4.5.4 Multiple Modes of Tissue Injury?

Hatschek and Witschi (1979) showed that a combination of inflammation and prevention of epithelial regeneration leads to fibrosis, consistent with the hypothesis that multiple hits are required to tip the balance from repair to fibrosis.

5 ROLE OF EXTRACELLULAR MATRIX IN AIRWAY REMODELING IN ASTHMA

A renewed emphasis on the structural changes that occur in asthma has led to the term ''remodeling'' to suggest that injury and repair processes cause functional alterations of asthmatic airways. We have reviewed and reanalyzed the quantitative morphometric data that exist on airway wall compartments (Roberts et al., 1997b), and concluded that fatal asthma involves a marked increase in airway wall thickness that involves all layers of the airway wall, and that patients with asthma who died of other reasons showed intermediate changes between persons with fatal asthma and normal persons. We have also reviewed in detail the mechanisms by which both geometric and biomechanical changes consequent to airway wall remodeling may lead to functional consequences in asthma (Roberts et al., 1997b). Functional consequences can include excessive airway narrowing to a contractile agonist; decreased bronchodilator responses to physiological stimuli, such as a big breath, or to a smooth muscle relaxant, such as a β-agonist; and persistent irreversible airway obstruction in some cases.

Although this concept of functional alterations caused by injury, and in some cases to overexuberant repair processes, forms a helpful framework, it is limited by a multitude of factors, some beyond our present ability to adequately evaluate, and there are considerable conflicting data on parameters that we can measure (see reviews by Fish and Peters, 1999; Busse et al., 1999). The term *remodeling* is very narrowly defined by some investigators, sometimes reflecting no more than the thickness of the collagen deposition beneath the basal lamina. Correlations between a specific structural property and in vivo determinants of pulmonary function are of limited benefit in understanding the pathophysiological processes involved and, as a result, it is not surprising that conflicting results arise when evaluating a complex disease at different time points and degrees of disease severity. However, these studies provide valuable information and suggest that alterations in extracellular matrix elements are key factors in pathophysiological changes described, as outlined in the following.

5.1 Epithelial Integrity and Function

Changes in epithelium in asthma have been noted by many investigators and the various functions of epithelium that could be altered in asthma do make this an important area of research. The major focus has related to desquamation of epithelium found in autopsy samples, sputum, and biopsies (Dunnill, 1960; Naylor, 1962; Laitinen et al., 1985). Limitations of these observations relate to the concern of artifact from damage in obtaining biopsies and our knowledge about epithelial function during injury and repair. Epithelium rapidly regenerates following injury, as demonstrated in both in vivo studies in guinea pigs (Erjefält et al., 1995) and in vitro airway explants following mechanical removal (Loewen et al., 1997). Although some investigators have found correlations of epithelial loss with airway hyperresponsiveness (Beasley et al., 1989; Jeffrey et al., 1989), others have not (Boulet et al., 1997). These studies reveal the limitations in evaluating only epithelial damage, rather than evaluating function, as the epithelium is a complex cellular milieu capable of secreting multiple factors, in addition to its barrier function (Boucher et al., 1988; Spina et al., 1994; Knight et al., 1994). A cytokine demonstrated to be upregulated in airway tissue of asthmatics is GM-CSF (Sousa et al., 1993) that has been demonstrated to lead to increased eosinophils, monocytes, and fibrosis when its gene is transfected into rat lung (Xing et al., 1996). It also primes eosinophils and decreases their apoptosis (Vignola et al., 1998a), and expression on the surface of progenitors may promote differentiation in atopic persons (Gavreau et al., 1998). Following antigen challenge of ragweed-allergic asthmatics, GM-CSF is produced for up to 2 weeks (Shaver et al., 1997), consistent with a role in repair.

5.2 ECM–Integrin Interactions

The importance of interactions of matrix proteins, such as fibronectin and tenascin, with integrin receptors in alterations of asthma has been highlighted in studies dealing especially with epithelial integrity. Human epithelial cells from nasal polyps, cultured on type I collagen, were dependent on fibronectin and $\alpha 5/\beta 1$-integrin for wound repair (Herard et al., 1996). With use of a similar system with the human epithelial cell line 16HBE145, other investigators demonstrated that antibodies to α-$_2$, α-$_3$, or α-$_6$ blocked wound repair of cells grown on type IV collagen, but not if grown on laminin-1 or -2 (White et al., 1999). This may be relevant to the disease state, for epithelial cells express integrins for laminin-1 and fibronectin present in basement membranes (Jeffrey et al., 1992; Albelda, 1995; Pilewski et al., 1997), but laminin-2 is expressed only in airways of patients with chronic asthma (Altraja et al., 1996). Blocking the β_1-integrin VLA-4 inhibited both early and late allergic reactions, plus airways hyperresponsiveness, in the rat (Rabb et al., 1994; Laberge et al., 1995), sheep (Abraham et al., 1994), and guinea pig (Pretolani et al., 1994). This did not affect eosinophilic infiltration, as would be anticipated. Further studies demonstrated that an antibody to VLA-4 strikingly inhibited mast cell mediator release (Hojo et al., 1998), raising the possibility that mediators altering ECM, possibly mast cell tryptase, may be important in induction of airway hyperresponsiveness. The complexity of integrin interactions in highlighted by the demonstration that TGF-β_1 latency-associated protein binds $\alpha v/\beta 6$, restricting activation of TGF-$\beta 1$ (Munger et al., 1999). Mice lacking this integrin develop exaggerated inflammation, but are protected from developing fibrosis. Relatively little information is available for asthmatic tissues but one study did demonstrate increased tenascin in airway basement membrane of asthmatics, a change that was decreased on treatment with inhaled steroid (Laitinen et al., 1997)

5.3 Subepithelial Collagen Deposition

A thickening of the layer below the basal lamina, consisting of collagens type I, III, and V, plus fibronectin (Roche et al., 1989), has received considerable attention as a hallmark of remodeling in asthma (Jeffrey et al., 1989; Brewster et al., 1990; Lundgren et al., 1988;

Ollerenshaw et al., 1992; Chetta et al., 1997; Wilson and Li, 1997; Boulet et al., 1997). This thickening appears to be associated with an increase in myofibroblasts (Brewster et al., 1990). Several studies have correlated the degree of thickening with airway hyperresponsiveness or disease severity (Jeffrey et al., 1989; Cho et al., 1996; Boulet et al., 1997; Chetta et al., 1997), but a recent study evaluating total collagen content by Sirius red staining as well as collagen types I and III by immunocytochemical analysis failed to demonstrate differences in samples from very severe asthmatics versus milder asthmatics or nonasthma controls (Chu et al., 1998). This study also failed to find increased collagen in the submucosal area, as did two other studies (Brewster et al., 1990; Godfrey et al., 1995), whereas this was found in one study (Wilson and Li, 1997).

The primary factor implicated in subepithelial fibrosis is TGF-β, in particular the β_1-isotype. Conflicting data exists on a correlation of mRNA expression or protein for TGF-β_1 with asthma disease activity or specific morphological changes. Using Northern blot analysis, one study found no difference between expression of TGF-β_1 in asthmatic versus in chronic obstructive pulmonary disease (COPD) airways (Aubert et al., 1994), and another study failed to detect differences in immunohistochemical detection of TGF-β_1 in biopsies of asthmatics versus normals (Hoshino et al., 1998). Conversely, in situ hybridization has demonstrated that a major source of TGF-β_1 is the eosinophil (Ohno et al., 1992; Minshall et al., 1997), and the latter study found a striking inverse correlation between either EG2+ cells or subepithelial fibrosis with forced expiratory volume in 1 sec (FEV_1). In agreement with this was a recent study demonstrating increased TGF-β^+ cells in biopsies of severe asthmatics demonstrating eosinophilia that also had increased subepithelial fibrosis compared with a group of severe asthmatics without eosinophilia who had neither of these changes (Wenzel et al., 1999). In contrast to the previous study, however, those subjects with eosinophilia had better FEV_1 values than those without. Still lacking are studies of TGF-β biological activity in bronchoalveolar lavage (BAL) or airway preparations from asthmatics. Fibroblasts isolated from asthmatic versus normal airways failed to show more procollagen I or III following stimulation with TGF-β_1 (Dube et al., 1998). However, this does not preclude increased expression of collagen genes in vivo, which may be due to increased fibroblast numbers, increased local concentrations of TGF-β_1 in vivo, or a phenotypic difference that does not persist in vitro.

Perhaps more important than the absolute amount of collagen is its organization. Electron microscopy evaluation suggests that this layer in asthmatics is not in normal fibrillar array, but is a disorganized reticulin mesh. This could have significant implications for airway narrowing. Whereas a thickened layer of fibrillar collagen might be expected to limit bronchoconstriction, a disorganized reticulin layer would be expected to be more compliant in compression and could additionally increased airway narrowing for a given degree of smooth-muscle contraction, owing to its thickness alone.

5.4 Airway Smooth Muscle

Many investigators have suggested that asthmatics have increased smooth muscle on the basis of evaluation of autopsy material (Huber and Koessler, 1922; Dunnill, 1960; Dunnill et al., 1969; Hossain, 1973, Heard and Hossain, 1973; Carroll et al., 1993; Ebina et al., 1993; Kuwano et al., 1993), and these data are reviewed and reanalyzed in Roberts et al. (1997b). Rather surprisingly, a study from our group did not demonstrate an increase in muscle in airways of two asthmatic subjects, whose airway wall tissue showed two- to threefold increases in force and shortening (Thomson et al., 1996). This has major implications for the defect in asthma because it clearly shows that amount of muscle cannot account for the unique mechanical properties of these airways, because the muscle stress (kg/cm^2) in these asthmatic tissue samples was two to three times greater than for nonasthmatic tissues. A host of studies have evaluated the proliferation and properties of isolated airway smooth-muscle cells (Panettieri and Kotlikoff, 1998; Panettieri and Grunstein, 1997). Such studies are helpful in defining intracellular-signaling mechanisms and cell surface determinants, but have limitations in terms of modulating factors present in the normal tissue milieu. This is due to the rapid differentiation of cultured cells to a noncontractile phenotype, with loss of muscle myosin and α-smooth-muscle actin (Halayko et al., 1996; 1997). Although conceivable that this might happen in asthma to increase muscle mass, these cells would have to later redifferentiate to a contractile phenotype.

Extracellular matrix elements may limit smooth-muscle proliferation, and degradation of these allow increases in muscle. A recent study demonstrated, by immunocytochemistry and biological activity, that matrix matalloprotease-1 (MMP-1), but not MMP-2, -3, or -9, was increased in asthmatic smooth muscle (Rajah et al., 1999). In addition to cleaving collagen, which surrounds smooth-muscle cells in vivo, MMP-1 has proteolytic activity for insulin-like growth factor (IGF)-binding proteins that inhibit cell growth. In isolated smooth-muscle cell cultures, leukotriene-D_4 is mitogenic (Cohen et al., 1995) and modulates the IGF axis by inducing MMP-1 (Rajah et al., 1996). Therefore, the increased MMP-1 activity could lead to increased amounts of smooth muscle. Whether this occurs in vivo remains to be demonstrated. In studies that we have performed with airway explants, factors shown to induce proliferation of isolated airway cells (including leukotrienes) have had no effect on the amount of muscle measured morphometrically or by bromodeoxyuridine (B*rd*U) incorporation, nor had increases in muscle force generation. This emphasizes the importance of the normal cellular milieu, including extracellular matrix elements, in modulating myocyte proliferation and likely also function.

5.4.1 Collagen

Human airway myoctes are intimately associated with fibrillar collagen (Fig. 12). The extent of collagen between individual muscle cells and bundles is best appreciated by the color photographs shown in the manuscript by Thomson et al., 1996. An electron micrograph of this association is shown in Figure 13. Although it would be difficult to quantify changes in this element morphologically, it is easy to appreciate how altered collagen at this site could dramatically change airway smooth-muscle function. This was demonstrated in our study of the mechanical properties of human airway smooth muscle before and following treatment with 20 U/mL collagenase (Fig. 14) (Bramley et al., 1995). As passive tension of the airway preparation decreased, the degree of shortening and force generation increased. Collagen degradation would decrease the load on the muscle, thereby allowing greater shortening. This treatment could also decrease the radial constraint to myocyte expansion and allow greater shortening and force generation as suggested by studies of rabbit trachea (Meiss, 1999).

5.4.2 Elastin

Elastic fibers are present in the subepithelium as well as in the smooth-muscle layer of airways. Studies of asthmatic airways has suggested a disruption and loss of the thinner fibers that normally lie perpendicular to the smooth muscle and appear anchored to the

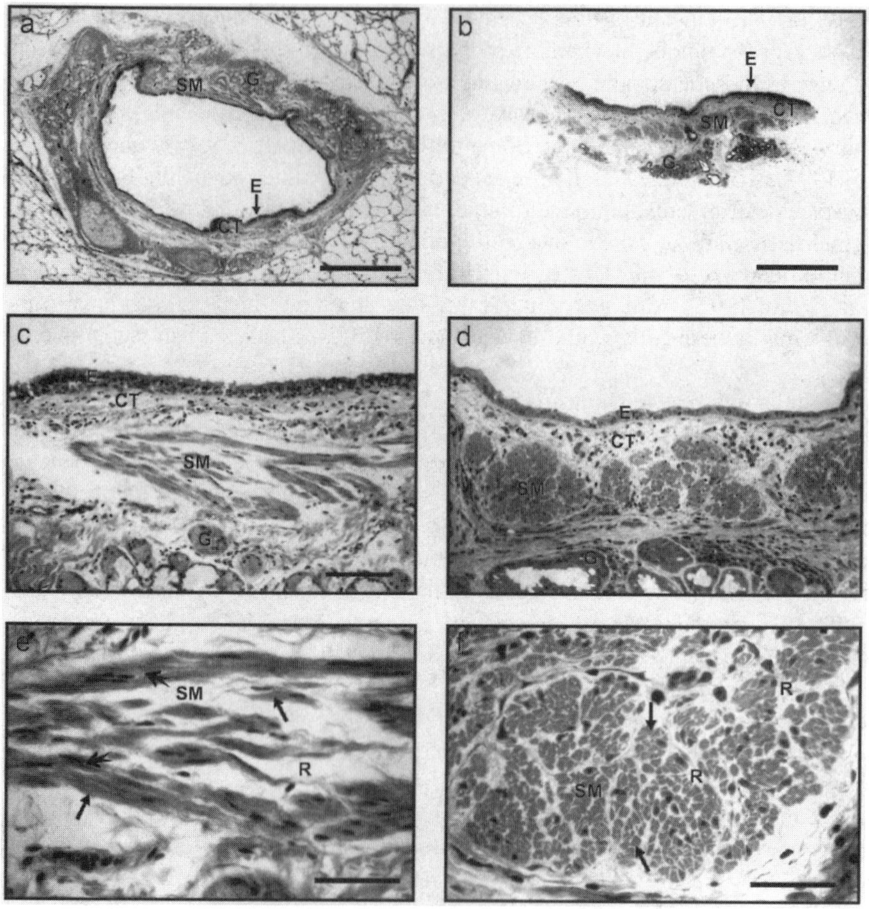

Figure 12 Comparative samples of a human airway revealing the abundance of extracellular matrix within the total wall, between smooth-muscle bundles and even between individual myocytes. Left-hand panels (a, c, e) show 5-μm–thick cross sections of paraffin-embedded Masson's trichrome-stained tissue, and the right-hand panels (b, d, f) show 1.5-μm–thick axial sections of glycol methacrylate-embedded, toluidine blue-O-stained tissue. Paired micrographs show low- (a and b; scale bars represent 1.0 mm), medium- (c and d; scale bars represent 0.1 mm) and high- (e and f; scale bars represent 0.05 mm) magnification views. Sections show epithelium (E), subepithelial glands (G), connective tissue elements (CT), smooth-muscle bundles (SM), smooth-muscle cells (thin arrows), extracellular matrix between smooth-muscle cells (thick arrows), and connective tissue ribbons within smooth-muscle bundles (R). (From Thomson et al., 1996.)

basement membrane (Bousquet et al., 1996; Mauad et al., 1999). Loss of this normal structure may allow the development of excessive inward folding of the inner wall into the lumen. Loss of these elastic fibers might also dissociate the inner airway structures from the smooth muscle so that relaxation of the muscle would have less effect on dilating the lumen. Increased levels of elastase have been detected in induced sputum samples of asthmatics (Vignola et al., 1998b), which suggests that even transient neutrophil infiltration in asthmatics may be more detrimental than the far greater numbers of eosinophils present.

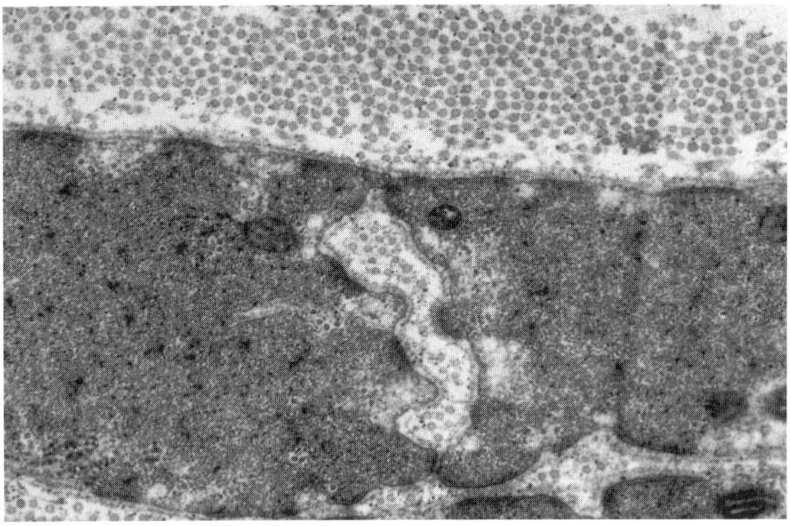

Figure 13 Transmission electron micrograph demonstrating the fibrillar collagen between two myocytes in the airway.

5.4.3 Proteoglycans

Matrix proteoglycans influence tissue mechanics, matrix assembly, cell growth and maturation; bind and influence the biological activities of growth factors (Roberts, 1997a; Iozzo, 1998). Increased amounts of several proteoglycans have been found in human asthmatic airways. Deposition of versican, biglycan, and hyaluronan were greater in autopsy samples from fatal asthma cases (Roberts, 1995) and versican, biglycan, and lumican were increased in the submucosa of asthmatic airway biopsies, with the amount correlating with the degree of airway hyperresponsiveness (Huang et al., 1999). Loss of proteoglycan (primarily aggrecan) from airway cartilage in fatal asthma has been described (Roberts, 1995; Roberts et al., 1997b). A recent study has evaluated perichondrial thickening in patients with asthma and chronic lung diseases and found a correlation with this and the degree of eosinophilia (Haraguchi et al., 1999), which would fit with the previously mentioned studies of TGF-β_1. This study also evaluated the proportion of degenerated cartilage that was increased in airways of asthmatics and chronic bronchitics, and this parameter correlated with the number of neutrophils in the airway. This is of specific interest in light of the findings of increased neutrophils in severe those asthmatics who are refractory to steroid therapy (Wenzel et al., 1997)—consistent with neutrophilic proteases degrading matrix elements and eosinophil TGF-β_1 inducing collagen production.

5.4.4 Matrix-Degrading Enzymes

The major interest in asthma has been the role played by matrix metalloproteases (MMPs) and the tissue inhibitors of MMPs (TIMPs). The regulation of these enzymes, which are secreted as zymogens, is very complex, and it is likely that our measurements of activities provide us with limited information. As a result, some of the data are conflicting. The most striking elevations in MMP-9 (10- to 160-fold increases) were noted in BAL from ventilated subjects with status asthmaticus (Lemjabbar et al., 1999), who also had elevated

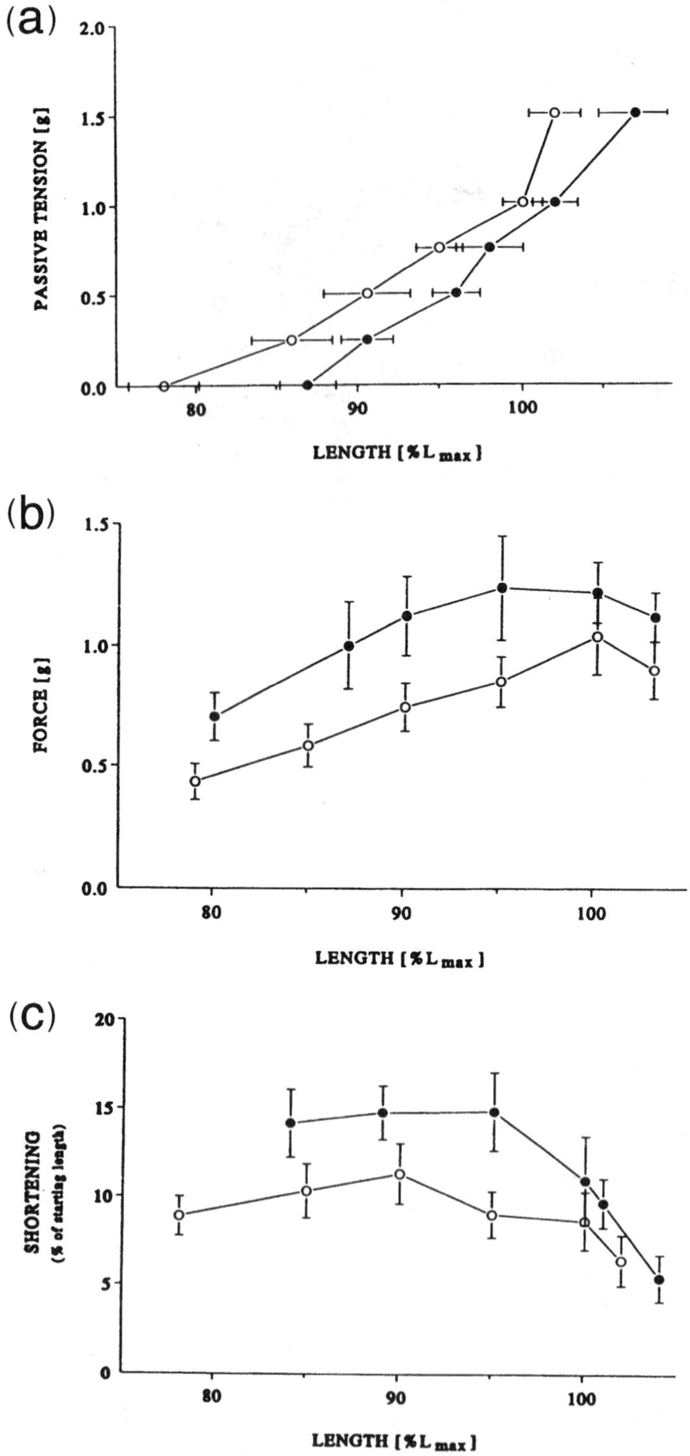

Figure 14 Collagenase treatment of human airway smooth-muscle preparations (closed circles) results in (a) increased length for a given passive tension, (b) increased force generation, and (c) increased shortening, compared with controls (open circles). (From Bramley et al., 1995.)

MMP-3 levels. No increases in these were determined in BAL of mild asthmatics. Another study found higher TIMP-1 levels in untreated asthmatics that correlated with IL-6 levels and numbers of alveolar macrophages (Mautino et al., 1997). Sputum MMP-9/TIMP-1 molar ratios were lower in asthmatics, with a correlation with FEV_1, neutrophils, and macrophages (Vignola et al., 1998c) in one study, and the serum MMP-9/TIMP-1 ratio correlated with a response to oral corticosteroids in a group of severe asthmatics in another (Bosse et al., 1999). These results are consistent with increased antiprotease effects associated with fibrosis, but conflict with a biopsy study that showed increased MMP-9/TIMP-1 relative amounts by image analysis (Hoshino et al., 1998).

These studies highlight the difficulty in determining primary versus secondary events in a pathophysiological process involving simultaneous inflammatory injury and tissue repair. Although most studies have concentrated on the deposition of new collagen as a detrimental component of remodeling (largely because this is a relatively easy parameter to evaluate with bronchial biopsies), the mechanical consequences of this are unknown. The relative contributions of geometric factors, quality of matrix, and structural changes in matrix to increased airway narrowing are as yet difficult to assess.

6 THERAPEUTIC MODULATION OF ECM IN ALLERGIC DISEASE

Inhibition of changes in lung architecture is the key future goal in therapy of inflammatory diseases that cause lung remodeling (Panos, 1994). Future therapeutic strategies include

1. Specific anti-inflammatory agents that would secondarily cause a decrease in the remodeling processes
2. Inhibition of growth factor synthesis, secretion, or biological activity
3. Inhibition of collagen secretion (e.g., colchicine) or assembly (e.g., prolyl hydroxylase inhibitors)
4. Agents that inhibit the expression of collagen genes
5. Agents that inhibit fibroblast proliferation, a process that may require expression or ligation of specific integrins, or the action of proteases.

Alterations in extracellular matrix components in allergic diseases, such as asthma and allergic alveolitis, involve both degradation and new synthesis. Both processes are ongoing simultaneously by the time the disease state is recognized and treatments with agents such as corticosteroids may alter many different elements, some limiting ECM degradation and some limiting repair. The main effect of corticosteroids in chronic inflammatory disease is limiting inflammation—and this can be clearly disease-modifying. For example, studies in bleomycin-induced injury and fibrosis show that corticosteroid treatment reduces the number of macrophages entering the lung, reducing the TGF-β burden with no effect on TGF-β concentration per cell (Khalil et al., 1993). Early intervention with corticosteroids could prevent irreversible changes through such a mechanism. Various approaches that antagonize cytokines and growth factors that are currently under development have the potential to be disease-modifying. These generally target TGF-β or TNF activation, or the biological activity of IL-10. An anticytokine approach directed against IL-4 can also alter fibrosis in an animal model of scleroderma, the Tsk mouse (Ong et al., 1998). If one accepts that the initial injury in allergic disease causing structural changes, is the release of proteolytic enzymes from mast cells and recruited inflammatory cells, then inhibition or release and inhibition of enzymic activities would be important therapeutic goals. Inhibition of protease release by agents inhibiting mast cell mediator release or IgE induction of release is discussed in other chapters in this volume.

Mast cell tryptase has striking effects on the ECM of human airways. In preliminary experiments in our laboratory, the addition of mast cell tryptase to human airway explants leads to a threefold increase in the shortening ability of the smooth muscle, comparable with the changes found in asthmatic tissues. Smaller changes have been reported with shorter incubations with guinea pig tissue (Barrios et al., 1998). Using the selective tryptase inhibitor 1,5-bis-{4-[(3-carbamimidoyl-benzenesulfonylamino)methyl]-phenoxyl}-pentane, Wright et al. (1999a) demonstrated inhibition of allergen-induced early- and late-phase bronchoconstriction, as well as airway hyperresponsiveness in sheep. This inhibitor has more selective activity on tryptase than the naturally produced secretory leukocyte protease inhibitor (SLPI), which is a potent inhibitor of cathepsin G, elastase, chymotrypsin, and trypsin, as well as mast cell tryptase (Wright et al., 1999b). SLPI inhibited antigen-induced responses in sheep and airway hyperresponsiveness induced by antigen in both sheep and guinea pigs (Wright et al., 1999b). Its broader action may be preferable in light of evidence for neutrophil-mediated changes in asthmatic airways. That mast cell tryptase may also influence collagen deposition in airways is suggested by the study by Cairns and Walls (1997) showing that it stimulates collagen synthesis in a fibroblast cell line. Whether this effect is seen in whole airway tissue remains to be determined.

Tumor necrosis factor-α (TNF-α) is synthesized and released from isolated mast cells (Gordon and Galli, 1990) and from alveolar macrophages following antigenic challenge (Gosset et al., 1991). Because TNF-α stimulates the release of numerous proteolytic enzymes from inflammatory cells, it will be interesting to determine if inhibitors of its action, such as the TNF receptor fusion protein (Mohler et al., 1994) or monoclonal chimeric antibody (Brennan et al., 1984), have effects on airway changes leading to hyperresponsiveness. Based on many similarities of ECM alterations in inflammatory arthritic conditions that respond to these therapies (Moreland et al., 1997; Maini et al., 1999) and asthma, these therapeutic agents warrant investigation.

Inhibitors of MMPs may also be of value in limiting the initial injury. Several specific inhibitors have been developed and await testing in animal models and human allergic disease. Although eosinophil transmigration across membranes appears to be dependent on MMP-9, this is not so for basophils or neutrophils. Thus, specific inhibitors of MMP-9 may selectively block eosinophil infiltration, which could be beneficial in allergic disease. However, recent studies with anti-IL-5 suggest that inhibiting eosinophil infiltration does not alter late-phase allergic reactions or airway hyperresponsiveness. Whether preventing eosinophilia decreases collagen deposition (e.g., secondary to TGF-β production) remains to be seen.

Some investigators have suggested that overproduction of TIMPs is the problem leading to fibrotic changes in the airway. Although this possibility cannot be ruled out, it seems likely that increased MMP activity–decreased TIMP activity are a regulated feature of the wound-healing process. MMP inhibitors are in clinical trials as potential therapeutic agents in neoplasia and inflammatory diseases (Marimastat; British Biotechnology). Agents that abrogate inhibitor (TIMP) activity, or enhance MMP activity, although a future possibility, are unlikely to be developed or applied clinically until the hypotheses that MMPs potentiate cancer spread and inflammation are disproved.

β-Adrenergic agonists may modulate ECM as well as inhibit mast cell mediator release. Increasing AMP in fibroblasts down-regulates collagen synthesis induced by

TGF-β by its effect on connective tissue growth factor (Duncan et al., 1999), making it conceivable that long-acting β-agonists have effects on extracellular matrix elements, in addition to the known action on smooth muscle.

It is likely that therapy for remodeling processes in chronic inflammatory lung disease will continue to center on corticosteroids, despite that these affect multiple components of airway inflammation, injury, and repair. More specific agents that antagonize cytokines and growth factors generated in the inflammatory process are in development, as are agents that may have the capacity to repress mesenchymal cell proliferation or matrix synthesis. Long-term suppression of extracellular matrix remodeling will be central to future therapeutic approaches to chronic inflammatory lung diseases.

ACKNOWLEDGMENTS

Work supported by grants from the British Columbia Lung Association, The Medical Research Council of Canada (MT-15171 and MT-8017), and The British Columbia Health Research Foundation. Dr. Clive Roberts is a Medical Research Council of Canada/British Columbia Lung Association Scientist.

REFERENCES

Abraham WM, Sielczak MW, Ahmed A, Cortes A, Lauredo IT, Kim J, Pepinsky B, Benjamin CD, Leone DR, Lobb RR, Weller PF. alpha 4-Integrins mediate antigen-induced late bronchial responses and prolonged airway hyperresponsiveness in sheep. J Clin Invest 93:776–787, 1994.

Adamson IYR, Hedgecock C, Bowden DH. Epithelial cell–fibroblast interactions in lung injury and repair. Am J Pathol 137:385–392, 1990.

Adamson IYR, Young L, King GM. Reciprocal epithelial:fibroblast interactions in the control of fetal and adult rat lung cells in culture. Exp Lung Res 17:821–835, 1991.

Albelda SM. Endothelial and epithelial cell adhesion molecules. Am J Respir Cell Mol Biol 4:195–203, 1995.

Altraja A, Laitinen A, Virtanen I, Kampe M, Simonsson BG, Karlsson S–E, Hakansson L, Venge P, Sillastu H, Laitinen LA. Expression of laminins in various types of asthmatic patients: a morphometric study. Am J Respir Cell Mol Biol 15:482–488, 1996.

Apsberg A, Binkert C, Ruoslahti E. The versican C-terminal lectin domain recognizes the adhesion protein tenascin-R. Proc Natl Acad Sci USA 92:10590–10594, 1995.

Assmann V, Marshall JF, Fieber C, Hoffmann M, Hart IR. The human hyaluronan receptor RHAMM is expressed as an intracellular protein in breast cancer cells. J Cell Sci 111:1685–1694, 1998.

Aubert JD, Dalal BI, Bai TR, Roberts CR, Hayashi S, Hogg JC. Transforming growth factor B1 gene expression in human airways. Thorax 49:225–232, 1994.

Bachhuber BG, Sarembock IJ, Owens GK. alpha-Thrombin induces transforming growth factor beta 1 mRNA and protein in cultured vascular smooth muscle cells via a proteolytically activated receptor. J Vasc Res 34:41, 1997.

Barrios VE, Middleton SC, Kashem MA, Havill AM, Toombs CF, Wright CD. Tryptase mediates hyperresponsiveness in isolated guinea pig bronchi. Life Sci 63:2295–2303, 1998.

Beasley R, Roche WR, Roberts JA, Holgate ST. Cellular events in the bronchi of mild asthma and after bronchial provocation. Am Rev Respir Dis 139:806–817, 1989.

Bedossa P, Houghlum K, Trautwein C, Holstege A, Chojkier M. Stimulation of collagen a1(I) gene expression is associated with lipid peroxidation in hepatocellular injury: a link to tissue fibrosis? Hepatology 19:1262–1271, 1994.

Behzad A, Chu F, Walker DC. Fibroblasts are in a position to provide directional information to migrating neutrophils during pneumonia in rabbit lungs. Microvasc Res 51:303–316, 1996.

Bensadoun ES, Burke AK, Hogg JC, Roberts CR. Proteoglycan deposition in lung fibrosis. Am J Respir Crit Care Med 154:1819–1828, 1996.

Bensadoun ES, Burke AK, Hogg JC, Roberts CR. Proteoglycans in granulomatous lung diseases. Eur Respir J 10:2731–2737, 1997.

Bissell MJ, Hall HG, Parry G. How does the extracellular matrix direct gene expression? J Theor Biol 99:31–68, 1982.

Böck P, Stockinger L. Light and electron microscopic identification of elastic, elaunin and oxytalin fibers in human tracheal and bronchial mucosa. Anat Embryol 170:145–153, 1994.

Bosse M, Chakir J, Rouabhia M, Boulet L–P, Audette M, Laviolette M. Serum matrix metalloproteinase-9:tissue inhibitor of metalloproteinase-1 ratio correlates with steroid responsiveness in moderate to severe asthma. Am J Respir Crit Care Med 159:596–602, 1999.

Boucher RC, Van Scott MR, Willumsen N, Stutts MJ. Epithelial injury. Mechanisms and cell biology of airway epithelial injury. Am Rev Respir Dis 138:S41–S44, 1988.

Boulet LP, Laviolette M, Turcotte H, Cartier A, Dugas M, Malo JL, Boutet M. Bronchial subepitheleial fibrosis correlates with airway responsiveness to methacholine. Chest 112:45:52, 1997.

Bourdoulous S, Orend G, McKenna DA, Pasqualini R, Ruoslahti E. Fibronectin matrix regulates activation of RHO and cdc 42 GTPases and cell cycle progression. J Cell Biol 143:267–276, 1998.

Bousquet J, Lacoste J, Chanez P, Vic P, Godard P, Michel F. Bronchial elastic fibers in normal subjects and asthmatic patients. Am Respir Crit Care Med 153:1648–1653, 1996.

Bramley AM, Roberts CR, Schellenberg RR. Collagenase increases shortening of human bronchial smooth muscle in vitro. Am J Respir Crit Care Med 152:1513–1517, 1995.

Brass DM, Hoyle GW, Poovey HG, Liu JY, Brody AR. Reduced tumor necrosis factor-alpha and transforming growth factor-beta1 expression in the lungs of inbred mice that fail to develop fibroproliferative lesions consequent to asbestos exposure. Am J Pathol 154:853–862, 1999.

Brennan FM, Chantry D, Jackson A, Maini R, Feldmann M. Inhibitory effect of TNFα antibodies on synovial cell interleukin-1 production in rheumatoid arthritis. Lancet 2:244–247, 1989.

Bretschneider E, Kaufmann R, Braun M, Wittpoth M, Glusa E, Nowak G, Schor K. Evidence for proteinase activated receptor-2 (PAR2)-mediated mitogenesis in coronary artery smooth muscle cells. Br J Pharmacol 126:1735–1740, 1999.

Brewster CEP, Howarth PH, Djukanovic R, Wilson J, Holgate ST, Roche WR. Myofibroblasts and subepithelial fibrosis in bronchial asthma. Am J Respir Cell Mol Biol 3:507–511, 1990.

Broekelmann TJ, Limper AH, Colby TV, McDonald JA. Transforming growth factor beta 1 is present at sites of extracellular matrix gene expression in human pulmonary fibrosis. Proc Natl Acad Sci USA 88:6642–6646, 1991.

Busse W, Elias J, Sheppard D, Banks–Schlegel S. Airway remodeling and repair. Am J Respir Crit Care Med. 160:1035–1042, 1999.

Cairns JA, Walls AF. Mast cell tryptase stimulates the synthesis of type I collagen in human lung fibroblasts. J Clin Invest 99:1313–1321, 1997.

Cantin AM, North SL, Fells GA, Hubbard RC, Crystal RG. Oxidant-mediated epithelial cell injury in idiopathic pulmonary fibrosis. J Clin Invest 79:1665, 1987.

Carroll N, Elliot J, Morton A, James A. The structure of large and small airways in nonfatal and fatal asthma. Am Rev Respir Dis 147:405–410, 1993.

Champion BR, Poole AR. Immunity to homologous cartilage proteoglycans in rabbits with chronic inflammatory arthritis. Coll Related Res 1:453–473, 1981.

Chapman HA, Allen CL, Stone OL. Abnormalities in pathways of alveolar fibrin turnover among patients with interstitial lung disease. Am Rev Respir Dis 133:437–444, 1986.

Chetta A, Foresi A, Donno D, Bertorelli G, Pesci A, Olivieri D. Airway remodeling is a distinctive feature of asthma and is related to severity of asthma. Chest 111:852–857, 1997.

Cho SH, Seo JY, Choi DC, et al. Pathological changes according to the severity of asthma. Clin Exp Allergy 26:1210–1219, 1996.

Chu HWC, Halliday JL, Martin RJ, Leung DYM, Szefler SJ, Wenzel SE. Collagen deposition in large airways may not differentiate severe asthma from milder forms of the disease. Am J Respir Crit Care Med 158:1936–1944, 1998.

Cohen P, Bhala A, Herrick D, Noveral J, Grunstein M. The effects of leukotriene D_4 on the proliferation of airway smooth muscle cells are mediated by modulation of the IGF axis. Am J Physiol 269:L151–L157, 1995.

Cotta–Pereira G, Rodrigo FG, Bittencourt–Sampaio S. Oxytalin, elaunin and elastic fibers in the human skin. J Invest Dermatol 66:143–148, 1976.

Cotta–Pereira G, Rodrigo FG, David–Ferreira JF. The elastic system fibers. In: Sandberg LB, Gray WR, Franzblau C, eds. International Conference on Elastin and Elastic Tissue, Alta, Utah, 1977:19–33.

Crystal RG. Pulmonary fibrosis. In: Crystal RG, West JB, Weibel ER, Barnes PJ, eds. The Lung: Scientific Foundations. 2nd ed. Philadelphia: Lippincott–Raven, 1997.

Damiano VV, Cohen A, Tsang Z, Batra B, Petersen R. A morphologic study of the influx of neutrophils into dog lung alveoli after lavage with sterile saline. Am J Pathol 100:349–364, 1980.

Desmouliere A, Redard M, Darby I, Gabbiani G. Apoptosis mediates the decrease in cellularity during the transition between granulation tissue and scar. Am J Pathol 146:56–66, 1995.

Dube J, Chakir J, Laviolette M, Saint Martin S, Boutet M, Desrochers C, Auger F. Fibroblasts from normal and asthmatic subjects. Lab Invest 78:297–307, 1998.

Duncan MR, Frazier KS, Abramson S, William HK, Huang X, Grotendorst GR. Connective tissue growth factor mediates transforming growth factor β-induced collagen synthesis: down-regulation by cAMP. FASEB J 13:1774–1786, 1999.

Dunnill MS. The pathology of asthma with special reference to changes in the bronchial mucosa. J Clin Pathol 13:27–33, 1960.

Dunnill MS, Massarella GR, Anderson JA. A comparison of the quantitative anatomy of the bronchi in normal subjects, in status asthmaticus, in chronic bronchitis and in emphysema. Thorax 24: 176–179, 1969.

Ebina M, Takahashi T, Chiba T, Motomiya M. Cellular hypertrophy and hyperplasia of airway smooth muscles underlying bronchial asthma. A 3D morphometric study. Am Rev Respir Dis 48:720–726, 1993.

Erickson HP, Bourdon MA: Tenascin: an extracellular matrix protein prominent in specialized embryonic tissues and tumours. Annu Rev Cell Biol 5:71–92, 1989.

Erjefält JS, Erjefält I, Sundler F, Persson CGA. In vivo restitution. Medicine 154:749–757, 1995.

Evans MJ, Guha SC, Cox RA, Moller PC. Attenuated fibroblast sheath around the basement membrane zone in the trachea. Am J Respir Cell Mol Biol 8:188–192, 1993.

Fahrenbach WH, Sandberg LB, Cleary EC. Ultrastructural studies on early elastogenesis. Anat Rec 155:563–576, 1966.

Fine J–D. Structure and antigenicity of the skin basement membrane zone. J Cutan Pathol 18:401–409, 1991.

Fish JE, Peters SP. Airway remodeling and persistent airway obstruction in asthma. J Allergy Clin Immunol 104:509–516, 1999.

Fraser RG, Pare JA, Pare PD, Fraser RS, Genereux GP. Diagnosis of Diseases of the Lung. 3rd ed. Philadelphia: WB Saunders, 1991.

Frisch SM, Ruoslahti E. Integrins and anoikis. Curr Opin Cell Biol 9:701–706, 1997.

Fukuda Y, Basset F, Ferrans VJ, Yamanaka N. Significance of early intra-alveolar fibrotic lesions and integrin expression in lung biopsy specimens from patients with idiopathic pulmonary fibrosis. Hum Pathol 26:53–61, 1995.

Gabbiani G, Hirschel, BJ, Ryan GB, Statkov PR, Maino G. Granulation tissue as a contractile organ. A study of structure and function. J Exp Med 135:719–734, 1972.

Gavreau GM, O'Byrne PM, Moqbel R, Velazquez J, Watson RM, Howie KJ, Denburg JA. Enhanced expression of GM-CSF in differentiating eosinophils of atopic and atopic asthmatic subjects. Am J Respir Cell Mol Biol 19:55–62, 1998.

Gawlik Z. Morphological and morphochemical properties of the elastic system in the motor organ of man. Folia Histochem Cytochem 3:223–251, 1965.

Giancotti FG, Ruoslahti E. Integrin signalling. Science 285:1028–1032, 1999.

Glant TT, Mikecz K, Arzoumanian A, Poole AR. Proteoglycan-induced arthritis in BALB/c mice. Clinical features and histopathology. Arthritis Rheum 30:201–212, 1987.

Godfrey RWA, Lorimer S, Majumdar S, Adelroth E, Johnston PW, Rogers AV, Johansson SA, Jeffery PK. Airway and lung elastic fiber is not reduced in asthma nor in asthmatics following corticosteroid treatment. Eur Respir J 8:922–927, 1995.

Gordon JR, Galli SJ. Mast cells as source of both preformed and immunologically inducible TNFα/cachectin. Nature 346:274–276, 1990.

Gosset P, Tsicopoulos A, Wallaert B, et al. Increased secretion of tumor necrosis factor α and interleukin-6 by alveolar macrophages consecutively to the late asthmatic reaction after bronchial allergen challenge. J Allergy Clin Immunol 88:561–571, 1991.

Greenlee TK, Ross R, Hartman JL. The fine structure of elastic fibers. J Cell Biol 30:59–71, 1966.

Guerassimov A, Zhang Y, Cartman A, Rosenberg LC, Esdaile J, Fitzcharles MA, Poole AR. Immune responses to cartilage link protein and the G1 domain of proteoglycan aggrecan in patients with osteoarthritis. Arthritis Rheum 42:527–533, 1999.

Halayko AJ, Rector E, Stephens NL. Characterization of molecular determinants of smooth muscle cell heterogeneity. Can J Physiol Pharmacol 75:917–929, 1997.

Halayko AJ, Salari H, Ma X, Stephens NL. Markers of airway smooth muscle phenotype. Am J Physiol 270:L1040–L1051, 1996.

Haraguchi M, Shimura S, Shirato K. Morphometric analysis of bronchial cartilage in chronic obstructive pulmonary disease and bronchial asthma. Am J Respir Crit Care Med 159:1005–1013, 1999.

Hatschek WM, Witschi HP. Pulmonary fibrosis—a possible mechanism. Toxicol Appl Pharmacol 51:475–487, 1979.

Hautmann MB, Madsen Cort S, Owens GK. A transforming growth factor beta (TGF beta) control element drives TGF beta-induced stimulation of smooth muscle actin-gene expression in concert with two CArG elements J Biol Chem 272:10948, 1997.

Heard BE, Hossain S. Hyperplasia of bronchial muscle in asthma. J Pathol 110:319–331, 1973.

Herard A–L, Pierrot D, Hinnrasky J, Kaplan H, Sheppard D, Puchelle E, Zahm J–M. Fibronectin and its α5β1-integrin receptor are involved in the wound-repair process of airway epithelium. Am J Physiol 271:L726–L733, 1996.

Hoffmann M, Fieber C, Assmann V, Gottlicher M, Sleeman J, Plug R, Howells N, von Stein O, Ponta H, Herrlich P. Identification of HABP, a 95 kDa intracellular hyaluronate binding protein. J Cell Sci 111:1673–1684, 1998.

Hojo M, Maghni K, Issekutz TB, Martin JG. Involvement of a-4 integrins in allergic airway responses and mast cell degranulation in vivo. Am J Respir Crit Care Med 158:1127–1133, 1998.

Hollister DW, Godfrey M, Sakai LY, Pyeritz RE. Immunohistologic abnormalities of microfibrillar fiber system in the Marfan syndrome. N Engl J Med 323:152–159, 1990.

Hoshino M, Nakamura Y, Sim J–J, Shimojo J, Isogai S. Bronchial subepithelial fibrosis and expression of matrix metalloproteinase-9 in asthmatic airway inflammation. J Allergy Clin Immunol 102:783–788, 1998.

Hoshino M, Nakamura Y, Sim JJ. Expression of growth factors and remodelling of the airway wall in bronchial asthma. Thorax 53:21–27, 1998.

Hossain S. Quantitative measurement of bronchial muscle in men with asthma. Am Rev Respir Dis 107:99–109, 1973.

Huang J, Olivenstein R, Taha R, Hamid Q, Ludwig M. Enhanced proteoglycan deposition in the airway wall of atopic asthmatics. Am J Respir Crit Care Med 160:725–729, 1999.

Huber HL, Koessler KK. The pathology of bronchial asthma. Arch Intern Med 30:689–760, 1922.

Iozzo RV. Matrix proteoglycans: from molecular design to cellular function. Annu Rev Biochem 67:609–652, 1998.

Isogai Z, Shinomura T, Yamakawa N, Takeuchi J, Tsuji T, Heinegard D, Kimata K. 2B1 Antigen characteristically expressed on extracellular matrices of human malignant tumours is a large chondroitin sulfate proteoglycan, PG-M/versican. Cancer Res 56:3902–3908, 1996.

Jeffrey PK, Godfrey RW, Adelroth E, Nelson F, Johansson SA. Effects of treatment on airway inflammation and thickening of the basement membrane reticular collagen in asthma: a quantitative and electron microscopic study. Am Rev Respir Dis 145:890–899, 1992.

Jeffrey PK, Wardlaw AJ, Nelson FC, Collins JV, Kay AB. Bronchial biopsies in asthma: an ultrastructural, quantitative study and correlation with hyperactivity. Am Rev Respir Dis 140:1745–1753, 1989.

Jones AW, Barson AJ. Elastogenesis in the developing chick lung: a light and electron microscopical study. J Anat 110:1–15, 1971.

Junqueira LCU, Montes GS, Martins JEC, Joazeiro PP. Dermal collagen, distribution. A histochemical and ultrastructural study. Histochemistry 79:397–403, 1983.

Karlinsky JB, Goldstein RH. Regulation of sulfated glycosaminoglycan production by prostaglandin E_2 in cultured lung. J Lab Clin Med 114:176–184, 1989.

Kawanami O, Ferrans VJ, Crystal RG. Anchoring fibrils in the normal canine respiratory system. Am Rev Respir Dis 120:595–611, 1979.

Khalil N, O'Connor RN, Unruh HW, Warren PW, Flanders KC, Kemp A, Bereznay OH, Greenberg AH. Increased production and immunohistochemical localization of transforming growth factor-beta in idiopathic pulmonary fibrosis. Am J Respir Cell Mol Biol 5:155–162, 1991.

Khalil N, Whitman C, Zuo L, Danielpour D, Greenberg A. Regulation of macrophage transforming growth factor beta secretion by corticosteroids in bleomycin-induced pulmonary inflammation in the rat. J Clin Invest 92:1812–1818, 1993.

Khalil N, Corne S, Whitman C, Yacyshyn H. Plasmin regulates the activation of cell-associated latent transforming growth factor-beta 1 secreted by rat alveolar macrophages after in vivo bleomycin injury. Am J Respir Cell Mol Biol 15:252–260, 1996.

Knight DA, Stewart GA, Thompson PJ. The respiratory epithelium and airway smooth muscle homeostasis: its relevance to asthma. Clin Exp Allergy 24:698–706, 1994.

Komuro T, Hashimoto Y. Three-dimensional structure of the rat intestinal wall (mucosa and submucosa). Arch Histol Cytol 53:1–21, 1990.

Kuhn C, Mason RJ. Immunolocalization of SPARC, tenascin and thrombospondin in pulmonary fibrosis. Am J Pathol 147:1759–1769, 1995.

Kuhn C, McDonald JA. The roles of the myofibroblast in idiopathic pulmonary fibrosis. Ultrastructural and immunohistochemical features of sites of active extracellular matrix synthesis. Am J Pathol 138:1257–1265, 1991.

Kuhn C, Boldt J, King TE Jr, Crouch E, Vartio T, McDonald JE. An immunohistochemical study of architectural remodeling and connective tissue synthesis in pulmonary fibrosis. Am Rev Respir Dis 140:1693–1703, 1989.

Kuwano K, Bosken CH, Pare PD, Bai TR, Wiggs BR, Hogg JC. Small airways dimensions in asthma and in chronic obstructive pulmonary disease. Am Rev Respir Dis 148:1220–1225, 1993.

Laberge S, Rabb H, Issekutz TB, Martin JG. The role of VLA-4 and LFA-1 in allergen-induced airway hyperresponsiveness and lung inflammation in the rat. Am J Respir Crit Care Med 151: 822–829, 1995.

Laitinen A, Altaja A, Kampe M, Linden M, Virtanen I, Laitinen LA. Tenascin is increased in airway basement membrane of asthmatics and decreased by an inhaled steroid. Am J Respir Crit Care Med 156:951–958, 1997.

Laitinen LA, Heino W, Laitinen A, Kava T, Haahtela T. Damage of the airway epithelium and bronchial reactivity in patients with asthma. Am Rev Respir Dis 131:599–606, 1985.

Laurie GW, Leblond CP. What is known of the production of basement membrane components. J Histochem Cytochem 31:159–163, 1983.

Laurie GW, Rada JA, Chakravarti S, Hassell JR. Perlecan. In: Kreis T, Vale R, eds. Guidebook to the Extracellular Matrix and Adhesion Proteins. Oxford University Press, Oxford, 1993:35–37.

Lee EY, Parry G, Bissell MJ. Modulation of secreted proteins of mouse mammary epithelial cells by the collagenous substrata. J Cell Biol 98:146–155, 1984.

Leick–Maldonado EA, Lemos M. Differential distribution of elastic system fibers in control and bronchoconstricted intraparenchymatous airways in the guinea-pig lung. J Submicrosc Cytol Pathol 29:427–434, 1997.

Lemjabbar H, Gosset P, Lamblin C, Tillie I, Hartmann D, Wallaert B, Tonnel AB, Lafuma C. Contribution of 92 kDa gelatinase/type IV collagenase in bronchial inflammation during status asthmaticus. Am J Respir Crit Care Med 159:1298–1307, 1999.

Lesley J, Hyman R, Kincade PW. CD44 and its interaction with extracellular matrix. Adv Immunol 54:271–335, 1993.

Limper AH, Broekelmann TJ, Colby TV, Malizia G, McDonald JA. Analysis of local mRNA expression for extracellular matrix proteins and growth factors using in situ hybridization in fibroproliferative lung disorders. Chest 99:55S–56S, 1991.

Liu JY, Morris GF, Lei WH, Hart CE, Lasky JA, Brody AR. Rapid activation of PDGF-A and -B expression at sites of lung injury in asbestos-exposed rats. Am J Respir Cell Mol Biol 17:129–140, 1997.

Loewen DAJ, Pare PD, Schellenberg RR. Prolonged effects of epithelial injury and repair on the mechanical properties and proliferation of airway smooth muscle (ASM). Am J Respir Crit Care Med 155:A369, 1997.

Lundgren R, Soberberg M, Herstedt P, Stenling R. Morphological studies on bronchial mucosal biopsies from asthmatics before and after ten years treatment with inhaled corticosteroids in asthma. Eur Respir J 1:883–889, 1988.

MacDonell SD, Chu FSF, Walker DC. The role of fibroblasts in eosinophil and neutrophil migration through the conducting airway interstitium. FASEB J 12:A180, 1998.

Macklin CC. A note on the elastic membrane of the bronchial tree of mammals, with an interpretation of its functional significance. Anat Rec 24:119–135, 1922.

Maini R, St Clair EW, Breedveld E, et al. Infliximab (chimeric anti-tumor necrosis factor α monoclonal antibody) versus placebo in rheumatoid arthritis patients receiving concomitant methotrexate: a randomized phase III trial. Lancet 354:1932–1939, 1999.

Martinet Y, Rom WN, Grotendorst GR, Martin GR, Crystal RG. Exaggerated spontaneous release of platelet-derived growth factor by alveolar macrophages from patients with idiopathic pulmonary fibrosis. N Engl J Med 317:202–209, 1987.

Mauad T, Xavier ACG, Saldiva PHN, Dolhnikoff M. Elastosis and fragmentation of fibers of the elastic system in fatal asthma. Am J Respir Crit Care Med 160:968–975, 1999.

Mautino G, Oliver N, Chanez P, Bousquet J, Capony F. Increased release of matrix metalloproteinase-9 in bronchoalveolar lavage fluid and by alveolar macrophages of asthmatics. Am J Respir Cell Mol Biol 17:583–592, 1997.

McCourt PA, Ek B, Forsberg N, Gustavso S. Intercellular adhesion molecule-1 is a cell surface receptor for hyaluronan. J Biol Chem 269:30081–30084, 1994.

McDonald JA. Idiopathic pulmonary fibrosis. A paradigm for lung injury and repair. Chest 99:87S–93S, 1991.

McDonald JA. The yin and yang of fibrin in the airways [editorial; comment]. N Engl J Med 322:929–931, 1990.

Meiss RA. Influence of intercellular tissue connections on airway muscle mechanics. J Appl Physiol 86:5–15, 1999.

Mercer RR, Crapo JD. Spatial distribution of collagen and elastin fibers in the lungs. J Appl Physiol 69:756–765, 1990.

Miller WS. The Lung. Springfield, IL: Charles C Thomas, 1937:222.

Minshall EM, Leung DYM, Martin RJ, Song YL, Cameron L, Ernst P, Hamid Q. Eosinophil-associated TGF-B1 mRNA expression and airways fibrosis in bronchial asthma. Am J Respir Cell Mol Biol 17:326–333, 1997.

Mohler KM, Sleath PR, Fitzner JN, Cerretti DP, Alderson M, Kerwar SS, Torrance DS, Otten-Evans C, Greenstreet T, Weerawarna K. Protection against a lethal dose of endotoxin by an inhibitor of tumor necrosis factor processing. Nature 370(6486):218–220, 1994.

Montes GS, Bezerra MSF, Junqueira LCU. Collagen distribution in tissues. In: Ruggeri A, Motta PM, eds. Ultrastructure of the Connective Tissue Matrix. Boston: Martinus Nijhoff 1984:65–88.

Montes GS. Distribution of oxytalan, elaunin and elastic fibres in tissues. J Brazil Assoc Adv Sci 44:224–233, 1992.

Montes GS, Krisztan RM, Shigihara KM, Tokoro R, Mourao PAS, Junqueira LCU. Histochemical and morphological characterization of reticular fibers. Histochemistry 65:131–141, 1980.

Moreland LW, Baumgartner SW, Schiff MH, et al. Treatment of rheumatoid arthritis with a recombinant human tumor necrosis factor receptor (p75)–Fc fusion protein. N Engl J Med 337:141–147, 1997.

Morris GF, Liu JY, Lei WH, Brody AR. Expression of genes coding for growth factors in experimental pneumoconiosis. Chest 109(3 suppl):45S–49S, 1996.

Munger JS, Huang X, Kawakatsu H, Griffiths MJD, Dalton SL, Wu J, Pittet J–F, Kaminski N, Garat C, Mathay MA, Rifkin DB, Sheppard, D. The integrin αVβ6 binds and activates latent TGFB1: a mechanism for regulating pulmonary inflammation and fibrosis. Cell 96:319–328, 1999.

Murdoch AD, Dodge GR, Cohen I, Tuan RS, Iozzo RV. Primary structure of the human heparan sulfate proteoglycan from basement membrane. J Biol Chem 267:8544–8557, 1992.

Naylor B. The shedding of the mucosa of the bronchial tree in asthma. Thorax 17:69–72, 1962.

Ohno I, Lea RG, Flanders KC, Clark DA, Banwatt D, Dolovich J, Denburg J, Harley CB, Gauldie J, Jordana M. Eosinophils in chronically inflamed airway tissues express transforming growth factor B1 gene (TGF-B1). J Clin Invest 89:1662–1668, 1992.

Ollerenshaw SL, Woolcock AJ. Characteristics of the inflammation in biopsies from large airways of subjects with asthma and subjects with chronic airflow limitation. Am Rev Respir Dis 145: 922–927, 1992.

Olsen BR, Ninomiya Y. Basement membrane collagens (type IV). In: Kreis T, Vale R, eds. Guidebook to the Extracellular Matrix and Adhesion Proteins. Oxford University Press, Oxford, 1993: 32–48.

Ong C, Wong C, Roberts CR, Teh H–S, Jirik FR. Anti-interleukin 4 treatment prevents progression of dermal fibrosis in the tight-skin mouse model of scleroderma. Eur J Immunol 28:2619–2629, 1998.

Palacek SP, Loftus JC, Ginsberg MH, Lauffenberger DA, Horwitz AF. Integrin–ligand binding properties govern cell migration speed through cell–substratum adhesiveness. Nature 385:537–540, 1997 (erratum 388:210, 1997).

Panettieri RA, Grunstein MM. Airway smooth muscle hyperplasia and hypertrophy. In: Barnes PJ, Grunstein MM, Leff AR, Woolcock AJ, eds. Asthma. New York: Lippincott-Raven 1997:823–842.

Panettieri RA, Kotlikoff MI. Cellular and molecular mechanisms regulating airway smooth muscle cell physiology and pharmacology. In: Fishman AP, Elias JA, Fishman JA, Grippi MA, Kaiser LR, Senior RM, eds. Fishman's Pulmonary Diseases and Disorders. 3rd ed. New York: McGraw-Hill, 1998:107–117.

Panos RJ. Therapy and management of idiopathic pulmonary fibrosis. Comp Ther 20:289–293, 1994.

Papakonstantinou E, Karakiulakis G, Roth M, Block LH. Platelet-derived growth factor stimulates secretion of hyaluronic acid by proliferating human vascular smooth muscle cells. Proc Natl Acad Sci USA 92:9881–9885, 1995.

Parker FG, Barnes EV, Kaye GI. The pericryptal fibroblast sheath IV. Replication, migration and differentiation of the subepithelial fibroblasts of the crypt and villus of the rabbit jejunum. Gastroenterology 67: 607–621, 1974.

Pierce JA, Ebert RV. Fibrous network of the lung and its change with age. Thorax 20:469–476, 1965.

Pilewski JM, Latoche JD, Arcasoy SM, Albelda SM. Expression of integrin cell adhesion receptors during human airway epithelial repair in vivo. Am J Physiol 273:L256–L263, 1997.

Pretolani M, Ruffie C, Lapa e Silva JR, Joseph D, Lobb RR, Vargafting BB. Antibody to very late antigen 4 prevents antigen- induced bronchial hyperreactivity and cellular infiltration in the guinea pig airways. J Exp Med 180:795–805, 1994.

Prockop DJ. Marrow stromal cells as stem cells for nonhematopoietic tissues. Science 276:71–73, 1997.

Rabb HA, Olivenstein R, Issekutz TB, Renzi PM, Martin JG. The role of leukocyte adhesion molecules VLA-4, LFA-1, and Mac-1 in allergic airway responses in the rat. Am J Respir Crit Care Med 149:1186–1191, 1994.

Raghu G, Striker LJ, Hudson LD, Striker GE. Extracellular matrix in normal and fibrotic human lungs. Am Rev Respir Dis 131:281–289, 1985.

Rajah R, Nachajon RV, Collins MH, Hakonarson H, Grunstein MM, Cohen P. Elevated levels of the IGF-binding protein protease MMP-1 in asthmatic airway smooth muscle. Am J Respir Cell Mol Biol 20:199–208, 1999.

Rajah R, Nunn S, Herrick D, Grunstein MM, Cohen P. LTD-4 induces matrix metalloproteinase-1 which functions as an IGFBP protease in airway smooth muscle cells. Am J Physiol 271: L1014–L1022, 1996.

Rhodin JAG. Histology, a Text and Atlas. New York: Oxford University Press. 1974:803.

Roberts CR. Is asthma a fibrotic disease? Chest 107:111S–117S, 1995.

Roberts CR, and Burke AK. Synthesis of the proteoglycan versican in pulmonary fibrosis. Int J Exp Pathol 81:A21, 2000.

Roberts CR, Wight TN, Hascall VC. Proteoglycans in the lung. In: Crystal RG, West JB, Weibel ER, Barnes PJ. eds. The Lung: Scientific Foundations. 2nd ed. Philadelphia: Lippincott–Raven, 1997a:757–767.

Roberts CR, Okazawa M, Wiggs BR, Pare PD. Airway wall thickening. In: Barnes PJ, Grunstein MM, Leff AR, Woolcock AJ, eds. Asthma. Philadelphia: Lippincott–Raven, 1997b:925–935.

Roche WR, Beasley R, Williams JH, Holgate ST. Sub-epithelial fibrosis in the bronchi of asthmatics. Lancet 1:520–524, 1989.

Rochester CL, Elias JA. Semin Respir Med 14:389–416, 1993.

Ross R, Raines EW, Bowen–Pope DF. The biology of platelet-derived growth factor. Cell 46:155–169, 1986.

Ross R. Wound healing. Sci Am 220:40–50, 1969.

Ruoslahti E. RGD and other recognition sequences for integrins. Annu Rev Cell Dev Biol 12:697–715, 1996.

Ryan GB, Cliff WJ, Gabbiani G, Irle C, Montandon D, Statkov PR, Majno G. Myofibroblasts in human granulation tissue. Hum Pathol 5:55–67, 1974.

Sage H. Collagens of basement membranes. J Invest Dermatol 79:51–59, 1982.

Sakai LY, Keene DR, Engvall E. Fibrillin, a new 350 kDa glycoprotein is a component of extracellular microfibrils. J Cell Biol 103:2499–2509, 1986.

Sampson PM, Rochester CL, Freundlich B, Elias J. Cytokine regulation of human lung fibroblast hyaluronan (hyaluronic acid) production. Evidence for cytokine-regulated hyaluronan (hyaluronic acid) degradation and human lung fibroblast-derived hyaluronidase. J Clin Invest 90: 1492–1503, 1992.

Schonherr E, Jarvelainen HT, Sandell LJ, Wight TN. Effects of platelet-derived growth factor and transforming growth factor-beta 1 on the synthesis of a large versican-like chondroitin sulfate proteoglycan by arterial smooth muscle cells. J Biol Chem 266:17640–17647, 1991.

Schultz–Cherry S, Chen H, Mosher DF, Misenheimer TM, Krutzsch HC, Roberts DD, Murphy–Ullirch JE. Regulation of transforming growth factor-beta activation by discrete sequences of thrombospondin 1. J Biol Chem 270:7304–7310, 1995.

Scott PG. Macromolecular constituents of basement membranes: a review of current knowledge on their structure and function. Can J Biochem Cell Biol 61:942–948, 1983.

Shaver JR, Zangrilli JG, Cho S–K, Cirelli RA, Pollice M, Hastie AT, Fish JE, Peters SP. Kinetics of the development and recovery of the lung from IgE-mediated inflammation: dissociation of pulmonary eosinophilia, lung injury, and eosinophil-active cytokines. Am J Respir Crit Care Med 155:442–448, 1997.

Shinomura T, Jensen K, Yamagata M, Kimata K, Solursh M. The distribution of mesenchyme proteoglycan (PG-M) during wing bud outgrowth. Anat Embryol 181:227–233, 1990.

Sousa AR, Poston RN, Lane SJ, Nakhosteen JA, Lee TH. Detection of GM-CSF in asthmatic bronchial epithelium and decrease by inhaled corticosteroids. Am Rev Respir Dis 147:1557–1561, 1993.

Soyombo AA, DiCorleto PE. Stable expression of platelet derived growth factor b chain by bovine aortic endothelial cells. Matrix association and selective proteolytic cleavage by thrombin. J Biol Chem 269:17734–17740, 1994.

Spina D. Epithelium-dependent regulation of airways smooth muscle tone. In: Raeburn D, Giembycz MA, eds. Airway Smooth Muscle: Development and Regulation of Contractility. Basel: Birkhauser-Verlag, 1994:259–289.

Sundberg C, Ivarrson, M, Gerdin B, Rubin K. Pericytes as collagen-producing cells in excessive dermal scarring. Lab Invest 74:452–466, 1996.

Svee K, White J, Vaillant P, Jessurun J, Roongta U, Krumwiede M, Johnson D, Henke C. Acute lung injury fibroblast migration and invasion of a fibrin matrix is mediated by CD44. J Clin Invest 98:1713–1727, 1996.

Thomson RJ, Bramley AM, Schellenberg RR. Airway muscle stereology: implications for increased shortening in asthma. Am J Respir Crit Care Med 154:749–757, 1996.

Tremble P, Chiquet–Ehrismann R, Werb Z. The extracellular matrix ligands fibronectin and tenascin collaborate in regulating collagenase gene expression in fibroblasts. Mol Biol Cell 5:439–453, 1994.

Turley EA. Hyaluronic acid stimulates protein kinase activity in intact cells and in an isolated protein complex. J Biol Chem 264:8951–8955, 1989.

Vaccaro CA, Brody JS. Structural features of alveolar wall basement membrane in the adult rat lung. J Cell Biol 91:427–438, 1981.

van der Rest M, Garrone R. Collagen family of proteins. FASEB J 5:2814–2823, 1991.

Vignola AM, Chanez P, Chiappara G, Gagliardo R, Bonsignore G, Bousquet J. Growth factors in the remodeling of asthma. Allergy Clin Immunol Int 10:149–153, 1998a.

Vignola AM, Bonanno A, Mirabella A, Riccobono L, Mirabella F, Profita M, Bellia V, Bousquet J, Bonsignore G. Increased levels of elastase and α_1-antitrypsin in sputum of asthmatic patients. Am J Respir Crit Care Med 157:505–511, 1998b.

Vignola AM, Riccobono L, Mirabella A, Profita M, Chanez P, Bellia V, Mautino G, D'Accardi P, Bousquet J, Bonsignore G. Sputum metalloproteinase-9/tissue inhibitor of metalloproteinase-1 ratio correlates with airflow obstruction in asthma and chronic bronchitis. Am J Respir Crit Care Med 158:1945–1950, 1998c.

Vracko R. Significance of basal lamina for regeneration of injured lung. Virchows Arch A Pathol Anat 355:264–274, 1972.

Walker DC, Behzad AR, Chu F. Neutrophil migration through pre-existing holes in the basal laminae of alveolar capillaries and epithelium during streptococcal pneumonia. Microvasc Res 50:397–416, 1995.

Wasano K, Yamamoto T. Microthread-like filaments connecting the epithelial basal lamina with underlying fibrillar components of the connective tissue in the rat trachea. Cell Tissue Res 239: 485–495, 1985.

Wenzel SE, Schwarz LB, Langmack EL, Halliday JL, Trudeau JB, Gibbs RL, Chu HW. Evidence that severe asthma can be divided pathologically into two inflammatory subtypes with distinct physiologic and clinical characteristics. Am J Respir Crit Care Med 160:1001–1008, 1999.

Wenzel SE, Szefler SJ, Leung DYM, Sloan SI, Rex MD, Martin RJ. Bronchoscopic evaluation of severe asthma: persistent inflammation associated with high dose glucocorticoids. Am J Respir Crit Care Med 156:737–743, 1997.

Westergren–Thorsson G, Sarnstrand B, Fransson LA, Malmstrom A. TGF-beta enhances the production of hyaluronan in human lung but not in skin fibroblasts. Exp Cell Res 186:192–195, 1990.

White SR, Dorsheid DR, Rabe KF, Wojcik KR, Hamann KJ. Role of very late adhesion integrins in mediating repair of human airway epithelial cell monolayers after mechanical injury. Am J Respir Cell Mol Biol 20:787–796, 1999.

Wilson JW, Li X. The measurement of reticular basement membrane and submucosal collagen in the asthmatic airway. Clin Exp Allergy 27:363–371, 1997.

Wright CD, Havill AM, Middleton SC, Kashem MA, Dripps DJ, Abraham WM, Thomson DS, Burgess LE. Inhibition of allergen-induced pulmonary responses by the selective tryptase inhibitor 1,5-bis {4-[(3-carbamimidoyl-benzenesulfonylamino)-methyl]-phenoxyl-pentane (AMG-126737). Biochem Pharmacol 58:1989–1996, 1999a.

Wright CD, Havill AM, Middleton SC, Kashem MA, Lee PA, Dripps DJ, O'Riordan TG, Bevilacqua MP, Abraham WM. Secretory leukocyte protease inhibitor prevents allergen-induced pulmonary responses in animal models of asthma. J Pharmacol Exp Ther 289:1007–1014, 1999b.

Wright RR. Elastic tissue of normal and emphysematous lungs. Am J Pathol 39:355–363, 1961.

Xing Z, Ohkawara Y, Jordana M, Graham F, Gauldie J. Transfer of granulocyte–macrophage colony-stimulating factor gene to rat lung induces eosinophilia, monocytosis, and fibrotic reactions. J Clin Invest 97:1102–1110, 1996.

Yamada KM. Fibronectin. In: Hay ED, ed. Cell Biology of Extracellular Matrix. New York: Plenum, 1991.

Yamagata M, Yamada KM, Suzuki S, Kimata K. Chondroitin sulfate proteoglycan (PG-M-like proteoglycan) is involved in the binding of hyaluronic acid to cellular fibronectin. J Biol Chem 261:13526–13535, 1986.

Yang B, Yang BL, Savani RC, Turley EA. Identification of a common hyaluronan binding motif in the hyaluronan binding proteins RHAMM, CD44 and link protein. EMBO J 13:286–296, 1994.

Yayon A, Klagsbrun M, Esko JD, Leder P, Ornitz D. Cell surface heparin-like molecules are required for binding basic fibroblast growth factor to its high affinity receptor. Cell 64:841–848, 1991.

Yeo T–K, Brown L, Dvorak HF. Alterations in proteoglycan synthesis common to healing wounds and tumours. Am J Pathol 138:1437–1450, 1991.

Yokosaki Y, Palmer EL, Prieto AL, Crossin KL, Bourdon MA, Pytela R, Sheppard D. The integrin alpha 9 beta 1 mediates cell attachment to a non RGD site in the third fibronectin type III repeat of tenascin. J Biol Chem 269:26691–26696, 1994.

Yurchenko PD, Ruben GC. Basement membrane structure in situ: evidence for lateral associations in the type IV collagen network. J Cell Biol 105:2559–2568, 1987.

Zhang K, Rehkter MD, Gordon D, Phan SH. Myofibroblasts and their role in lung collagen gene expression during pulmonary fibrosis—a combined immunohistochemical and in situ hybridization study. Am J Pathol 145:114–125, 1994.

8

The Regulation of IgE Synthesis

DONATA VERCELLI

University of Arizona, Tucson, Arizona

1 INTRODUCTION

Immunoglobulin (Ig) E plays a key role in the pathogenesis of asthma and allergy, diseases that affect a considerable proportion of the population worldwide. The cellular basis for IgE regulation has been worked out in detail. More recently, the molecular events underlying IgE synthesis have been actively investigated, both to understand the specific requirements of the IgE isotype, and because they represent an ideal model to characterize signals involved in Ig class switching.

In this chapter, the role of cells and cytokines, as well as the molecular mechanisms involved in human IgE synthesis, will be discussed.

2 THE ROLE OF CELLS AND CYTOKINES

2.1 The Two-Signal Model for the Induction of IgE Synthesis

During an immune response, a B lymphocyte can express different immunoglobulin heavy-chain classes, or isotypes, sharing the same variable (VDJ) region. This phenomenon (isotype switching) allows a single B-cell clone to produce antibodies with the same fine specificity, but different effector functions. Different immunoglobulin classes are found in most vertebrates, suggesting the importance of having different effector functions.

To switch to a particular isotype, a B cell needs to receive two signals (Fig. 1): signal 1 is cytokine-dependent, results in the activation of transcription at a specific region of the immunoglobulin locus, and thus determines isotype specificity. Signal 2 activates the recombination machinery, resulting in DNA switch recombination (1). The two signals required for switching to IgE are delivered to B cells by T cells through a complex series of interactions. A B cell that expresses IgM specific for the allergen binds the allergen

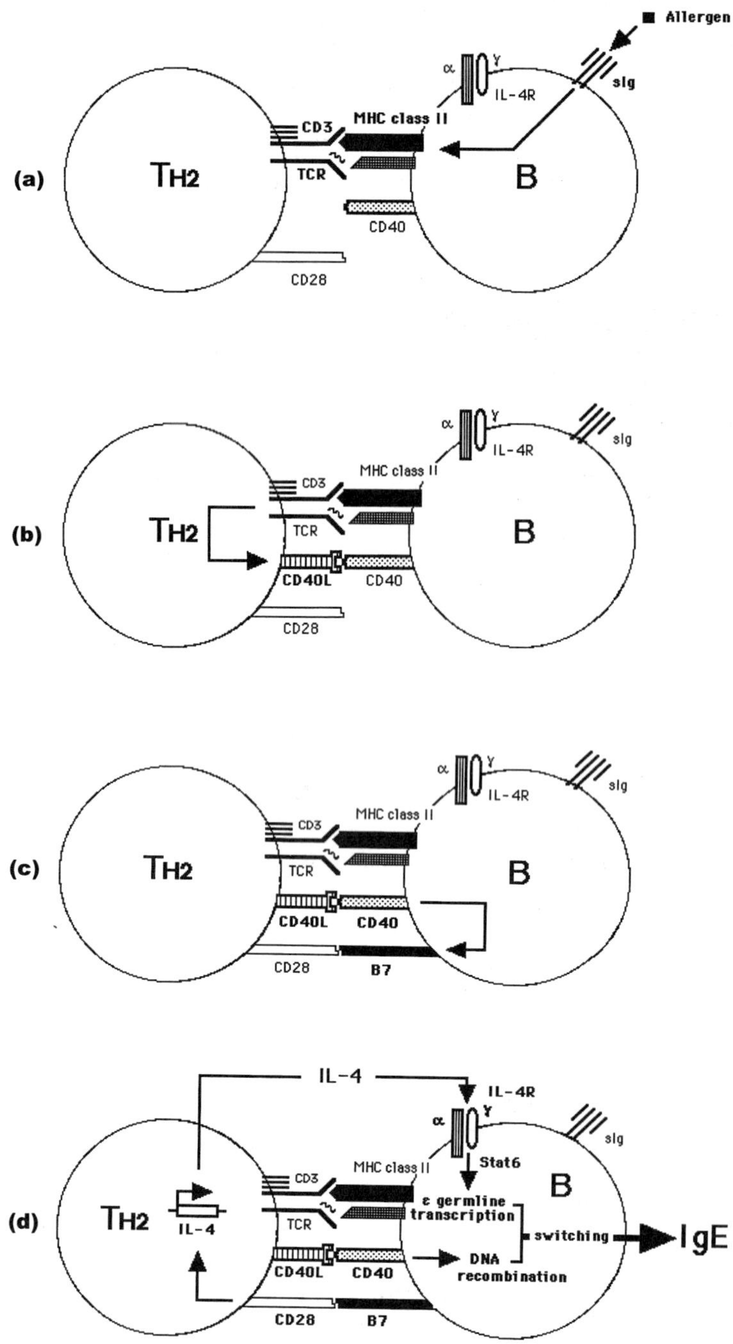

Figure 1 The two-signal model for the induction of human IgE synthesis: the different steps in the IgE induction process are schematically indicated by letters (a–d) and individually discussed in the text.

through surface immunoglobulins (sIg), processes it, and presents it to an allergen-specific Th2-like T cell; that is, a T cell programmed to secrete interleukin (IL)-4, but not interferon (IFN)-γ (see Fig. 1a). Engagement of the T-cell receptor–CD3 complex by major histocompatibility complex (MHC) class II molecules results in the rapid expression of CD40 ligand (CD40L, CD154), that engages CD40, the counterreceptor constitutively expressed on B cells (see Fig. 1b). T–B-cell interactions mediated by CD40/CD40L are amplified by interactions between accessory molecules, particularly the CD28–B7 ligand–receptor pair. Engagement of CD40 results in B7 expression on B cells (see Fig. 1c). B7 engages CD28, inducing high-rate secretion of IL-4. IL-4 binds the heterodimeric IL-4 receptor (IL-4R) that consists of an α-chain (shared with the IL-13R) and a γ-chain (shared with the receptors for IL-2, IL-7, IL-9, and IL-15). At this stage, the B cell is receiving both signals required for IgE switching: IL-4 triggers ε-germline transcription, thereby targeting the ε-switch region for recombination. Cross-linking of CD40 by CD40L activates DNA recombination to the targeted ε-switch region, leading to IgE isotype switching and IgE secretion (see Fig. 1d).

2.1.1 Signal 1: IL-4 and IL-13

Interleukin-4–IL-4R interactions deliver the first signal for switching to IgE. Evidence from different lines of inquiry indicates that IL-4 is essential for IgE production:

1. IL-4 was the only cytokine able to induce IgE synthesis in vitro, when added in recombinant form; injection of an anti-IL-4 antibody abolished IgE production in parasite-infected mice (2).
2. IL-4R exist in vivo not only as cell-bound molecules, but also in a soluble, circulating form. A recombinant extracellular IL-4R domain blocked switching to IgE by blocking IL-4–IL-4R interactions (3).
3. The same result was obtained using an IL-4 mutant in which a tyrosine at position 124 was replaced by aspartic acid (4). The mutation preserves the ability to bind IL-4R, but destroys the capacity to transmit a signal after receptor binding (5). Both these experiments show that it is sufficient to block the IL-4 signal to block isotype switching to IgE, and IgE production.
4. The most compelling evidence for the central role of IL-4 in IgE induction came from gene-targeting experiments. Mice in which the IL-4 gene had been knocked out by homologous recombination (IL-4 knockout mice) were unable to mount significant IgE responses; the IgG1 response was also suppressed, although to a lesser extent, whereas the production of other isotypes was unaffected (6).

More recently, it has become clear that another cytokine, IL-13, shares many of the functional properties of IL-4, including the ability to induce IgE synthesis by B cells. However, IL-13 does not induce IgE switching in murine B cells (7). Although the sequence homology between IL-13 and IL-4 is only about 30%, all residues that contribute to the hydrophobic core of IL-4 are conserved, or have conservative hydrophobic replacements in IL-13 (5). Furthermore, the IL-4R α-chain is a component of both the IL-4R (IL-4Rα:γc) and the IL-13R (IL-4Rα:IL-13Rα1 and IL-13Rα1:IL-13Rα2) (8). However, IL-4 and IL-13, as well as their receptors, are by no means identical. IL-13 does not bind to cells transfected either with cDNAs for the IL-4R α-chain or the γ-chain (9) and, most importantly, unlike IL-4, has no effects on human T cells (10). Furthermore, naive $CD4^+CD45RO^-$ human T cells develop into effector cells that secrete IL-13, IL-5, and

IFN-γ, but not IL-4 after T-cell receptor cross-linking. These cells are able to efficiently help IgE production (11). These findings suggest the intriguing possibility that, at least at certain stages of T-helper differentiation, the production of IL-13 and IL-4 may be independently regulated.

2.1.2 Signal 2: CD40–CD40L Interactions

The engagement of CD40 on B cells by CD40L expressed on T cells provides the second signal required for switching to IgE. CD40L can be replaced in vitro by anti-CD40 monoclonal antibodies (MAbs). Indeed, this was the first experimental system in which the B-cell–activating signal for human IgE synthesis was delivered by antibody-induced engagement of a discrete B-cell surface antigen (12).

CD40 is a 50-kDa glycoprotein expressed on human B lymphocytes, cytokine-activated monocytes, follicular dendritic cells, epithelial cells (including thymic epithelium), and certain carcinomas and melanomas, but not by T cells (13). CD40 plays a key role in the survival, growth, and differentiation of B cells. Signaling through CD40 triggers proliferation of resting B cells (14) and rescues B cells from apoptosis induced by Fas/CD95 or sIgM complex cross-linking (15,16).

CD40 belongs to the tumor necrosis factor receptor (TNFR) superfamily, which includes TNFRI and TNFRII, NGFR, CD30, CD27, and Fas (CD95) (13). Members within this family share sequence similarity through their extracellular regions that contain multiple cysteine-rich repeats. The common structural framework of the extracellular domain is reflected by the ability of the TNFR superfamily members to interact with a parallel family of TNF-related molecules, which includes the ligands for CD40, CD27, and CD30, TNF-α and lymphotoxin. CD40L is a 261-amino acid type 2 membrane glycoprotein, transiently expressed on activated, but not resting, Th1 and Th2 cells (17). Cells transfected with CD40L induced IgE synthesis by human B cells in the presence of IL-4, whereas a soluble CD40–Ig fusion protein inhibited IL-4-dependent IgE synthesis in human peripheral blood mononuclear cells (PBMC) (18). These results clearly indicated that CD40–CD40L interactions are critical in delivering the second signal required for IgE production. The central role of the CD40–CD40L pathway in IgE synthesis and, more generally, in isotype switching, was confirmed by the finding that defective switching in patients with X-linked hyper-IgM (HIM) syndrome is due to mutations in CD40L that result in impaired CD40–CD40L interactions (19). In addition to an inability to switch to T-cell–dependent isotypes, antibodies from HIM patients do not undergo affinity maturation, and B-cell memory does not develop. Likewise, no IgG, IgA, nor IgE response to thymus-dependent antigens was detectable in CD40 (20,21) and CD40L (22) knockout mice, and no germinal centers were recognizable in lymphoid organs. In contrast, responses to thymus-independent antigens were preserved. IgE expression in vivo appears to be completely dependent on CD40L. Interestingly, the inability of human newborn B cells to switch, and the consequent transient immunodeficiency observed in human neonates, has been ascribed to the decrease observed in both CD40L expression (23) and responses to CD40 agonists (24). Overall, these data point to a crucial role of CD40–CD40L interactions in germinal center formation, B-cell activation, isotype switching, and antibody production. The molecular events that lead to isotype switching following CD40 engagement will be discussed in Section III.C.

The interactions between CD40 and CD40L are tightly regulated. T cells become competent to activate B cells through CD40 only after they express CD40L, and this, in turn, requires T-cell receptor-dependent T-cell activation. The latter process seems to be anatomically constrained (i.e., CD40L is expressed in secondary lymphoid tissues only at the site of cognate T–B-cell interactions. Interestingly, a subset of $CD4^+$ memory T cells in germinal centers contains preformed CD40L that is rapidly (within minutes), but transiently, expressed on the cell surface after T-cell receptor-mediated activation (25). Rapid expression of CD40L on the T-cell surface may be critical for germinal center events because centrocytes either leave the light zone within a few hours of activation, or die by apoptosis in situ. On the other hand, the availability of CD40L is drastically limited, because the interaction with CD40 induces rapid endocytosis of surface CD40L (26).

2.2 B7–CD28 Interactions

Interactions between CD40 and CD40L are by no means sufficient to trigger DNA recombination and isotype switching. Studies in animal models have conclusively proved that the CD28–B7 ligand–receptor pair plays a major accessory role. CD28 knockout mice have reduced basal immunoglobulin levels, and decreased class switching after infection with viruses (27). Even more strikingly, mice deficient in both B7.1 and B7.2 failed to generate antigen-specific antibody responses and lacked germinal centers when immunized by several routes and even in the presence of complete Freund's adjuvant (28). Notably, the class-switching defect in these animals is similar to the phenotype observed in both the CD40- and the CD40L-deficient mice. Several studies have indicated an important interrelation between the CD40–CD40L and B7–CD28 pathways. Engagement of CD40 up-regulates B7.1 and B7.2 expression on B cells (29,30). On the other hand, engagement of CD28 results in increased expression of CD40L on T cells (31) and, most importantly, increases IL-4 secretion (31) and Th2 differentiation (32). IL-4, in turn, up-regulates B7 expression (33). Thus, CD28–B7 interactions appear to be required for both full T-cell activation into IL-4 secretion, and CD40-mediated B-cell activation.

2.3 Amplification of IgE Synthesis

Human basophils and mast cells have recently been reported to secrete IL-4 and IL-13 (34,35), and to express CD40L (36). Thus, in principle, basophils and mast cells may provide both signal 1 and signal 2 for IgE synthesis. However, these non-T cells are likely to be involved in IgE amplification more than induction. The optimal physiological stimulus for secretion of IL-4 and IL-13 appears to be allergen-dependent cross-linking of receptor-bound, allergen-specific IgE (34,35). Thus, cytokine secretion is predicated on the availability of allergen-specific IgE, which, in turn, requires the signals and the cells (including allergen-specific T cells) discussed in the foregoing. Once IgE has been produced, it can arm basophils and mast cells by binding to their IgE receptors, and induce IL-4/IL-13 secretion and CD40L expression after FcεR1 cross-linking. Only at this point may non-T cells trigger an IgE response, which would not necessarily be allergen-specific, but may also be polyclonal. Indeed, a significant proportion of the IgE response in hyper-IgE states is polyclonal, rather than allergen-specific.

2.4 Caveat: From a B Cell's Point of View

The complexity in the interplay between T cells, B cells, and cytokines involved in IgE induction makes it difficult to unambiguously establish a chronology of the events leading to IgE synthesis. On the other hand, the molecular studies discussed in the following point to a hierarchy in the signals that trigger IgE production. The initial event in switching to IgE appears to be the determination of isotype specificity through cytokine (IL-4, IL-13)-dependent induction of ε-germline transcription. This is followed by CD40-mediated DNA switch recombination. Our terminology of "signal 1" and "signal 2" thus reflects a B-cell–centered perspective, even though full T- and B-cell activations most likely develop as parallel processes.

3 MOLECULAR EVENTS IN THE INDUCTION OF IgE SYNTHESIS

3.1 The Role of Germline Transcripts in Isotype Switching

The ability of B cells to express immunoglobulins with identical antigen specificity, but different effector functions, results from their capacity to undergo isotype switching. The main steps of this process are shown in Figure 2. Isotype switching consists of an intrachromosomal DNA recombination event that involves repetitive switch (S) regions located 5′ to each C_H gene except C_δ, and results in the juxtaposition of different downstream C_H genes to the expressed VDJ gene (37). The S region involved in recombination is not targeted at random. Rather, switching appears to be directed by cytokines in conjunction with the regulation of B-cell proliferation and differentiation (38). Molecular analysis has shown that cytokine-dependent induction of isotype switching to a particular C_H gene almost invariably correlates with the transcriptional activation of the same gene in germline (i.e., unrearranged) configuration. Several murine and human germline (GL) transcripts have been cloned, and share structural similarities. GL, or switch, transcripts initiate from TATAA-less promoters a few kilobases upstream of the S region, proceed through short exons (I_H exons), the S regions and C_H exons, and are polyadenylated near the normal poly(A) site for mature IgH mRNAs. The I_H exon is then spliced to the normal acceptor site in the first exon of the C_H gene. During recombination, the region containing the GL promoter and the I_H exon is deleted as part of a switch circle (1,39).

In vivo, isotype switching occurs within germinal centers and is most likely initiated after B cells have undergone affinity maturation by somatic mutation and positive selection. This would allow the acquisition of distinct immunoglobulin isotypes (which confer specific effector functions), while keeping the high affinity for the selecting antigen. Notably, somatic mutation and isotype switching are two independent processes (i.e., somatic mutation can occur within germinal centers without triggering isotype switching, and isotype switching can occur in B-cell clones that have not undergone somatic mutation).

Expression of GL transcripts is thought to play a key role in modulating the accessibility of a particular S region to a putative common switch recombinase, thereby directing switching to the corresponding isotype. The role of GL transcription in the regulation of isotype switching has been recently tested by gene knockout experiments (37). Deletion of the Iγ1 or Iγ2b exons and their promoter resulted in inhibition of class switching to the corresponding genes, indicating that transcription in the S region is necessary to direct switch recombination. However, it is apparently insufficient: replacement of Iε with a B-cell–specific promoter cassette containing the murine Eμ intronic enhancer and a V_H promoter, without the Iε splice donor site, resulted in only marginal switch recombination to IgE, in spite of abundant amounts of large, probably unspliced transcripts (40). In contrast, replacement of all known IL-4–inducible control elements in the Sγ1 region with the heterologous human metallothionein IIA promoter did not impair switch recombination

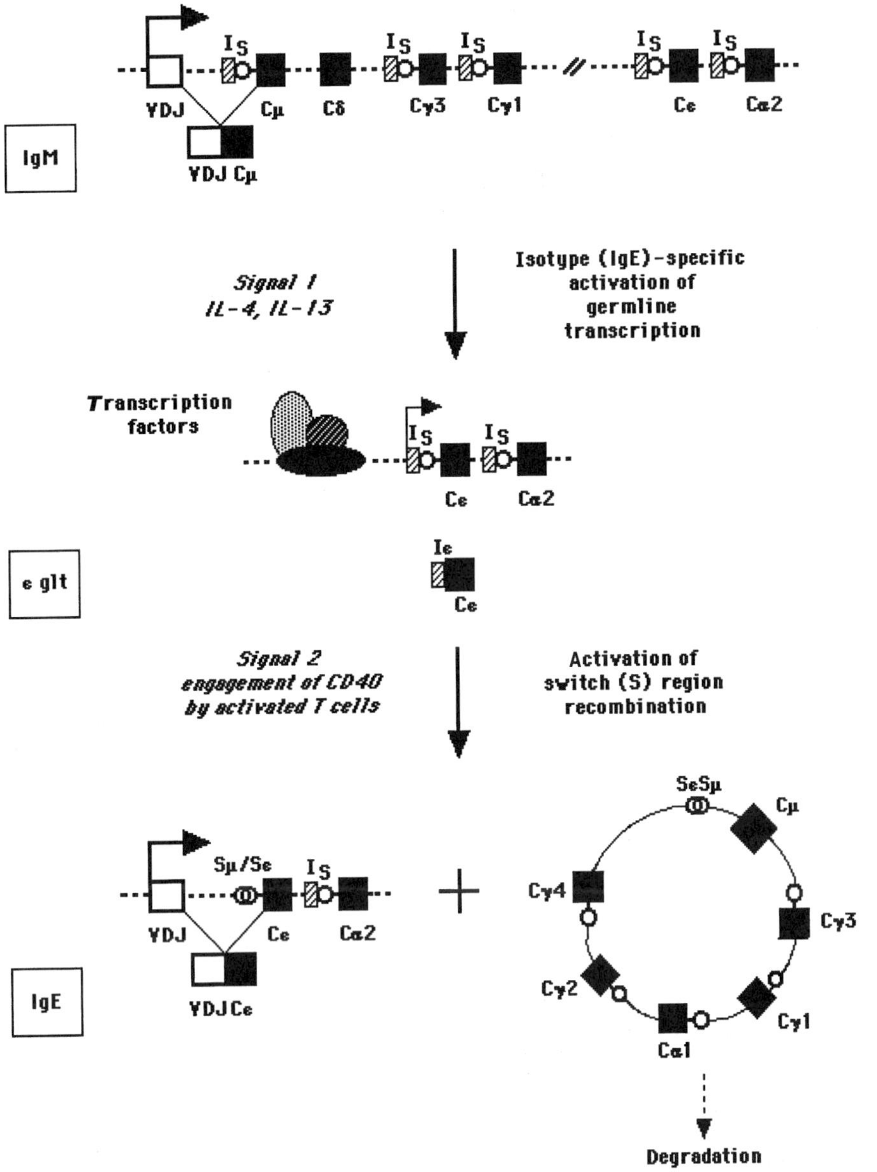

Figure 2 Signals and events involved in IgE isotype switching: cytokine (IL-4, IL-13: signal 1) stimulation of B cells results in the activation of ε-germline transcription and increased chromatin accessibility upstream from the switch (S) ε-region. CD40 cross-linking (signal 2) activates recombination between the Sμ region and the targeted Sε region, with formation of a hybrid Sμ–Sε region. Intervening DNA is looped out as a circle and is subsequently degraded.

to IgG1, provided that a 114-bp fragment spanning the 3′-section of Iγ1 and the 5′ section of Sγ1, with the splice donor site, was included in the construct, thereby allowing the induction of artificial, but processed, GL transcripts (41). These data indicate that artificial induction of structurally conserved, spliced GL transcripts can target switch recombination, whereas transcription in the S region, as such, cannot. Therefore, spliced switch transcripts (or the process of splicing) appeared to have a functional role in switch recombination. However, it was possible that the 114-bp Iγ1 fragment, containing the splice donor site, provided a binding site for a protein complex required for switch recombination. This issue was directly addressed by replacing the entire endogenous Iγ1 exon with an artificial I exon, with or without an adenoviral splice donor site. Switching to IgG1 was preserved only when the adenoviral splice site was included. These experiments conclusively proved that processing of GL transcripts, or the processed GL transcripts themselves, are required for switch recombination. Splicing may be important because splicing factors may be involved in switch recombination, or perhaps because splicing cuts the transcript, releasing the intron to associate with the DNA of the S region (42).

The importance of GL transcription for S region targeting is further reiterated by the finding that the Iμ GL promoter is constitutively active in B cells before and after the Sμ region sequence has undergone a primary recombination event (43). Because Cμ is deleted at switch recombination, the Iμ-containing GL transcript, generated after a primary switching event, is a hybrid that includes Iμ correctly spliced to the now-juxtaposed downstream C_H exon (e.g., Iμ–Cγ2b). These findings are consistent with a model in which simultaneous GL transcription of both the 5′ and 3′ genes involved in a given switch recombination event is needed to target them. The specificity of primary or sequential switching events would come from cytokine-induced GL transcription of the involved 3′ C_H gene.

GL transcripts have also been proposed to play a major role in interchromosomal RNA trans-splicing, whereby transcripts from rearranged VDJ exons are joined to C_H GL transcripts (44). This process, which would result in heavy-chain class switching in the absence of deletional DNA rearrangement in the C_H locus, underlies the production of multiple immunoglobulin isotypes in transgenic mice (45). Furthermore, multiple types of chimeric GL transcripts (Iμ–Cε, Iε–Cμ, Iμ–Cγ4, Iγ–Cμ, Iγ–Cε, Iε–Cγ, and Iγ4–Cα1) were detected in human B cells stimulated with IL-4 alone. Sequence analysis revealed that these transcripts contained the I exons from one locus spliced to the C_H exons from another locus by using consensus sequences for splicing donor and acceptor sites, suggesting that they were generated through the splicing machinery (46). Trans-splicing involving GL transcripts may potentially be of general importance for class switching. However, the role played by this mechanism under physiological conditions remains unclear.

3.2 Regulation of the εGL Promoter

Nuclear factors specifically bind to relatively short (10- to 20-bp) DNA sequences, functionally defined as responsive elements (RE). The general paradigm for promoters is that all slots for nuclear transcription factors need to be filled for a gene to fire. This implies a level of tight combinatorial control. Similar to all weak promoters, the GL promoters are likely to be limited at multiple steps of the transcription initiation reaction. Thus, different transcription factors have an influence on different limiting steps in the reaction.

Because transcription through the I_H exon and the S region seems to be required to target the appropriate S region for recombination and switching, the induction of GL transcription is a key step in determining the isotype specificity of the switching event. Different cytokines specifically induce different nuclear factors that activate transcription at the appropriate GL promoter. In particular, IL-4 induces εGL transcripts in murine (47–49) and human (50,51) B cells. IL-4-dependent εGL transcription is strongly up-regulated at CD40 engagement (52), an effect that is believed to be critical for the efficiency of switching. Of note, the synergism between IL-4 and CD40 cross-linking is essential not only for GL transcription, but also for the induction of switch recombinase activity (53).

Full activation of the εGL promoter in response to IL-4 and CD40 engagement requires a constellation of nuclear factors (NFs) that are either constitutively expressed or recruited to the promoter by specific activating signals. The murine εGL promoter has been extensively dissected, and several *cis*-acting elements have been characterized that regulate its activation in response to IL-4 and CD40 engagement. A highly conserved DNA sequence 5′ to the major initiation sites for murine ε-transcripts contains an IL-4RE that binds STAT6, members of the CCAAT/enhancer-binding protein (C/EBP) family of transcriptional regulators, and NF-κB/Rel proteins. Mutation of any of the binding sites for these factors abolished or strongly reduced promoter activity (54,55). Binding of B-cell–specific activator protein (BSAP) to a region closer to the cluster of transcription initiation sites was also essential for activation of the murine εGL promoter (56,57).

Binding elements for C/EBP, STAT6, NF-κB/Rel, and BSAP were identified in the homologous region of the human εGL promoter (58–61) (Fig. 3). In particular, the −109/−80 region represents an IL-4RE that binds recombinant C/EBPβ and STAT6, and is sufficient to confer IL-4 inducibility to a heterologous promoter in transient transfection studies (61,62). However the role of C/EBP proteins in the regulation of human εGL transcription remains unclear. Because sites for C/EBP and STAT6 proteins are often adjacent or overlapping in the promoters of IL-4–regulated genes, this arrangement was suggested to serve a functional purpose (63). Although both factors can bind DNA independently, C/EBPβ would stabilize STAT6 binding, thereby synergistically activating IL-4–dependent transcription (61). However, different groups found no evidence for interac-

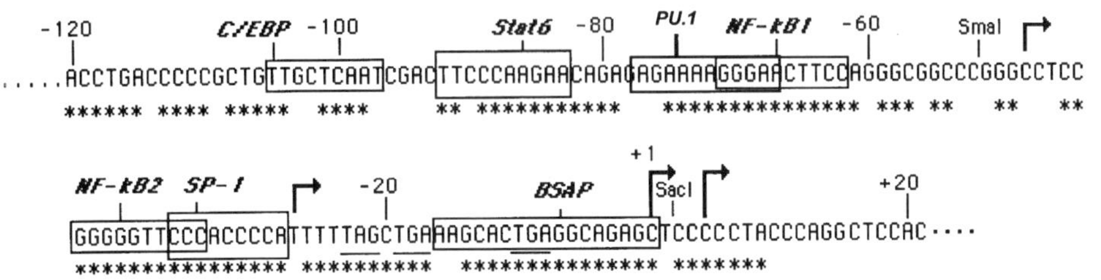

Figure 3 Map of the proximal region of the human ε-germline promoter: position −291 (not shown) corresponds to the A in an RsaI site (nucleotide 241 in Genbank accession no. X56797). The major transcription start sites are indicated by arrows. Position +1 corresponds to the major ε-RNA start site in BL-2 cells. The binding sites for transcription factors identified in the promoter are boxed. The asterisks mark the evolutionarily conserved sequence, a segment highly (> 80%) homologous between human and murine sequences. Stop codons are underlined.

tions with endogenous members of this family (64,65). Of note, production of IgE, after stimulation with IL-4 and a trimeric CD40 ligand, was normal in C/EBPβ-deficient mice (66). Transcription of εGL was not specifically assessed in this model; however, these findings suggest that C/EBPβ may not be necessary for IL-4–induced IgE switching in vivo. No data are as yet available an the role of C/EBPγ in IgE regulation, because deletion of the gene by homologous recombination is embryonically lethal (67). However, C/EBPγ lacks an activation domain, and it has been implicated in suppression, rather than activation, of transcription of genes triggered by other C/EBP family members, including CEBPβ (68). Even the synergism between STAT6 and C/EBPβ allows for exceptions. Indeed, no binding of endogenous C/EBP could be detected in the regions flanking the STAT6 site in the murine CD23a promoter (66).

The εGL promoter is exquisitely IL-4-inducible (69). Transduction of the IL-4 signal to the nucleus is critically dependent on the phosphorylation, dimerization, and activation of the transcription factor STAT6, the essential role of which in IL-4-dependent εGL transcription and IgE switching is well established (70). Indeed, STAT6-deficient mice do not express IgE (66,71,72). STAT6 belongs to the recently identified family of signal transducers and activators of transcription (STAT) (73). Binding of IL-4 to its receptor leads to activation by tyrosine phosphorylation of two receptor-associated cytoplasmic tyrosine kinases, Janus kinase (JAK)-3 and JAK-1 (74). These kinases are believed to rapidly (within minutes) induce phosphorylation of critical tyrosine residues in the intracellular domain of the IL-4R α-chain. These phosphorylated tyrosine residues provide docking sites for the latent cytosolic transcription factor STAT6. STAT6 binds to these docking sites by its SH2 domain and, in turn is tyrosine-phosphorylated by the receptor-associated JAKS. Phosphorylated STAT6 then homodimerizes, translocates to the nucleus, and binds to the promoter of several genes, contributing to the activation of transcription (75). STAT6 preferentially binds dyad symmetrical half-sites separated by four base pairs (TTC-N_4-GAA) (76). DNA binding specificity is localized to a region of 180 amino acids at the N-terminal side of the putative SH3 domain (77). The discovery of JAKs and STATS finally provided an explanation for the apparent paradox that the IL-4R, as well as several other cytokine receptors, lack kinase domains, but still couples ligand binding to tyrosine phosphorylation. STAT6 is not B-cell–specific, and is induced by IL-4 in monocytes, in which it participates in the transcriptional regulation of the IL-4–inducible CD23b promoter (78), and possibly of the FcγR1 promoter (79). STAT6-binding sites have been identified in the promoters of various other IL-4–responsive genes, such as the γ1 GL promoter (69) and MHC class II. The presence of a homologous RE in the promoter of different genes underlies the concerted regulation of these genes by a single cytokine. Thus, the concerted modulation in the expression of εGL transcripts, CD23 and MHC class II in B cells stimulated with IL-4, is mediated by IL-4RE located in the promoters of these genes.

The NF-κB/Rel proteins bind two distinct sites in the εGL promoter and play an essential role in IL-4–dependent responses, cooperating with STAT6 for the synergistic activation of human εGL transcription. Consistent with the well-known ability of CD40 signaling to induce NF-κB activation (80,81), these nucleoproteins appeared to be critical for the CD40-dependent enhancement of IL-4-induced εGL transcription. Interestingly, however, NF-κB activity was also essential for IL-4 responsiveness in the absence of antibody-mediated CD40 cross-linking. Both effects are likely to reflect the physical association between NF-κB/Rel proteins and STAT6 (55,82). After interaction with NF-κB, STAT6 appears to undergo critical quantitative and functional changes: DNA-binding affinity is substantially enhanced and, most importantly, transactivating ability is induced (82). Thus, direct STAT6–NF-κB interactions are necessary for the synergistic activation of transcription from promoters containing both cognate sites. Notably, activation of neither STAT6 nor NF-κB requires de novo protein synthesis, permitting the rapid transmission of the IL-4/CD40 signal to the nucleus.

The upstream NF-κB site overlaps with a PU.1-binding motif. Abrogation of DNA binding of both PU.1 and NF-κB resulted in loss of IL-4 inducibility of IgE GL promoter constructs even in the presence of a functional C/EBP site (64). This result suggested that PU.1 as well as NF-κB factors may cooperate functionally with STAT6 to mediate IL-4 induction of the IgE GL promoter. Thus, the PU.1–NF-kB1 unit may play a key role in defining a minimal IL-4 response element together with STAT6, whereas C/EBP would exert an amplifying function.

The B-cell–specific activator protein (BSAP, Pax-5) is a homeodomain-class transcription factor specifically expressed in the B-cell lineage from the pro-B to the mature B-cell stage. However, BSAP is not found in terminally differentiated plasma cells (83). Binding sites for BSAP have been found in a variety of promoters of B-cell–related genes, including CD19, V_{preB1}, λ5, and the tyrosine kinase *blk* and, furthermore, in the immunoglobulin gene locus (84). Interestingly, although BSAP binding positively regulates transcription from various promoters, binding of BSAP to sites in the immunoglobulin 3′ α-enhancer has a negative effect (85). BSAP binds to a highly conserved region immediately upstream from the major Iε transcription initiation site in both murine (56) and human (60) B cells. Reporter assays, with constructs containing a luciferase gene driven by the εGL promoter, with or without mutations in the BSAP-binding site, showed that BSAP plays a role in both IL-4–dependent induction and CD40-mediated up-regulation of human εGL transcription. Notably, among the transcription factors that regulate εGL expression, BSAP is unique, in that it is B-cell–specific, and it is at the merging point of two signaling pathways that are distinct, but both critical, for the induction of IgE switching.

BSAP may contribute to the specificity of isotype switching through a differential regulation of GL transcription. Indeed, overexpression of BSAP under the control of a tetracycline-regulated promoter inhibits αGL transcription and switching to IgA in $sIgM^+$ I.29μ cells, but enhances εGL transcription and switching to IgE (57). Proliferation of I.29μ cells was not affected in this system. The opposite effects of BSAP on ε- and αGL transcription exemplify the ability of this factor to activate or inhibit transcription, depending on which protein it interacts with at a particular binding site (86,87). The affinity of BSAP for its different binding motifs is also a critical variable. During a B-cell immune response, BSAP maintains its activator functions, but is relieved of its repressor functions. This selective targeting of BSAP activities is regulated by a concentration-dependent mechanism whereby activator motifs for BSAP had a 20-fold higher-binding affinity than repressor motifs. An exchange of activator and repressor motifs, however, showed that the context of the motif, rather than the affinity, determined whether BSAP operated as an activator or repressor (87).

3.3 DNA Switch Recombination

Although IL-4 (signal 1) is, by itself, sufficient for the initiation of transcription through the ε-locus, switching and expression of mature C_ε transcripts (containing VDJ spliced to C_ε1-4) require signal 2 (engagement of CD40 by CD40 ligand). The molecular events that follow the delivery of the second signal for switching to IgE have been characterized only recently. The classic model, according to which switching occurs by loop-out and deletional recombination between highly repetitive S regions, was challenged in the late 1980s, at least for the IgE isotype. Indeed, it was reported that IgE could be produced by B cells in which the immunoglobulin locus was retained in germline configuration (88). Thus, it became important to characterize the molecular mechanisms that underlie the expression of mature VDJ–Cε mRNA in normal human B cells. This issue was investigated using polymerase chain reaction (PCR)-based approaches that permit amplification, cloning, and sequencing of chimeric Sμ/Sε switch fragments composed of the 5′-Sμ joined to the 3′-portion of the targeted Sε-region, or of switch circles, their reciprocal products. DNA sequencing of Sμ/Sε switch fragments, amplified from IgE-producing B-cell cultures, formally proved that deletional switch recombination had occurred. Most of the switch fragments represented direct joining of Sμ to Sε (52,89,90). The finding of IgE synthesis in B-cell lines, with an unrearranged immunoglobulin locus probably reflected transplicing.

Interestingly, some fragments amplified from B cells stimulated with IL-4 and hydrocortisone contained insertions at the Sμ/Sε junction which were derived from Sγ4 (90). The presence of an Sγ4-derived insertion suggested that some B cells had undergone sequential isotype switching from IgM, to IgG4, to IgE. Indeed, IL-4 induces isotype switching to IgG4 (91) as well as to IgE, and single B cells can give rise to clones that secrete IgG4 and IgE (92).

Sequential switching and direct switching coexist. Sequencing of switch circles generated in B cells triggered a switch to IgE by IL-4 and anti-CD40 MAb showed the presence of μ–γ–ε switching, and of sequential events even more complex (μ–α1–γ–ε). However, μ–ε circles representing direct-switching events were also found, at high frequency (93). More recently, was shown that a chimeric Sμ/Sγ1 region resulting from a switching event between μ and γ1 can undergo a secondary recombination between the very 5′-end of Sμ and the very 3′-end of Sγ1. The secondary recombination removes essentially all the tandemly repeated S-region sequences from the corresponding chromosome (94). The mechanisms responsible for secondary recombination events in previously rearranged, chimeric S regions are still unknown. In particular, it is unclear whether secondary recombination requires retargeting of the recombinase. This would be problematic, because of the deletion of the region encompassing the I_H exon and the GL promoter. Secondary recombination, however, may represent a mechanism to prevent continued switching to downstream isotypes and to ensure isotype stabilization of switched B cells. After secondary recombination, in fact, the S sequences retained by the active immunoglobulin gene may be insufficient to serve as a substrate for further S–S recombination.

The importance of sequential switching in vivo was investigated by examining switching to IgE in mutant mice that lacked the Sγ1 region (95), and, therefore, were unable to support sequential switching by IgG1. In these mice, the frequency of switching to IgE was not affected (96). These results indicated that sequential switching may merely reflect the simultaneous accessibility of two acceptor S-regions for switch recombination induced by one cytokine. The apparent dominance of sequential switching observed in the generation of murine IgE-expressing cells, following IL-4 stimulation, may be due to the parallel activation of Sγ1 and Sε by IL-4: Sγ1 being intrinsically more accessible to recombination with Sμ. Thus, the overall low frequency of IgE switching is an autonomously determined intrinsic feature of Sε and its control elements. This may explain why, in vitro, in the presence of saturating concentrations of IL-4, the frequency of IgE switching reaches at most 10% of the frequency of switching to IgG1, which is also induced by IL-4.

4 A PERSPECTIVE FOR THE FUTURE: APPLYING TO ALLERGY WHAT WE LEARNED FROM PARASITIC INFECTIONS

Immunoglobulin E-mediated hypersensitivity reactions are rare in patients with chronic helminth infections, even though FcεRI-bearing cells are sensitized with antiparasite IgE and are exposed—often continuously—to parasite antigens. This inhibition of allergic reactivity is mainly due to IgG4-blocking antibodies. IgG4 molecules are unusually predominant among antifilarial antibodies (50–95% of the total IgG response) (97,98). Depletion of IgG4 specifically removes the blocking activity from the sera of microfilaremic patients (99). IgG4 with blocking activity have also been detected in patients receiving immunotherapy for insect venom and house dust mite hypersensitivity (100). Interestingly, IL-10, a cytokine reported to play a crucial role in the induction of peripheral tolerance associated with successful immunotherapy, suppresses allergen-specific IgE but enhances allergen-specific IgG4 (101).

Blocking IgG4 competes with cell-bound IgE for allergen binding (102). Because the IgG4 molecule is functionally monovalent, does not fix complement, and binds weakly to Fcγ receptors (103,104), antigen binding by IgG4 has no, or minimal, harmful consequences. However, competition between IgG4 and IgE can occur only if the two antibody isotypes have at least in part the same fine antigen specificity. Such a property was indeed observed for antifilarial IgE and IgG4 (102). A molecular mechanism for this overlap in specificity was provided by the demonstration that isotype switching can occur sequentially from IgM to IgE through IgG4 (see Sec. III.C). This finding proved that two functionally antagonistic immunoglobulin isotypes, IgE and IgG4, can be induced by the same cytokine: IL-4; and provided a rationale for the observation that IgE and IgG4 levels appear to be coregulated in vivo. Once the molecular mechanisms of IgG4 and IgE coregulation are thoroughly understood, it may become possible to apply to allergy the lesson we learned from helminth infections, and redirect IL-4-dependent responses to favor IgG4 over IgE.

REFERENCES

1. Vercelli D, Geha RS. Regulation of isotype switching. Curr Opin Immunol 1992; 4:794–797.
2. Finkelman FD, Katona IM, Urban JF, Snapper CM, Ohara J, Paul WE. Suppression of in vivo polyclonal IgE responses by monoclonal antibody to the lymphokine B-cell stimulatory factor 1. Proc Natl Acad Sci USA 1986; 83:9675–9678.
3. Garrone P, Djossou O, Galizzi J–P, Banchereau J. A recombinant extracellular domain of the human interleukin 4 receptor inhibits the biological effects of interleukin 4 on T and B lymphocytes. Eur J Immunol 1991; 21:1365–1369.
4. Aversa G, Punnonen J, Cocks BG, Vega F, Zurawski S, Zurawski G, de Waal Malefyt R, de Vries JE. An IL-4 mutant protein inhibits IL-4 or IL-13 induced human IgG4 and IgE synthesis and B cell proliferation: support for a common component shared by IL-4 and IL-13 receptors. J Exp Med 1993; 178:2213–2216.
5. Zurawski SM, Vega F, Huyghe B, Zurawski G. Receptors for interleukin-13 and interleukin-4 are complex and share a novel component that functions in signal transduction. EMBO J 1993; 12:2663–2670.
6. Kühn R, Rajewsky KR, Müller W. Generation and analysis of interleukin-4 deficient mice. Science 1991; 254:707–710.
7. de Vries J. The role of IL-13 and its receptor in allergy and inflammatory responses. J Allergy Clin Immunol 1998; 102:165–169.

8. Nelms K, Keegan AD, Zamorano J, Ryan JJ, Paul WE. The IL-4 receptor: signaling mechanisms and biological functions. Annu Rev Immunol 1999; 17:701–738.
9. Vita N, Lefort S, Laurent P, Caput D, Ferrara P. Characterization and comparison of the interleukin 13 receptor with the interleukin 4 receptor on several cell types. J Biol Chem 1995; 270:3512–3517.
10. Zurawski G, de Vries JE. Interleukin 13, an interleukin 4-like cytokine that acts on monocytes and B cells, but not on T cells. Immunol Today 1994; 15:19–26.
11. Brinkmann V, Kristofic C. TCR-stimulated naive human $CD4^{+}45RO^{-}$ T cells develop into effector cells that secrete IL-13, IL-5, and IFN-γ, but no IL-4, and help efficiently IgE production by B cells. J Immunol 1995; 154:3078–3087.
12. Jabara HH, Fu SM, Geha RS, Vercelli D. CD40 and IgE: synergism between anti-CD40 MAb and IL-4 in the induction of IgE synthesis by highly purified human B cells. J Exp Med 1990; 172:1861–1864.
13. Banchereau J, Bazan F, Blanchard D, Briére F, Galizzi JP, van Kooten C, Liu YJ, Rousset F, Saeland S. The CD40 antigen and its ligand. Annu Rev Immunol 1994; 12:881–922.
14. Gruber MF, Bjorndahl JM, Nakamura S, Fu SM. Anti-CD45 inhibition of human B cell proliferation depends on the nature of activation signals and the state of B cell activation. J Immunol 1989; 142:4144–4152.
15. Garrone P, Neidhardt E–M, Garcia E, Galibert L, van Kooten C, Banchereau J. Fas ligation induces apoptosis of CD40-activated human B lymphocytes. J Exp Med 1995; 182:1265–1273.
16. Tsubata T, Wu J, Honjo T. B-cell apoptosis induced by antigen receptor crosslinking is blocked by a T-cell signal through CD40. Nature 1993; 364:645–648.
17. Armitage RJ, Fanslow WC, Strockbine L, Sato TA, Clifford KN, Macduff BM, Anderson DM, Gimpel SD, Davis–Smith T, Maliszewski CR, Clark EA, Smith CA, Grabstein KH, Cosman D, Spriggs MK. Molecular and biological characterization of a murine ligand for CD40. Nature 1992; 357:80–82.
18. Fanslow WC, Anderson DM, Grabstein KH, Clark EA, Cosman D, Armitage RJ. Soluble forms of CD40 inhibit biologic responses of human B cells. J Immunol 1992; 149:655–660.
19. Fuleihan R, Ramesh N, Loh R, Jabara H, Rosen FS, Chatila T, Fu SM, Stamenkovic I, Geha RS. Defective expression of the CD40 ligand in X-chromosome–linked immunoglobulin deficiency with normal or elevated IgM. Proc Natl Acad Sci USA 1993; 90:2170–2173.
20. Castigli E, Alt FW, Davidson L, Bottaro A, Mizoguchi E, Bhan AK, Geha RS. CD40 deficient mice generated by RAG-2 deficient blastocyst complementation. Proc Natl Acad Sci USA 1994; 91:12135–12139.
21. Kawabe T, Naka T, Yoshida K, Tanaka T, Fujiwara H, Suematsu S, Yoshida N, Kishomoto T, Kikutani H. The immune responses in CD40-deficient mice: impaired immunoglobulin class switching and germinal center formation. Immunity 1994; 1:167–178.
22. Xu J, Foy TM, Laman JD, Elliott EA, Dunn JJ, Waldschmidt TJ, Elsemore J, Noelle RJ, Flavell RA. Mice deficient for the CD40 ligand. Immunity 1994; 1:423–431.
23. Fuleihan R, Ahern D, Geha RS. Decreased expression of the ligand for CD40 in newborn lymphocytes. Eur J Immunol 1994; 24:1925.
24. Durandy A, de Saint Basile G, Lisowska–Grospierre B, Gauchat J–F, Forveille M, Kroczek RA, Bonnefoy J–Y, Fischer A. Undetectable CD40 ligand expression on T cells and low B cell responses to CD40 binding agonists in human newborns. J Immunol 1995; 154:1560–1568.
25. Casamayor–Palleja M, Khan M, MacLennan ICM. A subset of $CD4^{+}$ memory T cells contains preformed CD40 ligand that is rapidly but transiently expressed on their surface after activation through the T cell receptor complex. J Exp Med 1995; 181:1293–1301.
26. Yellin MJ, Sippel K, Inghirami G, Covey LR, Lee JJ, Sinning J, Clark EA, Chess L, Lederman S. CD40 molecules induce down-modulation and endocytosis of T cell surface T cell–

B cell activating molecule/CD40 ligand. Potential role in regulating helper effector function. J Immunol 1994; 152:598–608.

27. Shahinian A, Pfeffer K, Lee KP, Kündig TM, Kishihara K, Wakeham A, Kawai K, Ohashi PS, Thompson CB, Mak TW. Differential T cell costimulatory requirements in CD28-deficient mice. Science 1993; 261:609–612.
28. Borriello F, Sethna MP, Boyd SD, Schweitzer AN, Tivol EA, Jacoby D, Strom TB, Simpson EM, Freeman GJ, Sharpe AH. B7-1 and B7-2 have overlapping, critical roles in immunoglobulin class switching and germinal center formation. Immunity 1997; 6:303–313.
29. Roy M, Aruffo A, Ledbetter J, Linsley P, Kehry M, Noelle R. Studies on the interdependence of gp39 and B7 expression and function during antigen-specific immune responses. Eur J Immunol 1995; 25:596–603.
30. Ranheim EA, Kipps TJ. Activated T cells induce expression of B7/BB1 on normal or leukemic B cells through a CD40-dependent signal. J Exp Med 1993; 177:925–935.
31. Klaus SJ, Pinchuk LM, Ochs HD, Law C–L, Fanslow WC, Armitage RJ, Clark EA. Costimulation through CD28 enhances T cell-dependent B cell activation via CD40–CD40L interaction. J Immunol 1994; 152:5643–5652.
32. King CL, Stupi RJ, Craighead N, June CH, Thyphronitis G. CD28 activation promotes Th2 subset differentiation by human $CD4^+$ cells. Eur J Immunol 1995; 25:587–595.
33. Vallé A, Aubry J–P, Durand I, Banchereau J. IL-4 and IL-2 upregulate the expression of antigen B7, the B cell counterstructure to T cell CD28: an amplification mechanism for T–B cell interactions. Int Immunol 1991; 3:229–235.
34. Schroeder JT, MacGlashan DW, Kagey–Sobotka A, White JM, Lichtenstein LM. IgE-dependent IL-4-secretion by human basophils—the relationship between cytokine production and histamine release in mixed leukocyte cultures. J Immunol 1994; 153:1808–1817.
35. Burd PR, Thompson WC, Max EE, Mills FC. Activated mast cells produce interleukin-13. J Exp Med 1995; 181:1373–1380.
36. Gauchat J–F, Henchoz S, Mazzei G, Aubry J–P, Brunner T, Blasey H, Life P, Talabot D, Flores–Romo L, Thompson J, Kishi K, Butterfield J, Dahinden C, Bonnefoy J–Y. Induction of human IgE synthesis in B cells by mast cells and basophils. Nature 1993; 365:340–343.
37. Stavnezer J. Molecular processes that regulate class switching. Curr Top Microbiol Immunol 2000; 245:127–168.
38. Lundgren M, Ström L, Bergquist L–O, Skog S, Heiden T, Stavnezer J, Severinson E. Cell cycle regulation of immunoglobulin class switch recombination and germ-line transcription: potential role of Ets family members. Eur J Immunol 1995; 25:2042–2051.
39. Stavnezer J. Immunoglobulin class switching. Curr Opin Immunol 1996; 8:199–205.
40. Bottaro A, Lansford R, Xu L, Zhang J, Rothman P, Alt FW. S region transcription per se promotes basal IgE class switch recombination but additional factors regulate the efficiency of the process. EMBO J 1994; 13:665–674.
41. Lorenz M, Jung S, Radbruch A. Switch transcripts in immunoglobulin class switching. Science 1995; 267:1825–1828.
42. Reaban ME, Griffin JA. Induction of RNA-stabilized DNA conformers by transcription of an immunoglobulin switch region. Nature 1990; 348:342–344.
43. Li SC, Rothman PB, Zhang J, Chan C, Hirsh D, Alt FW. Expression of Iμ–Cγ hybrid germline transcripts subsequent to immunoglobulin heavy chain class switching. Int Immunol 1994; 6:491–497.
44. Durdik J, Gerstein RM, Rath S, Robbins PF, Nisonoff A, Selsing E. Isotype switching by a microinjected μ immunoglobulin heavy chain gene in transgenic mice. Proc Natl Acad Sci USA 1989; 86:2346–2350.
45. Shimizu A, Nussenzweig MC, Han H, Sanchez M, Honjo T. Trans-splicing as a possible molecular mechanism for the multiple isotype expression of the immunoglobulin gene. J Exp Med 1991; 173:1385–1393.

46. Fujieda S, Lin YQ, Saxon A, Zhang K. Multiple types of chimeric germ-line Ig heavy chain transcripts in human B cells. J Immunol 1996; 157:3450–3459.
47. Stavnezer J, Radcliffe G, Lin Y–C, Nietupski J, Berggren L, Sitia R, Severinson E. Immunoglobulin heavy-chain switching may be directed by prior induction of transcripts from constant-region genes. Proc Natl Acad Sci USA 1988; 85:7704–7708.
48. Rothman P, Lutzker S, Cook W, Coffman R, Alt FW. Mitogen plus interleukin 4 induction of Cε transcripts in B lymphoid cells. J Exp Med 1988; 168:2385–2389.
49. Severinson E, Fernandez C, Stavnezer J. Induction of germ-line immunoglobulin heavy chain transcripts by mitogens and interleukins prior to switch recombination. Eur J Immunol 1990; 20:1079–1084.
50. Gauchat J–F, Lebman DA, Coffman RL, Gascan H, de Vries JE. Structure and expression of germline ε transcripts in human B cells induced by interleukin 4 to switch to IgE production. J Exp Med 1990; 172:463–473.
51. Jabara HH, Schneider LC, Shapira SK, Alfieri C, Moody CT, Kieff E, Geha RS, Vercelli D. Induction of germ-line and mature Cε transcripts in human B cells stimulated with rIL-4 and EBV. J Immunol 1990; 145:3468–3473.
52. Shapira SK, Vercelli D, Jabara HH, Fu SM, Geha RS. Molecular analysis of the induction of IgE synthesis in human B cells by IL-4 and engagement of CD40 antigen. J Exp Med 1992; 175:289–292.
53. Kinoshita K, Tashiro J, Tomita S, Lee C–G, Honjo T. Target specificity of immunoglobulin class switch recombination is not determined by nucleotide sequences of S regions. Immunity 1998; 9:849–858.
54. Delphin S, Stavnezer J. Characterization of an IL-4 responsive region in the immunoglobulin heavy chain germline ε promoter: regulation by NF-IL-4, a C/EBP family member, and NF-κB/p50. J Exp Med 1995; 181:181–192.
55. Iciek LA, Delphin SA, Stavnezer J. CD40 cross-linking induces Igε germline transcripts in B cells via activation of NF-κB: synergy with IL-4 induction. J Immunol 1997; 158:4769–4779.
56. Liao F, Birshtein BK, Busslinger M, Rothman P. The transcription factor BSAP (NF-HB) is essential for immunoglobulin germ-line ε transcription. J Immunol 1994; 152:2904–2911.
57. Qiu G, Stavnezer J. Overexpression of BSAP/Pax5 inhibits switching to IgA and enhances switching to IgE in the I.29μ B cell line. J Immunol 1998; 161:2906–2918.
58. Albrecht B, Peiritsch S, Woisetschläger M. A bifunctional control element in the human IgE germline promoter involved in repression and IL-4 activation. Int Immunol 1994; 6:1143–1151.
59. Messner B, Stütz AM, Albrecht B, Peiritsch S, Woisetschläger M. Cooperation of binding sites for STAT6 and NFκB/rel in the IL-4-induced up-regulation of the human IgE germline promoter. J Immunol 1997; 159:3330–3337.
60. Thienes CP, De Monte L, Monticelli S, Busslinger M, Gould HJ, Vercelli D. The transcription factor B cell-specific activator protein (BSAP) enhances both IL-4- and CD40-mediated activation of the human ε germline promoter. J Immunol 1997; 158:5874–5882.
61. Mikita T, Kurama M, Schindler U. Synergistic activation of the germline ε promoter mediated by Stat6 and C/EBPβ. J Immunol 1998; 161:1822–1828.
62. Mikita T, Campbell D, Wu P, Williamson K, Schindler U. Requirements for interleukin-4–induced gene expression and functional characterization of Stat6. Mol Cell Biol 1996; 16: 5811–5820.
63. Lundgren M, Larsson C, Femino A, Xu M, Stavnezer J, Severinson E. Activation of the Ig germ-line γ1 promoter. Involvement of C/enhancer-binding protein transcription factors and their possible interactions with an NF–IL-4 site. J Immunol 1994; 153:2983–2995.
64. Stutz AM, Woisetschlager M. Functional synergism of STAT6 with either NF-κB or PU.1 to mediate IL-4-induced activation of IgE germline gene transcription. J Immunol 1999; 163: 4383–4391.

65. Monticelli S, Vercelli D. Molecular regulation of class switch recombination to IgE through germline transcription. Allergy 2001; 56:270–278.
66. Tinnell SB, Jacobs–Helber SM, Sterneck E, Sawyer ST, Conrad DH. STAT6, NF-κB and C/EBP in CD23 expression and IgE production. Int Immunol 1998; 10:1529–1538.
67. Henderson A, Calame K. Transcriptional regulation during B cell development. Annu Rev Immunol 1998; 16:163–200.
68. Cooper CL, Henderson A, Artandi S, Avitahl N, Calame K. Ig/EBP (C/EBPγ) is a transdominant negative inhibitor of C/EBP family transcriptional activators. Nucleic Acids Res 1995; 23:4371–4377.
69. Linehan LA, Warren WD, Thompson PA, Grusby MJ, Berton MT. STAT6 is required for IL-4-induced germline Ig gene transcription and switch recombination. J Immunol 1998; 161:302–310.
70. Shimoda K, van Deursen J, Sangster MY, Sarawar SR, Carson RT, Tripp RA, Chu C, Quelle FW, Nosaka T, Vignali DAA, Doherty PC, Grosveld G, Paul WE, Ihle JN. Lack of IL-4-induced Th2 response and IgE class switching in mice with disrupted Stat6 gene. Nature 1996; 380:630–633.
71. Takeda K, Tanaka T, Shi W, Matsumoto M, Minami M, Kashiwamura S-I, Nakanishi K, Yoshida N, Kishimoto T, Akira S. Essential role of Stat6 in IL-4 signalling. Nature 1996; 380:627–630.
72. Kaplan MH, Schindler U, Smiley ST, Grusby MJ. Stat6 is required for mediating responses to IL-4 and for the development of Th2 cells. Immunity 1996; 4:313–319.
73. Ihle JN, Kerr IM. Jaks and Stats in signaling by the cytokine receptor superfamily. Trends Genet 1995; 11:69–74.
74. Leonard WJ, O'Shea JJ. Jaks and Stats: biological implications. Annu Rev Immunol 1998; 16:293–322.
75. Hou J, Schindler U, Henzel WJ, Ho TC, Brasseur M, McKnight SL. An interleukin-4-induced transcription factor: IL-4 Stat. Science 1994; 265:1701–1706.
76. Seidel HM, Milocco LH, Lamb P, Darnell JE, Stein RB, Rosen J. Spacing of palindromic half sites as a determinant of selective STAT (signal transducers and activators of transcription) DNA binding and transcriptional activity. Proc Natl Acad Sci USA 1995; 92:3041–3045.
77. Schindler U, Wu P, Rothe M, Brasseur M, McKnight SL. Components of a Stat recognition code: evidence for two layers of molecular selectivity. Immunity 1995; 2:689–697.
78. Köhler I, Rieber EP. Allergy-associated Iε and Fcε receptor II (CD23b) genes activated via binding of an interleukin-4-induced transcription factor to a novel responsive element. Eur J Immunol 1993; 23:3066–3071.
79. Kotanides H, Reich NC. Requirement of tyrosine phosphorylation for rapid activation of a DNA binding factor by IL-4. Science 1993; 262:1265–1267.
80. Francis DA, Sen R, Rice N, Rothstein TL. Receptor-specific induction of NF-κB components in primary B cells. Int Immunol 1998; 10:285–293.
81. Lin S–C, Wortis HH, Stavnezer J. The ability of CD40L, but not lipopolysaccharide, to initiate immunoglobulin switching to immunoglobulin G1 is explained by differential induction of NF-κB/Rel proteins. Mol Cell Biol 1998; 18:5523–5532.
82. Shen C–H, Stavnezer J. Interaction of Stat6 and NF-κB: direct association and synergistic activation of interleukin-4–induced transcription. Mol Cell Biol 1998; 18:3395–3404.
83. Adams B, Dörfler P, Aguzzi A, Kozmik Z, Urbanek P, Maurer–Fogy I, Busslinger M. Pax-5 encodes the transcription factor BSAP and is expressed in B lymphocytes, the developing CNS, and adult testis. Genes Dev 1992; 6:1589–1607.
84. Neurath MF, Stüber ER, Strober W. BSAP: a key regulator of B-cell development and differentiation. Immunol Today 1995; 16:564–569.
85. Singh M, Birshtein BK. Concerted repression of an immunoglobulin heavy-chain enhancer, 3′αE(hs1,2). Proc Natl Acad Sci USA 1996; 93:4392–4397.
86. Neurath MF, Max EE, Strober W. Pax5 (BSAP) regulates the murine immunoglobulin 3′α

enhancer by suppressing binding of NF-αP, a protein that controls heavy chain transcription. Proc Natl Acad Sci USA 1995; 92:5336–5340.

87. Wallin JJ, Rinkenberger JL, Rao S, Gackstetter ER, Koshland ME, Zwollo P. B cell-specific activator protein prevents two activator factors from binding to the immunoglobulin J chain promoter until the antigen-driven stages of B cell development. J Biol Chem 1999; 274: 15959–15965.
88. MacKenzie T, Dosch HM. Clonal and molecular characteristics of the human IgE-committed B cell subset. J Exp Med 1989; 169:407–430.
89. Shapira SK, Jabara HH, Thienes CP, Ahern DJ, Vercelli D, Gould HJ, Geha RS. Deletional switch recombination occurs in IL-4 induced isotype switching to IgE expression by human B cells. Proc Natl Acad Sci USA 1991; 88:7528–7532.
90. Jabara HH, Loh R, Ramesh N, Vercelli D, Geha RS. Sequential switching from μ to ε via γ4 in human B cells stimulated with IL-4 and hydrocortisone. J Immunol 1993; 151:4528–4533.
91. Lundgren M, Persson U, Larsson P, Magnusson C, Smith CIE, Hammarström L, Severinson E. Interleukin 4 induces synthesis of IgE and IgG4 in human B cells. Eur J Immunol 1989; 19:1311–1315.
92. Gascan H, Gauchat J–F, Roncarolo MG, Yssel H, Spits H, de Vries JE. Human B cell clones can be induced to proliferate and to switch to IgE and IgG4 synthesis by interleukin 4 and a signal provided by activated $CD4^+$ T cell clones. J Exp Med 1991; 173:747–750.
93. Zhang K, Mills FC, Saxon A. Switch circles from IL-4-directed ε class switching from human B lymphocytes—evidence for direct, sequential and multiple step sequential switch from μ to ε Ig heavy chain gene. J Immunol 1994; 152:3427–3435.
94. Zhang K, Cheah H–K, Saxon A. Secondary deletional recombination of rearranged switch region in Ig isotype-switched B cells. A mechanism for isotype stabilization. J Immunol 1995; 154:2237–2247.
95. Jung S, Rajewsky K, Radbruch A. Shutdown of class switch recombination by deletion of a switch region control element. Science 1993; 259:984–987.
96. Jung S, Siebenkotten G, Radbruch A. Frequency of immunoglobulin E class switching is autonomously determined and independent of prior switching to other classes. J Exp Med 1994; 179:2023–2026.
97. Ottesen EA, Kumaraswami V, Paranjape R, Poindexter RW, Tripathy SP. Naturally occurring blocking antibodies modulate immediate hypersensitivity responses in human filariasis. J Immunol 1981; 127:2014.
98. Ottesen EA, Skvaril F, Tripathy SR, Poindexter RW, Hussain R. Prominence of IgG4 in the IgG antibody response to human filariasis. J Immunol 1985; 134:2707–2712.
99. Hussain R, Poindexter RW, Ottesen EA. Control of allergic reactivity in human filariasis—predominant localization of blocking antibody to the IgG4 subclass. J Immunol 1992; 148: 2731–2737.
100. AAAI Board of Directors. Measurement of specific and nonspecific IgG4 levels as diagnostic and prognostic tests for clinical allergy. J Allergy Clin Immunol 1995; 95:652–654.
101. Akdis CA, Blesken T, Akdis M, Wütrich B, Blaser K. Role of interleukin 10 in specific immunotherapy. J Clin Invest 1998; 102:98–106.
102. Hussain R, Ottesen EA. IgE responses in human filariasis. IV. Parallel antigen recognition of IgE and IgG4 subclass antibodies. J Immunol 1986; 136:1859–1863.
103. Kurniawan A, Yazdanbakhsh M, van Ree R, Aalberse R, Selkirk ME, Partono F, Maizels RM. Differential expression of IgE and IgG4 specific antibody responses in asymptomatic and chronic human filariasis. J Immunol 1993; 150:1941–1950.
104. Schuurman J, van Ree R, Perdok GJ, van Doorn HR, Tan KY, Aalberse RC. The apparent monovalency of human IgG4 is due to bispecificity. Int Arch Allergy Immunol 1999; 118: 187–189.

9

Effector Roles of IgE Antibodies: Targeting Allergen to the High-Affinity IgE Receptor for FcεRI-Dependent Signaling and Antigen Presentation

BRIDGET S. WILSON and JANET M. OLIVER

University of New Mexico Health Sciences Center, Albuquerque, New Mexico

1 INTRODUCTION

Immunoglobulin E antibodies play key roles in an array of acute and chronic human allergic reactions, including asthma, allergic rhinitis, atopic dermatitis, urticaria, and anaphylaxis. The biological activity of IgE is mediated principally through its interaction with the high-affinity receptor FcεRI. In rodents, this receptor is found only on basophils and mast cells. In humans, the FcεRI is expressed not only on basophils and mast cells, but also, at lower density, on monocytes, macrophages, eosinophils, and a range of dendritic cells (DC) including those in blood, lung, dermis, and epidermis.

This chapter focuses on the roles of allergen and IgE in two principal activities: FcεRI-mediated signal transduction; and the FcεRI-mediated internalization, processing, and presentation of antigen. As an introduction to these major topics, we first review the properties of the FcεRI on the basophils and mast cells of mouse and humans; on human dendritic cells, monocytes, and macrophages; and the mechanism and consequences of the IgE–FcεRI interaction on these various cell types. We also review properties of the cytoplasmic granules that are the focus of many FcεRI-dependent activities of basophils and mast cells.

We hope to convey the functional diversity of the human FcεRI. Over three decades of literature on the basophil and mast cell FcεRI has emphasized its role in the generation of mediators and cytokines responsible for acute inflammation. The more recent literature on the FcεRI of dendritic cells and monocytes emphasizes its ability to focus antigen for processing and presentation to T cells. However, there is evidence that cross-linking the FcεRI of dendritic cells, monocytes, and macrophages can provide mediators and cytokines that may contribute to acute allergic inflammation. Conversely, recent studies indicate that mast cells are capable of presenting antigen by a FcεRI-dependent mechanism. Future control of the allergic phenotype is likely to be accomplished by treatments that block antigen-stimulated FcεRI signaling in combination with treatments that block the FcεRI-mediated processing and presentation of antigen.

At the outset, we note that humans express a second, low-affinity IgE receptor, FcεRII (CD23), on B cells, eosinophils, monocytes, and macrophages. CD23 has a 100- to 1000-fold lower affinity for IgE than FcεRI (K_a = 10^6 to 10^7 M^{-1} vs. 10^9 to 10^{10} M^{-1}). As well as binding IgE, CD23 binds CD21 (also known as complement receptor 2; CR2), CD11b-CD18 (CR3) and CD11c-CD18 (CR4) (1). Recent reviews consistently suggest that CD23 serves principally as a regulator of B-cell IgE production (1–3). CD23 may yet be found to play important roles in the regulation of IgE function as well as in the regulation of IgE levels.

2 FcεRI COMPOSITION AND DISTRIBUTION

In 1989, members of the Metzger Laboratory at the National Institutes of Health (NIH) published a complete description of the FcεRI complex cloned from RBL-2H3 rat tumor mast cells (4). This work, and the preceding decade of detailed biochemical characterization (5), revealed three subunits: FcεRI α, a member of the immunoglobulin superfamily that binds IgE; FcεRI β that has four membrane-spanning domains; and FcεRI γ that is present as a homodimer. Assembled, these subunits yield the tetrameric ($\alpha\beta\gamma_2$) receptor illustrated in Figure 1a. Whereas the α-subunit is unique to the FcεRI, the β- and γ-subunits are shared with several other immunoreceptors. Thus, FcεRI γ is a subunit not only of

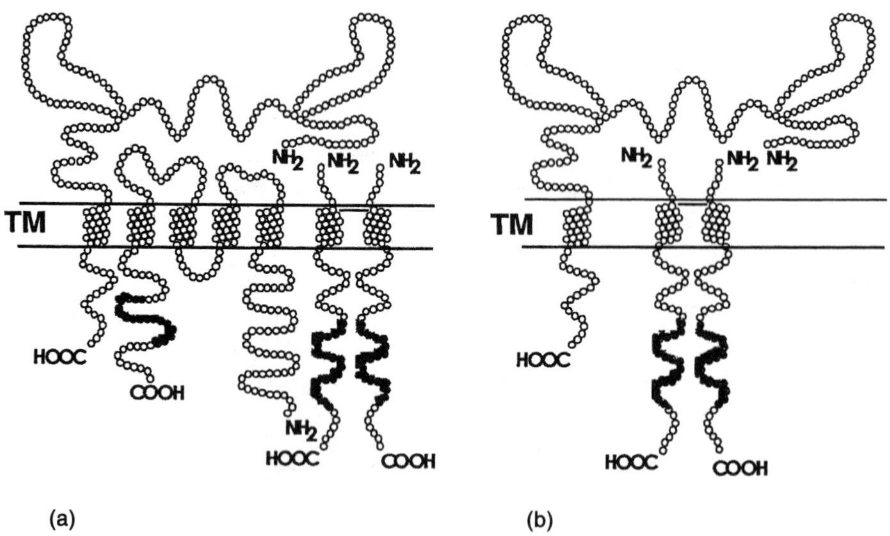

Figure 1 Comparison of the $\alpha\beta\gamma_2$ FcεRI that is the principal isoform expressed on (a) basophils and mast cells, with (b) the $\alpha\gamma_2$ FcεRI that is the principal isoform expressed on monocytes, macrophages and dendritic cells. (From Ref. 9.)

Table 1 Composition and Cellular Distribution of FcεRI in Mouse and Humans

Cells	Mice	Humans
Mast cells	$\alpha\beta\gamma_2$	$\alpha\beta\gamma_2$
Basophils	$\alpha\beta\gamma_2$	$\alpha\beta\gamma_2$
Monocytes–macrophages	—	$\alpha\gamma_2$
Langerhans–dendritic cells	—	$\alpha\gamma_2$

the FcεRI, but also of the IgG receptors, FcγRI and FcγRIII, found in many myeloid cells of some T-cell receptors, and of the platelet collagen receptor. In mast cells, FcγRIII also incorporates the FcεRI β subunit (6–9).

The complete characterization of the rodent receptor provided tools to characterize the FcεRI in the less accessible cells of humans. As predicted, the FcεRI of human basophils and mast cells is a tetrameric complex that is essentially identical with the rodent receptor (10). Despite some continued controversy (11), recent work indicates that FcεRI β transcripts are undetectable in monocytes, macrophages, Langerhans cells, and dendritic cells (9,12). It thus appears that the human FcεRI can be expressed in the $\alpha\beta\gamma_2$ form on cell types that are FcεRI-positive in rodents and, additionally, in an $\alpha\gamma_2$ form (see Fig. 1b; Table 1) on cells that are not FcεRI-positive in rodents. The explanation may lie in an additional endoplasmic reticulum (ER) retention signal in the rodent, but not the human FcεRI α-subunit that prevents the transit of FcεRI α that is not complexed with FcεRI β from the ER to the Golgi complex (9). Supporting this interpretation, Kinet and colleagues recently generated a transgenic mouse expressing the human FcεRI α gene and showed that the transgene induces expression of human FcεRI α in a complex with rodent FcεRI β and γ on basophils and mast cells and, additionally, in a complex with just rodent FcεRI γ on monocytes, macrophages, Langerhans cells, and eosinophils (9,13). One obvious consequence of this difference in FcεRI distribution between species is that FcεRI function may be substantially more diverse in humans than in the mouse.

3 INTERACTIONS OF IgE WITH THE FcεRI

Immunoglobulin E shares the overall structure of the other classes of antibody, but is distinguished from them by the structure of its (ε)-heavy chain constant region that consists of four domains, Cε1–Cε4, one more than in IgG, IgA, or IgD. The Cε3 domain of IgE is critical in FcεRI α binding (2), and Cε3, when expressed as a single domain, retains FcεRI α-binding activity (14,15). Site-directed mutagenesis within Cε3 has identified two ''patches'' of surface residues important in FcεRI α binding. One area incorporates residues from the CD, EF, and FG loops (16). The other involves residues in the Cε2–Cε3 linker region and D strand (17,16). When visualized within an IgE–Cε3–Cε4 model (18), these regions can be viewed as forming a coherent binding surface for FcεRI α (17).

Although IgE has two Cε3 domains, each with potential to bind FcεRI α, numerous laboratories have demonstrated a 1 : 1 stoichiometry of interaction between the two proteins (19–21). IgE and IgE–Fc adopt a ''bent'' conformation both in solution and when bound to FcεRI α (22–24), with the most significant bending occurring between the Cε2 and Cε3 domains (24). This bent structure was originally thought to preclude binding of a second FcεRI α to the concave face of IgE (14). However, recent work has revealed that a covalent dimer of Cε3–Cε4, which lacks the bending formed at the Cε2–Cε3 junction, also complexes with sFcεRI α in a 1 : 1 ratio (25). A conformational change that distorts the second-binding site within IgE on establishment of the primary interaction with FcεRI α provides an alternative, but not universally supported, explanation for the 1 : 1 ratio of IgE binding to FcεRI (25,26).

Immunoglobulin E binding is localized entirely to the FcεRI α ectodomain (27,28) although the γ-subunits may modulate the receptor's affinity for ligand (29), as previously described for homologous Fcγ receptors (30). FcεRI α comprises two C2 immunoglobulin-like domains, for which the more C-terminal α2-domain contains the principal IgE-binding site and the α1-domain is required to retain native affinity for IgE (31). Modeling studies based on similar proteins of known structure have identified candidate IgE-binding regions within the α2-domain (32–34). Amino acid modification within these regions have implicated specific residues within the B-C, C-C′, and F-G loops of α2 in IgE binding (33,34). Involvement of the C-C′ region was particularly highlighted by the ability of an 11-mer cyclized peptide, based on the sequence of the C-C′ loop of α2, to inhibit IgE binding to FcεRI α (33,36). Perhaps surprisingly, considering the naturally high affinity of FcεRI α for IgE, it is also possible to elevate receptor affinity for IgE through specific mutagenesis (34,35). Soluble FcεRI α, or receptor-based peptides, incorporating these higher-affinity mutant residues could provide a means of more effectively competing with endogenous FcεRI α for IgE and could thus be of interest for their therapeutic usefulness (31).

The newly defined crystal structure of soluble FcεRI α has enabled the rationalization of the binding data and has generally confirmed their validity (37,38). Many of the amino acids highlighted from mutagenesis studies as being contact residues are surface-exposed and form a contiguous binding surface. Interestingly, other implicated residues are buried, and so their effects on binding may relate to structural perturbations (37). One of the striking features of the genuine structure is the disposition of α1- and α2-domains relative to each other. The two domains are bent acutely, presumably reflecting the extensive interdomain interactions that exist. This feature is shared by the homologous IgG receptors, FcγRIIa and FcγRIIb (39,40). It has been suggested that the cleft formed between the FcεRI α domains may offer a binding surface to the extracellular regions of FcεRI β or γ (37,38). The FcεRI α crystal structure provides a platform for further analysis of potential FcεRI α residues that are involved in interacting with IgE. Amino acids within domain α1, which lie proximal to the major binding site within domain α2 (37), may contribute to complex formation, a possibility also suggested when the two receptor-binding patches within IgE were found to span more than a single domain of FcεRI α (36). A successful structural determination of the complex formed between FcεRI α and IgE will provide conclusive answers to these issues.

4 CONSEQUENCES OF IgE BINDING TO FcεRI

Binding of IgE to FcεRI is commonly represented as an essentially passive event preparing the cell for allergen-induced responses. However, studies in the late 1970s in the Lichtenstein laboratory first noted a correlation between serum IgE levels and human basophil FcεRI levels (41). More recent studies in the mouse and humans have shown clearly that the presence of increased IgE induces an increase in FcεRI expression levels both in vivo and in vitro in basophils and mast cells, and also in vivo in human monocytes, macrophages, the dendritic cells of blood, dermis and epidermis, and in eosinophils (11,42–50). Importantly, MacGlashan and colleagues have discovered that treating patients with the recombinant humanized anti-IgE MAb, rHum-E25, to reduce serum IgE levels (51), causes a rapid, extensive (from about 250,000 receptors per cell to fewer than 10,000 receptors per cell) and reversible reduction in basophil FcεRI expression levels (52,53; see Chap. 24). These changes in basophil properties are correlated with the reduction and return of symptomatic disease (53,54). It remains to be shown if IgE binding increases FcεRI expression by inhibiting the constitutive process of FcεRI internalization and recycling, resulting in an increase in receptor expression at the cell surface, as suggested from studies in RBL-2H3 cells (55), or, alternatively, by signaling to the de novo synthesis of FcεRI subunits. Recent evidence linking the low levels of FcεRI surface expression on Langerhans cells from nonatopic donors with low serum IgE to the low expression of FcεRI γ in these cells supports a link between serum IgE levels and FcεRI subunit synthesis (50). In either case, these data make it clear that IgE binding to the FcεRI is not just a passive sensitization event, but indeed, is an event with its own significant sequelae for the cell.

5 DEVELOPMENT AND COMPOSITION OF MAST CELL AND BASOPHIL GRANULES

An understanding of the effector roles of IgE–receptor complexes on basophils and mast cells requires an introduction not only to IgE and FcεRI, but also to the granules that characterize these cells and are the focus of many of their FcεRI-dependent activities.

Early morphological work identified the granules of many leukocytes as specialized lysosomes (56), and lysosomal components were localized to basophil and mast cell granules more than 20 years ago (57). Nevertheless, the dense appearance of the mature mast cell granule of rat peritoneum (Fig. 2A) and of human lung and iliac mucosa (58) has led to a generally poor appreciation of these granules as secretory lysosomes. Indeed, their origin as an intersection of the endocytic and secretory pathways is more apparent in the appearance of granules in developing murine mast cells derived by culture of bone marrow progenitors in IL-3 (BMMC; see Fig. 2B, C) and of RBL-2H3 mast cells (see Fig. 2D). In these actively proliferating and endocytosing cells, granules are typically heterogeneous and contain little dense-core proteoglycan matrix material. Instead, the granule lumen is often filled with internal vesicles and multilamellar membranes. From work in other hematopoietic cells (59,60), the multivesicular bodies are most likely acquired by fusion of a lysosomal compartment with tubular endosomes that had previously formed inclusions by invagination. The secretory lysosome may also actively pinch vesicles inward from its own limiting membrane, as suggested by the frequent appearance of inwardly oriented ''cups'' in the granules of BMMC (see arrow, Fig. 2C). Adding to the complexity, there is evidence that histamine can be stored in cytoplasmic vesicles distinct from either mature or immature granules of mast cells and basophils (61,62; our unpublished results). All of the mast cell granules shown in Figure 2 look different from the typical granules of human basophils (Fig. 3A), further emphasizing the structural diversity of these organelles. For a comprehensive treatment of granule morphology in various types of mast cells and basophils, the reader is referred to the work of Ann Dvorak (58,61,63).

The best-characterized granule constituents are histamine, serotonin (in rodents), mast cell- and basophil-specific proteases, and lysosomal enzymes, all implicated in acute allergic responses (see Chap. 2). Recent studies have additionally localized molecules implicated in sustained inflammatory responses to granules. In particular, mast cells and basophils contain interleukins predominately of the Th2 type (IL-4, IL-5, IL-6, IL-8, IL-13), as well as tumor necrosis factor-α (TNF-α) and vascular endothelial growth factor–vascular permeability factor (VEGF–VPF) (64–70; see Chap. 11). Some, but not all, of

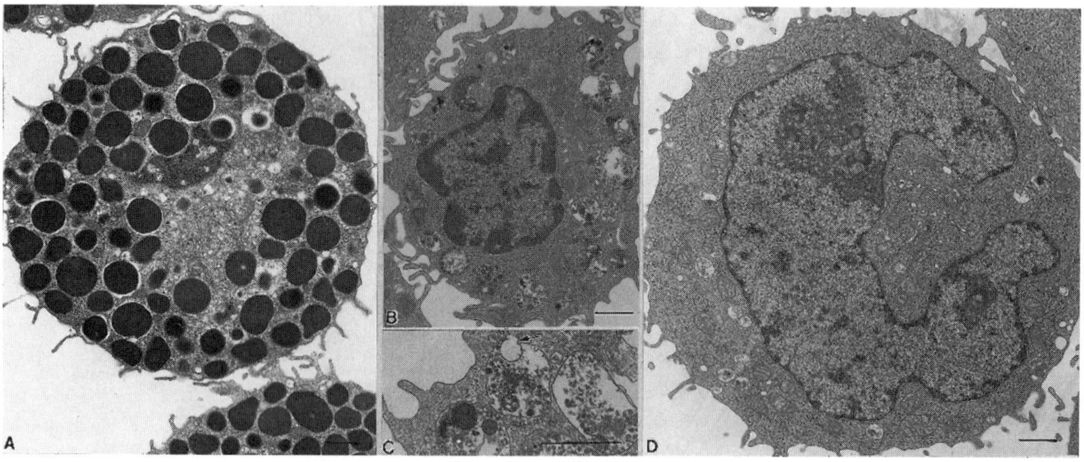

Figure 2 Ultrastructural heterogeneity of mast cells: These micrographs compare the typical morphology and relative sizes of (A) rat peritoneal mast cells, (B,C) mouse BMMC, and (D) RBL-2H3 mast cells. Peritoneal mast cells are characterized by large numbers of extremely dense granules. The small dense vesicles in the Golgi region very likely represent carriers en route to these mature granules. In contrast, the granules of BMMC and RBL-2H3 cells are less abundant, contain relatively little dense-core material and instead are characterized by the presence of internal vesicles and multilamellar membranes. The arrowhead in (C) points to an immature BMMC granule that appears to be pinching material inward from its limiting membrane. Bars, 1 μm.

these have been localized by immunoelectron microscopy to the secretory granule. Synthesis of many of these factors is up-regulated after IgE-mediated antigen stimulation (discussed later). There is little information as yet about the route of cytokines either to the cell surface or to the granule. Because the secretory lysosome receives a fraction of its cargo from the endosomal pathway, it is possible that some factors reach the granule by macropinocytosis of products released by neighboring immune cells, in addition to a more direct route as newly synthesized material on the exocytic pathway.

In addition to their possible role in the storage of cytokines, chemokines, and growth factors, mast cell granules may serve as sites for antigen processing and formation of peptide–MHC complexes. Raposo et al. (71) recently localized MHC II molecules to two distinct granule populations within BMMC: type I granules, with many internal membrane-bounded vesicles; and type II granules that possess both multivesicular structures and an incompletely formed electron-dense core. These two types of granules probably represent distinct stages in the maturation of the dense-core granule, relative to receipt of inward traffic from the endosomal pathway. The type I granules bear striking resemblance to the antigen-processing compartments of human B lymphocytes, in which there is a dramatic enrichment of MHC II molecules, costimulatory molecules and tetraspan proteins, including CD63, on internal vesicles (72). The role of the secretory lysosome in processing and presentation of antigen by mast cells and basophils is described later in this chapter.

The importance of a charged proteoglycan matrix as the ''glue'' for condensation and packing of mast cell granule contents was recently emphasized by studies in mice with a targeted disruption of the NDST-2 gene, the product of which is required for synthesis of heparin glycosaminoglycan. These animals have mast cells with abnormally large vacuoles

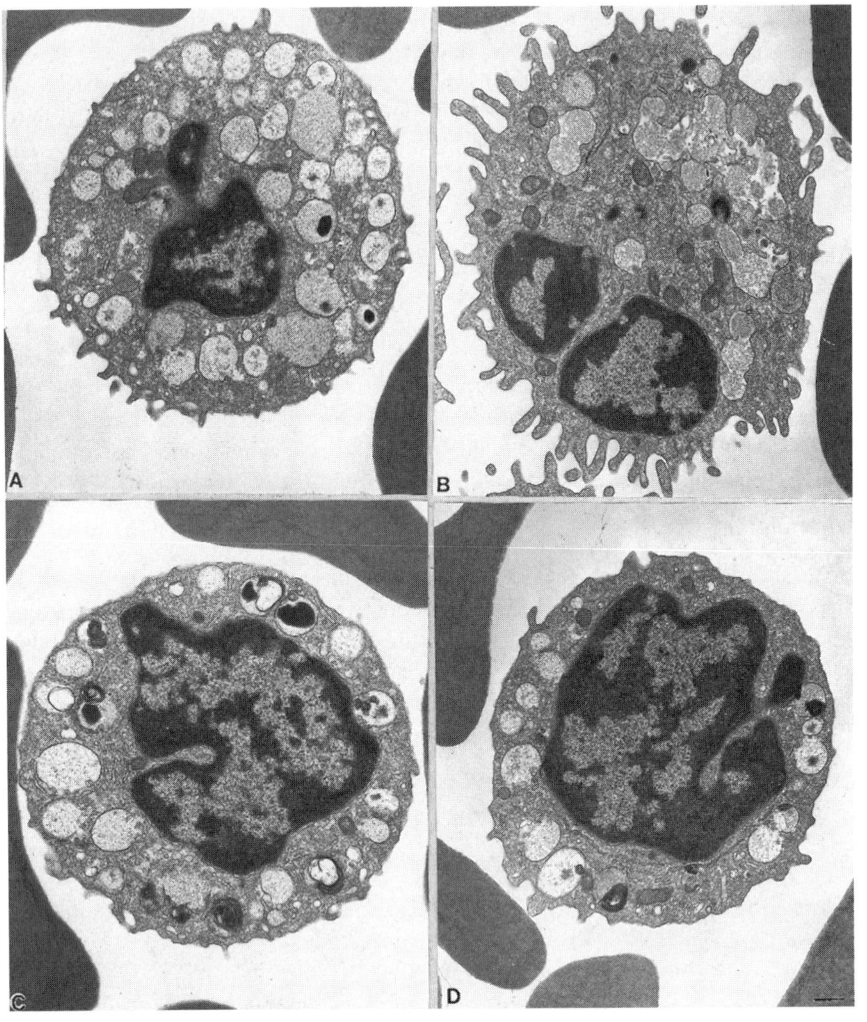

Figure 3 FcεRI-mediated degranulation and ruffling in human basophils: (A,B) IgE-primed releaser and (C,D) nonreleaser basophils were incubated for 15 min at 37°C without (A,C) or with (B,D) 1 μg/mL of anti-IgE antibody, then fixed and examined by transmission electron microscopy. (A,C) Resting cells show numerous granules, with a variable content of dense-core material, a multilobed nucleus, relatively sparse endoplasmic reticulum and mitochondria, and a fairly smooth plasma membrane. FcεRI cross-linking causes the intracellular fusion of granules and extracellular release of (B) granule contents in releaser, but not (D) nonreleaser basophils. FcεRI cross-linking also induces a dramatic membrane ruffling response in the releaser but not in the nonreleaser cells. Bars, 1 μm. (From Ref. 98.)

and severely reduced stores of histamine and mast cell proteases (73,74). Mucosal mast cells, that contain chondroitin sulfate instead of heparin, are unaffected in the NDST-2 null mice (73). In addition, studies of several genetic diseases will likely reveal details of the assembly not only of basophil and mast cell granules, but also of the related secretory lysosomes responsible for accumulating clotting factors in platelets, lytic enzymes in cytotoxic T cells, bone-resorbing hydrolases in osteoclasts, and pigment in melanocytes (75). As examples, Chediak–Higashi, Griscelli's, and Hermansky–Pudlak syndromes are all human genetic diseases linked to abnormal formation of secretory lysosomes, or acquisition of their cargo, in mast and other cells. These inherited diseases are associated with multiple symptoms, including partial albinism, bleeding disorders, and immunodeficiencies (76).

6 SIGNALING THROUGH THE FcεRI OF BASOPHILS AND MAST CELLS

6.1 Physiological Responses

FcεRI-positive basophils and mast cells are typically activated by the addition of multivalent antigen or anti-IgE antibodies to IgE-primed cells. The resulting cross-linking of adjacent IgE–FcεRI complexes initiates the cascade of biochemical, ionic, and physiological responses shown schematically in Figure 4 (see also previous reviews in Refs. 77–81).

6.1.1 Degranulation

Despite the variability between the granules of different basophils and mast cells, FcεRI cross-linking consistently causes the release of histamine and other inflammatory mediators by fusion of cytoplasmic granules with the plasma membrane. Degranulation is also

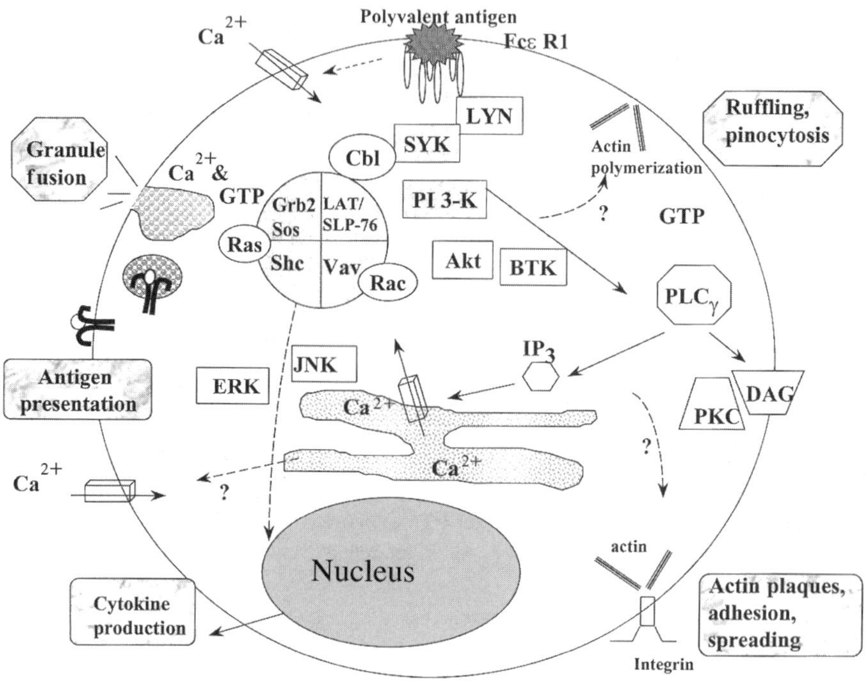

Figure 4 An overview of FcεRI signaling in basophils and mast cells. Boxes outside the "cell" show the principal physiological responses induced by FcεRI cross-linking. A subset of the biochemical and ionic events linking FcεRI cross-linking to these physiological responses are illustrated inside the "cell."

consistently induced by Ca^{2+} ionophores, demonstrating that Ca^{2+} mobilization is one key event tying FcεRI cross-linking to secretion. The time course of the release varies with stimulus and cell type, but is typically rapid (in seconds to minutes). The process of release is also variable. Granule fusion with the plasma membrane is often preceded or accompanied by homotypic fusion of granules, as shown for the activated human basophil in Figure 3B. In contrast, the series of micrographs from a movie of degranulation induced by FcεRI cross-linking in an RBL-2H3 cell expressing GFP–Fas ligand clearly shows the trajectory of a single granule as it translocates to the cell surface for fusion (Fig. 5A–C).

Many laboratories are actively seeking to define the proteins that regulate the mast cell secretory process. Our understanding is complicated by 1) the knowledge that different model systems contain granules at different stages of maturation or fusion competency; 2) the probability that distinct mechanisms regulate heterotypic fusion (granule with plasma membrane) and homotypic fusion (granule to granule); and 3) by the apparent existence

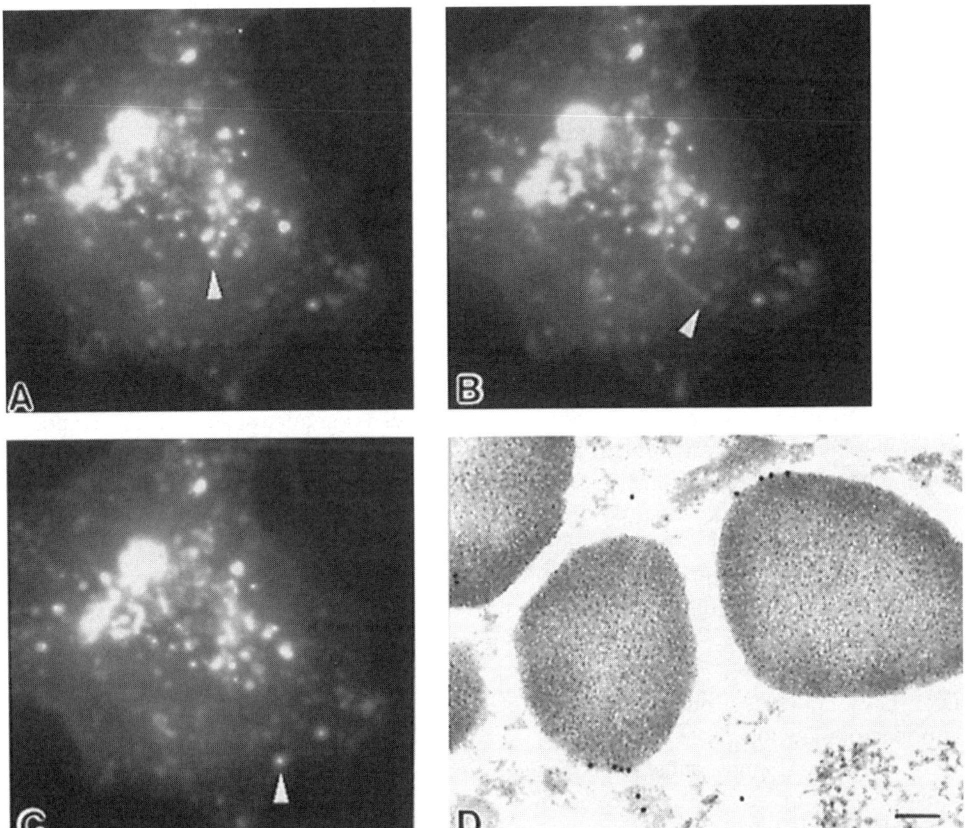

Figure 5 FcεRI-mediated degranulation in RBL-2H3 cells: (A–C) RBL-2H3 cells expressing transfected GFP-Fas ligand, a marker for granule membranes, were stimulated with DNP–BSA, and granule distribution was followed by fluorescence video microscopy. Three frames taken at 1-sec intervals show the movement of one granule from the cell center to the periphery. (D) Frozen sections of rat peritoneal mast cells were labeled with anti-Rab3D antibody conjugated with 5-nm protein A–gold. Rab 3D, a GTPase, is associated with the granule membrane. Bar in D, 0.1 μm. (Courtesy of A Smith and BS Wilson.)

of stimulus-responsive, histamine-containing cytoplasmic vesicles, for which the target membrane (either the plasma membrane or the granule) is unknown. A limited number of molecules have now been implicated in mast cell secretion, opening the way for a detailed analysis of this complex system. These include *S*oluble *N*-ethylmaleinside sensitive *A*ttachment *P*rotein (SNAP)-23, a *t*arget-SNAP *r*eceptor (t-SNARE) that may be principally involved in granule–granule fusion (82); *v*esicle-*a*ssociated *m*embrane *p*rotein (VAMP)2, a candidate vesicle (v)-SNARE (83); syntaxins 3 and 4, candidate t-SNAREs that localize to granules and plasma membrane, respectively (82); and a host of GTP-binding (G) proteins.

Gomperts and colleagues were the first to demonstrate a role for GTP in mast cell secretion (84). For many years, the search focused on identification of a putative single G protein, G_E, responsible for GTP-dependent exocytosis. It is now clear that multiple GTP-dependent steps participate in the signaling cascades that initiate stimulus–secretion coupling, as well as the docking or fusion processes themselves. A partial list of the players presently implicated in mast cell degranulation includes the heterotrimeric G proteins, $G_{i\alpha 3}$ and $G_{s\alpha}$ (85) and their $\beta\gamma$-subunits (86), and members of the Ras superfamily including Rac and Cdc42 (86,87), and Rab3D (88–92). Of these, only the GTPase Rab3D has been specifically localized to the mast cell granule (91; see Fig. 5D). However, multiple proteins in the range of 20–25 kDa bind radiolabeled GTP following sodium dodecylsulfate–polyacrylamide gel electrophoresis (SDS–PAGE) and blotting of solubilized mast cell granules (Wilson BS, Martinez AM, unpublished results). These proteins are likely to include additional members of the Ras superfamily that directly associate with mast cell and basophil granules.

6.1.2 Membrane and Cytoskeletal Responses

As well as causing degranulation, FcεRI cross-linking in both human and rodent basophils and mast cells induces the polymerization of F-actin (77,93,94) and the deployment of this actin to support dramatic membrane and cytoskeletal changes. The ruffling response of human basophils to multivalent antigen is demonstrated in Figure 3B. Figure 6A and B demonstrates the same transition of RBL-2H3 mast cell membrane topography from microvillous to lamellar in response to FcεRI cross-linking. One clear consequence of ruffling is a substantial increase in fluid uptake by macropinocytosis induced by FcεRI cross-linking (93). Ruffling and pinocytosis are consistently induced by phorbol myristate acetate (PMA; see Fig. 6D), suggesting a role for PMA-sensitive protein kinase C isoforms in the pathway linking FcεRI cross-linking to membrane remodeling. Conversely, inhibitors of the enzyme phosphatidylinositol 3-kinase (PI 3-kinase), described in more detail later, have little effect on FcεRI-induced actin polymerization, but abolish both ruffling and macropinocytosis (see Fig. 6C; 95).

In RBL-2H3 mast cells, IgE-mediated F-actin assembly also contributes to a characteristic spreading response linked to the formation of novel adhesion structures called actin plaques (Fig. 7; 96). TEM studies revealed actin plaques as distinct, actin-rich structures that link the mast cell membrane to the underlying substratum. In human blood-derived macrophages, the assembly of comparable dynamic adhesion structures, called podosomes, is partly regulated by Wiskott–Aldrich syndrome protein (WASP) in cooperation with the Rho family GTPase, CDC42Hs (97). Although their function is not known with certainty, we anticipate that actin plaques contribute to the localization and migration of mast cells within tissues. Actin plaques have not been observed in human basophils.

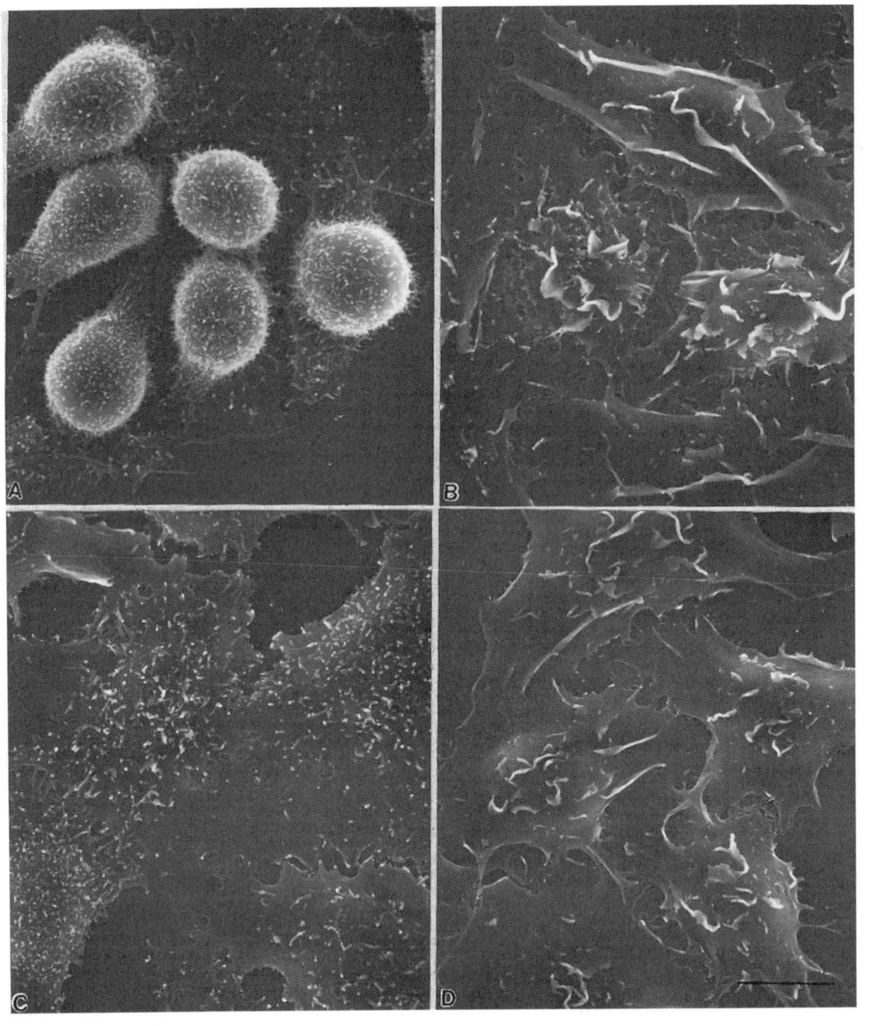

Figure 6 FcεRI-mediated ruffling in RBL-2H3 cells: Monolayers of IgE-primed RBL-2H3 cells on glass coverslips were incubated for 5 min at 37°C with (A) no addition; (B) 1 μg/mL DNP-BSA for 5 min; (C) 1 μg/mL DNP-BSA following 15 min with 10 ng/mL wortmannin; or (D) with 25 nM PMA. Cells were fixed and membrane topography observed by SEM. Antigen and PMA both induce ruffling and spreading; wortmannin inhibits ruffling but not spreading. Bar, 10 μm.

6.1.3 Adhesion

Both basophils (98) and RBL-2H3 mast cells (78) additionally upregulate the activity of their primary integrin, VLA-4 (CD49d/CD29) (99), in response to FcεRI cross-linking. We determine VLA-4 adhesive activity from the ability of basophils or mast cells to form conjugates with CHO cells transfected with VCAM-1 (CD106), the physiological ligand for VLA-4 on endothelial cells. The basophils or mast cells and VCAM–CHO cells are prelabeled separately with nonoverlapping fluorochromes, and the formation of dual color conjugates is measured by flow cytometry. The lower limit of VLA-4–mediated adhesion

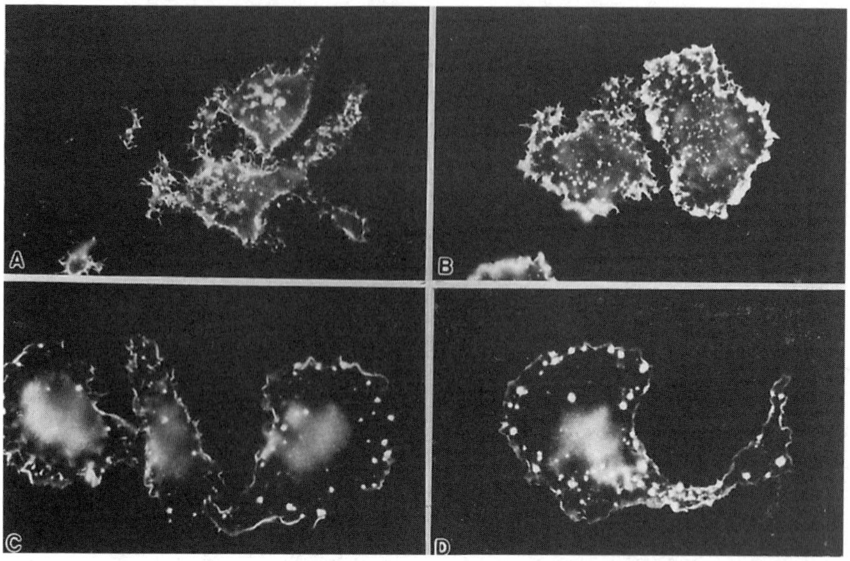

Figure 7 FcεRI-mediated actin plaque assembly in RBL-2H3 cells: (A) Monolayers of IgE-primed RBL-2H3 cells on glass coverslips were incubated at 37°C, with no addition or after adding 1 μg/mL DNP–BSA for (B) 2, (C) 5, and (D) 15 min. Cells were fixed and F-actin observed using rhodamine–phalloidin. Actin plaques are present at 2 min and prominent after 5 min of activation. (From Ref. 96.)

is set by including EDTA or antibodies to VLA-4 in the assay mixture, and the upper limit by including the VLA-4–activating MAb 8A2, together with the VLA-4–activating cation Mn^{2+}, in the incubation mixture. The results in Figure 8 (Andrews RP, Oliver JM, unpublished) show that the proportion of blood basophils that form conjugates during a 15-min rolling assay with VCAM–CHO cells is approximately doubled when the cells are activated by FcεRI cross-linking. Similar data were obtained with RBL-2H3 cells (78). We suppose that this adhesive response is linked to the membrane and cytoskeletal responses and jointly involved in basophil and mast cell recruitment from blood to inflamed tissues and migration within tissues.

6.1.4 De Novo Synthesis of Cytokines and Inflammatory Mediators

Within minutes of FcεRI cross-linking, mast cells release newly synthesized leukotrienes (LCs) and prostaglandins (PGs), notably LTC_4 and PGD_2. The synthesis and release of these mediators is described in a recent review (100; see also Chap. 10).

Several hours after FcεRI cross-linking, basophils and mast cells additionally begin to produce cytokines, including IL-4, IL-5, and IL-13 strongly implicated in the recruitment of other immune cells (eosinophils, lymphocytes) to sites of inflammation, in the proliferation of the Th2 (proinflammatory) subset of T cells and in the stimulation of B cells to produce more IgE (101–106). The peak production of IL-4 occurs after 2 hr of FcεRI cross-linking in RBL-2H3 cells and after 4 hr of FcεRI cross-linking in basophils (98,107). IL-4 production is also consistently induced by Ca^{2+} ionophores, suggesting that Ca^{2+} mobilization is one key event linking FcεRI cross-linking to the synthesis of cytokines. The discovery that activated basophils and mast cells are important sources of Th2

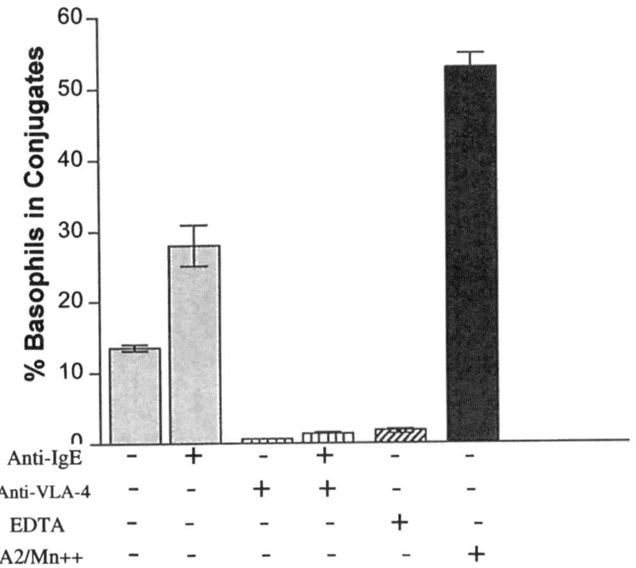

Figure 8 FcεRI-mediated VLA-4 up-regulation in human basophils: Fluorescence-labeled VLA-4–positive basophils were rolled for 15 min with VCAM–CHO cells, with no addition, or with the addition of anti-IgE, anti-VLA-4 (without and with anti-IgE), EDTA, and MAb 8A2 plus Mn^{2+}. The cells were fixed and VLA-4 adhesive activity was estimated from the proportion of basophil–VCAM-CHO conjugates measured by flow cytometry. EDTA and MAb 8A2 and Mn^{2+}, respectively, set the adhesion minima and maxima. Basophil VLA-4–dependent adhesion is substantially up-regulated by FcεRI cross-linking. (From Ref. 98.)

cytokines has led to a greater appreciation of these cells not only as effectors of symptomatic disease, but also as important contributors to the maintenance and exacerbation of the allergic phenotype.

6.2 Signal Initiation

6.2.1 The Discovery of FcεRI-Associated Tyrosine Kinases

One disappointment in learning the complete sequence of FcεRI was the lack of recognizable catalytic domains in any of the three FcεRI subunits. Nevertheless, circumstantial evidence implicated tyrosine kinases in FcεRI signaling. In particular, early biochemical studies (108) had shown phosphotyrosines in both the FcεRI β and FcεRI γ cytoplasmic tails; Benhamou et al. (109) had shown that FcεRI cross-linking induces the tyrosine phosphorylation of several proteins, including a 72-kDa species, in RBL-2H3 cells; and Deanin et al. (110,111) had reported that FcεRI-mediated secretion, and cytoskeletal responses could be inhibited in permeabilized RBL-2H3 mast cells by tyrosine kinase inhibitors and mimicked by tyrosine phosphatase inhibitors. Further studies confirmed that FcεRI signaling occurs by a tyrosine kinase-dependent pathway and identified the kinases and a series of their substrates. Among these early studies, the Kinet group (112) showed that multivalent antigen causes the tyrosine phosphorylation of the FcεRI β- and γ-subunits of cross-linked, but not monomeric receptors; Eiseman and Bolen (113) identified Lyn as the principal Src kinase family member in RBL-2H3 cells and showed its activation by

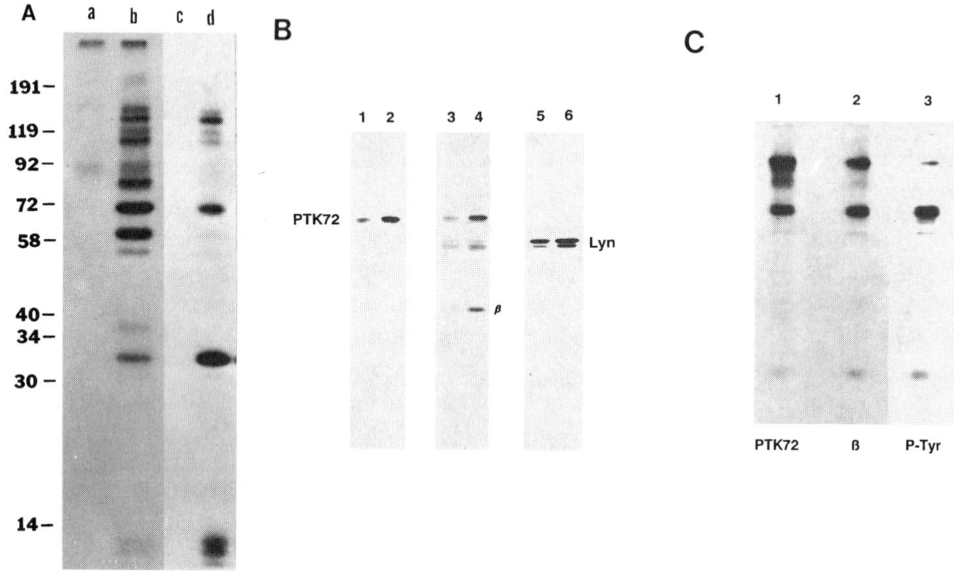

Figure 9 Identifying Syk as a FcεRI-associated protein tyrosine kinase: (A) [^{32}P] *ortho*phosphate-labeled IgE-primed RBL-2H3 cells were incubated for 2 min, without or with 0.1 μg/mL DNP–BSA, then lysed in Triton-containing buffer and the clarified lysates immunoprecipitated with either (lanes a and b) antiphosphotyrosine or (lanes c,d) anti-FcεRI β antibodies. (B) there is very little phosphoprotein in resting cells (lanes 1 and 3). FcεRI cross-linking causes the tyrosine phosphorylation of multiple proteins (lane 2), including a prominent FcεRI-associated 72-kDa phosphoprotein (lane d). (B) Lysates of resting and activated cells were immunoprecipitated with antibodies to PTK72–Syk (lanes 1,2). FcεRI β (lanes 3,4), and Lyn (lanes 5,6). The presence and activities of precipitated kinases was determined by adding [^{32}P]ATP to the immune complexes. FcεRI cross-linking increases the in vitro kinase activities of both Lyn and PTK72–Syk. Kinase activity, very likely mediated by coprecipitated Lyn and Syk, was also detected in antireceptor immune complexes from activated cells. (C) The 72-kDa proteins that are phosphorylated in anti-PTK72 (lane 1), anti-FcεRI β (lane 2) and antiphosphotyrosine (lane 3) immune complex kinase assays were eluted from the gels and are compared by one-dimensional peptide mapping. These studies identified the 72-kDa FcεRI-associated protein as PTK72, later renamed Syk. (From: A, Ref. 114; B,C, Ref. 115.)

FcεRI cross-linking; and we (114) demonstrated that a 72-kDa phosphoprotein is strongly associated with the phosphorylated FcεRI $\beta\gamma_2$-complex of activated RBL-2H3 cells (Fig. 9A). In 1992, we identified the 72-kDa protein tyrosine kinase PTK72 (115) in RBL-2H3 mast cells. PTK72 was originally purified from B cells (116). It was renamed Syk after the porcine gene, *Syk*, cloned by Taniguchi et al. (117), and encodes a protein tyrosine kinase identical with PTK72. Figure 9B is an in vitro kinase assay (115), that illustrates the activation of Lyn and PTK72/Syk induced by FcεRI cross-linking in RBL-2H3 cells. Peptide mapping studies (see Fig. 9C; 115) confirmed that the 72-kDa proteins that are phosphorylated in anti-PTK72/Syk and in anti-FcεRI β immune complex kinase assays are both PTK72/Syk.

The critical role of Syk in FcεRI signaling was established by studies with the Syk-selective tyrosine kinase inhibitor, piceatannol, that had no effect on the FcεRI-mediated tyrosine phosphorylation of Lyn and the FcεRI β- and γ-subunits, but abolished FcεRI-mediated Syk activation and all signaling responses both in RBL-2H3 mast cells (118) and in human blood basophils (119). A second inhibitor, ER-27319, that inhibits Syk, not by blocking its catalytic domain, but by blocking its interaction with FcεRI subunits, also spared Lyn activation and subunit phosphorylation, but inhibited downstream responses (120). These and other Syk inhibitors have been considered for the treatment of allergic inflammation. However, their potential as therapeutic tools is probably limited because of the critical role of Syk, its family member, ZAP-70, and its activating subunit FcεRI γ (see later) in many immune cells, in addition to basophils and mast cells. The pivotal role of Syk in rodent FcεRI signaling was further established by evidence that degranulation can be activated in transfected rat mast cells simply by cross-linking a chimeric receptor expressing full-length Syk as a cytoplasmic chain (121) and, conversely, by evidence that there is no IgE-mediated signaling in mast cells matured from the fetal liver of Syk knockout mice (122) or in a RBL-2H3 variant lacking Syk (123).

An ''experiment of nature'' may guide efforts to develop treatments for allergic inflammation based on Syk inactivation. Basophils from between 10 and 20% of nonallergic blood donors are structurally normal (see Fig. 3C), but do not degranulate in response to FcεRI cross-linking (103,124–126). As shown in Figure 3D, nonreleaser basophils also fail to ruffle in response to FcεRI cross-linking. Similar to other ''nonreleaser'' basophils, the nonreleaser basophils from five healthy donors identified by C. Kepley and L. Youssef in our laboratory expressed FcεRI and showed normal secretion and cytokine synthesis responses to Ca^{2+} ionophore, phorbol ester, and formyl peptide, all stimuli that bypass the FcεRI. These basophils contained Lyn protein. However, Syk protein was consistently undetectable (Fig. 10; for additional data see Ref. 98, 127). Although the basophils from all five donors lack Syk protein, they do contain Syk mRNA, suggesting that the abnormality in Syk is at the level of protein expression or stability. Furthermore, Syk is present in normal amounts in B cells, eosinophils, and neutrophils isolated from these donors, indicating that the defect is lineage-specific (see Fig. 10). Importantly, the Syk-negative phenotype is reversible in vivo and in vitro. Basophils from one nonreleaser converted spontaneously to the releaser phenotype, accompanied by Syk protein expression, and reverted back to the nonreleaser phenotype in the course of a 12-month study. Basophils from all five nonreleasers expressed low levels of Syk and showed modest degranulation after incubation for 4 days in medium with IL-3. There seems little doubt that understanding the lineage-specific suppression of Syk expression in nonreleaser basophils, and learning to replicate this property in patients with allergic asthma, would be a powerful way to protect these individuals against symptomatic disease while preserving essential Syk-mediated activities of their lymphoid and myeloid cells.

6.2.2 The Activation of FcεRI-Associated Kinases

The recognition of sequences called ITAMs, for immunoreceptor tyrosine-based activation motifs (6), was a critical event toward understanding both the family affiliations of the FcεRI and the sequence and mechanisms of Lyn and Syk activation induced by FcεRI cross-linking. ITAMs are 26- or 27-amino acid sequences that include two YxxL motifs separated by 9 or 10 amino acids. ITAMs are found in single copy in the C-terminal domains of both the FcεRI β- and γ-subunits. They occur additionally in the BCR Igα and Igβ subunits, and in the TCR CD3ε chain and in triplicate in the TCR ζ- and η-subunits. These receptors, together with FcγRI and FcγRIII, that share the ITAM-containing FcεRI γ-subunit, make up a new receptor family, the multichain immune recognition receptors (MIRRs) (Fig. 11). Work in the Metzger laboratory (128–130) showed that the FcεRI β- and γ-ITAMs are both targets for Lyn-mediated phosphorylation. Studies by

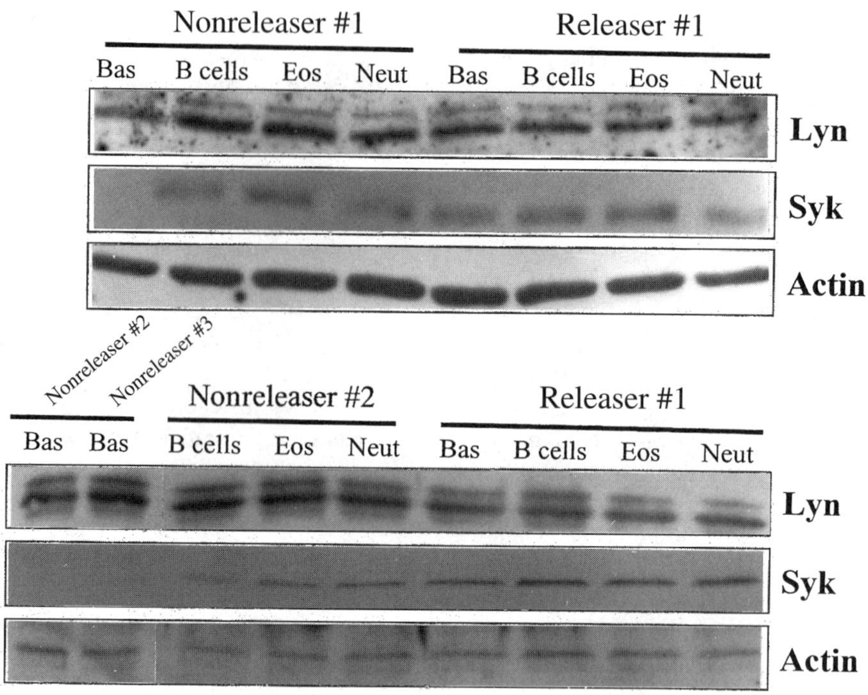

Figure 10 Nonreleaser basophils lack Syk: Lysates of highly purified releaser and nonreleaser basophils (Bas) as well as B cells, eosinophils (Eos), neutrophils (Neut) from the same donors, were analyzed by Western blotting for Lyn, Syk, and actin expression. (Upper panel) equal amounts of protein (13 μg) were added to the gel; (lower panel) equal numbers of cell equivalents (2×10^5 cells per lane) were used. (From Ref 127.)

Shuie et al. (131) showed that Syk is directly activated by the interaction of its tandem SH2 domains with the doubly phosphorylated ITAMs of the FcεRI γ-subunit (see Fig. 1). These and other data suggested that Lyn and Syk activation are sequential events in the FcεRI signaling cascade. They failed to clarify why the FcεRI has both β- and γ-subunit ITAMs when, perhaps, a single ITAM could support signaling.

The separate activities of the FcεRI β- and γ-subunit ITAMs in signaling were established by studies in transfected RBL-2H3 cells expressing chimeric receptors in which the full-length FcεRI β- and γ-cytoplasmic tails were linked to the extracellular and transmembrane sequences of the Tac antigen (132). Cross-linking the isolated FcεRI γ-tail activated Syk and elicited all of the signaling responses of the intact FcεRI, although to a lesser extent. In contrast, cross-linking the isolated FcεRI β-tail elicited no Syk activation or signaling responses. Furthermore, it inhibited subsequent Syk activation and signaling though the intact FcεRI on the same cells (Fig. 12). These data suggested that full-signaling activity resides in the FcεRI γ-subunit and that FcεRI β may function primarily as a regulator of FcεRI γ-mediated Syk activation and downstream signaling. Because FcεRI β binds Lyn (133), it was proposed that this regulation may occur in part by determining the availability of Lyn for FcεRI γ phosphorylation. The concept of FcεRI β as a regulator of FcεRIγ signaling was strongly supported by the Kinet group, who first showed in transfected NIH 3T3 cells and, subsequently, in transgenic mice that fibroblasts, basophils,

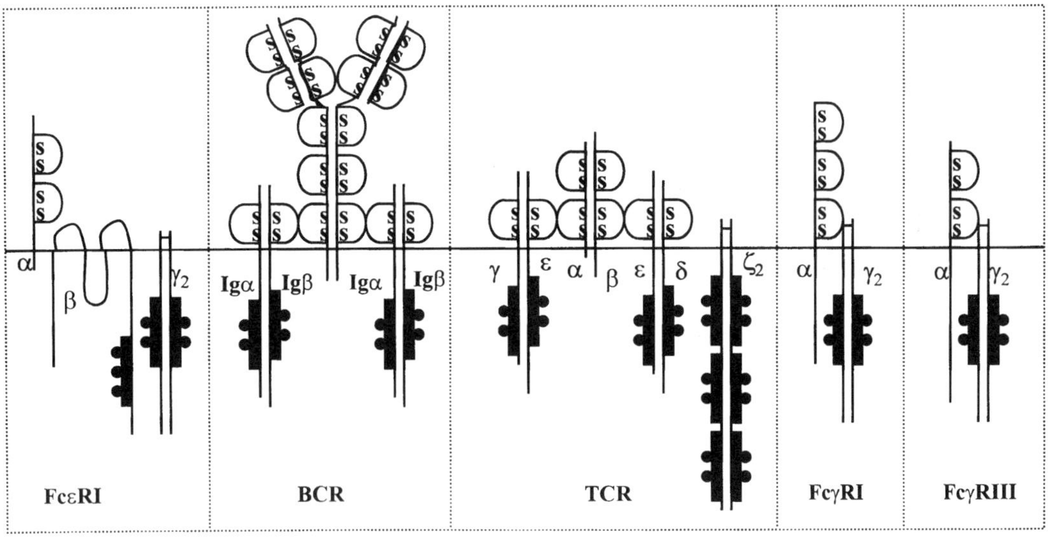

Figure 11 The multichain immune recognition receptor (MIRR) family: The FcεRI is shown in the context of its related family members. Semicircles represent immunoglobulin domains; solid bars represent ITAMs; balls show the location of tyrosine residues in the ITAMs.

and mast cells expressing an $\alpha\gamma_2$ FcεRI have a full range of normal-signaling activities, but all at a lower extent than the responses elicited by the $\alpha\beta\gamma_2$ FcεRI (13,134).

Recent studies have emphasized the importance not only of Lyn-mediated FcεRI subunit phosphorylation, but also of the subsequent dissociation of Lyn for Syk recruitment and signal progression. In general, anti-FcεRI α MAbs that induce formation of FcεRI dimers are almost as effective as multivalent antigen at triggering degranulation (135). An unusual anti-FcεRI α MAb, H10, was investigated that induced FcεRI dimer formation and initiated β- and γ-subunit phosphorylation, but failed to induce strong Syk activation and signaling responses. The impaired signaling properties of MAb H10–FcεRI dimers were linked to the formation of stable complexes of Lyn with incompletely phosphorylated subunits (136). Lyn dissociation, Syk activation, and signaling responses were all restored by cross-linking the dimers with goat anti-mouse IgG (137), raising the possibility that the signal curtailing properties of MAb H10–FcεRI dimers results from an unfavorable dimer orientation that is overcome by further cross-linking. A similarly incomplete phosphorylation of TCR subunits has been linked to the impaired signaling induced by certain altered peptide ligands (APLs) in T cells (138–142). Furthermore, it has been established that cytokine receptor signaling depends critically on orientational properties of the receptor dimer (143).

Recent work has clearly established that Lyn is rate-limiting for FcεRI signaling (144–147). Thus cross-linkers such as MAb H10, that sequester Lyn through the formation of stable complexes between Lyn and receptor dimers, should not only block the subset of ligated receptors, but also be strong inhibitors of allergen-induced FcεRI signaling through other receptors.

The diagram in Figure 13 shows a simplified model of the initiation of the FcεRI-signaling cascade. In resting cells (left), two FcεRIs are not cross-linked and not phosphorylated. FcεRI cross-linking (middle) induces the Lyn-mediated phosphorylation of

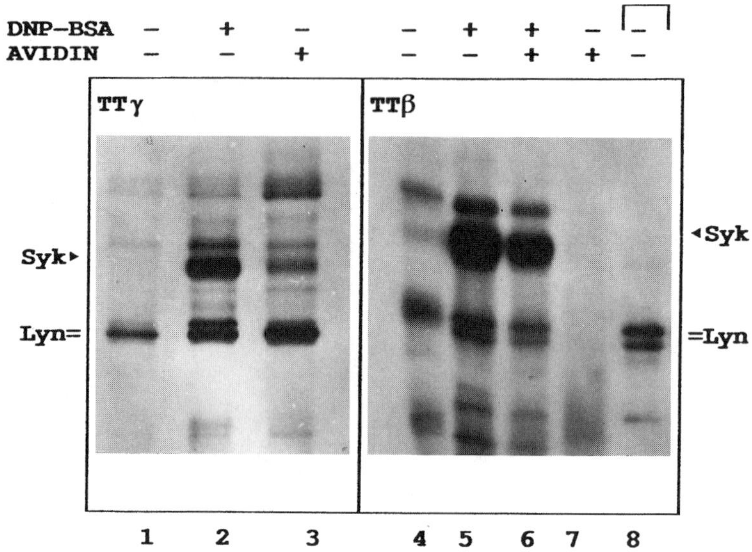

Figure 12 Distinct roles for FcεRI β and FcεRI γ in signal transduction: This experiment uses RBL-2H3 cells expressing both the native FcεRI and transfected chimeric receptors, consisting of the extracellular and transmembrane domains of the Tac antigen linked to the cytoplasmic tails of either FcεRI γ (TTγ) or FcεRI β (TTβ). The separate receptors were primed independently with IgE and with biotinylated anti-Tac antibody. FcεRI was cross-linked with antigen (DNP–BSA) and chimeric receptor with avidin. After 2-min activation through one or both receptors, cells were lysed and antiphosphotyrosine immune complexes were assayed for their in vitro kinase activities. (Left box) results show that cross-linking TTγ (lane 3) causes Lyn and Syk activation resembling the kinase activation induced by FcεRI cross-linking (lane 2). (Right box) results show that cross-linking TTβ (lane 7) causes no independent Lyn and Syk activation and, furthermore, partially inhibits the kinase activation induced by simultaneously cross-linked FcεRI (compare lanes 5 and 6). Lane 8 shows activated Lyn obtained from an in vitro kinase assay performed on immunoprecipitable Lyn. (From Ref. 132.)

FcεRI subunits. The dissociation of Lyn from fully phosphorylated subunits, in turn, permits Syk recruitment and signal propagation (right).

6.3 Signal Propagation

6.3.1 FcεRI Signal Propagation

Signaling from $Fc_{\varepsilon}RI$ cross-linking to Lyn and Syk activation brings us to a series of branch points from which secondary signaling cascades proliferate. A sampling of these is shown in Figure 4. Proteins that are phosphorylated as an apparently direct consequence of Syk activation include two phospholipase Cγ isoforms, PLCγ1 and PLCγ2, that link FcεRI cross-linking to Ca^{2+} mobilization implicated strongly in both degranulation and cytokine production; Vav (148), a GTP exchange factor (GEF) implicated in activating members of the Rho family of GTPases to initiate membrane and cytoskeletal responses; Grb2 that may couple FcεRI cross-linking to the activation of Sos and Ras; SLP-76, which is also implicated in coupling FcεRI cross-linking to GTPase cascades; and several PKC isoforms that may be upstream of Ras-independent pathways to MAP

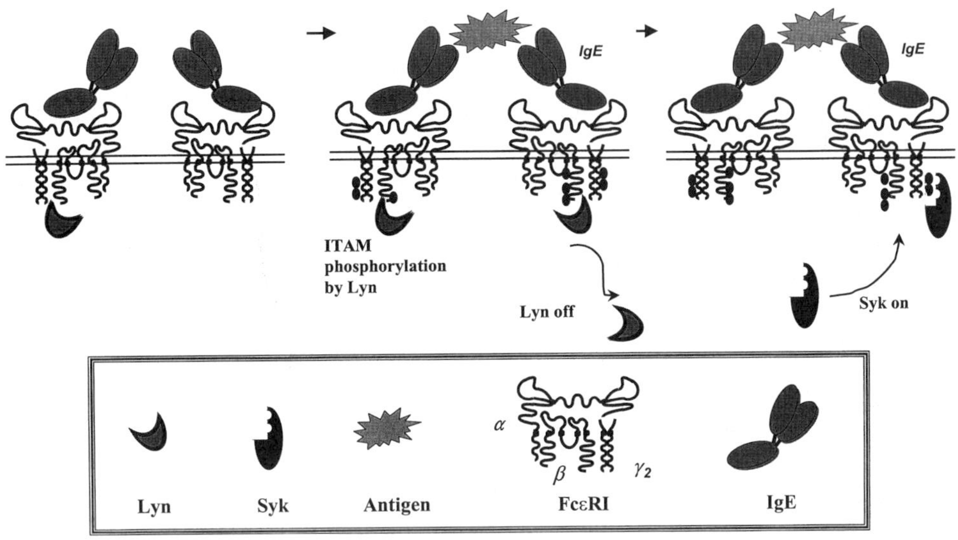

Figure 13 Initiating the FcεRI-signaling cascade in basophils and mast cells: (left) in resting cells, two FcεRIs are not cross-linked and not phosphorylated; (middle) FcεRI cross-linking induces the Lyn-mediated phosphorylation of ITAMs in the FcεRI β- and γ-subunits; (right) the dissociation of Lyn from fully phosphorylated subunits permits Syk recruitment and signal propagation.

kinase activation and gene expression. Curiously, we discovered that inactivating Ras by treatment with the farnesyl-specific prenylation inhibitor BZA-5B does not block the Raf/MEK/ERK activation pathway in RBL-2H3 cells (107). Thus, Ras-independent pathways to MAP kinase activation may be particularly important in mast cells. Other Syk substrates include Cbl, a ubiquitin ligase that forms complexes with Syk in resting cells and was recently implicated in the regulation of Syk degradation (149,150) and LAT (linker for the activation of T cells; 151,152) a transmembrane protein with no catalytic activity but multiple sites for Syk/ZAP-70–mediated tyrosine phosphorylation. In activated T cells, LAT is localized in TCR-signaling microdomains and provides binding sites for the recruitment and tyrosine phosphorylation of SH2 domain-containing signaling molecules. SLP-76, which interacts with LAT in TCR signaling, has also been implicated in FcεRI signaling based on a block in IL-6 production and secretion in SLP-76–deficient BMMCs (153). FcεRI cross-linking in mast cells also leads to activation of additional protein and lipid kinases, of which the class IA forms of PI 3-kinase, BTK (a member of the Tec family of cytoplasmic protein tyrosine kinases) (154) and Akt, a serine-threonine kinase downstream of the PI 3-kinase pathway (155), are only a partial list.

The role of PI 3-kinase, that converts phosphatidylinositol(4,5)P_2 to phosphatidylinositol (3,4,5)P_3, is of particular interest because it contributes at multiple levels to the signaling pathways downstream from FcεRI cross-linking and Syk activation. Of the physiological and biochemical responses to antigen stimulation, secretion, changes in cell surface topography, macropinocytosis, Akt activation, and Ins(1,4,5)P_3 synthesis, all are dependent on PI 3-kinase activity (95,156–159). No single mechanistic step, beyond the production of D3-phosphorylated phosphatidylinositols, is likely to provide a simple explanation to link these outcomes. Nowhere are the complexities of PI 3-kinase–dependent signaling more apparent than in the regulation of PLCγ isoforms and their production of

$Ins(1,4,5)P_3$. In antigen-stimulated RBL-2H3 cells, a primary means for increasing enzymatic activity of PLCγ enzymes is by their phosphorylation on activating tyrosine residues. In addition, both PLCγ1 and PLCγ2 are directly activated by $PtdIns(3,4,5)P_3$ (160) in a manner that is independent of the phosphorylation state of these enzymes (158). However, only the PLCγ1 isoform requires PI 3-kinase activity for translocation to the mast cell plasma membrane and partial activation by tyrosine phosphorylation (157). There are at least three candidate tyrosine kinases—Lyn, Syk, and BTK—that may be responsible for phosphorylation of the two different PLCγ isoforms. Although all three of these kinases are capable of phosphorylating the PLCγs in vitro (161; our unpublished observations), and Syk and BTK both appear to be critical upstream regulators of PLCγ activity and calcium mobilization (118,121–123,162), the precise sequence of events remains to be elucidated. Of particular interest is the interplay between the production of $PtdIns(3,4,5)P_3$ and BTK, that binds $PtdIns(3,4,5)P_3$ through its pleckstrin homology domain (163). Kinet and colleagues found an essential role for BTK in calcium mobilization that was PI 3-kinase dependent (162). The connection of BTK to PI 3-kinase is unlikely to be solely based upon a need for $PtdIns(3,4,5)P_3$ for BTK translocation and phosphorylation, as we found that wortmannin fails to block BTK phosphorylation in antigen-stimulated RBL-2H3 cells (157). Interestingly, kinase-dead BTK is capable of elevating $PtdIns(3,4,5)P_3$ levels, suggesting that one of BTK's roles may be to protect newly synthesized $PtdIns(3,4,5)P_3$ from degradation by phosphatases. A recent review of these issues is available (158).

A sustained increase in intracellular calcium is a critical event supporting both degranulation and transcriptional regulation in mast cells. A historical perspective spanning three decades of contributions in this field was recently published (164). It is generally recognized that the activation of PLCγ isoforms yields $Ins(1,4,5)P_3$, targeting IP_3 receptors that function as ligand-gated channels to permit the release of stored Ca^{2+}. Release of calcium from stores occurs within seconds after antigen stimulation and is followed by a sustained influx of extracellular calcium. Although the precise identity of the voltage-independent Ca^{2+} influx channel(s) remains elusive, new evidence in mast cells and other nonexcitable cells has recently reenergized the search. Early in this decade, critical patch-clamping experiments using T cells and mast cells identified a Ca^{2+} current that is activated by the emptying of intracellular stores (165–167; reviewed in Ref. 168). Because the properties of Ca^{2+}-conducting channels are similar in cells treated with antigen or with thapsigargin, which causes store depletion when the store's leak pathway is unopposed by constitutive uptake through the Sarco-Endoplasmic Reticulum Calcium-ATPase (SERCA) pump, Penner and colleagues named the putative channel, I_{CRAC} (CRAC = Ca^{2+} release-activated Ca^{2+} current). However, other studies suggested that different channels may mediate Ca^{2+} influx in antigen-stimulated cells and in cells where stores are passively depleted. First, the I_{CRAC} is poorly permeable to Ba^{2+} and Sr^{2+} ions, that readily enter the antigen-induced Ca^{2+} influx pathway (166,169). Second, a modest but measurable influx of Ca^{2+} precedes and supports Ca^{2+} stores release (170). Third, the PI 3-kinase inhibitor, wortmannin, consistently dampens antigen-stimulated Ca^{2+} influx, despite that Ca^{2+} stores are effectively depleted (158). Further studies of the new family of *trp* genes, that includes several candidates fitting the criteria for capacitative calcium channels (171,172), may resolve this dilemma. RBL-2H3 cells express multiple members of the Trp family, including Trp 1, 2, and 5 (173; Smith A, Wilson BS, unpublished results), opening the possibility that channels composed of distinct homo- or heterooligomers from members of this family are evoked with thapsigargin versus antigen stimulation. The profile of Trp family members expressed in human mast cells and basophils remains to be characterized.

7 SIGNALING THOUGH THE FcεRI OF DENDRITIC CELLS, MONOCYTES, AND MACROPHAGES

Until recently, it was thought that FcεRII/CD23 was the primary IgE-binding structure on cells other than basophils and mast cells. Pioneering work has now established not only that FcεRI is expressed in humans on dendritic cells, monocytes, and macrophages (as well as platelets and eosinophils), but also through studies with blocking antibodies to CD23 and FcεRI, that FcεRI is likely to be the primary receptor responsible for IgE-mediated signaling and antigen presentation on these cells (11,43,46,47,174–179; see Ref. 180 for evidence favoring CD23). As already described, FcεRI expression levels on these cells are typically 10- to 100-fold lower than on basophils and mast cells, with the highest levels occurring in atopic individuals with high serum IgE concentrations. Also, most investigators find that FcεRI is expressed on cells other than basophils and mast cells as an $\alpha\gamma_2$-trimer, rather than the familiar $\alpha\beta\gamma_2$-tetramer (9,43); however, there is evidence of FcεRI β expression in human alveolar macrophages (11).

Very few systematic studies of FcεRI signaling in cells other than basophils and mast cells have been reported. Nevertheless, there are multiple reports of the IgE-dependent release of lysosomal enzymes, active oxygen species, cytokines, chemokines and leukotrienes, and other arachidonate metabolites from alveolar macrophages (181–183) and of IgE-dependent cytokine and PGE_2 production by monocytes (184,185). Furthermore, Maurer et al. (176) and Jurgens et al. (186) have demonstrated FcεRI-mediated Ca^{2+} mobilization, respectively in adherent blood monocytes and in epidermal Langerhans cells from atopic donors, and work in the Bieber laboratory has shown that Langerhans cells contain multiple Src kinases, including Lyn, Fyn, and Lck, and that FcεRI cross-linking on these cells induces the rapid tyrosine phosphorylation of multiple proteins, including Syk (43,186).

Human peripheral blood monocytes and alveolar macrophages are relatively easy to obtain from blood and bronchioalveolar lavage fluid respectively, and recent studies have defined straightforward procedures to isolate dendritic cells from blood (111,187) and Langerhans cells from skin (186). Based on these technical advances, it now seems reasonable to predict a rapid growth in systematic knowledge of FcεRI signaling in human cells other than basophils and mast cells.

8 FcεRI-DEPENDENT ALLERGEN UPTAKE, PROCESSING, AND ANTIGEN PRESENTATION

Antigen-presenting cells (APC) are defined as cells with the capacity to take up and process antigen and subsequently present peptide–MHC class II complexes on the cell surface to T cells. This creates binding sites for allergen-specific T cells and, in conjunction with an appropriate range of contact-dependent and humoral costimulatory molecules, causes naïve T cells to proliferate and differentiate and memory T cells to proliferate and secrete effector molecules (188). The most effective APCs are dendritic cells, that originate in bone marrow and can be found in the peripheral blood, in the lungs, in lymphoid tissues, and in skin (dermal dendritic cells and epidermal Langerhans cells). Monocytes, macrophages, and B cells also synthesize MHC class II, express contact-dependent costimulatory molecules and cytokines, internalize and process antigen, and have APC activity. Additionally, mast cells are now recognized as having APC activity based on evidence 1) that they synthesize MHC class II molecules and express them both on the plasma membrane and in the secretory granules–secondary lysosomes; 2) that they express appropriate co-stimulatory molecules; and 3) that they synthesize Th2-polarizing cytokines (71,189–191). Most importantly, both rodent and human mast cells present antigen to T cells, resulting in IL-2 production by the T cells (189–193).

Antigen-presenting cells are capable of antigen uptake through both fluid phase pinocytosis and receptor-mediated endocytosis. Among these antigen capture methods, receptor-mediated endocytosis, which concentrates the antigen at the cell surface before internalization and allows the capture of rather large antigens and of antigens present in small amounts, should be the most efficient. Until recently, studies of receptor-mediated antigen uptake focused mainly on mannose receptors and low-affinity IgG receptors. The FcεRI was implicated among the receptors mediating antigen uptake through studies in monocytes and peripheral blood dendritic cells (12,43,46,177) and in Langerhans cells (43). These investigators showed that adding antigen to FcεRI-positive APC armed with specific IgE indeed results in a substantially better stimulation of both naïve and memory T cells than the stimulation that occurs in the absence of IgE–FcεRI complexes. Furthermore, evidence has been obtained (43) that cryptic antigen epitopes could be unmasked in the proteolytic compartment accessed by antigen–IgE–receptor complex and loaded onto MHC class II molecules. Figure 14 is a model (43) of the processing and presentation of antigen internalized by fluid pinocytosis (bottom) and by endocytosis as part of an antigen–IgE–FcεRI complex (top).

In mast cells, recent work (194,195) has shown that IFN-γ–treated mouse BMMC express high levels of MHC class II, but do not generate immunogenic peptides from soluble antigen (OVA) internalized by fluid-phase pinocytosis. The same cells become efficient APC when the antigen is internalized as an antigen–IgE-FcεRI complex. Two additional observations were particularly noteworthy. First, in addition to the dominant immunogenic peptide, several subdominant antigenic peptides were formed, creating conditions for the recruitment of naïve as well as memory T cells and for the expansion of the IgE repertoire, as already suggested (43) for antigen internalized by the FcεRI-dependent pathway of dendritic cells. Second, APC activity was inhibited by the Syk-selective tyrosine kinase inhibitor, piceatannol, and by the PI 3-kinase inhibitor, wortmannin, which both inhibit antigen-induced FcεRI signaling, but not the receptor-mediated endocytosis of bound antigen. These data suggest that the integrity of the FcεRI-signaling pathway is required for antigen presentation.

The pathways of FcεRI-mediated antigen uptake, processing, and presentation have not yet been well studied. We (93,196) have shown by immunogold-labeling studies in RBL-2H3 and P815 mast cells that the cross-linking of IgE–FcεRI complexes by multivalent antigen is followed within minutes by the redistribution of antigen–IgE–receptor complexes to clathrin-coated pits (Fig. 15A). The internalization process often involves the formation of tubular structures with clathrin-coated tips (see Fig. 15B). Once internalized, vesicles containing antigen are rapidly uncoated and delivered, very likely by an intermediate endosomal compartment, to cytoplasmic granules containing variable amounts of small vesicles, multilamellar membranes, and electron-dense core material (see Fig. 15C). As already described, these granules represent maturational stages of secretory lysosomes, the contents of which include proteolytic enzymes capable of degrading the allergen to immunogenic peptides, as well as MHC class II molecules, histamine, and lysosomal membrane markers (LAMPs). Because these granules can be released from activated mast cells, antigen-induced FcεRI cross-linking should permit not only the efficient uptake and processing of antigen for constitutive return to the cell surface as peptide–MHC class II

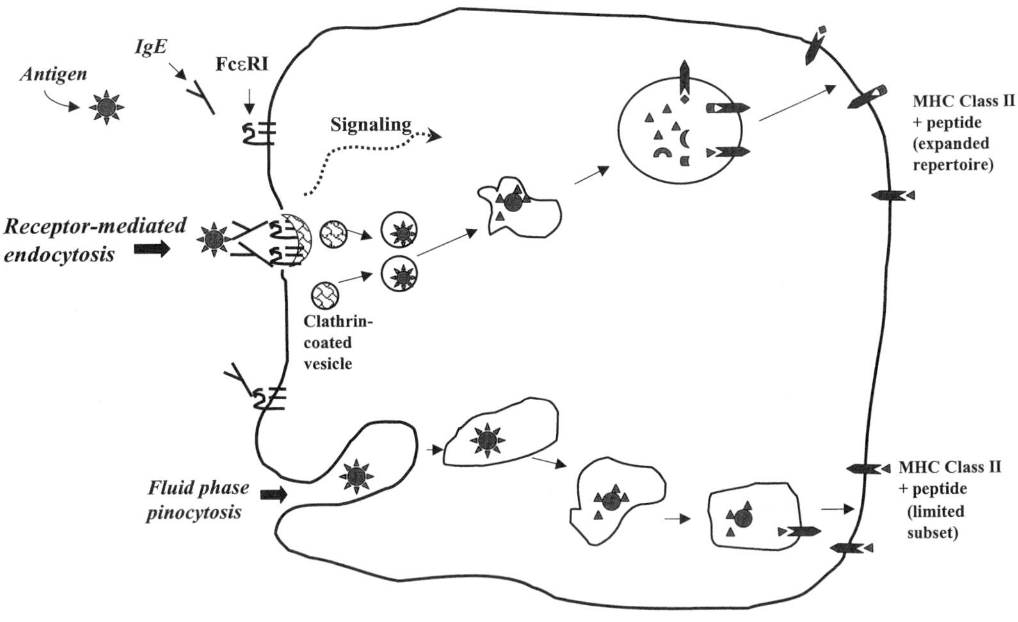

Figure 14 Different processing pathways for antigen taken up by fluid pinocytosis and by receptor-mediated endocytosis: This model suggests that antigen internalized by the clathrin-independent process of fluid pinocytosis is delivered to an endosomal compartment that supports rather limited processing for loading onto MHC class II molecules. In contrast, antigen internalized through coated pits as part of an antigen–IgE–receptor complex may be delivered to a separate endosomal–secretory lysosomal compartment that supports more efficient or extensive processing and MHC class II loading, leading to a stronger and more diverse T-cell response. Antigen-induced mast cell degranulation may additionally stimulate the insertion into the plasma membrane of peptide–MHC class II complexes generated during a previous cycle of receptor-mediated antigen uptake and processing, thereby, enhancing the presentation of processed peptides to T cells. (From Ref. 43.)

complexes, but also cause the rapid insertion into the plasma membrane of peptide–MHC class II complexes generated during a previous cycle of receptor-mediated antigen uptake and processing. Supporting this expectation, Raposo et al. (71) have demonstrated that antigen-induced FcεRI cross-linking stimulates the surface expression of peptide–MHC class II complexes during the process of degranulation. At the same time, degranulation results in the release of peptide-loaded MHC class II-containing internal vesicles, called ''exosomes.'' Although the physiological relevance of exosomes is not well understood, there is limited evidence that these small vesicles may represent a diffusible substitute for APCs in the stimulation of T cells (197). We anticipate that the internalization and trafficking pathways delivering antigen–IgE–receptor complexes to MHC class II-containing organelles in monocytes–macrophages and dendritic cells will be similar to or identical with the pathways observed in mast cells. It would not be surprising if FcεRI cross-linking also enhanced the presentation of peptide–MHC class II complexes on the surface of these cells.

Obviously, if FcεRI-mediated antigen uptake and processing contributes to the expression of new peptide–MHC class II complexes at the cell surface, with a subsequent widening of the IgE repertoire, treatments that inhibit the endocytosis or processing of

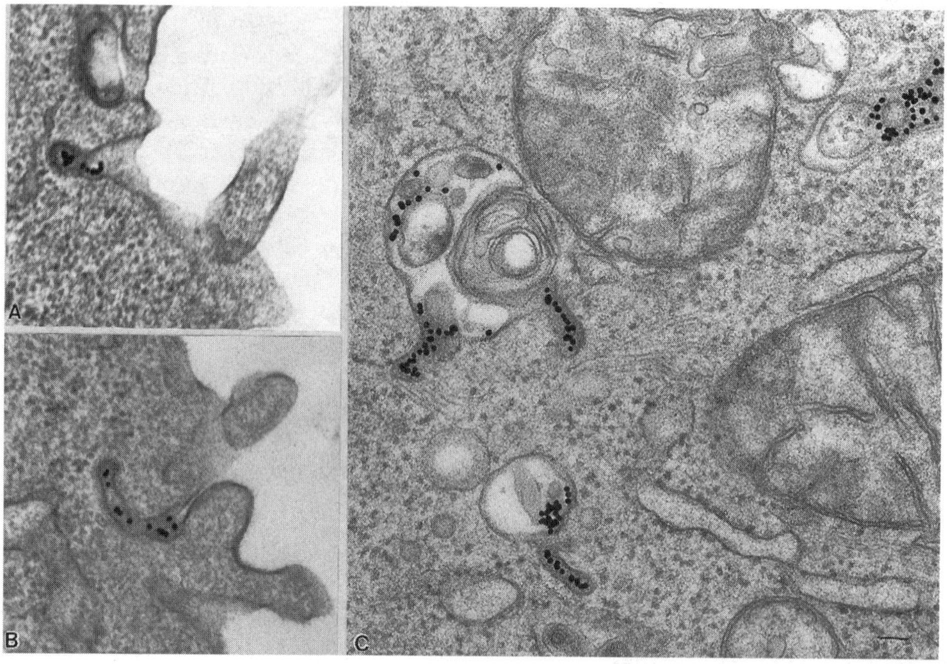

Figure 15 FcεRI-mediated antigen uptake in RBL-2H3 mast cells: IgE-primed RBL-2H3 cells were incubated for (A,B) 2 and (C) 10 min with DNP–BSA preconjugated to 15 nm colloidal gold particles. Cells were fixed and processed for transmission electron microscopy (93). Gold particles marking antigen–IgE–receptor complexes are internalized through (A) clathrin-coated pits, which (B) often elongate to form tubules with clathrin-coated tips. The particles are delivered to cytoplasmic granules that contain variable amounts of multilamellar membranes and internal vesicles. Bar, 1 μm.

antigen should contribute to the sustained relief of allergic inflammation by the decreased antigen-specific activation of both naïve and memory T cells. Supporting this, Maurer et al. (198) recently reported the delivery of antigen–IgE–FcεRI complexes of peripheral blood dendritic cells to acidic organelles containing MHC class II, lysosomal proteins, and cathepsin S, a cysteine protease required for the degradation of the invariant chain (Ii) of nascent MHC class II to allow loading with peptide. Importantly, cells treated with a specific active site-directed inhibitor of cathepsin S, *N*-morpholinurea-leucine-homophenylalanine-vinylsulfone-phenyl (LHVS), decreased the export of MHC class II to the cell surface and strongly reduced IgE–FcεRI-mediated antigen presentation. These studies suggest FcεRI trafficking pathways as promising targets for new therapies to block expansion of the repertoire of antigen-specific T cells in patients with allergic inflammation.

9 IMPLICATIONS FOR ALLERGIC INFLAMMATION

We have demonstrated that the IgE-dependent targeting of antigen to the human FcεRI may promote allergic inflammation by two distinct mechanisms. The first mechanism, dependent on FcεRI signaling, results in the acute induction of symptomatic disease by inflammatory mediators and the sustained maintenance of the allergic phenotype by the production of cytokines, such as IL-4, IL-5, and IL-13, that recruit other immune cells (eosinophils, lymphocytes) to sites of allergic inflammation, which stimulate the development of Th2 lymphocytes and promote IgE production by B cells. Treatments that inhibit FcεRI signaling are expected to reduce allergic inflammation partly by blocking both the acute symptoms of allergic diseases and the underlying immunological phenotype that favors the proliferation of Th2 lymphocytes and the production of IgE by B cells. The second mechanism, dependent on the endocytosis of antigen–IgE–receptor complexes, results in the more efficient delivery of antigen to MHC class II-containing granules for processing to peptide–MHC class II complexes. These complexes are then expressed on the cell surface and stimulate antigen-specific T-cell responses. Treatments that reduce FcεRI expression or inhibit the endocytosis and lysosomal processing of antigen–IgE–receptor complexes are expected to reduce allergic inflammation and to block the widening of the IgE repertoire, in part by reducing the activation of both naïve and memory T cells.

We have emphasized the functional diversity of the human FcεRI. In basophils and mast cells, a principal role of FcεRI is to generate mediators and cytokines responsible for acute inflammation. In dendritic cells and monocytes, a principal role of FcεRI is to focus antigen for processing and presentation to T cells. However, there is evidence that signaling through the FcεRI of dendritic cells, monocytes, and macrophages may contribute to the allergic phenotype through the production of inflammatory mediators and cytokines and, conversely, that FcεRI-enhanced antigen presentation by mast cells may contribute to the persistent T-cell activation that maintains and exacerbates allergic inflammation. Thus, FcεRI can serve both signaling and trafficking functions in the same cell type. Improved control of the allergic phenotype is likely to be accomplished by treatments that block FcεRI signaling in combination with treatments that block the FcεRI-mediated processing and presentation of antigen.

ACKNOWLEDGMENTS

We thank members of our laboratories for their many contributions to our analyses of basophil and mast cell signaling. Particular thanks go to Janet Pfeiffer for electron microscopy, Marina Martinez for biochemistry, Chris Kepley for expertise in human basophil purification, Chris Kepley, Lama Youssef, and Ron Andrews for studies of signaling in normal and nonreleaser human basophils, Alex Smith for video microscopy of RBL-2H3 degranulation, Rebecca Lee for studies of Ca^{2+} mobilization, and Graham Mackay for contributing the discussion of human FcεRI structure and IgE-binding properties. We also thank our collaborators Enrique Ortega and Martha Lara in Mexico City and Robert Geahlen at Purdue University for contributions to the work reviewed here. Finally, we thank Mary Lipscomb, Mark Schuyler, Barbara Masten, Julie Wilder, and other members of the UNM Asthma SCOR program and the UNM/ALA Asthma Research Center for supporting our transition to study FcεRI signaling in human cells and for sharing our fascination with the multiple contributions of IgE and FcεRI to the pathogenesis of allergic asthma. Work from our laboratories was supported in part by NIH grants RO1 GM49814, R29 GM50562, RO3 TW00440, and P50 HL56384 and by ACS grant RPG-99-233-0-CIM.

REFERENCES

1. Gould HJ, Beavil RI, Reljic R, Shi J, Ma CW, Sutton BJ, Chirlando R. IgE homeostasis: is CD23 the safety switch? In: Vercelli D, ed. IgE Regulation: Molecular Mechanisms. Chichester: John Wiley and Sons, 1997:37–59.

2. Sutton BJ, Gould HJ. The human IgE network. Nature 1993; 366:421–428.
3. Corry DB, Kheradmand F. Induction and regulation of the IgE response. Nature 1999; 402: B18–B23.
4. Blank U, Ra C, Miller L, White K, Metzger H, Kinet JP. Complete structure and expression in transfected cells of high-affinity IgE receptor. Nature 1989; 337:187–189.
5. Metzger H. The receptor with high-affinity for IgE. Immunol Rev 1992; 125:37–48.
6. Cambier JC. Antigen and Fc receptor signaling. The awesome power of the immunoreceptor tyrosine-based activation motif. J Immunol 1995; 15:3281–3285.
7. Tamir I, Cambier JC. Antigen receptor signaling: integration of protein–tyrosine kinase functions. Oncogene 1998; 17:1353–1364.
8. Watson SP, Gibbins J. Collagen receptor signaling in platelets: extending the role of the ITAM. Immunol Today 1998; 19:260–264.
9. Kinet JP. The high-affinity IgE receptor (FcεRI): from physiology to pathology. Anna Rev Immunol 1999; 17:931–972.
10. Kuster H, Zhang L, Brini AT, MacGlashan DW, Kinet JP. The gene and cDNA for the human high affinity immunoglobulin E receptor beta chain and expression of the complete human receptor. J Biol Chem 1992; 267:12782–12787.
11. Ochiai K, Kagami M, Umemiya K, Matsumura R, Kawashima T, Tomioka H. Expression of high affinity IgE receptor (FcεRI) on human alveolar macrophages from atopic and non-atopic patients. Int Arch Allergy Immunol 1996; 11(suppl 1):55–58.
12. Maurer D, Fiebiger E, Ebner C, Reininger B, Fischer GF, Wichlas S, Jouvin MH, Schmitt–Egenolf M, Kraft D, Kinet JP. Peripheral blood dendritic cells express FcεRI as a complex composed of FcεRI α- and FcεRI γ-chains and can use this receptor for IgE-mediated allergen presentation. J Immunol 1996; 157:607–616.
13. Dombrowicz D, Lin S, Flamand SV, Brini AT, Koller BH, Kinet JP. Allergy-associated FcRβ is a molecular amplifier of IgE- and IgG-mediated in vivo responses. Immunity 1998; 8:517–529.
14. Sutton BJ, Gould HJ. IgE and IgE receptors. In: Kay AB, ed. Allergy and Allergic Diseases. Boston: Blackwell Sciences, 1997.
15. Vangelista L, Laffer S, Turek R, Gronlund H, Sperr WR, Valent P, Pastore A, Valenta R. The immunoglobulin-like modules Cε3 and α2 are the minimal units necessary for human IgE–FcεRI interaction. J Clin Invest 1999; 103:1571–1578.
16. Presta L, Shields R, O'Connell L, Lahr S, Porter J, Gorman C, Jardieu P. The binding site on human immunoglobulin E for its high affinity receptor. J Biol Chem 1994; 269:26368–26373.
17. Henry AJ, Cook JP, McDonnell JM, Mackay GA, Shi J, Sutton BJ, Gould HJ. Participation of the N-terminal region of Cε3 in the binding of human IgE to its high-affinity receptor FcεRI. Biochemistry 1997; 36:15568–15578.
18. Helm BA, Ling Y, Teale C, Padlan EA, Brüggemann M. The nature and importance of the inter-ε chain disulfide bonds in human IgE. Eur J Immunol 1991; 21:1543–1548.
19. Robertson MW. Phage and *Escherichia coli* expression of the human high affinity immunoglobulin E receptor α-subunit ectodomain. Domain localization of the IgE-binding site. J Biol Chem 1993; 268:12736–12743.
20. Keown MB, Ghirlando R, Young RJ, Beavil AJ, Owens RJ, Perkins SJ, Sutton BJ, Gould HJ. Hydrodynamic studies of a complex between the Fc fragment of human IgE and a soluble fragment of the FcεRI α chain. Proc Natl Acad Sci USA 1995; 92:1841–1845.
21. Liu J, Ruppel J, Shire SJ. Interaction of human IgE with soluble forms of IgE high affinity receptors. Pharm Res 1997; 14:1388–1393.
22. Zheng Y, Shopes B, Holowka D, Baird B. Conformations of IgE bound to its receptor FcεRI and in solution. Biochemistry 1991; 30:9125–32.
23. Zheng Y, Shopes B, Holowka D, Baird B. Dynamic conformations compared for IgE and IgG1 in solution and bound to receptors. Biochemistry 1992; 31:7446–56.
24. Beavil AJ, Young RJ, Sutton BJ, Perkins SJ. Bent domain structure of recombinant human

IgE-Fc in solution by X-ray and neutron scattering in conjunction with an automated curve fitting procedure. Biochemistry 1995; 34:14449–61.

25. Keown MB, Henry AJ, Ghirlando R, Sutton BJ, Gould HJ. Thermodynamics of the interaction of human immunoglobulin E with its high-affinity receptor FcεRI. Biochemistry 1998; 37:8863–9.
26. Sechi S, Roller PP, Willette–Brown J, Kinet JP. A conformational rearrangement upon binding of IgE to its high affinity receptor. J Biol Chem 1996; 271:19256–63.
27. Hakimi J, Seals C, Kondas JA, Pettine L, Danho W, Kochan J. The α subunit of the human IgE receptor (FcERI) is sufficient for high affinity IgE binding. J Biol Chem 1990; 265: 22079–81.
28. Blank U, Ra CS, Kinet JP. Characterization of truncated α chain products from human, rat, and mouse high affinity receptor for immunoglobulin. Eur J Biol Chem 1991; 266:2639–46.
29. Suzuki K, Hirose T, Matsuda H, Hasegawa S, Okumura K, Ra C. The Fc receptor (FcR) γ subunit is essential for IgE-binding activity of cell-surface expressed chimeric receptor molecules constructed from human high-affinity IgE receptor (FcεRI) α and FcR γ subunits. Mol Immunol 1998; 35:259–70.
30. Miller KL, Duchemin AM, Anderson CL. A novel role for the Fc receptor γ subunit: enhancement of FcγR ligand affinity. J Exp Med 1996; 183:2227–33.
31. Sutton BJ, Gould HJ. Regulation of IgE-mediated inflammation by soluble fragments of the high affinity IgE receptor. In: Bousquet J, Yssel H, eds. Immunotherapy in Asthma. New York: Marcel Dekker, 1999:411–429.
32. Padlan EA, Helm BA. A modeling study of the α-subunit of human high-affinity receptor for immunoglobulin-E. Receptor 1992; 2:129–44.
33. McDonnell JM, Beavil AJ, Mackay GA, Jameson BA, Korngold R, Gould HJ, Sutton BJ. Structure based design and characterization of peptides that inhibit IgE binding to its high-affinity receptor. Nat Struct Biol 1996; 3:419–26.
34. Hulett MD, Brinkworth RI, McKenzie IF, Hogarth PM. Fine structure analysis of interaction of FcεRI with IgE. J Biol Chem 1999; 274:13345–52.
35. Cook JP, Henry AJ, McDonnell JM, Owens RJ, Sutton BJ, Gould HJ. Identification of contact residues in the IgE binding site of human FcεRI α. Biochemistry 1997; 36:15579–88.
36. McDonnell JM, Beavil AJ, Mackay GA, Henry AJ, Cook JP, Gould HJ, Sutton BJ. Structure-based design of peptides that inhibit IgE binding to its high-affinity receptor FcεRI. Biochem Soc Trans 1997; 25:387–92.
37. Garman SC, Kinet JP, Jardetzky TS. Crystal structure of the human high-affinity IgE receptor. Cell 1998; 95:951–61.
38. Garman SC, Kinet JP, Jardetzky TS. The crystal structure of the human high-affinity IgE receptor (FcεRI α). Annu Rev Immunol 1999; 17:973–6.
39. Maxwell KF, Powell MS, Hulett MD, Barton PA, McKenzie IF, Garrett TP, Hogarth PM. Crystal structure of the human leukocyte Fc receptor, FcγRIIa. Nat Struct Biol 1999; 6:437–42.
40. Sondermann P, Huber R, Jacob U. Crystal structure of the soluble form of the human Fcγ-receptor IIb: a new member of the immunoglobulin superfamily at 1.7 Å resolution. EMBO J 1999; 18:1095–103.
41. Malveaux FJ, Conroy MC, Adkinson NJF, Lichtenstein LF. IgE receptors on human basophils. Relationship to serum IgE concentration. J Clin Invest 1978; 62:176–181.
42. Hsu C, MacGlashan DW. IgE antibody upregulates high affinity IgE binding on murine bone marrow-derived mast cells. Immunol Lett 1996; 52:129–134.
43. Bieber T. FcεRI on antigen-presenting cells. Curr Opin Immunol 1996; 8:773–777.
44. Lantz CS, Yamaguchi M, Oettgen HC, Katona IM, Mayajima I, Kinet JP, Galli SJ. IgE regulates mouse basophil FcεRI expression in vivo. J Immunol 1997; 158:2517–2521.
45. Yamaguchi M, Lantz CS, Oettgen HC, Katona IM, Fleming T, Miyajima I, Kinet JP, Galli SJ. IgE enhances mouse mast cell FcεRI expression in vitro and in vivo: evidence for a novel amplification mechanism in IgE-dependent reactions. J Exp Med 1997; 185:663–672.

46. Stingl G, Maurer D. IgE-mediated allergen presentation via FcεRI on antigen-presenting cells. Int Arch Allergy Immunol 1997; 113:24–29.
47. Rajakulasingham K, Durham SR, O'Brien F, Humbert M, Barata LT, Reece L, Kay AB, Grant JA. Enhanced expression of high-affinity IgE receptor (FcεRI) α chain in human allergen-induced rhinitis with co-localization to mast cells, macrophages, eosinophils and dendritic cells. J Allergy Clin Immunol 1997; 100:78–86.
48. MacGlashan DW, Bochner BS, Adelman DC, Jardieu PM, Togias A, Lichtenstein LM. Serum IgE level drives basophil and mast cell IgE receptor display. Int Arch Allergy Immunol 1997; 113:45–47.
49. Ying S, Barata LT, Meng Q, Grant JA, Barkans J, Durham SR, Kay AB. High-affinity immunoglobulin E receptor (FcεRI)-bearing eosinophils, mast cells, macrophages and Langerhans' cells in allergen-induced late-phase cutaneous reactions in atopic subjects. Immunology 1998; 93:281–288.
50. Kraft S, Wessendorf JMH, Hanau D, Bieber T. Regulation of the high-affinity receptor for IgE on human epidermal Langerhans cells. J Immunol 1998; 161:1000–1006.
51. Heusser C, Jardieu P. Therapeutic potential of anti-IgE antibodies. Curr Opin Immunol 1997; 9:805–814.
52. MacGlashan DW, Bochner BS, Adelman DC, Jardieu PM, Togias A, McKenzie–White J, Sterbinsky SA, Hamilton RG, Lichtenstein LM. Down-regulation of FcεRI expression on human basophils during in vivo treatment of atopic patients with anti-IgE antibody. J Immunol 1997; 158:1438–1445.
53. Saini SS, MacGlashan DW, Sterbinsky SA, Togias A, Adelman DC, Lichtenstein LM, Bochner BS. Down-regulation of human basophil IgE and FcεRI surface densities and mediator release by anti-IgE-infusions is reversible in vitro and in vivo. J Immunol 1999; 162: 5624–5630.
54. Milgrom H, Fick RB, Su JQ, Reimann JD, Bush RK, Watrous ML, Metzger MJ. Treatment of allergic asthma with monoclonal anti-IgE antibody. N Engl J Med 1999; 341:1966–1973.
55. Furuichi K, Rivera J, Isersky C. The receptor for immunoglobulin-E on rat basophilic leukemia cells: effect of ligand-binding on receptor expression. Proc Natl Acad Sci USA 1985; 82:1522–1525.
56. Bainton DF, Nichols BA, Farquhar MG. Primary lysosomes of blood leukocytes. In: Dingle JT, Dean RT, eds. Lysosomes in Biology and Pathology. Vol 5. Amsterdam: North-Holland Publishing, 1976:3–32.
57. Bentfeld–Barker ME, Bainton DF. Cytochemical localization of arylsulfatase B in rat basophils and mast cells. J Histochem Cytochem 1980; 28:1055–1061.
58. Dvorak AM. Blood Cell Biochemistry 4. Basophil and Mast Cell Degranulation and Recovery. New York: Plenum Press, 1991.
59. Berger M, Wetzler E, August JT, Tartakoff AM. Internalization of type 1 complement receptors and de novo multivesicular body formation during chemoattractant-induced endocytosis in human neutrophils. J Clin Invest 1994; 94:1113–1115.
60. Heijnen HFG, Debili N, Vainchenchker W, Breton–Gorius J, Geuze HJ, Sixma JJ. Multivesicular bodies are an intermediate stage in the formation of platelet α-granules. Blood 1998; 7:2313–2325.
61. Dvorak AM, Morgan ES, Lichtensein LM, MacGlashan DW Jr. Activated human basophils contain histamine in cytoplasmic vesicles. Int Arch Allergy Immunol 1994; 105:8–11.
62. Baram D, Adachi R, Medalia O, Tuvim M, Dickey BF, Mekori YA, Sagi–Eisenberg R. Synaptotagmin II negatively regulates Ca^{2+}-triggered exocytosis of lysosomes in mast cells. J Exp Med 1999; 189:1649–1657.
63. Dvorak A. Ultastructural analysis of human mast cells and basophils. In: Marone G, ed. Human Basophils and Mast Cells: Biological Aspects. Chem Immunol 1995; 61:1–33.
64. Bradding P, Feather IH, Wilson S, Bardin PG, Heusser CH, Holgate ST, Howarth PH. Immu-

nolocalization of cytokines in the nasal mucosa of normal and perennial rhinitic subjects. J Immunol 1993; 1551:3853–3865.

65. Bradding P, Okayama Y, Howarth PH, Church MK, Holgate ST. Heterogeneity of human mast cells based on cytokine content. J Immunol 1995; 155:297–307.
66. Li H, Sim TC, Alam R. IL-13 released by and localized in human basophils. J Immunol 1996; 156:4833–4838.
67. Ying S, Humbert M, Barkans J, Corrigan CJ, Pfister R, Menz G, Larche M, Robinson DS, Durham SR, Kay AB. Expression of IL-4 and IL-5 mRNA and protein product by $CD4^+$ and $CD8^+$ T cells, eosinophils and mast cells in bronchial biopsies obtained from atopic and nonatopic (intrinsic) asthmatics. J Immunol 1997; 158:3539–3544.
68. Grutzkau A, Kruger–Krasagakes S, Kogel H, Moller A, Lippert U, Henz BM. Detection of intracellular interleukin-8 in human mast cell; flow cytometry as a guide for immunoelectron microscopy. J Histochem Cytochem 1997; 45:935–945.
69. Grutzkau A, Fruger–Krasagakes S, Baumeister H, Schwarz C, Kogel H, Welker P, Lippert U, Henz BM, Moller A. Synthesis, storage and release of vacular endothelial growth factor/vascular permeability factor (VEGF/VPF) by human mast cells: implications for the biological significance of $VEGF_{206}$. Mol Biol Cell 1998; 9:875–884.
70. Frangogiannis NG, Lindsey ML, Lloyd MH, Youker KA, Bressler RB, Mendoza LH, Spengler RN, Smith CW, Entman ML. Resident cardiac mast cells degranulate and release preformed TNF-α, initiating the cytokine cascade in experimental canine myocardial ischemia/reprefusion. Circulation 1998; 98:699–710.
71. Raposo G, Tenza D, Mecheri S, Peronet R, Bonnerot C, Desaymard C. Accumulation of major histocompatability complex class II molecules in mast cell secretory granules and their release upon degranulation. Mol Biol Cell 1997; 8:2631–2645.
72. Escola J–M, Kleijmeer MJ, Stoorvogel W, Griffith JM, Yoshie O, Geuze HJ. Selective enrichment of tetraspan proteins on the internal vesicles of multivesicular endosomes and on exosomes secreted by human B-lymphocytes. J Biol Chem 1998; 273:20121–20127.
73. Forsberg E, Pejler G, Ringvall M, Lunderius C, Tomasini–Johansson B, Kusche–Gullberg M, Eriksson I, Ledin J, Hellman L, Kjellen L. Abnormal mast cells in mice deficient in a heparin-synthesizing enzyme. Nature 1999; 400:773–776.
74. Humphries DE, Wong GW, Friend DS, Gurish MF, Qiu W–T, Huang C, Sharpe AH, Stevens RL Heparin in essential for the storage of specific granule protease in mast cells. Nature 1999; 400:769–772.
75. Stinchcombe JC, Griffiths GM. Regulated secretion from hemopoietic cells. J Cell Biol 1999; 147:1–5.
76. Odorizzi G, Cowles CR, Emr SD. The AP-3 complex: a coat of many colours. Trends Cell Biol 1998; 8:282–288.
77. Oliver JM, Seagrave JC, Stump RF, Pfeiffer JR, Deanin GG. Signal transduction and cellular response in RBL-2H3 mast cells. In: Becker EL, ed. Progress in Allergy. Basel: S Karger, 1988; 42:185–245.
78. Oliver JM, Pfeiffer JR, Wilson BS. Regulation and roles of the membrane, cytoskeletal and adhesive responses of RBL-2H3 rat tumor mast cells to FcεRI crosslinking. In: Hamawy MM, ed. IgE Receptor (FcεRI) Function in Mast Cells and Basophils. Austin, TX: RG Landes, 1997:139–172.
79. Beaven MA, Metzger H. Signal transduction by Fc receptors: the FcεRI case. Immunol Today 1993; 14:222–226.
80. Okazaki H, Siraganian RP. Signal transduction for secretion in basophils. ACII 1999; 3:86–92.
81. Turner H, Kinet JP. Signalling through the high-affinity IgE receptor, FcεRI. Nature 1999; 402:B24–B30.
82. Guo A, Turner C, Castle D. Relocation of the t-SNARE SNAP-23 from lamellipodia-like cell surface projections regulates compound exocytosis in mast cells. Cell 1998; 94:537–548.

83. Miesenbock G, De Angelis DA, Rothman JE. Visualizing secretion and synaptic transmission with pH-sensitive green fluorescent proteins. Nature 1998; 394:92–195.
84. Gomperts BD. Involvement of guanine nucleotide-binding protein in the gating of Ca^{2+} by receptors. Nature 1983; 306:64–67.
85. Sagi–Eisenberg R. Activation of heterotrimeric GTP-binding proteins. In: Razin E, Pecht I, Rivera J, eds. Signal Transduction in Mast Cells and Basophils. Austin, TX: Landes Bioscience, 1999:286–299.
86. Pinxteren JA, O'Sullivan AJ, Tatham PER, Gomperts BD. Regulation of exocytosis from rat peritoneal mast cells by G protein βγ subunits. EMBO J 1998; 17:6210–6218.
87. Brown AM, O'Sullivan AJ, Gomperts BD. Induction of exocytosis from permealized mast cells by the guanosine triphosphatases Rac and CDC42. Mol Biol Cell 1998; 9:1053–1063.
88. Oberhauser AF, Monck JR, Balch WE, Fernandez JM. Exocytotic fusion is activated by RAb3a peptides. Nature 1992; 360:270–273.
89. Kapp N, Barker S, Wilson BS. Identification of Rab3D in rat basophilic leukemia cells. Mol Biol Cell 1994; 5:447a.
90. Roa M, Paumet F, Le Mao J, David B, Blank U. Involvement of the ras-like GTPase rab3d in RBL-2H3 mast cell exocytosis following stimulation via high affinity IgE receptors. J Immunol 1997; 159:2815–2823.
91. Tumvin MJ, Adachi R, Chocano JF, Moore RH, Lampert RM, Zera E, Romero E, Knoll BJ, Dickey BF. Rab3D, a small GTPases, is localized on mast cell secretory granules and translocateds to the plasma membrane upon exocytosis. Am J Respir Cell Mol Biol 1999; 20:79–89.
92. Demo SD, Masuda E, Rossi AB, Throndset BT, Gerard AL, Chan EH, Armstrong RJ, Fox BP, Lorens JB, Payan, DG, Scheller RH, Fisher JM. Quantitative measurement of mast cell degranulation using a novel flow cytometric annexin-V binding assay. Cytometry 1999; 36: 340–348.
93. Pfeiffer JR, Seagrave JC, Davis BH, Oliver JM. Membrane and cytoskeletal changes associated with IgE-mediated serotonin release in rat basophilic leukemia cells. J Cell Biol 1985; 101:2145.
94. MacGlashan DW, Bochner BS, Warner JA. Graded changes in the response of individual human basophils to stimulation: distributional behavior of early activation events. J Leukoc Biol 1994; 55:13–23.
95. Barker SA, Caldwell KK, Hall A, Martinez AM, Pfeiffer JR, Oliver JM, Wilson BS. Wortmannin blocks lipid and protein kinase activities associated with PI 3-kinase and inhibits a subset of responses induced by FcεRI cross-linking. Mol Biol Cell 1995; 6:1145–1158.
96. Pfeiffer JR, Oliver JM. Tyrosine kinase-dependent assembly of actin plaques linking FcεRI cross-linking to increased cell–substrate adhesion in RBL-2H3 tumor mast cells. J Immunol 1994; 152:270–279.
97. Linder S, Nelson D, Weiss M, Aepfelbacher M. Wiskott–Aldrich syndrome protein regulates podosomes in primary human macrophages. Proc Natl Acad Sci USA 1999; 96:9648–9653.
98. Kepley CL, Youssef L, Andrews RP, Wilson BS, Oliver JM. Syk deficient non-releaser basophils show multiple functional defects in FcεRI signaling: partial recovery of Syk expression and signaling by incubation with IL-3. J Immunol 2000; 165:5913–5920.
99. Bochner BS, Sterbinsky SA, Briskin M, Saini SS, MacGlashan DW. Counter-receptors on human basophils for endothelial cell adhesion molecules. J Immunol 1996; 157:844–850.
100. Bingham CO III, Arm JP, Austen KF. Arachidonic acid metabolism in mast cells. In: Razin E, Pecht I, Rivera J, eds. Signal Transduction in Mast Cells and Basophils. Austin, TX: Landes Bioscience, 1999:350–361.
101. Plaut M, Pierce JH, Watson CJ, Hanley–Hyde J, Nordan RP, Paul WE. Mast cell lines produce lymphokines in response to cross-linkage of FcεRI or to calcium ionophores. Nature 1989; 339:64–67.
102. Schroeder JT, MacGlashan DW, Kagey–Sobotka A, White JM, Lichtenstein LM. IgE-depen-

dent IL-4 secretion by human basophils. The relationship between cytokine production and histamine release in mixed leukocyte cultures. J Immunol 1994; 153:1808–1817.

103. MacGlashan DW. Signal transduction and cytokine production by human basophils. In: Marone G, ed. Human Basophils and Mast Cells: Biological Aspects. Chem Immunol 1995; 61: 88–113.

104. Okayama Y, Bradding P, Tunon-de-Lara JM, Holgate ST, Church MK. Cytokine production by human mast cells. In: Marone G, ed. Human Basophils and Mast Cells: Biological Aspects. Chem Immunol 1995; 61:114–134.

105. Schroeder JT, MacGlashan DW. Updates on cells and cytokines. New concepts: the basophils. J Allergy Clin Immunol 1997; 99:429–433.

106. Sherman MA, Brown MA. Regulation of IL-4 expression in mast cells. In: Razin E, Pecht I, Rivera J, eds. Signal Transduction in Mast Cells and Basophils. Austin, TX: Landes Bioscience 1999:337–349.

107. Graham TE, Pfeiffer JR, Lee RJ, Kusewitt DF, Martinez AM, Foutz T, Wilson BS, Oliver JM. MEK and ERK activation in Ras-disabled RBL-2H3 mast cells and novel roles for geranylgeranylated and farnesylated proteins in FcεRI-mediated signaling. J Immunol 1998; 161: 6733–6744.

108. Quarto R, Metzger H. The receptor for immunoglobulin E: examination for kinase activity and as a substrate for kinases. Mol Immunol 1986; 23:1215–1223.

109. Benhamou M, Gutkind JS, Robbins KC, Siraganian RP. Tyrosine phosphorylation coupled to IgE receptor-mediated signal transduction and histamine release. Proc Natl Acad Sci USA 1990; 87:5327–5330.

110. Deanin GG, Pfeiffer JR, Cutts JL, Oliver JM. Isoprenoid pathway activity is required for IgE receptor-mediated, tyrosine kinase-coupled transmembrane signalling in permeabilized RBL-2H3 mast cells. Cell Regul 1991; 2:627–640.

111. Deanin GG, Martinez AM, Pfeiffer JR, Gardner ME, Oliver JM. Tyrosine kinase-dependent phosphatidylinositol turnover and functional responses in the FcεRI signalling pathway. Biochem Biophys Res Commun 1991; 179:551–557.

112. Paolini R, Jouvin MH, Kinet JP. Phosphorylation and dephosphorylation of the high affinity receptor for immunoglobulin E following receptor engagement and disengagement. Nature 1991; 353:855.

113. Eiseman E, Bolen JB. Engagement of the high affinity IgE receptor activates src protein-related tyrosine kinases. Nature 1992; 355:78–80.

114. Li W, Deanin GG, Margolis B, Schlessinger J, Oliver JM. FcεRI-mediated tyrosine phosphorylation of multiple proteins, including phospholipase Cγ1 and the receptor $\beta\gamma_2$-complex, in RBL-2H3 rat basophilic leukemia cells. Mol Cell Biol 1992; 12:3176–3182.

115. Hutchcroft JE, Geahlen RL, Deanin GG, Oliver JM. FcεRI-mediated tyrosine phosphorylation and activation of the 72 kDa protein–tyrosine kinase, PTK72, in RBL-2H3 rat tumor mast cells. Proc Natl Acad Sci USA 1992; 89:9107–9111.

116. Zioncheck TF, Harrison ML, Isaacson CC, Geahlen RL. Generation of an active protein–tyrosine kinase from lymphocytes by proteolysis. J Biol Chem 1988; 263:19195–19202.

117. Taniguchi T, Koboyashi T, Kondo J, Takahashi K, Nakamura H, Suzuki J, Nagai K, Yamada T, Nakamura S, Yamamura H. Molecular cloning of a porcine gene Syk that encodes a 72-kDa protein–tyrosine kinase showing high susceptibility to proteolysis. J Biol Chem 1991; 266:15790–15796.

118. Oliver JM, Burg DL, Wilson BS, McLaughlin J, Geahlen RL. Inhibition of mast cell FcεRI-mediated signaling and effector function by the Syk-selective inhibitor, piceatannol. J Biol Chem 1994; 269:29697–29703.

119. Kepley CL, Wilson BS, Oliver JM. Roles for the protein kinases Lyn, Syk and Zap70 in FcεRI-mediated human basophil degranulation. J Allergy Clin Immunol 1998; 102:304–315.

120. Moriya K, Rivera J, Odom S, Sakuma Y, Muramato K, Yoshiuchi T, Miyamoto M, Yamada

K. ER-27319, an acridone-related compound, inhibits release of antigen-induced allergic mediators from mast cells by selective inhibition of Fcε receptor I-mediated activation of Syk. Proc Natl Acad Sci USA 1997; 94:12539–12544.

121. Rivera VM, Brugge, JS. Clustering of Syk is sufficient to induce tyrosine phosphorylation and release of allergic mediators from rat basophilic leukemia cells. Mol Cell Biol 1995; 15:1582–1590.
122. Costello PS, Turner M, Walters AE, Cunningham CN, Bauer PH, Downward J, Tybulewicz VL. Critical role for the tyrosine kinase Syk in signalling through the high affinity IgE receptor of mast cells. Oncogene 1996; 13:2595–2605.
123. Zhang J, Berenstein EH, Evans RL, Siraganian RP. Transfection of Syk tyrosine kinase reconstitutes high affinity IgE receptor-mediated degranulation in a Syk-negative variant of rat basophilic leukemia RBL-2H3 cells. J Exp Med 1996; 184:71–79.
124. Ishizaka T, Soto CS, Ishizaka K. Mechanisms of passive sensitization III: numbers of IgE molecules and their receptor sites on human basophilic granulocytes. J Immunol 1973; 111: 500–511.
125. Nguyen KL, Gillis S, MacGlashan DW. A comparative study of releasing and nonreleasing human basophils: nonreleasing basophils lack an early component of the signal transduction pathway that follows IgE crosslinking. J Allergy Clin Immunol 1990; 85:1020–1029.
126. Knol EF, Mul FP, Kuijpers TW, Verhoeven AJ, Roos D. Intracellular events in anti-IgE nonreleasing human basophils. J Allergy Clin Immunol 1992; 90:92–103.
127. Kepley CL, Youssef L, Andrews RP, Wilson BS. Oliver JM. Syk deficiency in non-releaser basophils. J Allergy Clin Immunol 1999; 104:279–284.
128. Yamashita T, Mao SY, Metzger H. Aggregation of the high affinity IgE receptor and enhanced activity of p53/56lyn protein–tyrosine kinase. Proc Natl Acad Sci USA 1994; 91: 11251–11256.
129. Pribluda VS, Pribluda C, Metzger H. Biochemical evidence that the phosphorylated tyrosines, serines and threonines on the aggregated high affinity receptor for IgE are in the immunoreceptor tyrosine-based activation motifs. J Biol Chem 1997; 272:11185.
130. Pribluda VS, Pribluda C, Metzger H. Transphosphorylation as the mechanism by which the high-affinity receptor for IgE is phosphorylated upon aggregation. Proc Natl Acad Sci USA 1994; 91:11246.
131. Shiue L, Zoller MJ, Brugge JS. Syk is activated by phosphotyrosine-containing peptides representing the tyrosine-based activation motifs of the high affinity receptor for IgE. J Biol Chem 1995; 270:10498–10502.
132. Wilson BS, Kapp N, Lee RJ, Pfeiffer JR, Martinez AM, Platt Y, Letourneur JF, Oliver JM. Distinct functions of the FcεRI γ and β subunits in the control of FcεRI-mediated tyrosine kinase activation and signaling responses in RBL-2H3 mast cells. J Biol Chem 1995; 270: 4013.
133. Vonakis BM, Chen H, Haleem–Smith H, Metzger H. The unique domain as a site on Lyn kinase for its constitutive association with the high affinity receptor for IgE. J Biol Chem 1997; 272:24072–24080.
134. Lin S, Cicala C, Scharenberg AM, Kinet JP. The FcεRI β subunit functions as an amplifier of FcεRIγ-mediated cell activation signals. Cell 1996; 85:985.
135. Ortega E, Schweitzer–Stenner R, Pecht I. Possible orientational constraints determine secretory signals induced by aggregation of IgE receptors on mast cells. EMBO J 1988; 7:4101–4109.
136. Ortega E, Lara M, Lee R, Santana C, Martinez AM, Pfeiffer JR, Lee RJ, Wilson BS, Oliver JM. Lyn dissociation from phosphorylated FcεRI subunits: a new regulatory step in the FcεRI signaling cascade revealed by studies of FcεRI dimer signaling activity. J Immunol 1999; 162:176.
137. Lara M, Ortega E, Pecht I, Pfeiffer JR, Wilson BS, Oliver JM. Overcoming the signaling defect of Lyn-sequestering, signal-curtailing FcεRI dimers: crosslinking the dimers restores

Lyn dissociation from phosphorylated FcεRI subunits and the formation of Syk–FcεRI signaling domains. 2000. Submitted.

138. Sloan–Lancaster J, Shaw AS, Rothbard JB, Allen PM. Partial T cell signaling: altered phospho-ζ and lack of Zap70 recruitment in APL-induced T cell anergy. Cell 1994; 79:913–922.
139. Madrenas Y, Wange RL, Wang JL, Isakov N, Samelson LE, Germain RN. zeta-Phosphorylation without ZAP-70 activation induced by TCR antagonists or partial agonists. Science 1995; 267:515–518.
140. Smith JA, Tso JY, Clark MR, Cole MS, Bluestone JA. Nonmitogenic anti-CD3 monoclonal antibodies deliver a partial T cell receptor signal and induce clonal anergy. J Exp Med 1997; 185:1413–1422.
141. Kersh GK, Kersh EN, Fremont DH, Allen PM. High- and low-potency ligands with similar affinities for the TCR: the importance of kinetics in TCR signaling. Immunity 1998; 9:817–826.
142. Kersh EN, Shaw AS, Allen PM. Fidelity of T cell activation through multistep T cell receptor ζ phosphorylation. Science 1998; 281:572–575.
143. Jiang G, Hunter T. Receptor signaling: when dimerization is not enough. Curr Biol 1998; 9:R568–R571.
144. Wofsy C, Torigoe C, Kent UM, Metzger H, Goldstein B. Exploiting the difference between intrinsic and extrinsic kinases: implications for regulation of signaling by immunoreceptors. J Immunol 1997; 159:5984–5992.
145. Wofsy C, Vonakis BM, Metzger H, Goldstein B. One Lyn molecule is sufficient to initiate phosphorylation of aggregated high-affinity IgE receptors. Proc Natl Acad Sci USA 1999; 96:8615–8620.
146. Torigoe C, Goldstein B, Wofsy C, Metzger H. Shuttling of initiating kinase between discrete aggregates of the high affinity receptor for IgE regulates the cellular response. Proc Natl Acad Sci USA 1997; 94:1372.
147. Torigoe C, Inman JK, Metzger H. An unusual mechanism for ligand antagonism. Science 1998; 281:568–571.
148. Margolis B, Hu P, Katzav S, Li W, Oliver JM, Ullrich A, Weiss A, Schlessinger J. Tyrosine phosphorylation of *vav* proto-oncogene product containing SH2 domain and transcription factor motifs. Nature 1992; 356:71–74.
149. Ota Y, Samelson LE. The product of the protooncogene c-*cbl*: a negative regulator of the Syk tyrosine kinase. Science 1997; 276:418–420.
150. Joazeiro CA, Wing SS, Huang HK, Leverson JD, Hunter T, Liu YC. The tyrosine kinase negative regulator c-Cbl as a RING-type, E2-dependent ubiquitin-protein ligase. Science 1999; 286:309–312.
151. Zhang W, Trible RP, Samelson LE. LAT palymitoylation: its essential role in membrane microdomain targeting and tyrosine phosphorylation during T cell activation. Immunity 1998; 9:239–246.
152. Facchetti F, Chan JKC, Zhang WF, Tironi A, Chilosi M, Parolini S, Noatrangelo LD, Samelson LE. Linker for activation of T cells (LAT), a novel histochemical marker for T cells, NK cells, mast cells and megakaryocytes: evaluation in normal and pathological conditions. Am J Pathol 1999; 154:1037–1046.
153. Pivniouk VI, Martin TR, Lu-Kuo JM, Katz HR, Oettgen HC, Geha RS. SLP-76 deficiency impairs signaling via the high-affinity IgE receptor in mast cells. J Clin Invest 1999; 103: 1737–1743.
154. Kawakami Y, Yao LB, Miura T, Tsukada S, Witte ON, Kawakami T. Tyrosine phosphorylation and activation of Bruton's tyrosine kinase upon FcεRI crosslinking. Mol Cell Biol 1994; 14:5108–5113.
155. Barker SA. Wortmannin inhibits a subset of responses to FcεRI crosslinking. PhD dissertation, University of New Mexico, Albuquerque, NM, 1998.
156. Yano H, Nakanishi S, Kimura K, Hanai N, Saitoh Y, Fukui Y, Nonomura Y, Matsuda Y.

Inhibition of histamine secretion by wortmannin through the blockade of phosphatidylinositol 3-kinase in RBL-2H3 cells. J Biol Chem 1993; 268:25846–25856.
157. Barker SA, Caldwell KK, Hall A, Pfeiffer JR, Wilson BS. Wortmannin-sensitive phosphorylation, translocation and activation of PLCγ1, but not PLCγ2, in antigen-stimulated RBL-2H3 mast cells. Mol Biol Cell 1998; 9:483–496.
158. Barker SA, Lujan D, Wilson BS. Multiple roles for PI 3-kinase in the regulation of PLCγ activity and Ca^{2+} mobilization in antigen-stimulated mast cells. J Leukoc Biol 1999; 65:321–329.
159. Marquardt DL, Alongi JL, Walker LL. The phosphatidylinositol 3-kinase inhibitor wortmannin blocks mast cell exocytosis but not IL-6 production. J Immunol 1996; 156:1942–1945.
160. Bae YS, Cantley LG, Chen C–S, Kim S–R, Kwon K–S, Rhee SG. Activation of phospholipase Cγ by phosphatidylinositol 3,4,5-triphosphate. J Biol Chem 1998; 273:4465–4469.
161. Buhl AM, Cambier JC. Phosphorylation of CD19, Y484 and Y515, and linked activation of phosphatidylinositol 3-kinase, are required for B cell antigen receptor-mediated activation of Bruton's tyrosine kinase. J Immunol 1999; 162:4438–4446.
162. Sharenberg AM, El-Hillal O, Fruman DA, Beitz LO, Li A, Lin S, Gout I, Cantley LC, Rawlings DJ, Kinet J–P. Phosphatidylinositol-3,4,5-triphosphate (PtdIns-3,4,5-P_3)/Tec kinase-dependent calcium signaling pathway: a target for SHIP-mediated inhibitory signals. EMBO J 1998; 17:1961–1972.
163. Ferguson KM, Lemmon MA, Schlessinger J, Sigler PB. Structure of the high-affinity complex of inositol trisphosphate with a phospholipase-C pleckstrin homology domain. Cell 1995; 83:1037–1046.
164. McCloskey MA. New perspectives on Ca^{2+} influx in mast cells. In: Razin E, Pecht I, Rivera J, eds. Signal Transduction in Mast Cells and Basophils. Austin, TX: Landes Bioscience, 1999:227–246.
165. Lewis RS, Cahalan MD. Mitogen-induced oscillations of cytosolic Ca^{2+} and transmembrane Ca^{2+} current in human leukemic T cells. Cell Regul 1989; 1:99–112.
166. Hoth M, Penner R. Depletion of intracellular calcium stores activates a calcium current in mast cells. Nature 1992; 355:353–356.
167. Zwifach A, Lewis RS. Mitogen-regulated Ca^{2+} current of T lymphocytes is activated by depletion of intracellular Ca^{2+} stores. Proc Natl Acad Sci USA 1993; 90:6295–6299.
168. Mathes C, Mendez F, Fleig A, Peener R. Role of I^{CRAC} in the regulation of secretion. In: Razin E, Pecht I, Rivera J, eds. Signal Transduction in Mast Cells and Basophils. Austin, TX: Landes Bioscience, 1999:362–371.
169. Hide M, Beaven MA. Calcium influx in a rat mast cell (RBL-2H3) line. Use of multivalent metal ions to define its characteristics and role in exocytosis. J Biol Chem 1991; 266:15221–15229.
170. Lee RJ, Oliver JM. Roles for Ca^{2+} stores release and two Ca^{2+} influx pathways in the FcεRI-activated Ca^{2+} responses of RBL-2H3 mast cells. Mol Biol Cell 1995; 6:825–839.
171. Hardie RC. Calcium signaling: setting store by calcium channels. Curr Biol 1996; 93:15195–15202.
172. Putney JW, McKay RR. Capacitative calcium entry channels. Bioessays 1999; 21:38–46.
173. Garcia RL, Schilling WP. Differential expression of mammalian TRP homologues across tissues and cell lines. Biochem Biophys Res Commun 1997; 239:279–283.
174. Wang B, Rieger A, Kilgus O, Ochiai K, Maurer D, Fodinger D, Kinet JP, Stingl G. Epidermal Langerhans' cells from normal human skin bind monomeric IgE via FcεRI. J Exp Med 1992; 175:1353–1365.
175. Bieber T, de la Salle H, Wollenberg A, Hakimi J, Chizzonite R, Ring J, Hanau D, de la Salle C. Human epidermal Langerhans cells express the high-affinity receptor for immunoglobulin E (FcεRI). J Exp Med 1992; 175:1285–1290.
176. Maurer D, Fiebiger E, Reininger B, Wolffwiniski B, Jouvin MH, Kilgus O, Kinet JP, Stingl G. Expression of functional high affinity IgE receptors (FcεRI) on monocytes of atopic individuals. J Exp Med 1994; 179:745–750.

177. Maurer D, Ebner C, Reininger B, Fiebiger E, Kraft D, Kinet JP, Stingl G. The high affinity IgE receptor (FcεRI) mediates IgE-dependent allergen presentation. J Immunol 1995; 154: 6285–6290.
178. Sihra BS, Kon OM, Grant JA, Kay AB. Expression of high affinity immunoglobulin E receptors (FcεRI) on peripheral blood basophils, monocytes and esosinophils in atopic and nonatopic subjects: relationship to total serum immunoglobulin E (IgE) concentrations. J Allergy Clin Immunol 1997; 99:699–706.
179. Gosset P, Tillie–Leblond I, Oudin S, Parmentier O, Wallaert B, Joseph M, Tonnel AB. Production of chemokines and proinflammatory and anti-inflammatory cytokines by human alveolar macrophages activated by IgE receptors. J Allergy Clin Immunol 1999; 103:289–297.
180. Ten RM, McKinstry MJ, Bren GD, Paya CV. Signal transduction pathways triggered by the FcεRIIb receptor (CD23) in human monocytes lead to nuclear factor-kappa B activation. J Allergy Clin Immunol 1999; 104:376–387.
181. Rankin JA, Hitchcock M, Merrill W, Bach MK, Brashler JR, Ashkenase PW. IgE-dependent release of leukotriene C_4 from alveolar macrophages. Nature 1982; 297:329–331.
182. Joseph M, Tonnel AB, Torpier G, Capron A, Arnoux B, Benveniste J. Involvement of IgE in the secretory process of alveolar macrophages from asthmatic patients. J Clin Invest 1983; 71:221–230.
183. Gosset P, Tsicopoulos A, Wallaert W, Joseph M, Capron M, Tonnel. AB. Tumor necrosis factor alpha and interleukin-6 production by human mononuclear phagocytes from allergic asthmatics after IgE-dependent stimulation. Annu Rev Respir Dis 1992; 146:768–774.
184. Borish L, Mascali JJ, Rosenwasser LJ. IgE-dependent cytokine production by human peripheral blood mononuclear phagocytes. J Immunol 1991; 146:63–67.
185. Takenaka M, Tanaka Y, Anan S, Yoshida H, Ra C. High affinity IgE receptor-mediated prostaglandin E_2 production by monocytes in atopic dermatitis. Int Arch Allergy Immunol 1995; 108:247–253.
186. Jurgens M, Wollenberg A, Hanau D, de la Salle H, Bieber T. Activation of human epidermal Langerhans cells by engagement of the high affinity receptor for IgE, FcεRI. J Immunol 1995; 155:5184–5189.
187. Crawford C, Gabuzda D, Pantazopoulos V, Xu J, Clement C, Reinherz E, Alper CA. Circulating $CD2^+$ monocytes are dendritic cells. J Immunol 1999; 163:5920–5928.
188. Abbas AK, Lichtman AH, Pober JS. Cellular and Molecular Immunology, 3rd ed. Philadelphia: WB Saunders, 1997.
189. Fox CC, Jewell SD, Whitacre CC. Rat peritoneal mast cells present antigen to a PPD-specific T cell line. Cell Immunol 1994; 158:253–264.
190. Frandji P, Tkaczyk C, Oskeritzian C, Lapeyre J, Peronet R, David B, Guillet JG, Mecheri S. Presentation of soluble antigens by mast cells: upregulation by interleukin-4 and granulocyte/macrophage colony-stimulating factor and downregulation by interferon-γ. Cell Immunol 1995; 163:37–46.
191. Dimitriadou V, Mecheri S, Koutsilieris M, Fraser V, Aldaccak R, Mourad W. Expression of functional major histocompatibility complex class-II molecules on HMC-1 human mast cells. J Leukoc Biol 1998; 64:791–799.
192. Frandji P, Mourad W, Tkaczyk C, Singer M, Colle D, David B, Mecheri S. IL-4 messenger-RNA transcription is induced in mouse bone-marrow-derived mast-cells through an MHC class II-dependent signaling pathway. Eur J Immunol 1998; 28:844–854.
193. Poncet P, Arock M, David B. MHC class II-dependent activation of CD4(+) T cell hybridomas by human mast cells through superantigen presentation. J Leukoc Biol 1999; 66:105–112.
194. Tkaczyk C, Villa I, Peronet R, Mecheri S. FcεRI-mediated antigen endocytosis turns interferon-gamma–treated mouse mast cells from inefficient into potent antigen-presenting cells. Immunology 1999; 97:333–340.
195. Mecheri S, David B. Functional and ultrastructural insights into the immunobiology of mouse and human mast cells. 1999; Allergy Clin Immunol Int 11:226–233.

196. Mao S–Y, Pfeiffer JR, Oliver JM, Metzger H. Effect of subunit mutation on the coated pit localization and internalization of cross-linked IgE-receptor complexes. J Immunol 1993; 151:2760–2774.
197. Raposo G, Nijman HW, Stoorvogel W, Leijendekker R, Harding CV, Melief CJM, Geuze HJ. B lymphocytes secrete antigen-presenting vesicles. J Exp Med 1996; 183:1161–1172.
198. Maurer D, Fiebiger E, Reininger B, Ebner C, Petzelbauer P, Shing GP, Chapmand HA, Stingl G. Fcε receptor I on dendritic cells delivers IgE-bound multivalent antigens into a cathepsin S-dependent pathway of MHC class II presentation. J Immunol 1998; 161:2731–2739.

10

Lipid Inflammatory Mediators: Leukotrienes, Prostaglandins, Platelet-Activating Factor

PANDORA E. CHRISTIE and WILLIAM R. HENDERSON, JR.

University of Washington, Seattle, Washington

1 INTRODUCTION

Lipid inflammatory mediators including leukotrienes, prostaglandins, and platelet-activating factor have potent biological activities relevant to the pathogenesis of asthma and other allergic diseases. The chapter will review in vitro and in vivo studies of the role of these lipid mediators in allergic inflammatory diseases. Identification of the enzymes involved in synthesis of lipid mediators has led to the development of specific inhibitors that block their production; receptor blockers have also recently been developed that antagonize the biological actions of these potent mediators. These novel therapeutic agents have great potential to modulate the allergic inflammatory response.

2 BIOSYNTHESIS OF LIPID MEDIATORS

The specific enzymatic pathways that produce platelet-activating factor (PAF) and the lipid inflammatory mediators derived from arachidonic acid (AA), termed eicosanoids, are shown in Figure 1. Metabolism of AA through the 5-lipoxygenase (LO) pathway results in the production of leukotriene (LT)C_4, LTD_4, and LTE_4, which are collectively termed cysteinyl leukotrienes, and LTB_4 (1). Metabolism of AA by the cyclooxygenase (COX) pathway results in the production of prostaglandin (PG)D_2, PGE_2, prostacyclin (PGI_2), and thromboxane (TX)A_2 (2). Other eicosanoid products are the 12- and 15-LO products of AA (3). The lysophospholipid derived from membrane phospholipid after

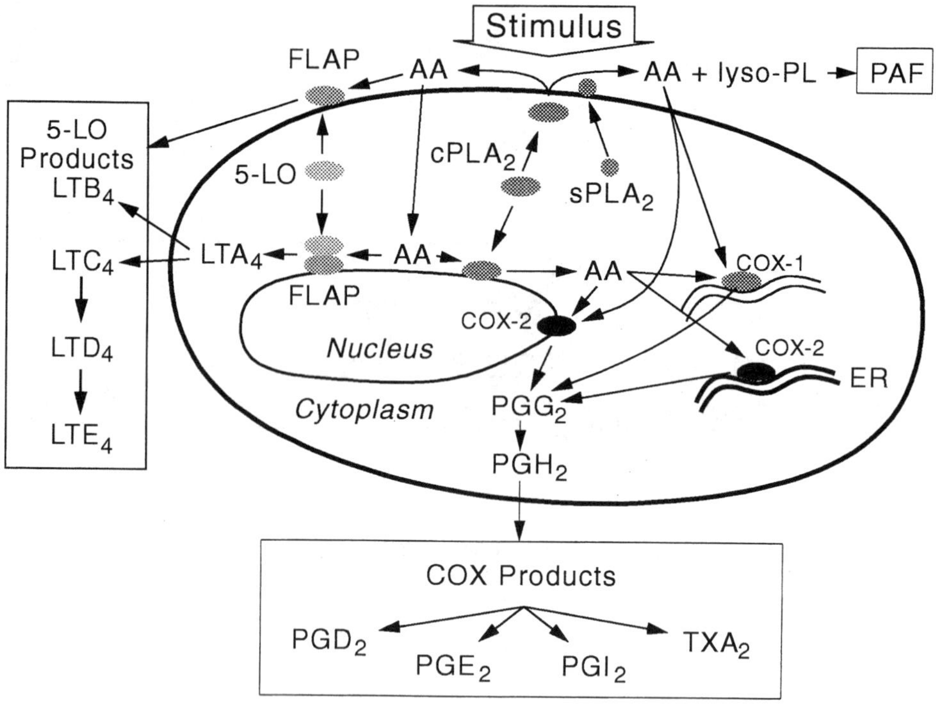

Figure 1 Lipid inflammatory mediators: 5-LO and COX AA products and PAF. (From Ref. 148.)

release of AA is acetylated by acetyltransferase to form platelet-activating factor (PAF) (2).

2.1 5-LO Pathway

The first step in leukotriene production occurs with phospholipase (PL)A_2 cleavage of AA from membrane phospholipids. Heterogeneity of PLA_2 enzymes exists including both cytosolic PLA_2 ($cPLA_2$) and secretory PLA_2 ($sPLA_2$) (1). The next step involves Ca^{2+}-dependent activation of 5-LO, which together with 5-LO-activating protein (FLAP) sequentially converts AA to 5-hydroperoxyeicosatetraenoic acid (5-HPETE) and LTA_4 (1). LTA_4 is metabolized by two different enzymes: a cytosolic protein LTA_4 hydrolase converts LTA_4 to the biologically active dihydroxy acid LTB_4, and a glutathione-*S*-transferase enzyme LTC_4 synthase converts LTA_4 to LTC_4 (1). γ-Glutamyl-transpeptidase converts LTC_4 to LTD_4, and a dipeptidase converts LTD_4 to LTE_4, each of which are biologically active. Oxidative degradation of LTB_4 and the cysteinyl leukotrienes results in less active metabolites (4).

2.2 COX Pathway

There are two isoenzymes, prostaglandin endoperoxide synthase-1 and -2 (PGHS-1 and PGHS-2), also referred to as COX-1 and COX-2, that catalyze the conversion of AA to prostaglandins and thromboxane (5). A dioxygenation reaction with AA by COX enzymes forms the unstable endoperoxide PGG_2, which is converted to another endoperoxide

PGH_2. PGH_2 is acted on by prostaglandin isomerases to form PGD_2, PGE_2, and $PGF_{2\alpha}$. Thromboxane and prostacyclin synthases convert PGH_2 to TXA_2 and PGI_2, respectively (2).

2.3 PAF Pathway

The metabolism of AA and PAF are closely linked (2). PLA_2 activation liberates long-chain fatty acids and AA from membrane phospholipids. The action of COA-dependent acetyltransferase on lysophosphocholine containing an ether-linked alkyl group on the first carbon forms PAF (1-*O*-alkyl-2 acetyl-*sn*-glycero-3-phosphocholine). Most phosphatidylcholine molecules contain an ester-linked acyl group on the first carbon and; consequently are not converted to PAF by this pathway. A 43-kDa protein known as PAF-acetylhydrolase (PAF-AH) is a group VII PLA_2 that hydrolyzes the *sn*-2 bond of PAF to form biologically inactive lyso-PAF (6); lyso-PAF can be reacylated with AA to form PAF.

3 REGULATION OF AA PATHWAY ENZYME EXPRESSION

Polymorphisms in the LTC_4 synthase gene and 5-LO have defined a potential role for these enzymes in mediating asthmatic inflammatory processes. In addition, AA products and cytokines have regulatory effects on specific enzymes of the AA metabolic pathway. The overall result is to alter lipid mediator production which, in turn, can modulate the inflammatory process.

3.1 $cPLA_2$ and $sPLA_2$

In allergic inflammatory processes, $cPLA_2$, an 85-kDa group IV PLA_2, is essential for the hydrolysis of phospholipids that contain AA at the *sn*-2 position, resulting in the release of AA. Allergic inflammatory cytokines may regulate $cPLA_2$ synthesis and release of AA products. $CD4^+$ T helper (Th) and $CD8^+$ T cytotoxic (Tc) cells infiltrate the airways in patients with asthma. These T cells secrete type 2 (Th2 and Tc2) cytokines IL-4, IL-5, and IL-13. In mouse peritoneal macrophages, IL-13 increases $cPLA_2$ gene and protein expression (7).

Eosinophilic infiltration is a key feature of the allergic inflammatory process in the lungs of asthmatics, and $cPLA_2$ plays a role in eosinophil migration into the lung. Eosinophil migration requires the interaction between surface adhesion receptors and ligands in pulmonary endothelium, extravascular tissue, and other inflammatory sites. The α_4-integrin subunit CD49d associates with either the β_1 (CD29) or β_7-subunit to form the integrin heterodimers very late antigen (VLA)-4 ($\alpha_4\beta_1$; CD49d/CD29) and $\alpha_4\beta_7$ (8). VLA-4 interaction with VCAM-1 is involved in eosinophil adherence to endothelium and transendothelial migration. A role for $cPLA_2$ in this process has been defined in studies using human eosinophil adherence to ICAM-1– or VCAM-1–coated plates (9). Integrin-dependent adhesion of human eosinophils in this system is blocked by the $cPLA_2$ inhibitor, arachidonyl trifluoromethylketone, indicating an essential role for $cPLA_2$ activation in this process. Because this effect on eosinophil adherence is blocked by the PAF receptor antagonist CV-6209, $cPLA_2$-induced eosinophil adhesion likely requires PAF (9).

Secretory PLA_2 (14-kDa protein, groups IIA, IIB, IIC, V PLA_2), unlike $cPLA_2$, hydrolyzes fatty acids independently of whether AA is present at the *sn*-2 position. $sPLA_2$ is found on the outer surface of monocytes, macrophages, mast cells, and other cells, and the AA it releases in inflammatory responses is a precursor for both leukotrienes (10) and prostaglandins (11). $sPLA_2$ induces hypersensitivity to muscarinic agonists in airway smooth muscle in vitro, a process mediated by TXA_2 (12). Tumor necrosis factor (TNF)-α, IL-1β, and lipopolysaccharide (LPS) increase $sPLA_2$ and COX-2 expression in rat tracheobronchial smooth-muscle cells, which may lead to increased lipid mediator production. This cytokine-induced increase in $sPLA_2$ expression is inhibited by dexamethasone (13). A role for $sPLA_2$ in the generation of AA in allergic processes is supported by increases of $sPLA_2$ in leukocytes and serum of asthmatics which correlate with asthma severity. Although $sPLA_2$ and AA levels in bronchoalveolar lavage (BAL) fluid do not differ between normal and asthmatic subjects; increases in BAL fluid $sPLA_2$ levels occur after inhaled antigen challenge in asthmatics (14).

3.2 5-LO and FLAP

5-Lipoxygenase and FLAP are typically found in cells of myeloid lineage: mast cells, basophils, neutrophils, eosinophils, monocytes, macrophages, and B lymphocytes. Lung inflammation results in expression of 5-LO and FLAP in pulmonary blood vessel endothelial cells, which do not express these proteins in basal states (15).

Heterogeneity in leukotriene production is observed in patients with asthma. To determine if 5-LO gene polymorphisms occur and account for variability in leukotriene production and clinical response to leukotriene modifier drugs, samples of genomic DNA, isolated from normal and asthmatic subjects, were analyzed for mutations in the known transcription factor-binding regions and protein-encoding region of the 5-LO gene. Mutations in the G+C-rich transcription factor-binding region of 5-LO consisted of the deletion of one, deletion of two, or addition of one of the five normally present zinc finger (*Sp1/ Egr-1*)-binding sites (16). Mutated binding regions were significantly less effective than the wild-type binding region as enhancers of 5-LO gene transcription. Thus, 5-LO gene polymorphisms may affect production of cysteinyl leukotrienes and LTB_4 in asthmatics. Furthermore, asthmatics with a mutant Sp1 enhancer region in the 5-LO gene are relatively resistant to treatment with the 5-LO inhibitor ABT-761, suggesting that these polymorphisms may help predict which patients will benefit from 5-LO inhibitors (17).

Similar to the cytokine stimulatory effects on $cPLA_2$ expression, cytokines also increase 5-LO and FLAP gene and protein expression. In vitro studies indicate that IL-5 increases expression of FLAP and translocates 5-LO to the nucleus in human blood eosinophils, enhancing LTC_4 synthesis (18). Allergic asthmatic patients have a greater proportion of circulating $FLAP^+$ eosinophils suggesting that allergic inflammatory processes may upregulate this key 5-LO pathway protein in vivo (18). Granulocyte–macrophage colony-stimulating factor (GM-CSF) and interleukin (IL)-3 increase 5-LO expression in monocytes (19). GM-CSF also increases leukotriene release by an eosinophilic substrain of HL-60 cells (20).

5-Lipoxygenase activation may be important in the increased asthma symptoms occurring after viral infection in asthmatic patients. Respiratory syncytial virus (RSV) infection in HEp-2 and BEAS-2B bronchial epithelial cell lines increases expression of 5-LO mRNA and protein; this increase in 5-LO expression is associated with increased leukotriene release in supernatants of the RSV-infected cells (21).

3.3 LTC_4 Synthase

Leukotriene C_4 synthase is an 18-kDa integral membrane protein expressed in eosinophils, mast cells, monocytes, macrophages, platelets, endothelial cells, and vascular smooth-muscle cells (22,23). LTC_4 synthase and FLAP belong to a gene family with a high degree of homology at the amino acid level. LTC_4 synthase has three hydrophobic domains and two hydrophilic loops that correspond to the predicted secondary structure of FLAP. AA binds at a 22-amino acid sequence at the C-terminus of the first hydrophilic loop of FLAP. FLAP inhibitors interact at this site to block leukotriene formation. LTC_4 synthase displays a high degree of amino acid identity at this hydrophilic region of FLAP (22). Recently, microsomal glutathione-*S*-transferase (GST-11) has been identified as a member of the same gene family, and the relative importance of LTC_4 synthase and GST-11 in LTC_4 synthesis has been investigated. Whereas LTC_4 synthase is the primary enzyme responsible for LTC_4 production in human lung membranes and platelet homogenates, GST-11 increases LTC_4 formation in endothelial cells, with a minor role in human lung membranes (24).

Eosinophils, key cells in allergic pulmonary inflammatory processes, produce predominantly cysteinyl leukotrienes (1). An in vitro study to define the expression of $cPLA_2$, 5-LO, FLAP, and LTC_4 synthase from cord blood progenitor cells indicates that AA pathway enzyme expression in eosinophils differs according to the stage of eosinophil maturation. During the development of eosinophils from cord blood mononuclear cells in vitro, mRNA for $cPLA_2$, 5-LO, and FLAP, but not LTC_4 synthase, is expressed at 7 days (25). At 14 days, when 94% of the cells are of eosinophil lineage, LTC_4 synthase mRNA and protein are present. Further increases in 5-LO, FLAP, and LTC_4 synthase protein occur with eosinophil maturation at 28 days. Thus, expression of $cPLA_2$, 5-LO, and FLAP occurs during the early stages of eosinophil development, whereas LTC_4 synthase expression occurs later in more mature cells (25). Cytokines also affect LTC_4 synthase activation. In the monocyte-like cell line THP-1, TGF-β_1, -β_2, and -β_3 increase LTC_4 synthase expression (26).

LTC_4 synthase is likely an important enzyme in the pathogenesis of aspirin-intolerant asthma (AIA). AIA is an acquired non–IgE-mediated reaction to aspirin and other COX inhibitors. The onset of AIA appears in patients with sinusitis, nasal polyps, and chronic severe asthma. After the ingestion of aspirin or other COX inhibitors, individuals with AIA develop bronchoconstriction, which can be life-threatening; AIA is associated with increased airway hyperreactivity to inhaled LTE_4. Increased cysteinyl leukotriene production occurs after aspirin ingestion in these patients, and this hypersecretion is associated with bronchoconstriction (27). Leukotriene receptor antagonists and 5-LO inhibitors attenuate aspirin-induced bronchospasm in AIA (28). The overproduction of cysteinyl leukotrienes in AIA may be partly attributable to increased expression of eosinophil LTC_4 synthase found in eosinophils in the lungs of patients with AIA (29). The increase in LTC_4 synthase correlates with the increased leukotriene release into BAL fluid observed in AIA patients after bronchial lysine–aspirin challenge (29). The mechanism for increased LTC_4 synthase activity in AIA patients compared with asthmatics tolerant to aspirin is unknown. An adenine to cytosine polymorphism at the promoter region of LTC_4 synthase, leading to increased enzyme transcription, is associated with AIA (30). LTC_4 synthase polymorphisms may account for differences in leukotriene production between different subgroups of asthmatics (e.g., AIA vs. aspirin-tolerant asthma).

Localization of the LTC_4 synthase gene to chromosome region 5q35 is of interest in asthma, because this area is in close proximity to the cytokine (i.e., GM-CSF, IL-3, IL-4, IL-5, IL-9, and IL-13) and the β_2-adrenergic and corticosteroid receptor gene sites implicated in asthma pathogenesis (23). It is unknown whether polymorphisms of the LTC_4 synthase gene occur alone or in conjunction with polymorphisms of other genes (e.g., IL-4) in this region or on different chromosomes (e.g., 5-LO gene polymorphism on chromosome 10). Polymorphisms resulting in altered cytokine, 5-LO, and LTC_4 synthase expression may significantly contribute to the heterogeneity of allergic inflammatory processes in asthma.

3.4 LTA_4 Hydrolase

Leukotriene-A_4 hydrolase (a 69-kDa enzyme) is a zinc-containing hydrolase with aminopeptidase activity (31). In contrast to 5-LO and FLAP proteins, LTA_4 hydrolase is found in erythrocytes, T-cell lines, fibroblasts, and airway epithelial cells. A 59-kDa LTA_4 hydrolase isoform has been identified that is constitutively expressed in cells along with the 69-kDa LTA_4 hydrolase isoform (32).

3.5 COX-1 and COX-2

Of current interest is identification of the role of the two pathways for prostaglandin synthesis (COX-1 and COX-2) in allergic inflammation. COX-1 is an enzyme constitutively expressed in most cells and accounts for the physiological generation of prostaglandins. COX-2 is expressed only in response to stimuli, such as growth factors, cytokines, lipopolysaccharide (LPS), and hormones, and accounts for inflammation-associated generation of prostaglandins (33). Expressions of COX-1 and of COX-2 enzymes are regulated differently by inflammatory stimuli.

In mouse bone marrow-derived mast cells, IL-1β and IL-10 induce COX-2 mRNA and protein expression, leading to synthesis of PGD_2 (34). In contrast, IgE and antigen stimulate PGD_2 production by COX-1 activation in these cells (34). COX-1 and COX-2 may be coupled to distinct phospholipases in mouse bone marrow-derived mast cells. In these cells, PGD_2 production has two phases: an immediate phase, within 15 min, and a delayed phase at 4–6 hr after mast cell activation. The immediate phase of PGD_2 production results from COX-1 acting on AA produced by $cPLA_2$ and $sPLA_2$, the delayed phase of PGD_2 production from COX-2 acting on AA produced by $cPLA_2$ (35). Although corticosteroids and cytokines do not affect COX-1 expression, dexamethasone, IL-10, and TGF-β inhibit COX-2 expression (36,37).

The possibility that COX-1 and COX-2 isoforms differ in the profile of generated products from AA has implications in allergic and other inflammatory processes. In resident rat peritoneal macrophages, which contain only COX-1, AA metabolism is converted primarily to PGI_2, TXA_2, PGD_2, and 12-hydroxyheptadecatrienoic acid. In contrast, blockade of COX-1 by aspirin and subsequent induction of COX-2 by LPS results in PGI_2 and PGE_2 synthesis by these cells (38). Differences in intracellular distribution of these enzymes involved in COX metabolism may explain the different metabolic fates of AA observed in these studies. COX-1 is found in the intracellular membrane system of cells, and COX-2 localizes to the nuclear envelope; PGD_2 synthase is present in the cytoplasm and PGE_2 synthase in the endoplasmic reticulum and nuclear envelope (38).

The regulation of AA metabolism by COX-1 versus COX-2 pathways within monocytes and macrophages depends on the stage of cell differentiation. Alveolar macrophages are derived from blood monocytes that migrate into the lung. IL-4 inhibits LPS-induced COX-2 activation and PGE_2 synthesis in human alveolar macrophages, whereas IL-10, IL-13, and IFN-γ have no effect on either COX-2 activity or PGE_2 release in these cells (39). In monocytes, IL-4, IL-10, and IL-13 suppress LPS-dependent COX-2 mRNA induction and PGE_2 synthesis (39). In studies using COX-1-deficient, COX-2-deficient, and wild-type mice, if one isoenzyme is inhibited pharmacologically or absent genetically, there is enhanced expression of both the $cPLA_2$ gene and the remaining functional COX isoenzyme gene, leading to increased production of PGE_2 (40).

4 CELLULAR SOURCE OF LIPID MEDIATORS

Because of the wide distribution of enzymes involved in AA metabolism, eicosanoid synthesis occurs in varied inflammatory and resident cells and tissues. Some cells produce both 5- LO and COX AA products. For example, monocytes and macrophages produce the 5-LO products LTC_4 and LTB_4 and the COX products PGE_2, PGI_2, and TXA_2 (41); mast cells release LTC_4 and PGD_2 as their predominant 5-LO and COX products, respectively. Other cells are more restricted in the type of AA metabolites they generate. Eosinophils and neutrophils generate nearly exclusively 5-LO products; eosinophils release LTC_4, and neutrophils release LTB_4 (1). $CD4^+$ T cells do not secrete leukotrienes. Other cells that lack 5-LO or FLAP enzymes may still participate in leukotriene synthesis by conversion of LTA_4 exported by other inflammatory cells. For example, neutrophil-derived LTA_4 may be used by erythrocytes that contain LTA_4 hydrolase to convert LTA_4 to LTB_4. Platelets that contain LTC_4 synthase can convert exogenously derived LTA_4 to LTC_4. PAF is produced by most cells involved in airway inflammation (i.e., monocytes, alveolar macrophages, mast cells, basophils, eosinophils, neutrophils, platelets, and endothelial cells) (2).

5 LIPID MEDIATOR RECEPTORS

Eicosanoids and PAF have distinct G-coupled receptors that mediate their biological actions. Specific antagonists of many of these receptors have been developed for clinical use in the treatment of allergic and other inflammatory diseases.

5.1 LTB_4 Receptors

The LTB_4 receptors are members of the rhodopsin-like receptor superfamily. LTB_4 interacts with an LTB_4 receptor at the cell surface (designated BLTR) and binds and activates the intranuclear transcription factor, peroxisome proliferator-activated receptor (PPAR)-α (42). LTB_4 receptors are identified on the surface of human neutrophils, alveolar macrophages, and eosinophils. LTB_4 receptors have been found in lymph nodes. Two forms of LTB_4 receptors have been characterized in neutrophils according to the affinity of LTB_4 for the receptors. The high-affinity LTB_4 receptor mediates chemotaxis, chemokinesis, aggregation, and adherence to endothelium; the low-affinity LTB_4 receptor mediates degranulation and oxygen radical release (1). Overexpression of BLTR in leukocytes leads to increased neutrophil influx into the lungs after ischemia–reperfusion in mice (43). Leukotriene formation is also required for neutrophil trafficking in this model of lung injury because 5-$LO^{-/-}$ mice have a significantly decreased infiltration of the airways by neutrophils after reperfusion (43).

5.2 Cysteinyl Leukotriene Receptors

The receptors for LTC_4, LTD_4, and LTE_4 are named CysLT receptors and are distinct from the LTB_4 receptors. Two classes of CysLT receptors have been identified: $CysLT_1$ and $CysLT_2$ according to their sensitivity to selective LT receptor antagonists (e.g., pobilukast, pranlukast, montelukast, and zafirlukast). The $CysLT_1$ receptor is sensitive to many

LT receptor antagonists, whereas the $CysLT_2$ receptor is resistant to most CysLT antagonists, with the exception of Bay u9773, a mixed $CysLT_1$ and $CysLT_2$ antagonist (44). The $CysLT_1$ receptor gene has been mapped to the X chromosome (45). In human endothelial kidney (HEK)-293 cells, the $CysLT_1$ receptor responds to leukotrienes C_4, D_4, and E_4 with a calcium mobilization response and a rank order of potency as follows: $LTD_4 > LTC_4 > LTE_4$ (46). The $CysLT_1$ receptor has been identified in human smooth-muscle cells, lung macrophages, and peripheral blood leukocytes (47). In human lung, $CysLT_2$ receptors are present in pulmonary veins (47).

5.3 Prostanoid Receptors

Prostanoid receptors are rhodopsin-type receptors with seven transmembrane domains consisting of many types and subtypes. Even though predominant prostanoid binding may be at receptors termed DP, EP, FP, IP, and TP (PGD_2, PGE_2, PGF_{2a}, PGI_2, and TXA_2, respectively), significant overlap occurs between these receptor-binding sites (48). For example, although PGD_2 interacts most selectively with DP receptors, it also has agonist activity at FP and TP receptor sites (48). Classes of prostanoid receptors are further subdivided; within these subdivisions, isoforms also exist [e.g., EP_{1-4}, EP_3 receptor isoforms, and FP isoforms FP(A) and FP(B)] (48). Many of these receptors have been cloned, such as the human PGE_2 receptor EP_2 (49). In rat fibroblasts, the action of PGE_2 on expression of COX-1 genes is mediated through the EP_2 receptor (50).

5.4 PAF Receptors

The receptor for PAF, also a seven-transmembrane domain receptor, has been cloned in humans (51). PAF receptors are identified in a variety of organs, including the heart, skeletal muscle, eye, skin, trachea, and aorta (51). Increases in PAF receptor mRNA levels in the lungs of patients with asthma support a role for PAF in allergic airway inflammation (52).

6 ROLE OF AA MEDIATORS IN ALLERGIC INFLAMMATION

Lipid mediators are elevated in many allergic inflammatory disorders. Most of the studies to elucidate the role of these mediators in allergic inflammation are in asthma and will be discussed in this section.

6.1 Asthma

The main inflammatory features of asthma include airway eosinophilia, edema, mucous hypersecretion, bronchial epithelial injury, subepithelial fibrosis, and bronchoconstriction. Bronchoalveolar lavage and biopsy data indicate increased numbers of $CD4^+$ and $CD8^+$ T cells and correlation of the amounts of the Th2 and Tc2 cytokines (IL-4, IL-5, IL-13), but not Th1 cytokines (IFN-γ, IL-2), with symptom severity and airway hyperresponsiveness (AHR). In vitro and in vivo studies indicate that lipid mediators are important mediators of allergic airway inflammation (Table 1). Inhaled allergen in asthmatic individuals provokes an early asthmatic response (EAR), which is followed in about 50% of patients by a late asthmatic response (LAR). The LAR is associated with increases in AHR to agents such as methacholine. The EAR is an IgE-mediated reaction to allergen characterized by lung mast cell degranulation and mediator release. The release of lipid mediators (5-LO

Table 1 Lipid Mediators Elevated in Inflammatory Diseases

Disease	Site/tissue	Lipid mediator	Ref.
Asthma			
Chronic	BAL fluid	LTB_4, TXB_2, PGD_2	57,103
	Nasal fluid	LTC_4	93
	Urine	LTE_4	57
	Blood	LTE_4	104
	Sputum	CysLTs	105
Allergen-induced	BAL fluid	PGD_2, TXB_2 LTC_4, LTE_4, LTB_4	55,56,99,106
	Urine	LTE_4, PGD_2	99,100,107
	Blood	PAF	108
Acute			
Exercise-induced	Urine	LTE_4, PGD_2	109,110
Cold air-induced	Urine	LTE_4	59
	Nasal lavage	CysLTs, PGD_2	111
Aspirin-induced	Urine	LTE_4, PGD_2	27,112
Nocturnal	BAL fluid	LTB_4, CysLTs	113
	Urine	LTE_4	113
Pulmonary			
Cystic fibrosis	BAL fluid	LTB_4, PGE_2, TXB_2, CysLTs	114
	Sputum	CysLTs	115
	Urine	LTE_4, PGE_2, TXB_2	116,117
ARDS	Blood	LTB_4	114
	BAL fluid	LTC_4, LTD_4, PAF	118–120
Idiopathic pulmonary fibrosis	Lung tissue	LTB_4, LTC_4	121
Rhinitis/sinusitis			
Chronic sinusitis	Sinus lavage fluid	CysLTs, PGD_2	122
Allergic rhinitis	Nasal lavage fluid	CysLTs	123
Skin			
Atopic dermatitis	Skin	LTB_4	124
	Urine	LTC_4, LTE_4	125,126
Cold urticaria	Blood	LTE_4	127
Psoriasis	Skin lesions	LTB_4, CysLTs, PAF	128,129
Anaphylaxis	Urine	LTE_4	130
Eye			
Giant papillary conjunctivitis	Tears	LTC_4	131
Vernal conjunctivitis	Tears	LTB_4	132
Allergen-induced conjunctivitis	Tears	PGD_2	133
Autoimmune			
Kawasaki	Urine	LTE_4	134
Henoch-Schonlein purpura	Blood	LTC_4, TXA_2, PGI_2	135,136
Behcet's disease	Blood	LTC_4, PGE_2	137
Rheumatoid arthritis (adult)	Synovial fluid	LTB_4, LTC_4, PGE_2	138,139
Rheumatoid arthritis (juvenile)	Blood	LTB_4	140
Gastrointestinal			
Ulcerative colitis	GI lavage	PAF, LTB_4, PGE_2, TXB_2	141
	Blood	PGE_2	142
	Colonic mucosa	LTB_4, PGE_2	142
	Rectal dialysis fluid	LTB_4	143
Crohn's disease	Colonic mucosa	LTB_4, PAF	144
	Jejunal perfusion	LTC_4	145
	GI lavage	LTB_4, PGE_2, TXB_2	142,146
	Urine	LTE_4	147

and COX AA products and PAF) during the EAR promotes the inflammatory influx of eosinophils, neutrophils, lymphocytes, and macrophages into the airways observed in the LAR. Eicosanoids and PAF are also released by the infiltrating inflammatory cells to further augment lung inflammation in the LAR.

6.2 Other Allergic Diseases

Lipid mediators are also important in the pathogenesis of other inflammatory diseases, including allergic rhinitis, atopic dermatitis, allergic conjunctivitis, vasculitis, and anaphylaxis (see Table 1).

7 BIOLOGICAL ACTIVITIES OF LIPID MEDIATORS

Although the lipid mediators are clearly important participants in the airway inflammatory process in asthma, their exact role in these complex inflammatory responses relative to other mediators has been unclear. Their role has been clarified recently with the development of (1) a mouse model of asthma, (2) mice deficient in specific eicosanoid pathway proteins (i.e., 5-LO$^{-/-}$, FLAP$^{-/-}$, COX-1$^{-/-}$, and COX-2$^{-/-}$ mice), and (3) specific synthesis inhibitors, receptor antagonists, and inactivators of these lipid mediators.

7.1 Leukotrienes

Leukotriene-B_4 induces chemokinesis and chemotaxis of human neutrophils and monocytes, aggregation of neutrophils, and enhanced expression of complement receptors on granulocytes. It also stimulates release of lysosomal enzymes from neutrophils and leukocyte adherence to endothelial cells. The LTB_4-induced increased adhesiveness of endothelial cells for neutrophils is secondary to increased expression of both specific domains of the CD54 adhesion molecule on endothelial cells and CD11/CD18 on the surface of neutrophils (8). LTB_4 has weak bronchoconstrictor activity through COX AA product release. Human monocyte IL-6 production is augmented by LTB_4, which increases IL-6 gene transcription and mRNA stabilization (53).

The cysteinyl leukotrienes LTC_4, LTD_4, and LTE_4 are potent bronchoconstrictors, mucous secretagogues, and inducers of eosinophil chemotaxis and vasopermeability (1). Patients with asthma are hyperresponsive to bronchial challenge with cysteinyl leukotrienes compared with histamine. The cysteinyl leukotrienes have great biological activity in stimulating release of mucus from human bronchial tissue with the following rank order of potency: cysteinyl leukotrienes $>$ LTB_4 $>$ COX AA products $>$ histamine (54). The increased adherence of leukocytes to vascular endothelium induced by cysteinyl leukotrienes is partly mediated by translocation of P-selectin (CD62P) to the luminal surface of endothelial cells from subcellular sites (8). Inhaled LTE_4 in patients with asthma causes bronchoconstriction, AHR, and pulmonary eosinophilia. In contrast, LTB_4 inhalation in asthmatics results in airway neutrophilia, with no effect on airway tone or AHR.

Increased LTB_4 and LTC_4 levels in BAL fluid, and LTE_4 levels in urine occur after endobronchial challenge with specific allergen in atopic asthmatics (55,56). Increased levels of LTB_4 are found in the BAL fluid of patients with severe asthma despite high-dose corticosteroid therapy. In these severe asthmatics, increased numbers of neutrophils are found in BAL fluid and in endobronchial and transbronchial biopsies (57). These data suggest that LTB_4 may play a major role in the influx of neutrophils into the lungs of patients with severe asthma. Leukotrienes are also implicated in the pathogenesis of acute, nocturnal, and aspirin-, exercise-, and cold air-induced asthma (see Table 1) (58,59).

An important role for leukotrienes in airway eosinophilia, mucus hypersecretion, and AHR has been demonstrated using a mouse model of asthma (60). Administration of ovalbumin (OVA) to normal BALB/c and C57 BL/6 mice induces a late-phase allergic response similar to that seen in patients with asthma. In this murine model of asthma, OVA sensitization and challenge induces OVA-specific IgE and increases total IgE levels. Also noted are release of 5-LO products in BAL fluid, eosinophil influx into the BAL fluid and lung interstitium, and airway mucus hypersecretion (60). OVA-treated mice have a Th2, but not Th1, cytokine profile in bronchial lymph nodes, and AHR to methacholine (61,62). In situ polymerase chain reaction (PCR) studies in the OVA-treated mice demonstrate increased FLAP and 5-LO gene and protein expression in the lungs (63). FLAP and 5-LO gene activation is primarily associated with eosinophils and macrophages in leukocytic infiltrates in the lung interstitium surrounding pulmonary blood vessels and in airway submucosal regions. Alveolar macrophages also exhibit prominent FLAP mRNA and protein in the OVA-sensitized challenged mice.

The development of knockout mice deficient in 5-LO (5-LO$^{-/-}$) and FLAP (FLAP$^{-/-}$) (64,65) has been important in understanding the role of the 5-LO pathway in allergic inflammation. 5-LO$^{-/-}$ murine macrophages after activation have a more increased release of COX AA products than similarly treated cells from 5-LO$^{+/+}$ littermates (65); these data suggest that in the absence of the 5-LO pathway, shunting of AA into the COX oxidative pathway occurs. When 5-LO$^{+/+}$ and 5-LO$^{-/-}$ mice are sensitized and challenged with OVA, the OVA-treated 5-LO$^{-/-}$ mice do not demonstrate AHR to methacholine compared with similarly treated 5-LO$^{+/+}$ mice (66). The absence of airway hyperresponsiveness is associated with reduced total cells and eosinophils in the lung interstitium and BAL fluid and airway mucus (Henderson et al., unpublished observations). The inability to develop AHR in the 5-LO deficient mice suggests a crucial role for 5-LO products in this process. In 5-LO$^{+/+}$ mice, to further indicate the importance of leukotrienes in mediating airway eosinophilia and mucus hypersecretion, the 5-LO inhibitor zileuton and the FLAP inhibitor MK-886 block the eosinophilia and release of mucus (60). In this mouse model of asthma, the CysLT$_1$ receptor antagonist, montelukast inhibits influx of eosinophils into the airways (Henderson et al., unpublished observations). Similarly, in allergic Brown–Norway rats, montelukast inhibits the LAR, airway eosinophilia, and IL-5 mRNA$^+$ cells (67).

In animal models, depletion of CD4$^+$ T cells by pretreatment with specific monoclonal antibodies after allergen sensitization, but before allergen challenge, prevents AHR and eosinophil recruitment. Although CD4$^+$ T cells do not secrete leukotrienes, in vitro studies show that leukotrienes have important effects on T-lymphocyte activation. 5-LO activation and LTE$_4$ release occur in Jurkat T cells after T-cell receptor (TCR/CD3) cross-linking (68). 5-LO activation and LTB$_4$ production are necessary for CD28-mediated NF-κB and IL-2 gene expression and T-cell activation, indicating a potential role for leukotrienes in T-cell function (69).

7.2 Prostaglandins

Cyclooxygenase products are important mediators of allergic inflammation and regulate immune responses mediated by mature B and T lymphocytes (2). PGE$_2$ relaxes bronchial smooth muscle and blocks antigen-induced EAR and LAR. PGE$_2$ inhibits the acute bronchoconstriction that occurs after ingestion of COX inhibitors in the subgroup of asthmatics with AIA. PGD_2, $PGF_{2\alpha}$, and TXA_2 constrict bronchial smooth muscle. PGD_2, the major COX AA product released by lung mast cells, is also a mucus secretagogue. PGI_2 has important vasoactive properties. PGI_2 dilates the pulmonary vasculature and relaxes bronchial smooth muscle and inhibits intrapulmonary platelet aggregation. Both constitutive COX-1 and inducible COX-2 isoforms are expressed in T cells in the absence of prostaglandin synthesis (70). Activation of COX-1 and COX-2 is important in T-cell development. Studies using COX-1- and COX-2-deficient mice and COX isoform-specific inhibitors demonstrate different roles for COX-1 and -2 in T-cell development. COX-1 is involved in the transition of $CD4^-CD8^-$ double-negative to $CD4^+CD8^+$ double-positive T cells (5). COX-2 is important for early thymocyte proliferation and differentiation and maturation of the $CD4^+$ helper T cell.

Peritoneal macrophages from COX-1-deficient mice form less than 1% PGE_2 from AA as substrate compared with COX-1 wild-type mice (71). COX-2 deficiency causes severe kidney disease and spontaneous peritonitis in some animals and modulates allergic lung responses (72,73). In OVA-sensitized and challenged COX-1- and COX-2–deficient mice compared with wild-type mice, COX-$1^{-/-}$–deficient mice have reduced PGE_2 recovery from BAL fluid compared with COX-$2^{-/-}$ or wild-type controls suggesting an important role for COX-1 in PGE_2 production (74). After OVA challenge, lung inflammatory indices are greater in COX-$1^{-/-}$ and -$2^{-/-}$ mice compared with wild-type mice. In contrast with 5-LO–deficient mice, allergic COX-$1^{-/-}$–deficient mice exhibit increased AHR to methacholine, and LTB_4 and cysteinyl leukotriene recovery from BAL fluid of allergic COX-$1^{-/-}$ mice compared with allergic wild-type and COX-$2^{-/-}$ mice (74). These results suggest that blockade of either 5-LO or COX shunts AA into the alternative pathway of metabolism and could explain the increase in leukotriene recovery observed in COX-1–deficient mice. It is unknown why allergic COX-2–deficient mice do not demonstrate rises in 5-LO AA products similar to the COX-1–deficient mice.

7.3 PAF

The biological activities of PAF also appear relevant to the pathogenesis of allergic inflammation. Many of the effects of PAF on vasculature, bronchial smooth muscle, and production of mucus are similar to those induced by cysteinyl leukotrienes, and in some cases, the biological actions of PAF are mediated by cysteinyl leukotrienes. Biological effects of PAF include increase in vascular permeability after intracutaneous administration, airway inflammatory cells (eosinophils and neutrophils), and release of mucus (2). The hemodynamic effects of PAF are mediated by leukotrienes, for 5-$LO^{-/-}$ mice do not undergo the lethal PAF-induced cardiovascular collapse observed in 5-$LO^{+/+}$ mice (64,65). Transgenic mice that overexpress PAF receptors have an increased bronchoconstrictor response to PAF and AHR to methacholine which is attenuated by thromboxane synthesis inhibitors and leukotriene receptor antagonists (75). The route of administration of PAF results in different patterns of cellular infiltration. In guinea pigs, intracutaneous and intratracheal administration of PAF causes tissue neutrophilia, whereas intravenous injection produces airway and parenchymal eosinophilia. In humans, PAF injection into the skin causes eosinophilia in atopic individuals and neutrophilia in nonatopic subjects (76).

The plasma protein PAF-acetylhydrolase (PAF-AH) cleaves PAF to its biologically inactive form lyso-PAF. A genetic mutation (V279F) has been identified in the PAF-AH gene which leads to deficiency of PAF-AH in approximately 4% of the Japanese population (77,78). It has been hypothesized that deficiency of PAF-AH may result in greater levels of PAF and PAF-induced inflammatory effects. An association between the V279F mutation and severity of asthma in children has been reported in one report (79), but not confirmed in another study (80). PAF-AH has been cloned and expressed as a human recombinant protein (rPAF-AH). After intravenous administration, rPAF-AH inhibits PAF-induced pleurisy and paw edema in rats (6). In OVA-sensitized and challenged mice, the administration of rPAF-AH reduces the late-phase pulmonary inflammatory response to allergen, with reduced influx of airway eosinophils, mucus hypersecretion, and AHR to methacholine (81). However, in mild asthmatics, intravenous rPAF-AH at a dose of 1 mg/kg does not affect the early or late response to antigen, induced sputum cell counts, nor sputum eosinophil cationic protein (ECP) and tryptase levels (82).

Despite the potential role of PAF as a key mediator in allergic inflammatory processes, the effects of PAF receptor antagonists in patients with asthma have been disappointing. Although several studies have suggested beneficial effects of PAF receptor antagonists on AHR and the LAR to allergen challenge in mild asthmatics (83,84), most studies have not found these agents to be clinically beneficial in patients with asthma (85–88).

8 ANTI-INFLAMMATORY EFFECTS OF INHIBITORS OF LIPID MEDIATORS

Various strategies have been developed to inhibit either the synthesis or biological action of eicosanoids and PAF. These approaches include pharmacological agents that inhibit 5-LO or FLAP to block leukotriene formation or antagonize the actions of LTB_4, cysteinyl leukotrienes, and PAF by selective receptor antagonists (1,89,90). Selective COX-2 inhibitors have recently been developed, but their effect on allergic airway inflammation is largely unexplored.

8.1 $CysLT_1$ Receptor Antagonists

In patients with asthma, treatment with $CysLT_1$ receptor antagonists has marked anti-inflammatory effects, including inhibition of airway eosinophil influx, secretion of mucus and cytokine and mediator release, supporting a critical role for cysteinyl leukotrienes in these inflammatory processes.

Pranlukast inhibits antigen-specific production of Th2 cytokines (eg., IL-3, IL-4, and GM-CSF), but not Th1 cytokines (e.g., IL-2) from human peripheral blood mononuclear cells in vitro (91). In patients with chronic asthma, montelukast therapy (10 mg q.h.s.) reduces sputum and peripheral blood eosinophilia (92) and nasal lavage fluid levels of LTC_4 (93). Forty-eight hours after segemental antigen challenge in asthmatics, zafirkulast (20 mg b.i.d. for 7 days) compared with placebo, significantly decreases the number of basophils and lymphocytes and levels of TNF-α in the BAL fluid (94). Alveolar macrophages from these zafirlukast-treated asthmatics also have reduced phorbol ester-induced superoxide release compared with cells from the same subjects after placebo treatment (94). In similar segmental allergen challenge studies, BAL fluid eosinophil levels are significantly reduced after treatment with a higher dose of zafirlukast (160 mg b.i.d.) (95). Compared with placebo, 4 weeks of treatment with pranlukast (225 mg b.i.d.) decreases the cellular infiltration in bronchial mucosa in mild–moderate asthmatics (96). $AA1^+$ ($tryptase^+$) mast cells, $EG2^+$ (activated eosinophils) cells, and $CD3^+$ and $CD4^+$ T cells are reduced in bronchial biopsies after pranlukast therapy, compared with baseline (96). In contrast, the numbers of EG1$^+$ (nonactivated eosinophils), CD68$^+$ (macrophages), or NP57$^+$ (neutrophils) cells in the airways of these subjects are not affected by pranlukast.

Leukotriene receptor antagonists have additive benefits to inhaled corticosteroids in patients with persistent asthma (97,98). A significant reduction of peripheral blood eosinophils is observed when montelukast and beclomethasone dipropionate (BDP) are used together compared with BDP treatment alone in patients with chronic asthma (98). An explanation for this finding is that leukotrienes constitute an inflammatory pathway in asthma that is not affected by corticosteroids given either systemically or by inhalation. Prednisone therapy (60 mg q.d. for 6–9 days) does not alter 5-LO AA product release into BAL fluid or LTE_4 urinary levels either at baseline or after allergen challenge in atopic asthmatics (99). Similarly, high-dose inhaled fluticasone (1000 μg q.d. for 2 weeks) compared with placebo has no effect on the increased urinary LTE_4 levels observed after allergen challenge in allergic asthmatics (100).

8.2 PAF Inhibitors

Although potent PAF receptor antagonists can block cellular and pulmonary effects of PAF aerosol challenge (101), these antagonists have been of limited clinical benefit in patients with either acute (102) or chronic (87,88) asthma. As discussed in the foregoing, rPAF-AH treatment fails to reduce either the EAR or LAR after allergen challenge in atopic asthmatics (82).

9 SUMMARY

The lipid mediators, leukotrienes, prostaglandins, and PAF play an important role in the complex inflammatory process of airway eosinophilia, edema hypersecretion of mucus, and AHR observed in patients with asthma. These mediators are also likely key participants in the pathogenesis of other allergic diseases. An important goal of future research is to clarify the complex interactions between the lipid mediators and the inflammatory stimuli that regulate their production. Novel inhibitors and antagonists of the lipid mediators, such as the $CysLT_1$ receptor antagonists, have recently been developed that have great promise in the treatment of allergic diseases.

REFERENCES

1. Henderson WR Jr. The role of leukotrienes in inflammation. Ann Intern Med 1994; 121: 684–697.
2. Henderson WR Jr. Eicosanoids and platelet-activating factor in allergic respiratory diseases. Am Rev Respir Dis 1991; 143:S86–S90.
3. Henderson WR. Products of 12 and 15 lipoxygenase. In: Henson PM, Murphy RC, eds. Handbook of Inflammation. Vol. 6. Mediators of the Inflammatory Process. Amsterdam: Elsevier Science, 1989:45–75.
4. Henderson WR. Formation and oxidative degradation of leukotrienes by eosinophils and neutrophils. In: Samuelsson B, Berti F, Folco GC, Velo GP, eds. Drugs Affecting Leukotrienes and Other Eicosanoid Pathways. New York: Plenum, 1985:339–349.
5. Smith WL, DeWitt DL. Prostaglandin endoperoxide H synthases-1 and -2. Adv Immunol 1996; 62:167–215.
6. Tjoelker LW, Wilder C, Eberhardt C, Stafforini DM, Dietsch G, Schimpf B, Hooper S, Trong HL, Cousens LS, Zimmerman GA, Yamada Y, McIntyre TM, Prescott SM, Gray PW. Anti-

inflammatory properties of a platelet-activating factor acetylhydrolase. Nature 1995; 374: 549–553.

7. Rey A, M'Rini C, Sozzani P, Lamboeuf Y, Beraud M, Caput D, Ferrara P, Pipy B. IL-13 increases the $cPLA_2$ gene and protein expression and the mobilization of arachidonic acid during an inflammatory process in mouse peritoneal macrophages. Biochim Biophys Acta 1998; 1393:244–252.
8. Carlos TM, Harlan JM. Leukocyte–endothelial adhesion molecules. Blood 1994; 84:2068–2101.
9. Zhu X, Munoz NM, Kim KP, Sano H, Cho W, Leff AR. Cytosolic phospholipase A_2 activation is essential for beta 1 and beta 2 integrin-dependent adhesion of human eosinophils. J Immunol 1999; 163:3423–3429.
10. Marshall LA, Bolognese B, Winkler JD, Roshak A. Depletion of human monocyte 85-kDa phospholipase A_2 does not alter leukotriene formation. J Biol Chem 1997; 272:759–765.
11. Balboa MA, Balsinde J, Winstead MV, Tischfield JA, Dennis EA. Novel group V phospholipase A_2 involved in arachidonic acid mobilization in murine P388D, macrophages. J Biol Chem 1996; 271:32381–32384.
12. Takata Y, Nishimura Y, Maeda H, Yokoyama M. Phospholipase A_2 augments contraction and intracellular calcium mobilization through thromboxane A_2 in bovine tracheal smooth muscle. Eur Respir J 1999; 14:396–404.
13. Vadas P, Stefanski E, Wloch M, Grouix B, Van Den BH, Kennedy B. Secretory non-pancreatic phospholipase A_2 and cyclooxygenase-2 expression by tracheobronchial smooth muscle cells. Eur J Biochem 1996; 235:557–563.
14. Bowton DL, Seeds MC, Fasano MB, Goldsmith B, Bass DA. Phospholipase A_2 and arachidonate increase in bronchoalveolar lavage fluid after inhaled antigen challenge in asthmatics. Am J Respir Crit Care Med 1997; 155:421–425.
15. Wright L, Tuder RM, Wang J, Cool CD, Lepley RA, Voelkel NF. 5-Lipoxygenase and 5-lipoxygenase activating protein (FLAP) immunoreactivity in lungs from patients with primary pulmonary hypertension. Am J Respir Crit Care Med 1998; 157:219–229.
16. In KH, Asano K, Beier D, Grobholz J, Finn PW, Silverman EK, Silverman ES, Collins T, Fischer AR, Keith TP, Serino K, Kim SW, De Sanctis GT, Yandava C, Pillari A, Rubin P, Kemp J, Busse W, Ledford D, Murray JJ, Segal A, Tinkelman D, Drazen JM. Naturally occurring mutations in the human 5-lipoxygenase gene promoter that modify transcription factor binding and reporter gene transcription. J Clin Invest 1997; 99:1130–1137.
17. Drazen JM, Yandava CN, Dube L, Szczerback N, Hippensteel R, Pillari A, Israel E, Schork N, Silverman ES, Katz DA, Drajesk J. Pharmacogenetic association between ALOX5 promoter genotype and the response to anti-asthma treatment. Nat Genet 1999; 22:168–170.
18. Cowburn AS, Holgate ST, Sampson AP. IL-5 increases expression of 5-lipoxygenase-activating protein and translocates 5-lipoxygenase to the nucleus in human blood eosinophils. J Immunol 1999; 163:456–465.
19. Ring WL, Riddick CA, Baker JR, Munafo DA, Bigby TD. Lymphocytes stimulate expression of 5-lipoxygenase and its activating protein in monocytes in vitro via granulocyte macrophage colony-stimulating factor and interleukin 3. J Clin Invest 1996; 97:1293–1301.
20. Scoggan KA, Ford–Hutchinson AW, Nicholson DW. Differential activation of leukotriene biosynthesis by granulocyte–macrophage colony-stimulating factor and interleukin-5 in an eosinophilic substrain of HL-60 cells. Blood 1995; 86:3507–3516.
21. Behera AK, Kumar M, Matsuse H, Lockey RF, Mohapatra SS. Respiratory syncytial virus induces the expression of 5-lipoxygenase and endothelin-1 in bronchial epithelial cells. Biochem Biophys Res Commun 1998; 251:704–709.
22. Penrose JF, Spector J, Baldasaro M, Xu K, Boyce J, Arm JP, Austen FK, Lam BK. Molecular cloning of the gene for human leukotriene C_4 synthase. J Biochem 1996; 271:11356–11361.
23. Penrose JF. LTC_4 synthase. Enzymology, biochemistry, and molecular characterization. Clin Rev Allergy Immunol 1999; 17:133–152.

24. Scoggan KA, Jakobsson PJ, Ford–Hutchinson AW. Production of leukotriene C_4 in different human tissues is attributable to distinct membrane bound biosynthetic enzymes. J Biol Chem 1997; 272:10182–10187.
25. Boyce JA, Lam BK, Penrose JF, Friend DS, Parsons S, Owen WF, Austen KF. Expression of LTC_4 synthase during the development of eosinophils in vitro from cord blood progenitors. Blood 1996; 88:4338–4347.
26. Riddick CA, Serio KJ, Hodulik CR, Ring WL, Regan MS, Bigby TD. TGF-beta increases leukotriene C_4 synthase expression in the monocyte-like cell line, THP-1. J Immunol 1999; 162:1101–1107.
27. Lee TH, Christie PE. Leukotrienes and aspirin induced asthma. Thorax 1993;48:1189–1190.
28. Israel E, Fischer AR, Rosenberg MA, Lilly CM, Callery JC, Shapiro J, Cohn J, Rubin P, Drazen JM. The pivotal role of 5-lipoxygenase products in the reaction of aspirin-sensitive asthmatics to aspirin. Am Rev Respir Dis 1993; 148:1447–1451.
29. Cowburn AS, Sladek K, Soja J, Adamek L, Nizankowska E, Szczeklik A, Lam BK, Penrose JF, Austen KF, Holgate ST, Sampson AP. Overexpression of leukotriene C_4 synthase in bronchial biopsies from patients with aspirin-intolerant asthma. J Clin Invest 1998; 101:834–846.
30. Sanak M, Simon HU, Szczeklik A. Leukotriene C_4 synthase promoter polymorphism and risk of aspirin-induced asthma. Lancet 1997; 350:1599–1600.
31. Mancini JA, Evans JF. Cloning and characterization of the human leukotriene A_4 hydrolase gene. Eur J Biochem 1995; 231:65–71.
32. Jendraschak E, Kaminski WE, Kiefl R, von Schacky C. The human leukotriene A_4 hydrolase gene is expressed in two alternatively spliced mRNA forms. Biochem J 1996; 314:733–737.
33. Pang L, Knox AJ. Effect of interleukin-1 beta, tumour necrosis factor-alpha and interferon-gamma on the induction of cyclo-oxygenase-2 in cultured human airway smooth muscle cells. Br J Pharmacol 1997; 121:579–587.
34. Murakami M, Matsumoto R, Austen KF, Arm JP. Prostaglandin endoperoxide synthase-1 and -2 couple to different transmembrane stimuli to generate prostaglandin D_2 in mouse bone marrow-derived mast cells. J Biol Chem 1994; 269:22269–22275.
35. Reddy ST, Herschman HR. Prostaglandin synthase-1 and prostaglandin synthase-2 are coupled to distinct phospholipases for the generation of prostaglandin D_2 in activated mast cells. J Biol Chem 1997; 272:3231–3237.
36. Kujubu DA, Herschman HR. Dexamethasone inhibits mitogen induction of the TIS 10 prostaglandin synthase/cyclooxygenase gene. J Biol Chem 1992; 267:7991–7994.
37. Reddy ST, Gilbert RS, Xie W, Luner S, Herschman HR. TGF-β 1 inhibits both endotoxin-induced prostaglandin synthesis and expression of the TIS 10/prostaglandin synthase 2 gene in murine macrophages. J Leukoc Biol 1994; 55:192–200.
38. Brock TG, McNish RW, Peters–Golden M. Arachidonic acid is preferentially metabolized by cyclooxygenase-2 to prostacyclin and prostaglandin E_2. J Biol Chem 1999; 274:11660–11666.
39. Endo T, Ogushi F, Kawano T, Sone S. Comparison of the regulations by Th2-type cytokines of the arachidonic-acid metabolic pathway in human alveolar macrophages and monocytes. Am J Respir Cell Mol Biol 1998; 19:300–307.
40. Kirtikara K, Morham SG, Raghow R, Laulederkind SJ, Kanekura T, Goorha S, Ballou LR. Compensatory prostaglandin E_2 biosynthesis in cyclooxygenase 1 or 2 null cells. J Exp Med 1998; 187:517–523.
41. Yong EC, Chi EY, Henderson WR Jr. *Toxoplasma gondii* alters eicosanoid release by human mononuclear phagocytes: role of leukotrienes in interferon-γ-induced antitoxoplasma activity. J Exp Med 1994; 180:1637–1648.
42. Yokomizo T, Izumi T, Chang K, Takuwa Y, Shimizu T. A G–protein-coupled receptor for leukotriene B_4 that mediates chemotaxis. Nature 1997; 387:620–624.
43. Chiang N, Gronert K, Clish CB, O'Brien JA, Freeman MW, Serhan CN. Leukotriene B_4

receptor transgenic mice reveal novel protective roles for lipoxins and aspirin-triggered lipoxins in reperfusion. J Clin Invest 1999; 104:309–316.
44. Back M, Jonsson EW, Dahlen SE. The cysteinyl-leukotriene receptor antagonist BAY u9773 is a competitive antagonist of leukotriene C_4 in the guinea-pig ileum. Eur J Pharmacol 1996; 317:107–113.
45. Lynch KR, O'Neill GP, Liu Q, Im DS, Sawyer N, Metters KM, Coulombe N, Abramovitz M, Figueroa DJ, Zeng Z, Connolly BM, Bai C, Austin CP, Chateauneuf A, Stocco R, Greig GM, Kargman S, Hooks SB, Hosfield E, Williams DL Jr, Ford–Hutchinson AW, Caskey CT, Evans JF. Characterization of the human cysteinyl leukotriene $CysLT_1$ receptor. Nature 1999; 399:789–793.
46. Sarau HM, Ames RS, Chambers J, Ellis C, Elshourbagy N, Foley JJ, Schmidt DB, Muccitelli RM, Jenkins O, Murdock PR, Herrity NC, Halsey W, Sathe G, Muir AI, Nuthulaganti P, Dytko GM, Buckley PT, Wilson S, Bergsma DJ, Hay DW. Identification, molecular cloning, expression, and characterization of a cysteinyl leukotriene receptor. Mol Pharmacol 1999; 56:657–663.
47. Nicosia S, Capra V, Accomazzo MR, Galbiati E, Ragnini D, Saponara R, Novarini S, Rovati GE. Receptors and second messengers for Cys-leukotrienes. In: Folco GC, Samuelsson B, Maclouf JA, Velo GP, eds. Eicosanoids: From Biotechnology to Therapeutic Applications. New York: Plenum, 1996:127–136.
48. Coleman RA. Prostanoid receptors. Classification, characterisation and therapeutic relevance. In: Folco GC, Samuelsson B, Maclouf J, Velo GP, eds. Eicosanoids: From Biotechnology to Therapeutic Applications. New York: Plenum, 1996:137–154.
49. Bastien L, Sawyer N, Grygorczyk R, Metters KM, Adam M. Cloning, functional expression, and characterization of the human prostaglandin E_2 receptor EP2 subtype. J Biol Chem 1994; 269:11873–11877.
50. Choung J, Taylor L, Thomas K, Zhou X, Kagan H, Yang X, Polgar P. Role of EP2 receptors and cAMP in prostaglandin E_2 regulated expression of type I collagen alpha1, lysyl oxidase, and cyclooxygenase-1 genes in human embryo lung fibroblasts. J Cell Biochem 1998; 71: 254–263.
51. Bito H, Shimizu T. Molecular characterization and physiological functions of PAF receptors. Adv Exp Med Biol 1997; 400A:215–221.
52. Shirasaki H, Nishikawa M, Adcock IM, Mak JC, Sakamoto T, Shimizu T, Barnes PJ. Expression of platelet-activating factor receptor mRNA in human and guinea pig lung. Am J Respir Cell Mol Biol 1994; 10:533–537.
53. Rola–Pleszczynski M, Stañková J. Leukotriene B_4 enhances interleukin-6 (IL-6) production and IL-6 messenger RNA accumulation in human monocytes in vitro: transcriptional and posttranscriptional mechanisms. Blood 1992; 80:1004–1011.
54. Larivée P, Levine SJ, Rieves RD, Shelhamer JH. Airway inflammation and mucous hypersecretion. In: Takishima T, Shimura S, eds. Airway Secretion. Physiological Bases for the Control of Mucous Hypersecretion. New York: Marcel Dekker, 1994:469–511.
55. Wenzel SE, Larsen GL, Johnston K, Voelkel NF, Westcott JY. Elevated levels of leukotriene C_4 in bronchoalveolar lavage fluid from atopic asthmatics after endobronchial allergen challenge. Am Rev Respir Dis 1990; 142:112–119.
56. Wenzel SE, Westcott JY, Larsen GL. Bronchoalveolar lavage fluid mediator levels 5 minutes after allergen challenge in atopic subjects with asthma: relationship to the development of late asthmatic responses. J Allergy Clin Immunol 1991; 87:540–548.
57. Wenzel SE, Szefler SJ, Leung DYM, Sloan SI, Rex MD, Martin RJ. Bronchoscopic evaluation of severe asthma. Persistent inflammation associated with high dose glucocorticoids. Am J Respir Crit Care Med 1997; 156:737–743.
58. Manning PJ, Watson RM, Margolskee DJ, Williams VC, Schwartz JI, O'Byrne PM. Inhibition of exercise-induced bronchoconstriction by MK-571, a potent leukotriene D_4-receptor antagonist. N Engl J Med 1990; 323:1736–1739.

59. Israel E, Dermarkarian R, Rosenberg M, Sperling R, Taylor G, Rubin P, Drazen JM. The effects of a 5-lipoxygenase inhibitor on asthma induced by cold, dry air. N Engl J Med 1990; 323:1740–1744.
60. Henderson WR Jr, Lewis DB, Albert RK, Zhang Y, Lamm WJE, Chiang GKS, Jones F, Eriksen P, Tien Y, Jonas M, Chi EY. The importance of leukotrienes in airway inflammation in a mouse model of asthma. J Exp Med 1996; 184:1483–1494.
61. Zhang Y, Lamm WJE, Albert RK, Chi EY, Henderson WR Jr, Lewis DB. Influence of the route of allergen administration and genetic background on the murine allergic pulmonary response. Am J Respir Crit Care Med 1997; 155:661–669.
62. Henderson WR Jr, Chi EY, Albert RK, Chu S–J, Lamm WJE, Rochon Y, Christie PE, Harlan JM. Blockade of CD49d (α_4 integrin) on intrapulmonary but not circulating leukocytes inhibits airway inflammation and hyperresposiveness in a mouse model of asthma. J Clin Invest 1997; 100:3083–3092.
63. Chu S–J, Tang LO, Chi EY, Henderson WR Jr. In situ amplification of 5-lipoxygenase and 5-lipoxygenase-activating protein in allergic airway inflammation and inhibition by leukotriene blockade. J Immunol 2000; 165:4640–4648.
64. Chen X–S, Sheller JR, Johnson EN, Funk CD. Role of leukotrienes revealed by targeted disruption of the 5-lipoxygenase gene. Nature 1994; 372:179–182.
65. Goulet JL, Snouwaert JN, Latour AM, Coffman TM, Koller BH. Altered inflammatory responses in leukotriene-deficient mice. Proc Natl Acad Sci USA 1994; 91:12852–12856.
66. Irvin CG, Tu YP, Sheller JR, Funk CD. 5-Lipoxygenase products are necessary for ovalbumin-induced airway responsiveness in mice. Am J Physiol 1997; 272:L1053–L1058.
67. Ihaku D, Cameron L, Suzuki M, Molet S, Martin J, Hamid Q. Montelukast, a leukotriene receptor antagonist, inhibits the late airway response to antigen, airway eosinophilia, and IL-5-expressing cells in Brown Norway rats. J Allergy Clin Immunol 1999; 104:1147–1154.
68. Cifone MG, Cironi L, Santoni A, Testi R. Diacylglycerol lipase activation and 5-lipoxygenase activation and translocation following TCR/CD3 triggering in T cells. Eur J Immunol 1995; 25:1080–1086.
69. Los M, Schenk H, Hexel K, Baeuerle PA, Droge W, Schulze–Osthoff K. IL-2 gene expression and NF-kappa B activation through CD28 requires reactive oxygen production by 5-lipoxygenase. EMBO J 1995; 14:3731–3740.
70. Pablos JL, Santiago B, Carreira PE, Galindo M, Gomez–Reino JJ. Cyclooxygenase-1 and -2 are expressed by human T cells. Clin Exp Immunol 1999; 115:86–90.
71. Langenbach R, Morham SG, Tiano HF, Loftin CD, Ghanayem BI, Chulada PC, Mahler JF, Lee CA, Goulding EH, Kluckman KD, Kim HS, Smithies O. Prostaglandin synthase 1 gene disruption in mice reduces arachidonic acid-induced inflammation and indomethacin-induced gastric ulceration. Cell 1995; 83:483–492.
72. Morham SG, Langenbach R, Loftin CD, Tiano HF, Vouloumanos N, Jennette JC, Mahler JF, Kluckman KD, Ledford A, Lee CA, Smithies O. Prostaglandin synthase 2 gene disruption causes severe renal pathology in the mouse. Cell 1995; 83:473–482.
73. Dinchuk JE, Car BD, Focht RJ, Johnston JJ, Jeffee BD, Covington MB, Contel NR, Eng VM, Collins RJ, Czerniak PM, Gorry SA, Trzaskos JM. Renal abnormalities and an altered inflammatory response in mice lacking cyclooxygenase II. Nature 1995; 378:406–409.
74. Gavett SH, Madison SL, Chulada PC, Scarborough PE, Qu W, Boyle JE, Tiano HF, Lee CA, Langenback R, Roggli VL, Zeldin DC. Allergic lung responses are increased in prostaglandin H synthase-deficient mice. J Clin Invest 1999; 104:721–732.
75. Nagase T, Ishii S, Katayama H, Fukuchi Y, Ouchi Y, Shimizu T. Airway responsiveness in transgenic mice overexpressing platelet-activating factor receptor. Roles of thromboxanes and leukotrienes. Am J Respir Crit Care Med 1997; 156:1621–1627.
76. Henocq E, Vargaftig BB. Skin eosinophilia in atopic patients. J Allergy Clin Immunol 1988; 81:691–695.
77. Miwa M, Miyake T, Yamanaka T, Sugatani J, Suzuki Y, Sakata S, Araki Y, Matsumoto

M. Characterization of serum platelet-activating factor (PAF) acetylhydrolase. Correlation between deficiency of serum PAF acetylhydrolase and respiratory symptoms in asthmatic children. J Clin Invest 1988; 82:1983–1991.

78. Stafforini DM, Satoh K, Atkinson DL, Tjoelker LW, Eberhardt C, Yoshida H, Imaizumi T, Takamatsu S, Zimmerman GA, McIntyre TM, Gray PW, Prescott SM. Platelet-activating factor acetylhydrolase deficiency. A missense mutation near the active site of an anti-inflammatory phospholipase. J Clin Invest 1996; 97:2784–2791.
79. Stafforini DM, Numao T, Tsodikov A, Vaitkus D, Fukuda T, Watanabe N, Fueki N, McIntyre TM, Zimmerman GA, Makino S, Prescott SM. Deficiency of platelet-activating factor acetylhydrolase is a severity factor for asthma. J Clin Invest 1999; 103:989–997.
80. Satoh N, Asano K, Naoki K, Fukunaga K, Iwata M, Kanazawa M, Yamaguchi K. Plasma platelet-activating factor acetylhydrolase deficiency in Japanese patients with asthma. Am J Respir Crit Care Med 1999; 159:974–979.
81. Henderson WR Jr, Lu J, Poole KM, Dietsch GN, Chi EY. Recombinant human platelet-activating factor-acetylhydrolase inhibits airway inflammation and hyperreactivity in mouse asthma model. J Immunol 2000; 164:3360–3367.
82. Henig NR, Aiken ML, Liu MC, Yu AS, Henderson WR Jr. Effect of recombinant human platelet-activating factor-acetylhydrolase on allergen-induced asthmatic responses. Am J Respir Crit Care Med 2000; 162:523–527.
83. Hozawa S, Haruta Y, Ishioka S, Yamakido M. Effects of a PAF antagonist, Y-24180, on bronchial hyperresponsiveness in patients with asthma. Am J Respir Crit Care Med 1995; 152:1198–1202.
84. Evans DJ, Barnes PJ, Cluzel M, O'Connor BJ. Effects of a potent platelet-activating factor antagonist, SR27417A, on allergen-induced asthmatic responses. Am J Respir Crit Care Med 1997; 156:11–16.
85. Freitag A, Watson RM, Matsos G, Eastwood C, O'Byrne PM. Effect of a platelet-activating factor antagonist, WEB 2086, on allergen induced asthmatic responses. Thorax 1993; 48: 594–598.
86. Kuitert LM, Hui KP, Uthayarkumar S, Burke W, Newland AC, Uden S, Barnes NC. Effect of the platelet-activating factor antagonist UK-74,505 on the early and late response to allergen. Am Rev Respir Dis 1993; 147:82–86.
87. Kuitert LM, Angus RM, Barnes NC, Barnes PJ, Bone MF, Chung KF, Fairfax AJ, Higenbotham TW, O'Connor BJ, Piotrowska B. Effect of a novel potent platelet-activating factor antagonist, modipafant, in clinical asthma. Am J Respir Crit Care Med 1995; 151:1331–1335.
88. Spence DPS, Johnston SL, Calverley PMA, Dhillon P, Higgins C, Ramhamadany E, Turner S, Winning A, Winter J, Holgate ST. The effect of the orally active platelet-activating factor antagonist WEB 2086 in the treatment of asthma. Am J Respir Crit Care Med 1994; 149: 1142–1148.
89. Henderson WR Jr. New modalities for the pharmacotherapy of asthma: leukotriene inhibitors and antagonists. Immunol Allergy Clin North Am 1996; 16:797–808.
90. Henig NR, Henderson WR Jr. Anti-leukotriene agents in the treatment of asthma. In: Kaliner MA, ed. Current Review of Allergic Diseases. Philadelphia: Current Medicine, Blackwell Science, 1999:67–78.
91. Tohda Y, Nakahara H, Kubo H, Haraguchi R, Fukuoka M, Nakajima S. Effects of ONO-1078 (pranlukast) on cytokine production in peripheral blood mononuclear cells of patients with bronchial asthma. Clin Exp Allergy 1999; 29:1532–1536.
92. Pizzichini E, Leff JA, Reiss TF, Hendeles L, Boulet LP, Wei LX, Efthimiadis AE, Zhang J, Hargreave FE. Montelukast reduces airway eosinophilic inflammation in asthma: a randomized, controlled trial. Eur Respir J 1999; 14:12–18.
93. Volovitz B, Tabachnik E, Nussinovitch M, Shtaif B, Blau H, Gil-Ad I, Weizman A, Varsano I. Montelukast, a leukotriene receptor antagonist, reduces the concentration of leukotrienes

in the respiratory tract of children with persistent asthma. J Allergy Clin Immunol 1999; 104:1162–1167.

94. Calhoun WJ, Lavins BJ, Minkwitz MC, Evans R, Gleich GJ, Cohn J. Effect of zafirlukast (Accolate) on cellular mediators of inflammation: bronchoalveolar lavage fluid findings after segmental antigen challenge. Am J Respir Crit Care Med 1998; 157:1381–1389.
95. Calhoun WJ, Williams KL, Simonson SG, Lavins BJ. Effect of zafirlukast (Accolate) on airway inflammation after segmental allergen challenge in patients with mild asthma [abstr]. Am J Respir Crit Care Med 1997; 155:A662.
96. Nakamura Y, Hoshino M, Sim JJ, Ishii K, Hosaka K, Sakamoto T. Effect of the leukotriene receptor antagonist pranlukast on cellular infiltration in the bronchial mucosa of patients with asthma. Thorax 1998; 53:835–841.
97. Virchow JC, Hassall SM, Summerton L, Harris A. Improved asthma control over 6 weeks with Accolate (zafirlukast) in patients on high-dose inhaled corticosteroids [abstr]. J Invest Med 1997; 45:286A.
98. Laviolette M, Malmstrom K, Lu S, Chervinsky P, Pujet JC, Peszek I, Zhang J, Reiss TF. Montelukast added to inhaled beclomethasone in treatment of asthma. Am J Respir Crit Care Med 1999; 160:1862–1868.
99. Dworski R, Fitzgerald GA, Oates JA, Sheller JR. Effect of oral prednisone on airway inflammatory mediators in atopic asthma. Am J Respir Crit Care Med 1994; 149:953–959.
100. O'Shaughnessy KM, Wellings R, Gillies B, Fuller RW. Differential effects of fluticasone propionate on allergen-evoked bronchoconstriction and increased urinary leukotriene E_4 excretion. Am Rev Respir Dis 1993; 147:1472–1476.
101. Gomez FP, Roca J, Barbera JA, Chung KF, Peinado VI, Rodriguez–Roisin R. Effect of a platelet-activating factor (PAF) antagonist, SR 27417A, on PAF-induced gas exchange abnormalities in mild asthma. Eur Respir J 1998; 11:835–839.
102. Gomez FP, Marrades RM, Iglesia R, Roca J, Barbera JA, Chung KF, Rodriguez–Roisin RM. Gas exchange response to a PAF receptor antagonist, SR 27417A, in acute asthma: a pilot study. Eur Respir J 1999; 14:622–626.
103. Liu MC, Bleeker R, Lichtenstein LM, et al. Evidence for elevated histamine prostaglandin D_2 and other bronchoconstricting prostaglandins in the airway of subjects with mild asthma. Am Rev Respir Dis 1990; 142:126–132.
104. Chavis C, Van Vyve T, Chanez P, Farce M, Bousquet J, Michel FB, Godard P. Leukotriene E_4 plasma levels in adult asthmatic patients with variable disease severity. Allergy 1997; 52: 589–592.
105. Pavord ID, Ward R, Woltmann G, Wardlaw AJ, Sheller JR, Dworski R. Induced sputum eicosanoid concentrations in asthma. Am J Respir Crit Care Med 1999; 160:1905–1909.
106. Evans DJ, Barnes PJ, Spaethe SM, van Alstyne EL, Mitchell MI, O'Connor BJ. Effect of a leukotriene B_4 receptor antagonist, LY293111, on allergen induced responses in asthma. Thorax 1996; 51:1178–1184.
107. Sladek K, Dworski R, Fitzgerald GA, Buitkus KL, Block FJ, Marney SR Jr, Sheller JR. Allergen-stimulated release of thromboxane A_2 and leukotriene E_4 in humans. Effect of indomethacin. Am Rev Respir Dis 1990; 141:1441–1445.
108. Chan–Yeung M, Lam S, Chan H, Tse KS, Salari H. The release of platelet-activating factor into plasma during allergen-induced bronchoconstriction. J Allergy Clin Immunol 1991; 87: 667–673.
109. Kikawa Y, Miyanomae T, Inoue Y, Saito M, Nakai A, Shigematsu Y, Hosoi S, Sudo M. Urinary leukotriene E_4 after exercise challenge in children with asthma. J Allergy Clin Immunol 1992; 89:1111–1119.
110. Nagakura T, Obata T, Shichijo K, Matsuda S, Sigimoto H, Yamashita K, Masaki T, Maekawa K. GC/MS analysis of urinary excretion of 9alpha, 11beta-PGF2 in acute and exercise-induced asthma in children. Clin Exp Allergy 1998; 28:181–186.
111. Togias AG, Naclerio RM, Peters SP, Nimmagadda I, Proud D, Kagey–Sobotka A, Adkinson

NF Jr, Norman PS, Lichtenstein LM. Local generation of sulfidopeptide leukotrienes upon nasal provocation with cold, dry air. Am Rev Respir Dis 1986; 133:1133–1137.

112. O'Sullivan S, Dahlen B, Dahlen SE, Kumlin M. Increased urinary excretion of the prostaglandin D_2 metabolite 9 alpha, 11 beta-prostaglandin F_2 after aspirin challenge supports mast cell activation in aspirin-induced airway obstruction. J Allergy Clin Immunol 1996; 98:421–432.
113. Wenzel SE, Trudeau JB, Kaminsky DA, Cohn J, Martin RJ, Westcott JY. Effect of 5-lipoxygenase inhibition on bronchoconstriction and airway inflammation in nocturnal asthma. Am J Respir Crit Care Med 1995; 152:897–905.
114. Konstan MW, Walenga RW, Hilliard KA, Hilliard JB. Leukotriene B_4 is markedly elevated in epithelial lining fluid of patients with cystic fibrosis. Am Rev Respir Dis 1993; 48:896–901.
115. Greally P, Hussein MJ, Cook AJ, Sampson AP, Piper PJ, Price JF. Sputum tumour necrosis factor-alpha and leukotriene concentrations in cystic fibrosis. Arch Dis Child 1993; 68:389–392.
116. Greally P, Cook AJ, Sampson AP, Coleman R, Chambers S, Piper PJ, Price JF. Atopic children with cystic fibrosis have increased urinary leukotriene E_4 concentrations and more severe pulmonary disease. J Allergy Clin Immunol 1994; 93:100–107.
117. Strandvik B, Svensson E, Seyberth HW. Prostanoid biosynthesis in patients with cystic fibrosis. Prostaglandins Leukot Essent Fatty Acids 1996; 55:419–425.
118. Nakos G, Kitsiouli EI, Tsangaris I, Lekka ME. Bronchoalveolar lavage fluid characteristics of early intermediate and late phases of ARDS. Alterations in leukocytes, proteins, PAF and surfactant components. Intensive Care Med 1998; 24:296–303.
119. Stephenson AH, Lonigro AJ, Hyers TM, Webster RO, Fowler AA. Increased concentrations of leukotrienes in bronchoalveolar lavage fluid of patients with ARDS or at risk for ARDS. Am Rev Respir Dis 1988; 138:714–719.
120. Antonelli M, Bufi M, De Blasi RA, Crimi G, Conti G, Mattia C, Vivino G, Lenti L, Lombardi D, Dotta A, Pontieri G, Gasparetto A. Detection of leukotrienes B_4, C_4 and of their isomers in arterial, mixed venous blood and bronchoalveolar lavage fluid from ARDS patients. Intensive Care Med 1989; 15:296–301.
121. Wilborn J, Bailie M, Coffey M, Burdick M, Strieter R, Peters–Golden M. Constitutive activation of 5-lipoxygenase in the lungs of patients with idiopathic pulmonary fibrosis. J Clin Invest 1996; 97:1827–1836.
122. Georgitis JW, Matthews BL, Stone B. Chronic sinusitis: characterization of cellular influx and inflammatory mediators in sinus lavage fluid. Int Arch Allergy Immunol 1995; 106:416–421.
123. de Graaf-in t Veld C, Garrelds IM, Koenders S, Gerth van Wijk R. Relationship between nasal hyperreactivity, mediators and eosinophils in patients with perennial allergic rhinitis and controls. Clin Exp Allergy 1996; 26:903–908.
124. Koro O, Furutani K, Hide M, Yamada S, Yamamoto S. Chemical mediators in atopic dermatitis: involvement of leukotriene B_4 released by a type I allergic reaction in the pathogenesis of atopic dermatitis. J Allergy Clin Immunol 1999; 103:663–670.
125. Miyoshi M, Sakurai T, Kodama S. Clinical evaluation of urinary leukotriene E_4 levels in children with atopic dermatitis. Arerugi 1999; 48:1148–1152.
126. Fauler J, Neumann C, Tsikas D, Frolich J. Enhanced synthesis of cysteinyl leukotrienes in atopic dermatitis. Br J Dermatol 1993; 128:627–630.
127. Maltby NH, Ind PW, Causon RC, Fuller RW, Taylor GW. Leukotriene E_4 release in cold urticaria. Clin Exp Allergy 1989; 19:33–36.
128. Fauler J, Neumann C, Tsikas D, Frolich J. Enhanced synthesis of cysteinyl leukotrienes in psoriasis. J Invest Dermatol 1992; 99:8–11.
129. Izaki S, Yamamoto T, Goto Y, Ishimaru S, Yudate F, Kitamura K, Matsuzaki M. Platelet-activating factor and arachidonic acid metabolites in psoriatic inflammation. Br J Dermatol 1996; 134:1060–1064.

130. Denzlinger C, Haberl C, Wilmanns W. Cysteinyl leukotriene production in anaphylactic reactions. Int Arch Allergy Immunol 1995; 108:158–164.
131. Irkec MT, Orhan M, Erdener U. Role of tear inflammatory mediators in contact lens-associated giant papillary conjunctivitis in soft contact lens wearers. Ocul Immunol Inflamm 1999; 7:35–38.
132. Nathan H, Naveh N, Meyer E. Levels of prostaglandin E_2 and leukotriene B_4 in tears of vernal conjunctivitis patients during a therapeutic trial with indomethacin. Doc Ophthalmol 1994; 85:247–257.
133. Proud D, Sweet J, Stein P, Settipane RA, Kagey–Sobotka A, Friedlaender MH, Lichtenstein LM. Inflammatory mediator release on conjunctival provocation of allergic subjects with allergen. J Allergy Clin Immunol 1990; 85:896–905.
134. Mayatepek E, Lehmann WD. Increased generation of cysteinyl leukotrienes in Kawasaki disease. Arch Dis Child 1995; 72:526–527.
135. Buyan N, Hasanoglu E, Oguz A, Ercan S. The role of plasma arachidonic acid metabolites in the pathogenesis and the prognosis of Henoch–Schonlein purpura. Prostaglandins Leukot Essent Fatty Acids 1994; 50:353–356.
136. Tonshoff B, Momper R, Schweer H, Scharer K, Seyberth HW. Increased biosynthesis of vasoactive prostanoids in Schonlein–Henoch purpura. Pediatr Res 1992; 32:137–140.
137. Gurer MA, Keskin N, Gulekon A, Karel L, Aksakal B, Baysal V. Arachidonic acid metabolites and colchicine in Behcet's disease (BD). Prostaglandins Leukot Essent Fatty Acids 1991; 43:257–259.
138. Grignani G, Zucchella M, Belai BN, Brocchieri A, Saporiti A, Cherie Ligniere EL. Levels of different metabolites of arachidonic acid in synovial fluid of patients with arthrosis or rheumatoid arthritis. Minerva Med 1996; 87:75–79.
139. Hishinuma T, Nakamura H, Sawai T, Uzuki M, Itabash Y, Mizugaki M. Microdetermination of prostaglandin E_2 in joint fluid in rheumatoid arthritis patients using gas chromatography/selected ion monitoring. Prostaglandins Other Lipid Mediat 1999; 58:179–186.
140. Gursel T, Firat S, Ercan ZS. Increased serum leukotriene B_4 level in the active stage of rheumatoid arthritis in children. Prostaglandins Leukot Essent Fatty Acids 1997; 56:205–207.
141. Guimbaud R, Izzo A, Martinolle JP, Vidon N, Couturier D, Benveniste J, Chaussade S. Intraluminal excretion of PAF, lysoPAF, and acetylhydrolase in patients with ulcerative colitis. Dig Dis Sci 1995; 40:2635–2640.
142. Hommes DW, Meenan J, de Haas M, ten Kate FJ, von dem Borne AE, Tytgat GN, van Deventer SJ. Soluble Fc gamma receptor III (CD 16) and eicosanoid concentrations in gut lavage fluid from patients with inflammatory bowel disease: reflection of mucosal inflammation. Gut 1996; 38:564–567.
143. Wiercinska–Drapalo A, Flisiak R, Prokopowicz D. Mucosal and plasma prostaglandin E_2 in ulcerative colitis. Hepatogastroenterology 1999; 46:2338–2342.
144. Laursen LS, Naesdal J, Bukhave K, Lauritsen K, Rask–Madsen J. Selective 5-lipoxygenase inhibition in ulcerative colitis. Lancet 1990; 335:683–685.
145. Sobhani I, Hochlaf S, Denizot Y, Vissuzaine C, Rene E, Benveniste J, Lewin MM, Mignon M. Raised concentrations of platelet activating factor in colonic mucosa of Crohn's disease patients. Gut 1992; 33:1220–1225.
146. Schmidt C, Baumeister B, Kipnowski J, Schiermeyer–Dunkhase B, Vetter H. Alteration of prostaglandin E_2 and leukotriene B_4 synthesis in chronic inflammatory bowel disease. Hepatogastroenterology 1996; 43:1508–1512.
147. Kim JH, Tagari P, Griffiths AM, Ford–Hutchinson A, Smith C, Sherman PM. Levels of peptidoleukotriene E_4 are elevated in active Crohn's disease. J Pediatr Gastroenterol Nutr 1995; 20:403–407.
148. Chilton FH, Fonteh AN, Surette ME, Triggiani M, Winkler JD. Control of arachidonate levels within inflammatory cells. Biochim Biophys Acta 1996; 1299:1–15.

11

Cytokines in Allergic Inflammation

RAFEUL ALAM

University of Texas Medical Branch, Galveston, Texas

GITA KAMPEN

National University Hospital, Copenhagen, Denmark

1 INTRODUCTION

Inflammation is an immune response that is designed to eliminate offending foreign antigens and microbes through the recruitment of effector cells. One of the important mechanisms of this immune response is the elaboration of cytokines and chemokines. Once secreted, cytokines recruit additional inflammatory cells and, thereby, augment the immune response. The recruitment of inflammatory cells is a complex process that involves the interaction of tissue cells with leukocytes, draining lymph nodes, and bone marrow.

2 CYTOKINES REGULATING Th2-TYPE IMMUNE RESPONSES

Allergen-specific $CD4^+$ T cells from allergic patients fall predominantly within the T-helper cell type 2 (Th2) subset (1,2). These cells are functionally defined and distinguished from other Th cells (i.e., Th0, Th1, and Th3) by the panel of cytokines they secrete on stimulation (3–7). Archetypical, or fully polarized, Th2 cells secrete interleukin (IL)-4, IL-5, IL-6, IL-10, and IL-13, but no or very little interferon (IFN)-γ. In contrast, fully polarized Th1 cells secrete IL-2 and IFN-γ (1,2,8–10).

The Th2 cytokines participate in regulation of several key features of allergic inflammation. Thus, IL-4 and IL-13, which share the signal-transducing receptor subunit IL-4Rα, and promote B-cell isotype-switch and IgE production (11,12). IL-4 further induces Th2 differentiation (13), whereas IL-13 (and only to a much lesser extent IL-4) has been reported to stimulate the production of the CC chemokine eotaxin in human airways

(14). Consequently, IL-13 may be important in the orchestration of the recruitment of eosinophils to relevant tissue sites.

Interleukin-5 also plays a pivotal role in the allergic inflammation. As discussed in the next sections, it is an important stimulator of eosinophil proliferation, differentiation (15), function (16,17), and survival (18), and along with IL-4 and IL-6, it further modulates mast cell differentiation and function (19).

In a murine model, IL-6 initiates Th2 polarization by a mechanism that may involve induction of IL-4 gene transcription (20). Furthermore, IL-6 could serve as a cofactor for B-cell IgE production, because IL-6 antisense oligonucleotides inhibit IgE-production from IL-4/CD40 antibody-stimulated human tonsillar B cells (21).

In humans, IL-10 is expressed by both Th1 and Th2 cells (22). In contrast to IL-4, -5, -6, and -13, IL-10 has broad inhibitory effects on Th2-type immune responses; moreover, it inhibits several aspects of Th1-type reactions (22,23).

Interleukin-4 and IL-6 act not only as Th2 effector molecules, but also induce Th2 polarization. Furthermore, IL-4 is involved in a cross-regulatory network of cytokines regulating the polarization of Th cells. Other key players in this network comprise IL-12, which is thought to be the principal cytokine inducing Th1 polarization, and the archetypical Th1 cytokine IFN-γ. In general, the Th1-type cytokines inhibit Th2-dominated immune responses, and vice versa (24–29). However, IL-4 also primes for IL-12 production from human peripheral blood mononuclear cells (PBMCs) (29), indicating the probable complexity of the cross-regulation between Th1- and Th2-type cytokines.

3 CYTOKINES CONTROLLING DIFFERENTIATION AND MATURATION OF EFFECTOR CELLS

The major effector-cells of the allergic inflammation, namely mast cells, eosinophils, and basophils, originate from bone marrow stem cells. However, circulating progenitors of all three cell types have been demonstrated in both human and murine systems. The progenitors are dependent on cytokines for proliferation and differentiation into mature effector cells (30–33).

3.1 Cytokines Involved in Differentiation and Maturation of Mast Cells

The circulating committed mast cell progenitor is a mononuclear, agranular, $Fc_{\varepsilon}RI$- and $CD34^+$ cell. The progenitor is believed to extravasate into relevant tissue sites and to undergo terminal differentiation and maturation in situ under the influence of locally secreted cytokines (33).

Stem cell factor (SCF), a cytokine released constitutively by stromal cells, appears crucial in the differentiation of mast cells. SCF induces chemotaxis, proliferation, and differentiation of mast cell progenitors. However, this cytokine alone is insufficient to induce full mast cell maturation (34–36).

Interestingly, several Th2-type cytokines appear to support and extend SCF-driven mast cell proliferation and differentiation. Thus, IL-5, IL-6, and to a lesser extent IL-4 increase the proliferation of immature human mast cells stimulated with SCF. In more mature cells, IL-4 lost this effect (37,38). In other systems, IL-4 and IL-6 inhibit mast cell proliferation, induce down-regulation of the SCF receptor, c-*kit*, and increase chymase and FcεRI expression, histamine content, and mast cell maturation (39–41), indicating that IL-4 and IL-6 may also support the differentiation of mast cells.

In transgenic mice that overexpress IL-9, IL-9 acts synergistically with SCF in inducing mast cell proliferation. However, the resultant mast cells did not appear fully differentiated, indicating that factors other than SCF and IL-9 are necessary for the normal development of mature mast cells (42). The comitogenic effect of IL-9 has been confirmed in a model based on human mast cells (38).

In the murine model, IL-3 stimulates mast cell development (43,44). In agreement with the mouse data, some groups have reported that IL-3 on its own, or in synergy with SCF, induces the proliferation of human mast cells (33,38). However, other investigators have found that IL-3 supports the development of only a small fraction of mast cells (32,45), or actually, in the longer run, suppresses mast cell development and survival (45,46). Thus, the effect of IL-3 on human mast cell development remains somewhat unclear, and it may be that IL-3 in humans is primarily a basophil–eosinophil differentiation factor (discussed in the following section).

3.2 Cytokines Involved in Differentiation and Maturation of Eosinophils and Basophils

Eosinophils and basophils are thought to differentiate from a common progenitor cell, which is believed to be distinct from the mast cell progenitor (47,48). However, circulating cells with a mast cell–basophil hybrid phenotype have been detected in the peripheral blood of patients with chronic myeloid leukemia (49) or allergy (50). This could indicate the existence of an alternative pathway of basophil differentiation.

The common eosinophil–basophil progenitor has been detected in human bone marrow (51) and peripheral blood (47). The bone marrow is the most important site of normal eosinophil–basophil differentiation (52). In allergic patients, however, increased numbers of committed eosinophil–basophil progenitors can be detected in the peripheral blood, and it is conceivable that these progenitors migrate into tissue sites of allergic inflammation and develop into mature effector cells under the influence of locally produced cytokines (53).

Interleukin-3, IL-5, and granulocyte–macrophage colony-stimulating factor (GM-CSF) are the major cytokines determining the differentiation of eosinophils and basophils. GM-CSF stimulates the proliferation of not only the eosinophil–basophil lineage, but also of neutrophil and monocyte progenitors (54,55). IL-3 is essential for the growth and proliferation of multiple hematopoietic lineages (51,55,56). It induces the formation and differentiation of colonies containing both eosinophils and basophils (51,57,58). In contrast to GM-CSF and IL-3, IL-5 is a more selective stimulator of the eosinophil–basophil progenitor (56,59). In mice, IL-5 induces the proliferation and terminal differentiation of eosinophils (60). Likewise, IL-5 stimulates selective proliferation and differentiation of eosinophils and basophils in humans (58,60,61), but appears to preferentially support the development of eosinophils (51). However, the exact mechanism of eosinophil differentiation from lineage-committed precursor cells is poorly understood. Existing evidence suggests that the commitment of stem cells to various lineages is stochastic (i.e., independent of known growth factors) (64). Once the committed cells begin to express IL-5 receptor ($CD34^+$, IL-5Rα^+), the differentiation process is driven by IL-5. This is demonstrated by the presence of low levels of eosinophils in IL-5 knockout mice, which are unable to increase eosinophil differentiation in response to allergic or other inflammatory stimuli (65). Although GM-CSF can stimulate eosinophil differentiation in vitro, it does so by stimulating IL-5 production from committed cells. IL-5 then acts as an autocrine obligatory growth factor (66).

Cytokines other than IL-3, IL-5, and GM-CSF may also be involved in the differentiation of eosinophils and basophils. Transforming growth factor (TGF)-β has been reported to enhance IL-3-driven generation of basophils, while suppressing the generation of eosinophils; accordingly, it may be involved in the differential regulation of these cell types (62). IL-12 and IFN-γ also suppress eosinophil differentiation. However, it is unclear whether this effect is direct or is mediated by their inhibitory effect on Th2 cytokine (e.g., IL-5) production. IL-9 transgenic mice show significant eosinophilia (63). Whether IL-9 has a direct effect on eosinophil differentiation from stem cells is unknown. IL-9 induces CC chemokine production by epithelial cells, which could explain the influx of eosinophils into the airways of the IL-9 transgenic animals.

The eosinophil is a terminally differentiated cell and undergoes apoptosis after a few days in the tissue. However, eosinophil apoptosis is delayed significantly by the growth factors IL-3, IL-5, and GM-CSF (67). IL-13 also promotes eosinophil survival (68). IFN-γ has variable effects on eosinophil survival. In short-term culture of eosinophils, IFN-γ enhances eosinophil survival (69), whereas IFN-γ induces apoptosis of differentiating eosinophils on prolonged culture (70). The survival of eosinophils is inhibited by TGF-β (71). Eosinophils are capable of producing both growth-promoting (IL-5, GM-CSF) and growth-inhibitory (e.g., TGF-β) cytokines. There is evidence that neutralization of TGF-β alone can prolong eosinophil survival (71). Thus, eosinophil survival is reciprocally regulated by IL-5/GM-CSF and TGF-β.

4 CYTOKINES AND ADHESION OF INFLAMMATORY CELLS

Adhesion molecules expressed on endothelial cells and their counterreceptors on leukocytes mediate adhesion and homing (72). The initial step of adhesion is rolling and tethering of leukocytes. Selectins play an important role in this step. P-selectin is critical for tethering of eosinophils from the circulation (73). Its transcription is regulated by the transcription factor STAT-6, which is induced by both IL-4 and IL-13 (74). The next step of cellular adhesion is dependent on activation of cells, which is followed by expression and activation of the integrin family of adhesion molecules. The integins—α4β1(VLA-4), α6β1, and α4β7—are expressed on eosinophils, basophils, and lymphocytes, but not on neutrophils (72). The counterreceptor for α4β1 is vascular cellular adhesion molecule (VCAM), which is also the counterreceptor for the β_2-integrin αDβ2 (75). Other β2-integrins (αMβ2, αLβ2) bind to intracellular adhesion molecule (ICAM). Inhibition of these adhesion molecules blocks leukocyte migration and airway inflammation in animal models (73,76). Major cytokines that regulate the expression of adhesion molecules include IL-1, IL-4, IL-13, tumor necrosis factor (TNF)-α, and IFN-γ. All these cytokines up-regulate the expression of ICAM and VCAM on endothelial cells (72). TNF-α, IL-4, and IL-13 are particularly important for up-regulation of VCAM (77,78). For these reasons, IL-4, IL-13, and TNF-α are thought to play a crucial role in allergic inflammation.

Many cytokines increase the expression of adhesion molecules on leukocytes. For example, eosinophil growth factors (e.g., GM-CSF) up-regulate β_2-integrins on eosinophils (79). Chemokines stimulate the expression (80) and avidity of β_2-integrins (81) and, thereby, promote their migration and homing in the tissue. Eotaxin and other CCR3 ligands cause arrest of eosinophils under shear stress (83), and eotaxin has further been shown to be important for homing of eosinophils in the gastrointestinal tract (82).

5 CHEMOTAXIS

Chemokines play a crucial role in the directed migration, or chemotaxis, and homing of lymphocytes to various organs. Lymphocytes express a variety of chemokine receptors based on their activation status (84). Naïve T cells express CXCR4. When activated, T cells additionally express CCR1 and CCR2. The functionally polarized Th1 and Th2 cells have different profiles of chemokine receptor expression. Thus, Th1 cells preferentially express CXCR3 (85) and CCR5 (86), whereas Th2 cells express CCR3 (87) and CCR4 (88). This differential expression of chemokine receptors determines chemotactic response of T cells to chemokines (Figs. 1 and 2).

Peripheral blood eosinophils express the CC chemokine receptor-3 (CCR3) and, to a lesser extent, CCR1 (89). All CCR3 ligands (eotaxin-1,-2,-3, RANTES, MCP-2, -3, and -4) stimulate eosinophil chemotaxis. Interestingly, eosinophils from inflammatory sites express additional chemokine receptors (e.g., CCR2, CCR4, and CCR5) (90), making them susceptible to additional chemokines (e.g., MDC; Fig. 3). C10 is also chemotactic for eosinophils (91); however, the receptor involved in its action is currently unknown. The CC chemokines activate Gi protein, which increases the generation of inositol triphosphates and influx of intracellular calcium (92). Furthermore, the signaling through CCR3 causes the activation of ERK and p38 MAP kinases (93,94), and PI_3 kinase (95). The foregoing signaling molecules play a critical role in eosinophil degranulation and chemotaxis. IL-16 is also a potent eosinophil chemotactic factor (96), but its intracellular signal transduction mechanism is unknown. IL-5 induces eosinophil chemokinesis (97), but is unable to induce chemotaxis.

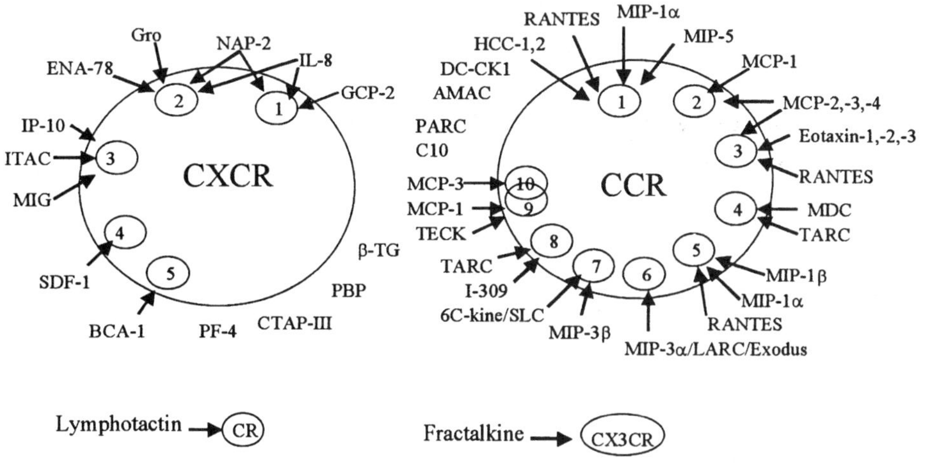

Figure 1 Chemokines and their receptors: CCR9 and CCR10 have identical amino acid sequences.

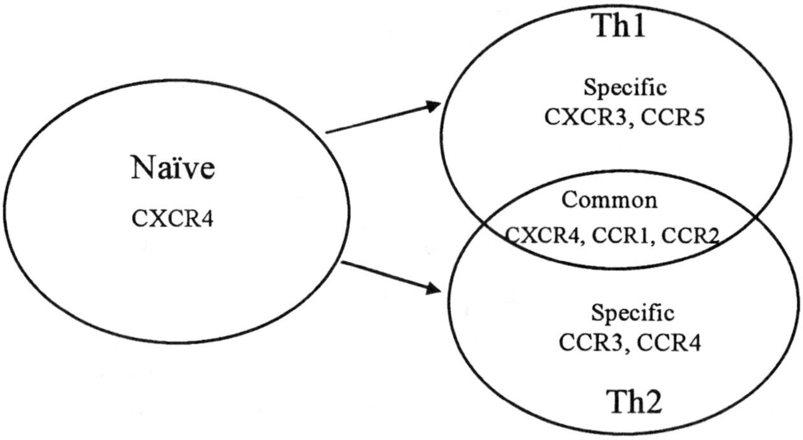

Figure 2 The expression of chemokine receptors on various T-cell populations.

6 ACTIVATION OF EFFECTOR CELLS

6.1 Eosinophils

Interleukin-3, IL-5, and GM-CSF prime eosinophils for multiple functions (67). Primed cells respond to lower concentrations of other stimuli. Exposure to these cytokines make eosinophils hypodense (98). Hypodensity represents a state of generalized activation of cells. Prolonged incubation of eosinophils with IL-3, IL-5, and GM-CSF induces degranulation (99), and thus causes the release of eosinophil cationic protein (ECP), eosinophil-derived neurotoxin (EDN), and other granular proteins, which then exert their toxic effect on airway epithelial cells. CC chemokines (e.g., RANTES and eotaxin) activate eosino-

	Blood Eosinophils			Tissue Eosinophils		
	FCM	Ca2+	Chemotaxis	FCM	Ca2+	Chemotaxis
CCR1	+	+	+	+	+	+
CCR2	-	-	-	+	+	+
CCR3	+	+	+	+	+	+
CCR4	-	-	-	+	+	+
CCR5	-	-	-	+	+	+

Figure 3 Chemokine receptor expression in peripheral blood and tissue-derived eosinophils. FCM indicates flow cytometry.

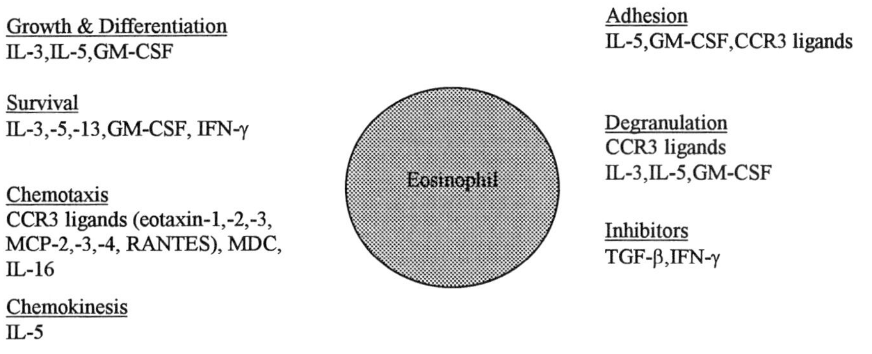

Figure 4 Cytokines regulating eosinophils.

phils and stimulate the release of ECP and EDN (80,94). Cytokines regulating major functions of eosinophils are shown in Figure 4.

6.2 Mast Cells

The activation of mast cells predominantly occurs through cross-linking of IgE receptors. SCF is the only cytokine identified, thus far, that augments IgE-mediated histamine release from mast cells (100). At high concentrations, SCF directly causes mast cell degranulation.

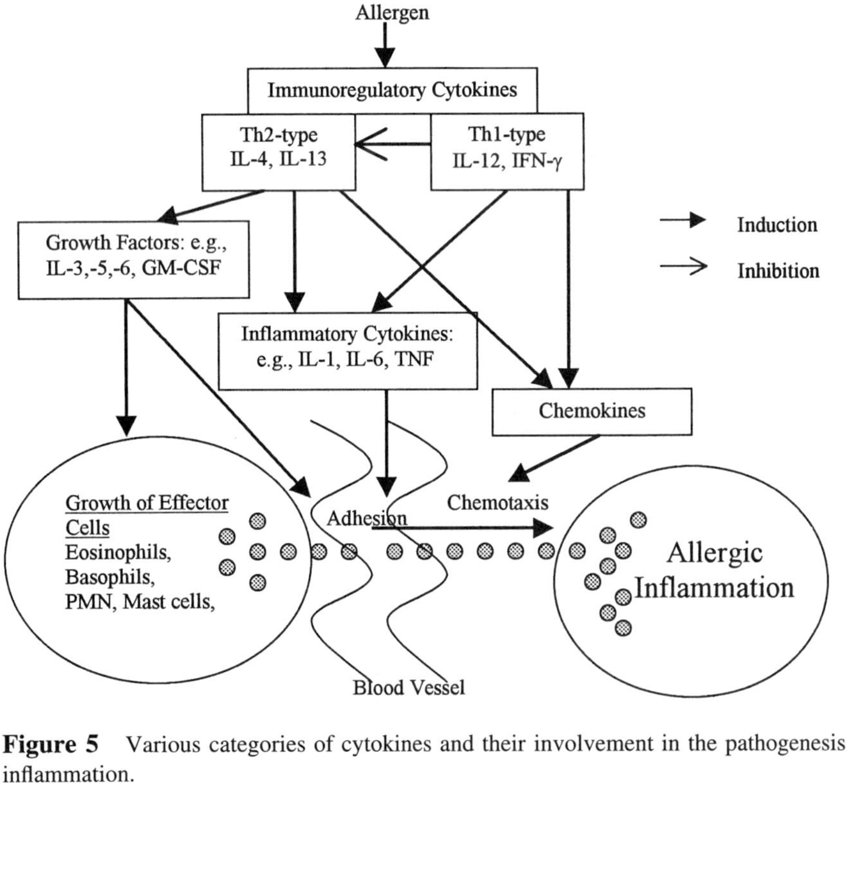

Figure 5 Various categories of cytokines and their involvement in the pathogenesis of allergic inflammation.

6.3 Basophils

Basophils express CCR2 (101), CCR3 (102), and CCR4 (103). The ligands for these receptors activate basophils and induce histamine release. Thus MCP-1 is one of the most potent secretagogues for basophils (104). Basophils also secrete leukotrienes in response to CC chemokines, especially if they are primed with IL-3, IL-5, and GM-CSF (105). In addition, the IgE-dependent histamine-releasing factor induces basophil activation (106).

In summary, cytokines affect the growth, differentiation, migration and activation of allergic inflammatory cells. A schematic presentation of cytokine regulation of inflammation is shown in Figure 5. To simplify the complexity of cytokines, they are divided into four types—immunoregulatory cytokines, growth factors, inflammatory cytokines, and chemokines. Although much attention has been paid to the role of immunoregulatory cytokines, it is becoming increasingly clear that inflammatory cytokines and chemokines play a crucial role in the induction of allergic inflammation. It should also be emphasized that eosinophilic inflammation is characteristic of, but not specific for, a Th2 immune response. CC chemokines are induced by Th1, Th2, and cells of innate immunity (e.g., macrophages). As a consequence, all these cell types can potentially induce an eosinophilic inflammation (Fig. 6). As a proof of concept, a recent study has shown that intracorneal application of IL-12, a Th1-inducer, causes eosinophilic inflammation (107). Similarly, eosinophilia has been reported in severe combined immunodeficiency (108). There is growing evidence that most pathological conditions actually represent a spectrum of all three types of immune responses (Th1, Th2, innate), although one may dominate in a particular environment. Clearly, the Th2 pathway plays a dominant role in the development of eosinophilic inflammation in most pathological conditions.

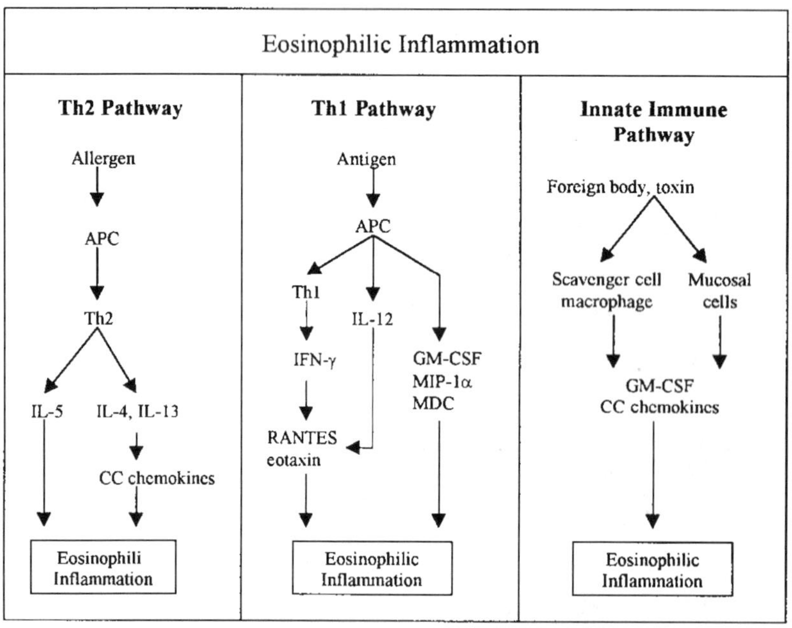

Figure 6 Three possible mechanisms of development of eosinophilic inflammation. The Th2 pathway is the dominant mechanism in most pathological conditions.

7 CYTOKINES AFFECTING EPITHELIAL WOUND HEALING AND REMODELING

Biopsy specimens from the airways of asthmatic patients frequently show significant desquamation and epithelial injury. Eosinophil granular proteins are very toxic to airway epithelial cells. Initially, ECP, EDN, and MBP cause ciliostasis, whereas sustained exposure induces epithelial sloughing. EGF, PDGF, and FGF are growth factors for epithelial cells. The production of EGF is increased in asthma (109), whereas the production of PDGF has been reported to be either increased (110) or normal (111). It is still unclear whether the action of these cytokines leads to significant regeneration of the airway epithelium. In addition to epithelial injury, asthma is characterized by thickening of the basement membrane and increased matrix protein synthesis. IL-4 (112) and TGF-β (113) stimulate fibroblast proliferation and matrix protein synthesis (e.g., collagen and tenascin). The production of these cytokines is increased in allergic inflammation (114), which is likely to contribute to the remodeling of the airway.

8 CYTOKINES AND ALLERGIC RHINITIS

The involvement of cytokines in allergic rhinitis has been studied either at the baseline or after an allergen challenge. Nasal biopsy studies from patients with allergic rhinitis show an increased production of IL-4, IL-5, IL-13, and eotaxin (115–118). An allergen challenge stimulates the synthesis of IL-1β, IL-8, IL-16, TNF-α, GM-CSF, MCP-1, MIP-1α, RANTES, and eotaxin (119–122). Most of the cytokines are recovered 3–7 hr after the allergen challenge, implying their importance in the development of the late-phase allergic reaction. Interestingly, the levels of TNF-α and MIP-1α also increase in the immediate-phase allergic reaction (119). The latter finding perhaps points to the mast cell origin of the cytokines. Natural exposure to allergens in seasonal allergic patients also increases the levels of cytokines. For example, MCP-1 production is upregulated in the ragweed season (123). The treatment of patients with topical glucocorticoids (119,121,122) or immunotherapy (124,125) results in a significant reduction in cytokine production in the nasal mucosa.

9 CYTOKINES AND BRONCHIAL ASTHMA

An increasing number of reports suggest that the levels of IL-1β, -2, -5, -6, -9, -13, and -16; GM-CSF; and TNF-α are elevated in the bronchoalveolar lavage (BAL) fluid from asthmatic patients (126–132). Biopsy studies of airway mucosa confirmed the foregoing findings and showed an increased number of cells expressing these cytokines (134). Furthermore, there was an increased expression of IL-3, IL-4, and IL-10 in airway mucosa (134–136). In situ hybridization and immunocytochemical studies show that T cells are the major source of IL-3, IL-4, and IL-5 in the airway mucosa from asthmatic patients. Resident mast cells and infiltrating eosinophils also produce a significant amount of IL-3, IL-4, IL-5, and other cytokines. An allergen challenge of the airways increases cytokine levels in the lavage fluid (132,133). Interestingly, the number of IL-5–producing T cells in bone marrow also increases following an allergen challenge, which results in accelerated eosinophilopoiesis (137). The result suggests that the bone marrow actively participates in the pathogenesis of allergen-induced inflammatory reactions. Steroid-resistant asthma represents an interesting model of allergic inflammation wherein very high doses of steroids are unable to inhibit the influx of inflammatory cells into the airways. T cells from steroid-resistant asthmatic patients produce exceedingly high quantities of IL-2 and IL-4 (138). In vitro studies suggest that a combination of IL-2 and IL-4 induces steroid resistance of lymphocytes.

In contrast to the foregoing cytokines the expression of IL-12 is not elevated in the airway mucosa from asthmatic patients (139). Interestingly, corticosteroid therapy increases IL-12 expression in asthmatic airways. The expression of IFN-γ in asthma has been a matter of controversy, and there are reports of both unchanged (128) and increased (140,141) expression of IFN-γ in airway cells from asthmatic patients.

The presence of chemokines in the airways from asthmatic patients has been investigated in several studies. The levels of MCP-1, MIP-1α, RANTES, and IL-8 are elevated in the BAL fluid from asthmatic patents as compared with healthy controls (142–145). An allergen challenge increases the concentration of eotaxin and RANTES in the BAL fluid from allergic asthmatic patients. The increased concentration of eotaxin and RANTES correlates with the eosinophil number (143). The eosinophil chemotactic activity of BAL fluid from asthmatic patients has been variably neutralized by antibodies against IL-5, eotaxin, RANTES, and MCP-3 (142,143,145). A higher number of bronchial mucosal cells from asthmatic patients expresses mRNA for eotaxin-1, RANTES, MCP-3, and MCP-4 when compared with those from normal and atopic controls (146–148). Interestingly, the expression of mRNA for these chemokines is higher in bronchial mucosa from nonatopic asthmatics than from atopic asthmatic patients (146). The expression of eotaxin correlates with eosinophil influx into the airways in asthmatic patients (147). An increase in eotaxin, MCP-1, MIP-1α, and IL-8 was also detected in the sputum from patients undergoing a natural exacerbation of asthma (149). The increased production of CC chemokines in asthma is associated with the heightened expression of CCR3 in airways of asthmatic patients (150). This heightened expression was correlated with bronchial hyperreactivity. Although most cells are capable of producing chemokines in vitro, the major source of chemokines in the airway mucosa are epithelium, macrophages, and to a lesser extent T cells. In contrast, vascular endothelium and macrophages predominantly produce chemokines in airway submucosa.

10 CYTOKINES AND ANIMAL MODELS OF ALLERGIC INFLAMMATION

Studies from animal models have provided evidence that cytokines are important in allergic inflammation of the airways. Antibodies against IL-4 (151) and IL-13 (152,153) block IgE antibody and eosinophilic inflammatory responses. Knockout mice for IL-5 are unable to mount an eosinophilic inflammatory response in the airways (154). Moreover, the mice lack airway hyperreactivity following an allergen challenge. Experiments with anti-IL-5 antibodies also produced similar results (155). Transgenic mice for IL-9 show many features of allergic inflammation, including eosinophilic inflammation and hyperplasia of mast cells and goblet cells (156,157). Knockout mice for eotaxin are unable to induce the early-phase of eosinophilic influx in the first 8–24 hr after an allergen challenge (158). However, the later (after 24 hr) influx of eosinophils into the airways was not impaired. The latter observation points to an important role of other CC chemokines in allergic inflammation, and indeed, this has been confirmed by experiments with neutralizing antibodies. In an ovalbumin sensitization model there was a significant increase in the expression of MCP-1, MCP-3, MIP-1α and eotaxin (159). Pretreatment of mice with an anti-

Table 1 Cytokines and Cytokine Receptors and Candidate Asthma Genes

Candidate	Chromosome	Function
IL-3	5q31-33	Growth and proliferation of hematopoietic cells
IL-4	5q31-33	Induction of Th2 response
IL-9	5q31-33	Growth factor for T cells and mast cells
TNF-α	6p21.3-2.3	Inducer of cellular adhesion, inflammatory cell activation
IL-4R_{α}	16p12	Induction of Th2 response
TGF-β_1	19q13.1-13.3	Wound healing, inhibition of specific immune response

MCP-3 antibody significantly abrogated the influx of eosinophils and other inflammatory cells into the airways (159). In a *Schistosoma mansoni* antigen sensitization model, an antibody against MCP-1 inhibited mononuclear cell influx and bronchial hyperreactivity (160). Antibodies against RANTES and MIP-1α blocked eosinophilic influx but did not affect bronchial hyperreactivity indicating a dichotomy between eosinophilic inflammation and bronchial hyperresponsiveness in this model.

The importance of cytokines in the pathogenesis of asthma is underscored by the recent findings that many putative asthma genes are associated with cytokine loci (161). Table 1 shows a list of asthma-associated cytokine genes. Many cytokines are being targeted for therapeutic interventions. There are several options to block cytokine functions in vivo. Examples include receptor antagonists, soluble receptor proteins, humanized neutralizing antibodies, and blockade of specific-signaling molecules. A soluble IL-4 receptor and an anti-IL-5 antibody are currently undergoing clinical trials. The former has significant steroid-sparing effects in patients with asthma (162).

REFERENCES

1. Umetsu DT, Jabara HH, DeKruyff RH, Abbas AK, Abrams JS, Geha RS. Functional heterogeneity among human inducer T cell clones. J Immunol 1988; 140:4211–4216.
2. Wierenga EA, Snoek M, de Groot C, Chretien I, Bos JD, Jansen HM, Kapsenberg ML. Evidence for compartmentalization of functional subsets of CD2$^+$ T lymphocytes in atopic patients. J Immunol 1990; 144:4651–4656.
3. Mosmann TR, Cherwinski H, Bond MW, Giedlin MA, Coffman RL. Two types of murine helper T cell clone. I. Definition according to profiles of lymphokine activities and secreted proteins. J Immunol 1986; 136:2348–2357.
4. Del Prete GF, De Carli M, Mastromauro C, Biagiotti R, Macchia D, Falagiani P, Ricci M, Romagnani S. Purified protein derivative of *Mycobacterium tuberculosis* and excretory–secretory antigen(s) of *Toxocara canis* expand in vitro human T cells with stable and opposite (type 1 T helper or type 2 T helper) profile of cytokine production. J Clin Invest 1991; 88: 346–350.
5. Firestein GS, Roeder WD, Laxer JA, Townsend KS, Weaver CT, Hom JT, Linton J, Torbett BE, Glasebrook AL. A new murine CD4$^+$ T cell subset with an unrestricted cytokine profile. J Immunol 1989; 143:518–525.
6. Paliard X, de Waal Malefijt R, Yssel H, Blanchard D, Chretien I, Abrams J, de Vries J, Spits H. Simultaneous production of IL-2, IL-4, and IFN-gamma by activated human CD4$^+$ and CD8$^+$ T cell clones. J Immunol 1988; 141:849–855.
7. Chen Y, Kuchroo VK, Inobe J, Hafler DA, Weiner HL. Regulatory T cell clones induced by oral tolerance: suppression of autoimmune encephalomyelitis. Science 1994; 265:1237–1240.

8. Zubiaga AM, Munoz E, Merrow M, Huber BT. Regulation of interleukin 6 production in T helper cells. Int Immunol 1990; 2:1047–1054.
9. Mosmann TR, Schumacher JH, Fiorentino DF, Leverah J, Moore KW, Bond MW. Isolation of monoclonal antibodies specific for IL-4, IL-5, IL-6, and a new Th2-specific cytokine (IL-10), cytokine synthesis inhibitory factor, by using a solid phase radioimmunoadsorbent assay. J Immunol 1990; 145:2938–2945.
10. Cherwinski HM, Schumacher JH, Brown KD, Mosmann TR. Two types of mouse helper T cell clone. III. Further differences in lymphokine synthesis between Th1 and Th2 clones revealed by RNA hybridization, functionally monospecific bioassays, and monoclonal antibodies. J Exp Med 1987; 166:1229–1244.
11. Pene J, Rousset F, Briere F, et al. IgE production by normal human lymphocytes is induced by interleukin 4 and suppressed by interferons gamma and alpha and prostaglandin E_2. Proc Natl Acad Sci USA 1988; 85:6880–6884.
12. Aversa G, Punnonen J, Cocks BG, de Waal Malefyt R, Vega F Jr, Zurawski SM, Zurawski G, de Vries JE. An interleukin 4 (IL-4) mutant protein inhibits both IL-4 or IL-13-induced human immunoglobulin G4 (IgG4) and IgE synthesis and B cell proliferation: support for a common component shared by IL-4 and IL-13 receptors. J Exp Med 1993; 178:2213–2218.
13. Swain SL, Weinberg AD, English M, Huston G. IL-4 directs the development of Th2-like helper effectors. J Immunol 1990; 145:3796–3806.
14. Li L, Yiyang X, Nguyen A, Lai HY, Feng L, Mosmann TR, Lo D. Effects of Th2 cytokines on chemokine expression in the lung: IL-13 potently induces eotaxin expression by airway epithelial cells. J Immunol 1999; 162:2477–2487.
15. Yamaguchi Y, Suda T, Suda J, Eguchi M, Miura Y, Harada N, Tominaga A, Takatsu K. Purified interleukin 5 supports the terminal differentiation and proliferation of murine eosinophilic precursors. J Exp Med 1988; 167:43–56.
16. Wang JM, Rambaldi A, Biondi A, Chen ZG, Sanderson CJ, Mantovani A. Recombinant human interleukin 5 is a selective eosinophil chemoattractant. Eur J Immunol 1989; 19:701–705.
17. Horie S, Gleich GJ, Kita H. Cytokines directly induce degranulation and superoxide production from human eosinophils. J Allergy Clin Immunol 1996; 98:371–381.
18. Yamaguchi Y, Suda T, Ohta S, Tominaga K, Miura Y, Kasahara T. Analysis of the survival of mature human eosinophils: interleukin-5 prevents apoptosis in mature human eosinophils. Blood 1991; 78:2542–2547.
19. Ochi H, Hirani WM, Yuan Q, Friend DS, Austen KF, Boyce JA. T helper cell type 2 cytokine-mediated comitogenic responses and CCR3 expression during differentiation of human mast cells in vitro. J Exp Med 1999; 190:267–280.
20. Rincon M, Anguita J, Nakamura T, Fikrig E, Flavell RA. Interleukin (IL)-6 directs the differentiation of IL-4-producing $CD4^+$ T cells. J Exp Med 1997; 185:461–469.
21. Bjorck P, Larsson S, Andang M, Ahrlund–Richter L, Paulie S. IL-6 antisense oligonucleotides inhibit IgE production in IL-4 and anti-CD40-stimulated human B-lymphocytes. Immunol Lett 1998; 61:1–5.
22. Del Prete G, De Carli M, Almerigogna F, Giudizi MG, Biagiotti R, Romagnani S. Human IL-10 is produced by both type 1 helper (Th1) and type 2 helper (Th2) T cell clones and inhibits their antigen-specific proliferation and cytokine production. J Immunol 1993; 150: 353–360.
23. Pretolani M, Goldman M. IL-10: a potential therapy for allergic inflammation. Immunol. Today 1997; 18:277–280.
24. Morris SC, Lees A, Finkelman FD. In vivo activation of naive T cells by antigen-presenting B cells. J Immunol 1994; 152:3777–3785.
25. Finkelman FD, Madden KB, Cheever AW, Katona IM, Morris SC, Gately MK, Hubbard BR, Gause WC, Urban JF Jr. Effects of interleukin 12 on immune responses and host protection in mice infected with intestinal nematode parasites. J Exp Med 1994; 179:1563–1572.

26. Wang ZE, Zheng S, Corry DB, Dalton DK, Seder RA, Reiner SL, Locksley RM. Interferon gamma-independent effects of interleukin 12 administered during acute or established infection due to *Leishmania major*. Proc Natl Acad Sci USA 1994; 91:12932–12936.
27. Koch F, Stanzl U, Jennewein P, Janke K, Heufler C, Kampgen E, Romani N, Schuler G. High level IL-12 production by murine dendritic cells: upregulation via MHC class II and CD40 molecules and downregulation by IL-4 and IL-10. J Exp Med 1996; 184:741–746.
28. Szabo SJ, Dighe AS, Gubler U, Murphy KM. Regulation of the interleukin (IL)-12R beta 2 subunit expression in developing T helper 1 (Th1) and Th2 cells. J Exp Med 1997; 185: 817–824.
29. D'Andrea A, Ma X, Aste–Amezaga M, Paganin C, Trinchieri G. Stimulatory and inhibitory effects of interleukin (IL)-4 and IL-13 on the production of cytokines by human peripheral blood mononuclear cells: priming for IL-12 and tumor necrosis factor alpha production. J Exp Med 1995; 181:537–546.
30. Denburg JA, Woolley M, Leber B, Linden M, O'Byrne P. Basophil and eosinophil differentiation in allergic reactions. J Allergy Clin Immunol 1994; 94:1135–1141.
31. Rodewald HR, Dessing M, Dvorak AM, Galli SJ. Identification of a committed precursor for the mast cell lineage. Science 1996; 271:818–822.
32. Kirshenbaum AS, Kessler SW, Goff JP, Metcalfe DD. Demonstration of the origin of human mast cells from $CD34^+$ bone marrow progenitor cells. J Immunol 1991; 146:1410–1415.
33. Rottem M, Okada T, Goff JP, Metcalfe DD. Mast cells cultured from the peripheral blood of normal donors and patients with mastocytosis originate from a $CD34^+$/Fc epsilon RI^- cell population. Blood 1994; 84:2489–2496.
34. Valent P, Spanblochl E, Sperr WR, Sillaber C, Zsebo KM, Agis H, Strobl H, Geissler K, Bettelheim P, Lechner K. Induction of differentiation of human mast cells from bone marrow and peripheral blood mononuclear cells by recombinant human stem cell factor/*kit*-ligand in long-term culture. Blood 1992; 80:2237–2245.
35. Hjertson M, Sundstrom C, Lyman SD, Nilsson K, Nilsson G. Stem cell factor, but not flt ligand, induces differentiation and activation of human mast cells. Exp Hematol 1996; 24: 748–754.
36. Nilsson G, Butterfield JH, Nilsson K, Siegbahn A. Stem cell factor is a chemotactic factor for human mast cells. J Immunol 1994; 153:3717.
37. Saito H, Ebisawa M, Tachimoto H, Shichijo M, Fukagawa K, Matsumoto K, Iikura Y, Awaji T, Tsujimoto G, Yanagida M, Uzumaki H, Takahashi G, Tsuji K, Nakahata T. Selective growth of human mast cells induced by Steel factor, IL-6, and prostaglandin E_2 from cord blood mononuclear cells. J Immunol 1996; 157:343–350.
38. Ochi H, Hirani WM, Yuan Q, Friend DS, Austen KF, Boyce JA. T helper cell type 2 cytokine-mediated comitogenic responses and CCR3 expression during differentiation of human mast cells in vitro. J Exp Med 1999; 190:267–280.
39. Toru H, Eguchi M, Matsumoto R, Yanagida M, Yata J, Nakahata T. Interleukin-4 promotes the development of tryptase and chymase double-positive human mast cells accompanied by cell maturation. Blood 1998; 91:187.
40. Xia HZ, Du Z, Craig S, Klisch G, Noben–Trauth N, Kochan JP, Huff TH, Irani AM, Schwartz LB. Effect of recombinant human IL-4 on tryptase, chymase, and Fc epsilon receptor type I expression in recombinant human stem cell factor-dependent fetal liver-derived human mast cells. J Immunol 1997; 159:2911–2921.
41. Kinoshita T, Sawai N, Hidaka E, Yamashita T, Koike K. Interleukin-6 directly modulates stem cell factor-dependent development of human mast cells derived from CD34(+) cord blood cells. Blood 1999; 94:496–508.
42. Godfraind C, Louahed J, Faulkner H, Vink A, Warnier G, Grencis R, Renauld JC. Intraepithelial infiltration by mast cells with both connective tissue-type and mucosal-type characteristics in gut, trachea, and kidneys of IL-9 transgenic mice. J Immunol 1998; 160:3989–3996.
43. Ihle JN, Keller J, Oroszlan S, Henderson LE, Copeland TD, Fitch F, Prystowsky MB, Goldwasser E, Schrader JW, Palaszynski E, Dy M, Lebel B. Biologic properties of homogeneous

interleukin 3. I. Demonstration of WEHI-3 growth factor activity, mast cell growth factor activity, p cell-stimulating factor activity, colony-stimulating factor activity, and histamine-producing cell-stimulating factor activity. J Immunol 1983; 131:282–287.
44. Nakahata T, Kobayashi T, Ishiguro A, Tsuji K, Naganuma K, Ando O, Yagi Y, Tadokoro K, Akabane T. Extensive proliferation of mature connective-tissue type mast cells in vitro. Nature 1986; 324:65–67.
45. Kempuraj D, Saito H, Kaneko A, Fukagawa K, Nakayama M, Toru H, Tomikawa M, Tachimoto H, Ebisawa M, Akasawa A, Miyagi T, Kimura H, Nakajima T, Tsuji K, Nakahata T. Characterization of mast cell-committed progenitors present in human umbilical cord blood. Blood 1999; 15:3338–3346.
46. Sillaber C, Sperr WR, Agis H, Spanblochl E, Lechner K, Valent P. Inhibition of stem cell factor dependent formation of human mast cells by interleukin-3 and interleukin-4. Int Arch Allergy Immunol 1994; 105:264–268.
47. Denburg JA, Telizyn S, Messner H, Lim B, Jamal N, Ackerman SJ, Gleich GJ, Bienenstock J. Heterogeneity of human peripheral blood eosinophil-type colonies: evidence for a common basophil–eosinophil progenitor. Blood 1985; 66:312–318.
48. Agis H, Willheim M, Sperr WR, et al. Monocytes do not make mast cells when cultured in the presence of SCF. Characterization of the circulating mast cell progenitor as a c-*kit*$^+$, CD34$^+$, Ly$^-$, CD14$^-$, CD17$^-$, colony-forming cell. J Immunol 1993; 151:4221–4227.
49. Zucker–Franklin D. Ultrastructural evidence for the common origin of human mast cells and basophils. Blood 1980; 56:534–540.
50. Li L, Li Y, Reddel SW, Cherrian M, Friend DS, Stevens RL, Krilis SA. Identification of basophilic cells that express mast cell granule proteases in the peripheral blood of asthma, allergy, and drug-reactive patients. J Immunol 1998; 161:5079–5086.
51. Saito H, Hatake K, Dvorak AM, Leiferman KM, Donnenberg AD, Arai N, Ishizaka K, Ishizaka T. Selective differentiation and proliferation of hematopoietic cells induced by recombinant human interleukins. Proc Natl Acad Sci USA 1988; 85:2288–2292.
52. Valent P. The phenotype of human eosinophils, basophils, and mast cells. J Allergy Clin Immunol 1994; 94:1177–1183.
53. Denburg JA. Bone marrow in atopy and asthma: hematopoietic mechanisms in allergic inflammation. Immunol Today 1999; 20:111–113.
54. Coutinho LH, Will A, Radford J, Schiro R, Testa NG, Dexter TM. Effects of recombinant human granulocyte colony-stimulating factor (CSF), human granulocyte macrophage-CSF, and gibbon interleukin-3 on hematopoiesis in human long-term bone marrow culture. Blood 1990; 75:2118–2129.
55. Ottmann OG, Abboud M, Welte K, Souza LM, Pelus LM. Stimulation of human hematopoietic progenitor cell proliferation and differentiation by recombinant human interleukin 3. Comparison and interactions with recombinant human granulocyte–macrophage and granulocyte colony-stimulating factors. Exp Hematol 1989; 17:191–197.
56. Ema H, Suda T, Nagayoshi K, Miura Y, Civin CI, Nakauchi H. Target cells for granulocyte colony-stimulating factor, interleukin-3, and interleukin-5 in differentiation pathways of neutrophils and eosinophils. Blood 1990; 76:1956–1961.
57. Valent P, Schmidt G, Besemer J, Mayer P, Zenke G, Liehl E, Hinterberger W, Lechner K, Maurer D, Bettelheim P. Interleukin-3 is a differentiation factor for human basophils. Blood 1989; 73:1763–1769.
58. Clutterbuck EJ, Hirst EM, Sanderson CJ. Human interleukin-5 (IL-5) regulates the production of eosinophils in human bone marrow cultures: comparison and interaction with IL-1, IL-3, IL-6, and GMCSF. Blood 1989; 73:1504–1512.
59. Lu L, Lin ZH, Shen RN, Warren DJ, Leemhuis T, Broxmeyer HE. Influence of interleukins 3, 5, and 6 on the growth of eosinophil progenitors in highly enriched human bone marrow in the absence of serum. Exp Hematol 1990; 18:1180–1186.
60. Denburg JA, Silver JE, Abrams JS. Interleukin-5 is a human basophilopoietin: induction of

histamine content and basophilic differentiation of HL-60 cells and of peripheral blood basophil–eosinophil progenitors. Blood 1991; 77:1462–1468.

61. Dvorak AM, Saito H, Estrella P, Kissell S, Arai N, Ishizaka T. Ultrastructure of eosinophils and basophils stimulated to develop in human cord blood mononuclear cell cultures containing recombinant human interleukin-5 or interleukin-3. Lab Invest 1989; 61:116–132.
62. Sillaber C, Geissler K, Scherrer R, Kaltenbrunner R, Bettelheim P, Lechner K, Valent P. Type beta transforming growth factors promote interleukin-3 (IL-3)-dependent differentiation of human basophils but inhibit IL-3–dependent differentiation of human eosinophils. Blood 1992; 80:634–641.
63. McLane MP, Haczku A, van de Rijn M, Weiss C, Ferrante V, MacDonald D, Renauld JC, Nicolaides NC, Holroyd KJ, Levitt RC. Interleukin-9 promotes allergen-induced eosinophilic inflammation and airway hyperresponsiveness in transgenic mice. Am J Respir Cell Mol Biol 1998; 19:713–20.
64. Shivdasani RA, Orkin SH. The transcriptional control of hematopoiesis. Blood 1996; 87: 4025–4039.
65. Foster PS, Hogan SP, Ramsay AJ, Matthaei KI, Young IG. IL-5 deficiency abolishes eosinophilia, airway hyperreactivity, and lung damage in a mouse asthma model. J Exp Med 1996; 183:195–201.
66. Robinson D, Tavernier J, Van der Heyden J, Verhee A, Brusselle G, Van Ostrade X, Vandekerckhove J, North J, Rankin SM, Kay AB. Interleukin-5 regulates the isoform expression of its own receptor alpha subunit. Blood 2000; 95:1600–1607.
67. Owen WF Jr, Austen KF. Cytokine regulation of eosinophil-mediated inflammatory reactions by modulation of eosinophil programmed cell death and subsequent priming for augmented function. In: Gleich GJ, Kay AB, eds. Eosinophils in allergy and inflammation. New York: Marcel Decker, 1994:239–253.
68. Luttmann W, Knoechel B, Foerster M, Matthys H, Virchow JC Jr, Kroegel C. Activation of human eosinophils by IL-13. Induction of CD69 surface antigen, its relationship to messenger RNA expression, and promotion of cellular viability. J Immunol 1996; 157:1678–1683.
69. Ochiai K, Kagami M, Matsumura R, Tomioka H. IL-5 but not interferon-gamma (IFN-gamma) inhibits eosinophil apoptosis by up-regulation of *bcl-2* expression. Clin Exp Immunol 1997; 107:198–204.
70. Morita M, Lamkhioued B, Soussi Gounni A, Aldebert D, Delaporte E, Capron A, Capron M. Induction by interferons of human eosinophil apoptosis and regulation by interleukin-3, granulocyte/macrophage colony-stimulating factor and interleukin-5. Eur Cytokine Network 1996; 7:725–732.
71. Alam R, Forsythe P, Stafford S, Fukuda Y. Transforming growth factor-β abrogates the effects of hematopoietins on eosinophils and induces their apoptosis. J Exp Med 1994; 179: 1041–1045.
72. Schleimer RP, Bochner BS. The role of adhesion molecules in allergic inflammation and their suitability as targets of antiallergic therapy [review]. Clin Exp Allergy 1998; 28(Suppl 3):15–23.
73. Broide DH, Sullivan S, Gifford T, Sriramrao P. Inhibition of pulmonary eosinophilia in P-selectin and ICAM-deficient mice. Am J Respir Cell Mol Biol 1998; 18:218–225.
74. Khew–Godall Y, Wadham C, Stein BM, Gamble JR, Vadas MA. STAT-6 activation is essential for IL-4 induction of P-selectin transcription in human umbilical vein endothelial cells. Arterioscler Thromb Vasc Biol 1999; 19:1421–1429.
75. Grayson MH, Van der Vieren M, Sterbinsky SA, Michael Gallatin W, Hoffman PA, Staunton DE, Bochner BS. alpha$_d$beta$_2$ Integrin is expressed on human eosinophils and functions as an alternative ligand for vascular cell adhesion molecule 1 (VCAM-1). J Exp Med 1998; 188:2187–2191.
76. Henderson WR, Chi EY, Albert RK, et al. Blockade of CD49d (alpha 4 integrin) on intrapul-

monary but not circulating leukocytes inhibits airway inflammation and hyperresponsiveness in a mouse model of asthma. J Clin Invest 1997; 100:13083–13092.
77. Fukuda T, Fukushima Y, Numato T, et al. Role of IL-4 and VCAM-1 in selective eosinophil migration into the airways in allergic asthma. Am J Respir Cell Mol Biol 1996; 14:84–94.
78. Ulfman LH, Kujiper PH, van den Linden JA. Lammers JW. Zwaginga JJ, Koenderman L. Characterization of eosinophil adhesion to TNF-alpha activated endothelium under flow conditions: alpha 4 integrins mediate initial attachment and E-selectin mediates rolling. J Immunol 1999; 163:343–350.
79. Nagata M, Sedgwick JB, Kita H, Busse WW. Granulocyte macrophage colony-stimulating factor augments ICAM-1 and VCAM-1 activation of eosinophil function. Am J Respir Cell Mol Biol 1998; 19:158–166.
80. Alam R, Stafford S, Forsythe P, Harrison R, Faubion D, Lett–Brown MA, Grant JA. RANTES is a chemotactic and activating factor for eosinophils. J Immunol 1993; 150:3442–3447.
81. Weber C, Kitayama J, Springer TA. Differential regulation of β1 and β2 integrin avidity by chemoattractants in eosinophils. Proc Natl Acad Sci USA 1998; 93:10939–10944.
82. Mishra A, Hogan SP, Lee JJ, Foster PS, Rothenberg ME. Fundamental signals that regulate eosinophil homing to the gastrointestinal tract. J Clin Invest 1999; 103:1719–1727.
83. Kitayam J, Mackay CR, Ponath PD, Springer TA. The CC chemokine receptor CCR3 participates in stimulation of eosinophil arrest on inflammatory endothelium in shear flow. J Clin Invest 1998; 101:2017–2024.
84. Ward SG, Bacon K, Westwick J. Chemokines and T lymphocytes: more than an attraction. Immunity 1998; 9:1–11.
85. Bonecchi R, Bianchi G, Bordignon RP, D'Ambrosio D, Lang R, Borsatti A, Sozzani S, Allavena P, Gray PA, Mantovani A, Sinigaglia F. Differential expression of chemokine receptors and chemotactic responsiveness of type 1 T helper cells (Th1s and Th2s). J Exp Med 1998; 187:129–134.
86. Loetscher P, Uguccioni M, Bordolli L, Baggiolini M, Moser B. CCR5 is characteristic of Th1 lymphocytes. Nature 1998; 391:344–345.
87. Sallusto F, MacKay CR, Lanzavecchia A. Selective expression of the eotaxin receptor CCR3 by human T helper 2 cells. Science 1997; 277:2005–2007.
88. D'Ambrosio D, Iellem A, Bonecchi R, Mazzeo D, Sozzani S, Mantovani A, Sinigaglia F. Selective up-regulation of chemokine receptors CCR4 and CCR8 upon activation of polarized human Th2 cells. J Immunol 1998; 161:5111–5115.
89. Heath H, Qin S, Rao P, Wu L, LaRosa G, Kassam N, Ponath PD, Mackay CR. Chemokine receptor usage by human eosinophils. The importance of CCR3 demonstrated using an antagonistic monoclonal antibody. J Clin Invest 1997; 99:178–84.
90. Lukacs NW, Oliveira SH, Hogaboam CM. Chemokines and asthma: redundancy of function or a coordinated effort? J Clin Invest 1999; 104:995–999.
91. Hogaboam CM, Gallinat CS, Taub DD, Strieter RM, Kunkel SL, Lukacs NW. Immunomodulatory role of C10 chemokine in a murine model of allergic bronchopulmonary aspergillosis. J Immunol 1999; 162:6071–6079.
92. Daugherty BL, Siciliano SJ, DeMartino JA, et al. Cloning, expression, and characterization of the human eosinophil eotaxin receptor. J Exp Med 1996; 183:2349–2354.
93. Boehme SA, Sullivan SK, Crowe PD, Santos M, Conlon PJ, Sriramrao P, Bacon KB. Activation of mitogen-activated protein kinase regulates eotaxin-induced eosinophil migration. J Immunol 1999; 163:1611–1618.
94. Kampen G, Stafford S, Adachi T, Jinquan T, Quan S, Grant JA, Skov P, Poulsen L, Alam R. Eotaxin induces degranulation and chemotaxis of eosinophils through the activation of ERK2 and p38 mitogen-activated protein kinases. Blood 2000; 95:1911–1917.
95. Coffer PJ, Schweizer RC, Dubois GR, Maikoe T, Lammers J–WJ, Koenderman L. Analysis of signal transduction pathways in human eosinophils activated by chemoattractants and the T-helper 2-derived cytokines IL-4 and IL-5. Blood 1998; 91:2547–2557.

96. Rand TH, Cruikshank WW, Center DM, et al. CD4-mediated stimulation of human eosinophils:lymphocyte chemoattractant factor and other CD4-binding ligands elicit eosinophil migration. J Exp Med 1991; 173:1521–1528.
97. Sehmi R, Wardlaw AJ, Cromwell O, Kurihara K, Waltmann P, Kay AB. Interleukin-5 selectively enhances the chemotactic response of eosinophils obtained from normal but not eosinophilic subjects. Blood 1992; 79:2952–2959.
98. Fukuda T, Gleich GJ. Heterogeneity of human eosinophils. J Allergy Clin Immunol 1989; 83:369–373.
99. Horie S, Gleich GJ, Kita H. Cytokines directly induce degranulation and superoxide production from human eosinophils. J Allergy Clin Immunol 1996; 98:371–381.
100. Bischoff SC, Sellge G, Schwengberg S, Lorentz A, Manns MP. Stem cell factor-dependent survival, proliferation and enhanced releasability of purified mature mast cells isolated from human intestinal tissue. Int Arch Allergy Immunol 1999; 118:104–107.
101. Garcia–Zepeda EA, Combadiere C, Rothenberg ME, Sarafi MN, Lavigne F, Hamid Q, Murphy PM, Luster AD. Human monocyte chemoattractant protein (MCP)-4 is a novel CC chemokine with activities on monocytes, eosinophils, and basophils induced in allergic and nonallergic inflammation that signals through the CC chemokine receptors (CCR)-2 and -3. J Immunol 1996; 157:5613–5626.
102. Uguccioni M, Mackay CR, Ochensberger B, Loetscher P, Rhis S, LaRosa GJ, Rao P, Ponath PD, Baggiolini M, Dahinden CA. High expression of the chemokine receptor CCR3 in human blood basophils. Role in activation by eotaxin, MCP-4, and other chemokines. J Clin Invest 1997; 100:1137–1143.
103. Power CA, Meyer A, Nemeth K, et al. Molecular cloning and functional expression of a novel CC chemokine receptor cDNA from a human basophilic cell line. J Biol Chem 1995; 270:19495–500.
104. Alam R, Lett–Brown MA, Forsythe PA, et al. Monocyte chemotactic and activating factor is a potent histamine-releasing factor for basophils. J Clin Invest 1992; 89:723–728.
105. Dahinden CA, Geiser T, Brunner T, et al. Monocyte chemotactic protein 3 is a most effective basophil- and eosinophil-activating chemokine. J Exp Med 1994; 179:751–756.
106. MacDonald SM, Rafnar T, Langdon J, Lichtenstein LM. Molecular identification of an IgE-dependent histamine-releasing factor. Science 1995; 269:688–690.
107. Pearlman E, Lass JH, Bardenstein DS, Diaconu E, Hazlett FE Jr, Albright J, Higgins AW, Kazura JW. IL-12 exacerbates helminth-mediated corneal pathology by augmenting inflammatory cell recruitment and chemokine expression. J Immunol 1997; 158:827–833.
108. Villa A, Santagata S, Bozzi F, Giliani S, Frattini A, Imberti L, Gatta LB, Ochs HD, Schwarz K, Notarangelo LD, Vezzoni P, Spanopoulou E. Partial V(D)J recombination activity leads to Omenn syndrome. Cell 1998; 93:885–896.
109. Amishima M, Munakata M, Nasuhara Y, Sato A, Takahashi T, Homma Y, Kawakami Y. Expression of epidermal growth factor and epidermal growth factor receptor immunoreactivity in the asthmatic human airway. Am J Respir Crit Care Med 1998; 157(6pt1):1907–1912.
110. Aubert JD, Hayashi S, Hards J, Bai TR, Pare PD, Hogg JC. Platelet-derived growth factor and its receptor in lungs from patients with asthma and chronic airflow obstruction. Am J Physiol 1994; 266(6pt1):L655–L663.
111. Chanez P, Vignola M, Stenger R, Vic P, Michel FB, Bousquet J. Platelet-derived growth factor in asthma. Allergy 1995; 50:878–883.
112. Makhluf HA, Stepniakowska J, Hoffman S, Smith E, LeRoy EC, Trojanowska M. IL-4 upregulates tenascin synthesis in scleroderma and healthy skin fibroblasts. J Invest Dermatol 1996; 107:856–859.
113. Zhao Y. Transforming growth factor-beta (TGF-beta) type I and type II receptors are both required for TGF-beta-mediated extracellular matrix production in lung fibroblasts. Mol Cell Endocrinol 1999; 150:91–97.
114. Vignola AM, Chanez P, Chiappara G, Merendino A, Pace E, Rizzo A, la Rocca AM, Bellia V, Bonsignore G, Bousquet J. Transforming growth factor-beta expression in mucosal biop-

sies in asthma and chronic bronchitis. Am J Respir Crit Care Med 1997; 156(2pt1):591–599.

115. Ying S, Durham SR, Jacobson MR, Rak S, Masuyama K, Lowhagen O, Kay AB, Hamid QA. T lymphocytes and mast cells express messenger RNA for interleukin-4 in the nasal mucosa in allergen-induced rhinitis. Immunology 1994; 82:200–206.
116. Masuyama K, Till SJ, Jacobson MR, Kamil A, Cameron L, Juliusson S, Lowhagen O, Kay AB, Hamid QA, Durham SR. Nasal eosinophilia and IL-5 mRNA expression in seasonal allergic rhinitis induced by natural allergen exposure: effect of topical corticosteroids. J Allergy Clin Immunol 1998; 102:610–617.
117. Ghaffar O, Laberge S, Jacobson MR, Lowhagen O, Rak S, Durham SR, Hamid Q. IL-13 mRNA and immunoreactivity in allergen-induced rhinitis: comparison with IL-4 expression and modulation by topical glucocorticoid therapy. Am J Respir Cell Mol Biol 1997; 17:17–24.
118. Minshall EM, Cameron L, Lavigne F, Leung DY, Hamilos D, Garcia–Zepada EA, Rothenberg M, Luster AD, Hamid Q. Eotaxin mRNA and protein expression in chronic sinusitis and allergen-induced nasal responses in seasonal allergic rhinitis. Am J Respir Cell Mol Biol 1997; 17:683–690.
119. Sim TC, Reece LM, Hilsmeier KA, et al. Secretion of chemokines and other cytokines in allergen-induced nasal responses: inhibition by topical steroid treatment. Am J Respir Crit Care Med 1995; 152:927–933.
120. Rajakulasingam K, Hamid Q, O'Brien F, et al. RANTES in human allergen-induced rhinitis. Am J Respir Crit Care Med 1997; 155:696–703.
121. Christodoulopoulos P, Wright E, Frenkiel S, Luster A, Hamid Q. Monocyte chemotactic proteins in allergen-induced inflammation in the nasal mucosa: effect of topical corticosteroids. J Allergy Clin Immunol 1999; 103:1036–1044.
122. Laberge S, Durham SR, Ghaffar O, Rak S. Center DM, Jacobson M, Hamid Q. Expression of IL-16 in allergen-induced late-phase nasal responses and relation to topical glucocorticosteroid treatment. J Allergy Clin Immunol 1997; 100:569–574.
123. Kuna P, Lazarovich M, Kaplan AP. Chemokines in seasonal allergic rhinitis. J Allergy Clin Immunol 1996; 97:104–112.
124. Durham SR, Ying S, Varney VA, Jacobson MR, Sudderick RM, Mackay IS, Kay AB, Hamid QA. Grass pollen immunotherapy inhibits allergen-induced infiltration of $CD4^+$ T lymphocytes and eosinophils in the nasal mucosa and increases the number of cells expressing messenger RNA for interferon-gamma. J Allergy Clin Immunol 1996; 97:1356–1365.
125. Durham SR, Walker SM, Varga EM, Jacobson MR, O'Brien F, Noble W, Till SJ, Hamid QA, Nouri–Aria KT. Long-term clinical efficacy of grass-pollen immunotherapy. N Engl J Med 1999; 341:468–475.
126. Broide DH, Lotz M, Cuomo AJ, et al. Cytokines in symptomatic asthmatic airways. J Allergy Clin Immunol 1992; 89:958–967.
127. Borish L, Mascali JJ, Dishuck J, et al. Detection of alveolar macrophage-derived IL-1 in asthma. Inhibition with corticosteroids. J Immunol 1992; 149:3078–3082.
128. Robinson DS, Hamid Q, Ying S, et al. Predominant Th2-type bronchoalveolar T-lymphocyte population in atopic asthma. N Engl J Med 1992; 326:298–304.
129. Robinson DS, Hamid Q, Bentley AM, et al. Activation of $CD4^+$ T cells and increased IL-4, IL-5 and GM-CSF mRNA positive cells in bronchoalveolar lavage fluid (BAL) 24 hours after allergen inhalation challenge of atopic asthmatic patients. J Allergy Clin Immunol 1993; 92:313–324.
130. Kips JC, Tavernier JH, Joos GF, et al. The potential role of TNF-α in asthma. Clin Exp Allergy 1993; 23:247–250.
131. Krishnaswamy G, Liu MC, Su SN, Kumai M, Xiao HQ, Marsh DG, Huang SK. Analysis of cytokine transcripts in the bronchoalveolar lavage cells of patients with asthma. Am J Respir Cell Mol Biol 1993; 9:279–286.

132. Cruikshank WW, Long A, Torpy RE, et al. Early identification of IL-16 and MIP-1α in bronchoalveolar lavage fluid of antigen-challenged asthma. Am J Respir Cell Mol Biol 1995; 13:738–747.
133. Ohnishi T, Kita H, Weiler D, et al. IL-5 is the predominant eosinophil-active cytokine in the antigen-induced pulmonary late-phase reaction. Am Rev Respir Dis 1993; 147:901–907.
134. Bradding P, Roberts JA, Britten KM, et al. IL-4, -5, and -6, TNF-α in normal and asthmatic airways: evidence for the human mast cell as a source of these cytokines. Am J Respir Cell Mol Biol 1994; 10:471–480.
135. Robinson DS, Tsicopolous A, Meng Q, et al. Increased IL-10 mRNA expression in atopic allergy and asthma. Am J Respir Cell Mol Biol 1996; 14:113–117.
136. Humbert M, Durham SR, Kimmitt P, et al. Elevated expression of mRNA encoding IL-13 in the bronchial mucosa of atopic and nonatopic subjects with asthma. J Allergy Clin Immunol 1997; 99:657–665.
137. Minshall EM, Schleimer R, Cameron L, et al. IL-5 expression in the bone marrow of sensitized BALB/c mice after allergen challenge. Am J Respir Crit Care Med 1998; 158:951–957.
138. Leung DY, Martin RJ, Szefler SJ, Sher ER, Ying S, Kay AB, Hamid Q. Dysregulation of interleukin 4, interleukin 5, and interferon gamma gene expression in steroid-resistant asthma. J Exp Med 1995; 181:33–40.
139. Naseer T, Minshall EM, Leung DY, et al. Expression of IL-12 and IL-13 mRNA in asthma and their modulation in response to steroid therapy. Am J Respir Crit Care Med 1997; 155: 845–851.
140. Cembrzynska–Nowak M, Szklarz E, Inglot AD, Teodorczy K, Injeyan JA. Elevated release of TNF-α and IFN-γ by bronchoalveolar leukocytes from patients with bronchial asthma. Am J Respir Dis 1993; 147:291–295.
141. Krug N, Madden J, Redington AE, Lackie P, Djukanobvic R, Schauer U, Holgate ST, Frew AJ, Howarth PH. T-cell cytokine profile evaluated at the single cell level in BAL and blood in allergic asthma. Am J Respir Cell Mol Biol 1996; 14:319–326.
142. Alam R, York J, Boyars M, Stafford S, Grant JA, Lee J, Forsythe P, Sim T, Ida N. Increased MCP-1, RANTES, and MIP-1α in bronchoalveolar lavage in allergic asthmatic patients. Am J Respir Crit Care Med 1996; 153:1398–1404.
143. Holgate ST, Bodey KS, Janezic A, et al. Release of RANTES, MIP-1α, and MCP-1 into asthmatic airways following endobronchial allergen challenge. Am J Respir Crit Care Med 1997; 156:1377–1383.
144. Venge J, Lampinen M, Hakansson L, et al. Identification of IL-5 and RANTES as the major eosinophil chemoattractants in the asthmatic lung. J Allergy Clin Immunol 1996; 97:1110–1115.
145. Sur S, Kita H, Gleich GJ, et al. Eosinophil recruitment is associated with IL-5, but not with RANTES, twenty four hours after allergen challenge. J Allergy Clin Immunol 1996; 97: 1272–1278.
146. Humbert M, Ying S, Corrigan C, Menz G, Barkans J, Pfister R, Meng Q, Van Damme J, Opdenakker G, Durham SR, Kay AB. Bronchial mucosal expression of the genes encoding chemokines RANTES and MCP-3 in symptomatic atopic and non-atopic asthmatics: relationship to the eosinophil-active cytokines IL-5, GM-CSF and IL-3. Am J Respir Cell Mol Biol 1997; 16:1–8.
147. Taha RA, Minshall EM, Miotto D, Shimbara A, Luster A, Hogg JC, Hamid QA. Eotaxin and monocyte chemotactic protein-4 mRNA expression in small airways of asthmatic and nonasthmatic individuals. J Allergy Clin Immunol 1999; 103(3pt1):476–483.
148. Lamkhioued B, Renzi PM, Abi-Younes S, Garcia–Zepada EA, Allakhverdi Z, Ghaffar O, Rothenberg MD, Luster AD, Hamid Q. Increased expression of eotaxin in bronchoalveolar lavage and airways of asthmatics contributes to the chemotaxis of eosinophils to the site of inflammation. J Immunol 1997; 159:4593–601.

149. Kurashima K, Mukaida N, Fijimura M, et al. Increase of chemokine levels in sputum precedes exacerbation of acute asthma attacks. J Leukoc Biol 1996; 59:313–316.
150. Ying S, Robinson DS, Meng Q, Rottman J, Kennedy R, Ringler DJ, Mackay CR, Daugherty BL, Springer MS, Durham SR, Williams TJ, Kay AB. Enhanced expression of eotaxin and CCR3 mRNA and protein in atopic asthma. Association with airway hyperresponsiveness and predominant co-localization of eotaxin mRNA to bronchial epithelial and endothelial cells. Eur J Immunol 1997; 27:3507–3516.
151. Lukacs NW, Strieter RM, Chensue SW, Kunkel SL. Interleukin-4-dependent pulmonary eosinophil infiltration in a murine model of asthma. Am J Respir Cell Mol Biol 1994; 10:526–532.
152. Wills-Karp M, Luyimbazi J, Xu X, Schofield B, Neben TY, Karp CL, Donaldson DD. Interleukin-13: central mediator of allergic asthma. Science 1998; 282:2258–2261.
153. Grunig G, Warnock M, Wakil AE, Venkayya R, Brombacher F, Rennick DM, Sheppard D, Mohrs M, Donaldson DD, Locksley RM, Corry DB. Requirement for IL-13 independently of IL-4 in experimental asthma. Science 1998; 282:2261–2263.
154. Foster PS, Hogan SP, Ramsay AJ, Matthaei KI, Young IG. IL-5 deficiency abolishes eosinophilia, airway hyperreactivity, and lung damage in a mouse asthma model. J Exp Med 1996; 183:195–201.
155. Hamelmann E, Cieslewicz G, Schwarze J, Ishizuka T, Joetham A, Heusser C, Gelfand EW. Anti-interleukin 5 but not anti-IgE prevents airway inflammation and airway hyperresponsiveness. Am J Respir Crit Care Med 1999; 160:934–941.
156. McLane MP, Haczku A, van de Rijn M, Weiss C, Ferrante V, MacDonald D, Renauld JC, Nicolaides NC, Holroyd KJ, Levitt RC. Interleukin-9 promotes allergen-induced eosinophilic inflammation and airway hyperresponsiveness in transgenic mice. Am J Respir Cell Mol Biol 1998; 19:713–720.
157. Temann UA, Geba GP, Rankin JA, Flavell RA. Expression of interleukin 9 in the lungs of transgenic mice causes airway inflammation, mast cell hyperplasia, and bronchial hyperresponsiveness. J Exp Med 1998; 188:1307–1320.
158. Rothenberg ME, MacLean JA, Pearlman E, Luster AD, Leder P. Targeted disruption of the chemokine eotaxin partially reduces antigen-induced tissue eosinophilia. J Exp Med 1997; 185:785–790.
159. Stafford S, Li H, Bravo R, et al. Monocyte chemotactic protein-3 in eosinophilic inflammation of the airways and the inhibitory effects of an anti-MCP-3 antibody. J Immunol 1997; 158:4953–4960.
160. Lukacs NW, Strieter RM, Warmington K, Lincoln P, Chensue SW, Kunkel SL. Differential recruitment of leukocyte populations and alteration of airway hyperreactivity by C-C family chemokines in allergic airway inflammation. J Immunol 1997; 158:4398–4404.
161. Rosenwasser LJ. Promoter polymorphism in the candidate genes, IL-4, IL-9, TGF-beta 1, for atopy and asthma. Int Arch Allergy Immunol 1999; 118:268–270.
162. Borish LC, Nelson HS, Lanz MJ, Claussen L, Whitmore JB, Agosti JM, Garrison L. IL-4 receptor in moderate atopic asthma. A phase I/II randomized, placebo-controlled trial. Am J Respir Crit Care Med 1999; 160:1816–1823.

12

Mechanisms of Allergic Rhinitis

YONG-JIN PARK

The Catholic University of Korea and St. Vincent's Hospital, Suwon, Korea

JAMES N. BARANIUK

Georgetown University, Washington, D.C.

1 REDUCTIONIST APPROACH TO THE HISTOLOGY AND PHYSIOLOGY OF THE HUMAN NASAL MUCOSA

The functions, capabilities, and pathophysiological changes of the human nasal mucosa can be appreciated from turbinate histology (Fig. 1). A reductionist approach has been developed that identifies four major compartments within the nasal mucosa that account for most of the signs and symptoms of rhinitis (Fig. 2). The superficial postcapillary venules are responsible for the endothelium-directed leakage of plasma that leads to local edema and watery rhinorrhea. These endothelial cells direct leukocyte traffic by the expression of chemoattractants and adhesion markers that recruit the unique sets of interstitial, epithelial, and lumenal cellular inflammation in various forms of rhinitis. The deep venous sinusoids control nasal patency on the minute-to-minute, and longer, ''nasal cycle'' schedules. These vasomotor processes are orchestrated by brain stem rhythms and enacted through autonomical nerves. Finally, the epithelial and glandular serous and mucous cells contribute the sol-phase antimicrobial defense factors (e.g., sIgA), sticky gel-phase mucopolysaccharide mucins, and ionic composition of the nasal epithelial lining fluid (1,2).

Factors modifying the responsiveness of each of these compartments within the mucosa are still under investigation. New immunopathological principles will likely lead to a restructuring of our understanding of the changes that occur during different phases of allergic rhinitis (AR) as we learn more about 1) the various subtypes of lymphocytes driving antigen-specific inflammation; 2) differentiation and restructuring of epithelial and other mucosal structures (e.g., adhesion markers on endothelial and epithelial cells, chemoattractants, or glandular changes); 3) neurogenic mechanisms responsible for irritant syndromes that may occur in the apparent absence of mucosal inflammation (3,4); and 4) the structure of the human genome. It is already clear that the genes expressed

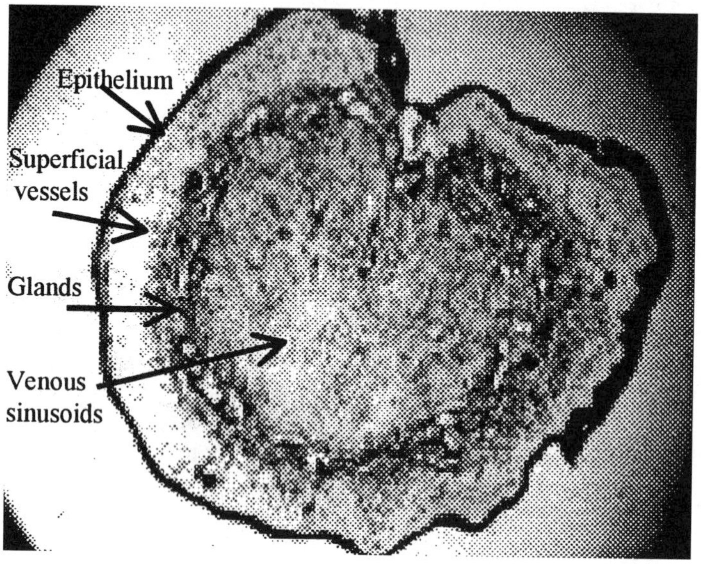

Figure 1 Normal nasal mucosa: This cross section of the inferior turbinate shows the outer layer of typical respiratory epithelium, its basement membrane, and the superficial region of fenestrated capillaries and postcapillary venules. The latter is the region of vascular permeability and inflammatory cell diapedesis. Deep to these superficial vessels are the submucosal glands. At the center of the turbinate are the deep venous sinusoids. Dilation of the sinusoids increases the diameter of the turbinate and reduces the available airspace. Constriction of these vessels leads to nasal patency.

on the distal portion of the long arm of the fifth chromosome (5q31.1-q33) play major roles in atopy, vernal keratoconjunctivitis (5), myelodysplastic (6) and other neoplastic syndromes (Table 1) (7,8). It is also of interest that the β_2-adrenergic, α_{1B}-adrenergic, dopamine type 1A, and glucocorticoid receptors are also clustered to this region (9). Genetic modification of the expression of these genes may become possible in the coming century.

2 OVERVIEW OF THE NASAL ALLERGEN RESPONSE

The standard allergen challenge model will be used to define the phases leading to chronic allergic rhinitis (Fig. 3). Circulating IgE binds to high-affinity Fcε-receptor I (FcεR1 on mast cells and basophils. It is unclear if mast cells circulate through regions of IgE production to pick up their IgE, or if they passively adsorb the IgE from plasma or tissue interstitial fluids. Mast cells exit in postcapillary venules in the mucosa and reside in the submucosal regions. Reexposure to allergen leads to cross-linking of these Fc receptors, and degranulation of these cells. The preformed and newly formed products will be described in the next section. Stimulation of type C ''itch'' fibers leads to neurogenic responses. After the immediate response abates, a ''recruitment phase'' (1) follows, with the infiltration of the tissue by eosinophils, basophils, and Th2 cells. Their activation and mediator release during the late-phase response (LPR) recapitulates much of the pathology of the immediate response. Continued allergen exposure heightens both the immediate- and late-phase responses, so that an exuberant chronic phase of inflammation develops (Fig. 4).

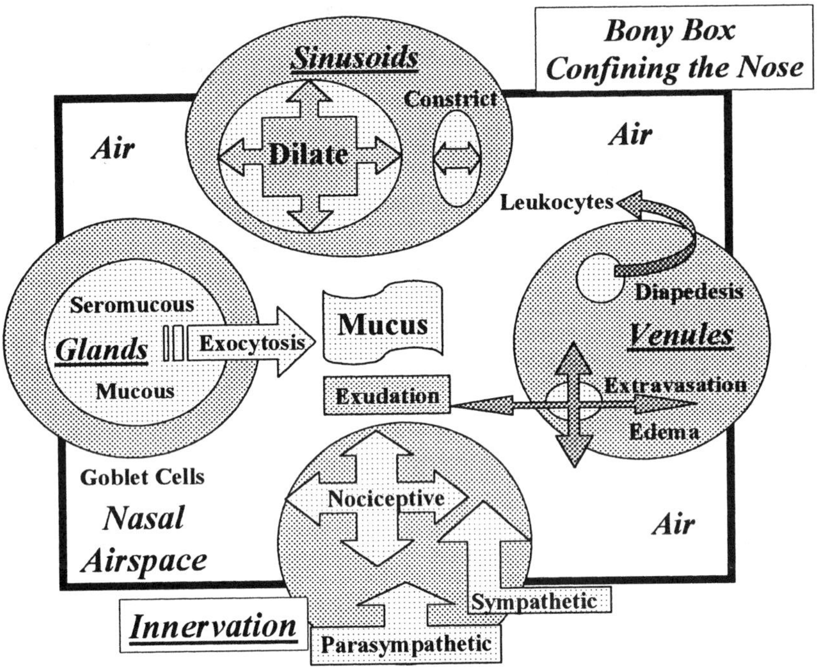

Figure 2 Reductionist view of the nasal mucosa: This schematic separates the four functional components of the nasal mucosa as invaginations into the nasal airspace. (1) The venous sinusoids swell and constrict in response to sympathetic tone and other mechanisms. They serve as the predominant mechanism to regulate nasal airflow and nasal patency. (2) Postcapillary venules are present in the superficial lamina propria and are the site of plasma extravasation and leukocyte diapedesis. Their endothelial cells respond to a wide range of blood-borne and interstitial mediators by contracting, which opens gaps on the basement membrane, expressing adhesion markers, and releasing nitric oxide, endothelin, and other mediators that regulate vascular tone. (3) The "exocytosis" domain comprises surface epithelial goblet, microvilli, and ciliated cells, as well as glandular seromucous and mucous cells. Seromucous cells release antimicrobial factors, such as lysozyme, lactoferrin, sIgA, hyaluronan, neutral mucins, and other factors. Mucous cells and goblet cells release acidic mucins expressing sialic acid and sulfate groups that make them exceedingly "sticky" and permit them to adsorb any particulate or irritant chemicals that may be present on the mucosal surface. (4) The final domain represents the innervation of these structures. Nonmyelinated type C nociceptive nerves are highly branched in the epithelium. There may be functional subsets mediating sensations of itch (H_1-receptors present) or burning pain (capsaicin-sensitive vanillyl receptor present). Parasympathetic nerves include cholinergic nerves, and possibly, a separate set of VIP–nitric oxide–substance P-containing neurons, as has been shown in ferret trachea. Sympathetic fibers are responsible for vasodilation of the venous sinusoids. These fibers contain either norepinephrine or norepinephrine plus neuropeptide Y (NPY). The predominant norepinephrine effect appears to be the vasoconstriction and collapse of the venous sinusoids, thinning of the mucosa, and an increase in nasal patency. NPY is unique in that it can reduce vascular permeability induced, for example, by bradykinin. (Copyright James N. Baraniuk, M.D.)

Table 1 Genes Expressed Along Human Chromosome 5q31.1-q33

IL-3
GM-CSF
IL-5
IL-13
IL-4
IL-9
M-CSF-receptor
IL-12B p40 (40 kDa) monomer
Anonymous gene that may control the maintenance of responsiveness to IL-12
Fibroblast growth factor (FGF-1) (''acidic'')
Early growth response gene 1 (EGRF-1)
Endothelial cell growth factor
Platelet-derived growth factor
Feline myosarcoma viral oncogene homologue (FMS, tyrosine kinase)
CD14 monocyte differentiation factors
Dopamine receptor type 1A
α_{1B}-Adrenergic receptor
β_2-Adrenergic receptor
Glucocorticoid receptor

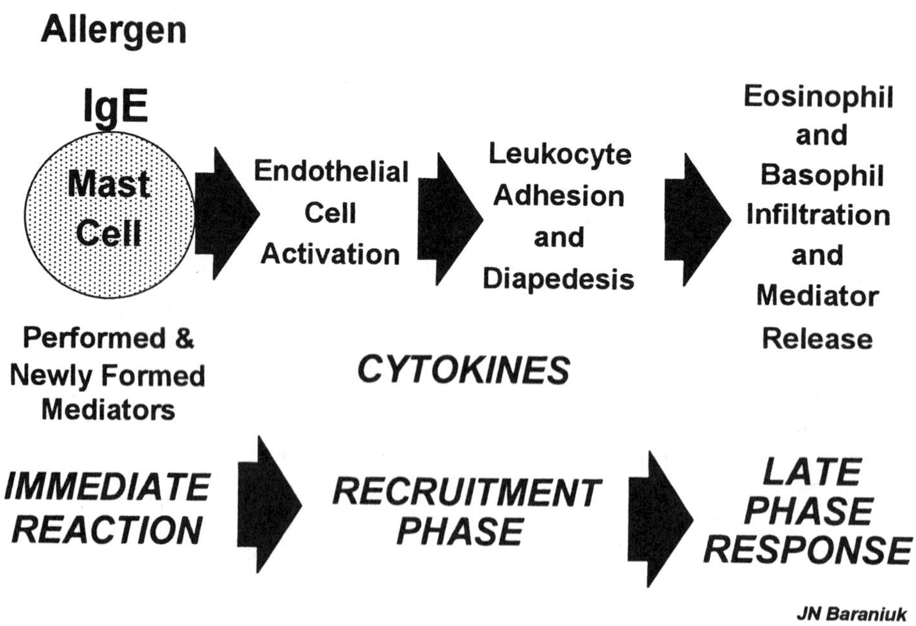

Figure 3 Nasal allergen challenge model: Allergen exposure leads to IgE-mediated mast cell degranulation and the immediate reaction. This is followed by the ''quiescent'' recruitment phase that leads to the inflammatory late-phase response (LPR). This chapter will follow this model to describe the various components of allergic rhinitis.

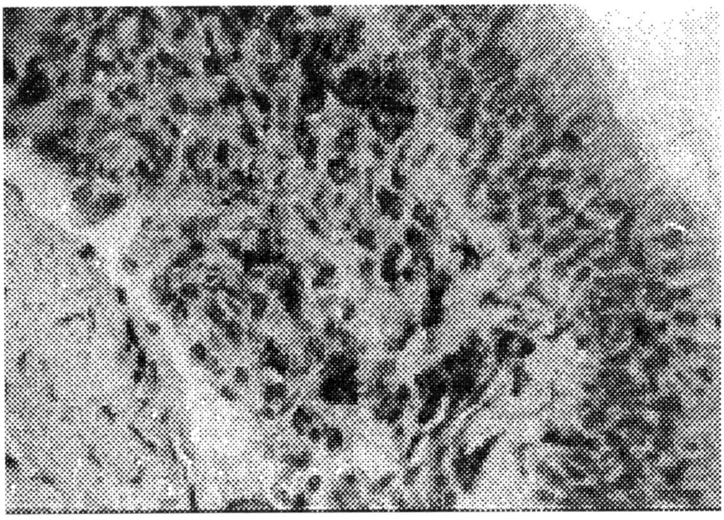

Figure 4 Eosinophilic infiltration during allergic rhinitis.

3 THE CONSEQUENCES OF IMMEDIATE PHASE MAST CELL MEDIATOR RELEASE

Deep-tissue mast cells express chymase, tryptase, and tumor necrosis factor-α (TNF-α) and are termed connective tissue mast cells (MC_{TC}) (10,11). This cell population represents 85% of the interleukin-4 (IL-4)-positive mast cells in the nasal lamina propria. Mast cells in the lamina propria also express IL-13, although it is unclear which subset is involved (12).

During allergen assault, there is an increase in the proportion of epithelial mast cells (13). These cells produce predominantly tryptase, without chymase, and are termed mucosal mast cells (MC_T). MC_T cells are thought to express IL-5, IL-6, and represent 15% of IL-4–positive mast cells (10,11). These cells proliferate in allergic rhinitis, perhaps under the influence of Th2 cytokines (14). Proliferation of MC_T cells appears to occur in the epithelium and most superficial layers of the lamina propria. Epithelial mast cells have a higher rate of cell division in allergic rhinitis than do those of nonallergic nasal mucosa. Epithelial mast cell density is decreased by topical nasal glucocorticoids (13).

The explosive degranulation of mast cells that follows application of allergen to the human nasal mucosa rapidly leads to itch, sneezing, nasal discharge, and mucosal swelling, with increased nasal airways resistance (1,15,16). Histamine plays the preeminent role in these immediate reactions. This is clear from antihistamine studies, because these drugs reduce immediate symptoms by 50–60% (15). Hence, the consequences of histamine release during the immediate phase are greater than the combined immediate effects of tryptase, prostaglandin (PGD_2), $PGF_{2\alpha}$, leukotrienes (LT)C4, LTD4, or LTE4, mast cell kininogenase-mediated production of bradykinin, tumor necrosis factor-α (TNF-α), interleukin-4 (IL-4), IL-5, IL-6, transforming growth factor-β (TGF-β), and IL-13 production (17). Histamine has synergistic effects with this melange of mediators. Leukotrienes and chymase stimulate glandular exocytosis and mucous secretion (18,19). Histamine, bradykinin, leukotrienes, and platelet-activating factor (PAF) activate the endothelial cells of postcapillary venules to induce vasodilation, vascular permeability, and cellular adhesion. Contraction of postcapillary venule endothelial cells opens gaps that permit the hydrostatic intravascular pressure to force plasma into the interstitial space. A pressure of 5 cm H_2O is capable of driving fluid from the vessels through the interstitium, across the epithelial basement membrane, and between epithelial cells' tight junctions, and into the nasal lumen (20). This is a nondamaging, reversible event that is driven by hydrostatic pressure. Plasma exudation may occur without significant tissue edema. Also, the nasal capillaries are fenestrated, which may allow the free exchange of plasma and interstitial fluids, leading to the rapid uptake of medications and mediators that enter the lamina propria.

Histamine activates H_1 receptors on nociceptive nerve fibers to induce the sensation of itching. Histamine receptors belong to the rhodopsin receptor family with seven transmembrane segments, extracellular N-terminal, three extracellular loops, three intracellular loops, and a C-terminal tail (15). These receptors generate intracellular messages by activating GTP-binding protein (G proteins). Three histamine receptors have been cloned. The H_1 receptor is the workhorse for histamine's allergic effects. The H_2 receptor participates in stomach acid production, but also plays a role in vasodilation, and possibly cardiac effects of histamine. H_3 receptors are present on neurons, on which they appear to act as ''inhibitory autoreceptors'' that reduce neural activity (''shut-off'' nerves), and in adipose tissue. H_3 inhibitory autoreceptor activity on nociceptive and parasympathetic nerves is currently subject to intense investigation in humans. Activation of these receptors may hyperpolarize these nerves and reduce the likelihood that they will be depolarized when stimulated by nocifers such as histamine acting through H_1-receptors or preganglionic neurotransmission.

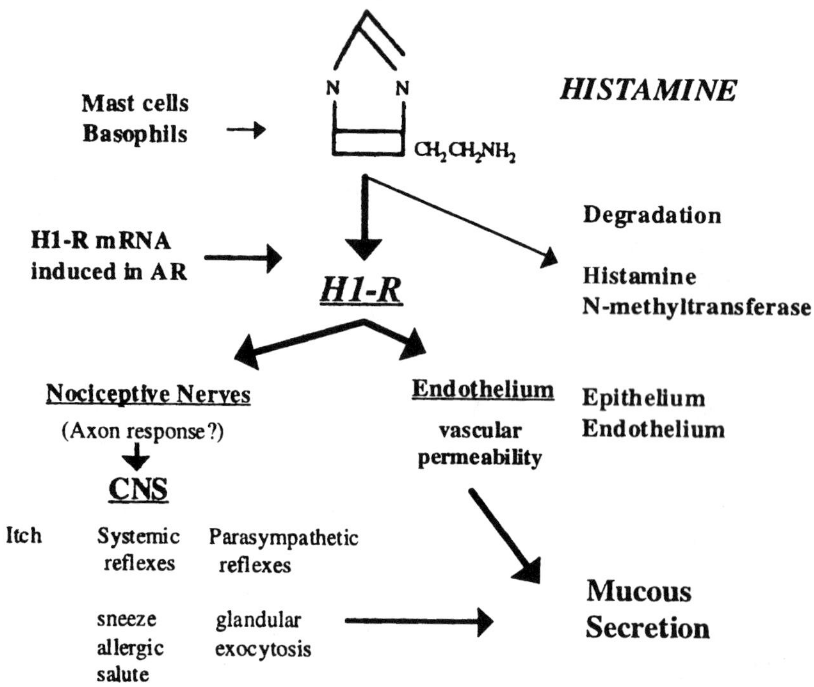

Figure 5 Histamine actions and metabolism.

Table 2 Histamine Releasing Factors

Direct agonists	Augment histamine release	Inhibit histamine release
IgE-dependent HRF	IL-1α, IL-1β	Cromolyn
IL-1	IL-3	Nedocromil
MCP-1	IL-5	TGF-β_1
MCP-3	IL-6	TGF-β_1 antisense oligonucleotides
MIP-1α	IL-7	
NAP-2	c-*kit* ligand	$Fc_\varepsilon R1\alpha$ antisense oligonucleotides
CTAP III		
C3a, C5a		Isoprenaline > salmeterol > albuterol
Opioids		"Sainte" and "Val d'Orb" waters
Vancomycin		
Intravenous contrast dye		Prolonged use of nonsedating antihistamines
High doses of substance P		
Mast cell degranulating peptide		

H_1-receptor mRNA is up-regulated in allergic rhinitis (21). These receptors are present on endothelial cells where they act to induce vascular permeability and the copious watery rhinorrhea of acute allergic rhinitis (22). Histamine has been thought to directly stimulate glandular production of mucus. However, histamine does not induce exocytosis in human nasal mucosal explants in vitro. Instead, histamine appears to activate afferent nociceptive itch nerves, leading to the appreciation of that sensation in the central nervous system, along with recruitment of brain stem parasympathetic reflexes that are responsible for the glandular secretion component. This reflex arc supplies the rational for using anticholinergic drugs in allergic rhinitis, and in other mucous hypersecretory states.

Histamine is degraded by epithelial and endothelial histamine *N*-methyltransferase (HMT; Fig. 5) (23). This action of HMT limits the duration of action of histamine in the mucosa, and explains why allergen provocation testing leads to self-limited vascular leak. Submucosal glands do not express HMT mRNA. The lack of H_1-receptors and HMT on nasal submucosal glands is consistent with the absence of histamine-induced exocytosis observed in vitro (2).

Mast cell mediator release also participates in nonatopic disorders. Anaphylactoid reactions caused by highly charged or ampiphilic molecules, such as intravenous contrast media and vancomycin (red man syndrome), cause immediate reactions, similar to those of IgE-mediated mast cell degranulation. A wide range of peptides, drugs, complement factors (e.g., C3a and C5a released by immune complex formation, as in serum sickness), and other IgE-independent mechanisms can trigger histamine, arachidonic acid metabolite, or cytokine release (Table 2). The difference between anaphylactic and anaphylactoid responses is the ability to demonstrate a reproducible IgE-mediated immediate mechanism.

4 NOCICEPTIVE NERVE RESPONSES

In addition to directly inducing vascular permeability, histamine binds to H_1-receptors on nociceptive type C nerves. Prostaglandins (PGs) and leukotrienes (LTs) increase the sensitivity of these nerves to histamine and other *nocifers* (agents that depolarize nociceptive nerves) (Fig. 6). These nociceptive neurons originate from the first and second divisions of the trigeminal nerve. They are extensively branched in the epithelium and submucosal regions (24). In the mucosa, depolarization of the neuron may lead to the release of neurotransmitters, such as substance P (SP), calcitonin gene-related peptide (CGRP), neurokinin A (NKA), gastrin-releasing peptide (GRP), and possibly others, by the axon response mechanism. These neuropeptides lead to local inflammatory responses termed "neurogenic inflammation." The axon response has been extensively studied in rodents and is thought to induce vascular permeability and leukocyte infiltration (25). However, in normal humans and pigs, the axon response appears to have little if any effect on vascular leak (26,27). The situation may differ in untreated severe allergic subjects who have an increase in basal plasma extravasation as a part of their allergic pathophysiology. The cause for this increase in basal vascular leak is unknown, but does not appear to be related to neurogenic mechanisms (27,28). This leak may be amenable to treatment with β_2-adrenergic agonists (29). Because of this disconnect between the vascular neurogenic responses of the animal models and their apparent absence in humans, the role of the nociceptive nerve axon response in human airway mucosa has been called into question (28). This discrepancy suggests that rodents are not a totally suitable model for human airway neurogenic inflammation.

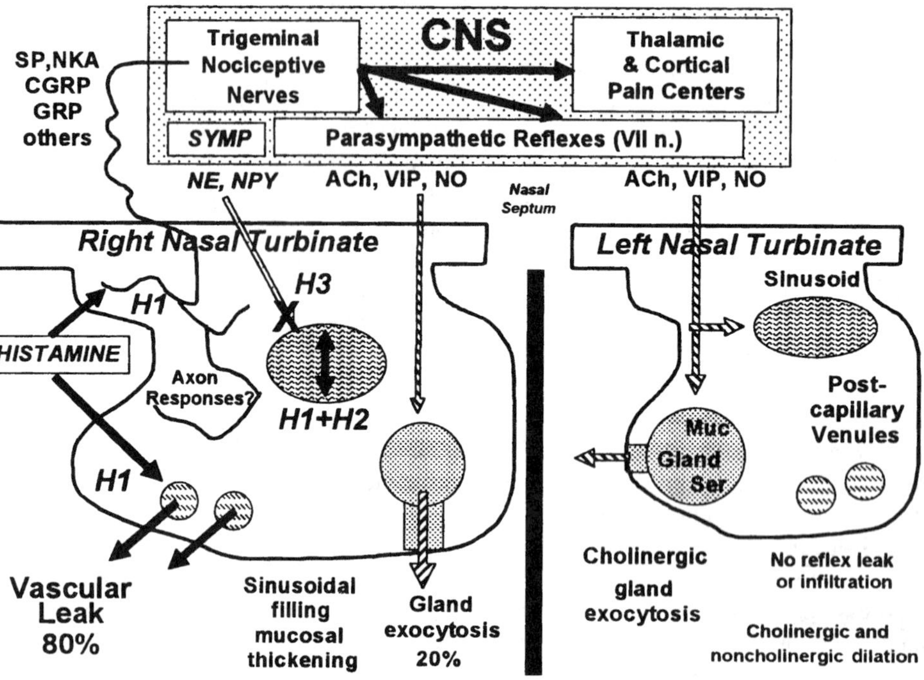

Figure 6 How the nose runs: Histamine acts on H_1-receptors to induce vascular permeability, and activate nociceptive nerves that recruit parasympathetic reflexes. Activation of nociceptive nerves may lead to axon–response-mediated release of neuropeptides, such as substance P and calcitonin gene-related peptide, but the most potent effects are to activate brain stem centers that recruit systemic reflexes, such as sneezing, and parasympathetic cholinergic reflexes that mediate glandular secretion in allergic rhinitis.

In humans, it is likely that neurogenic inflammation is present, as SP and CGRP are released within 3 min after allergen challenge (25) and after hypertonic saline nasal provocation (30). An alternative hypothesis is that human airway axon responses may generate other defensive effects, such as glandular secretion and endothelial adhesion marker expression, that are aimed at limiting an initial mucosal insult and for preparing for further potential nociceptive stimuli. Hypertonic saline provocation leads to pain, SP release, and glandular secretion, but does not cause changes in vascular permeability or dilation of venous sinusoids (31). These data indicate that, in normal humans, the airway mucosal axon response induces the secretion of serous cell antibacterial enzymes, such as lysozyme, lactoferrin, and secretory IgA, plus mucin mucoglycoproteins from mucous and perhaps goblet cells.

This controversy about the roles of the axon responses in normal and inflamed nasal and bronchial mucosa will likely rage until tachykinin antagonists that block the actions of SP and other peptides are investigated in human allergic rhinitis. Differences in neurogenic responses may be due to the degree of underlying mucosal inflammation, as SP does have more potent effects in severe, untreated allergic rhinitis than in normal subjects. Repeated SP application leads to vascular permeability, with an increase in albumin-rich plasma exudation detectable in nasal lavage fluids (32). The percentages of eosinophils in nasal secretions were also significantly increased after SP treatment, increasing from approximately 18 to 42%. In vitro, treatment of human nasal mucosal explants with SP leads to significant increases in IL-1β, IL-2, IL-3, IL-4, IL-5, IL-6, TNF-α, and interferon-γ (IFN-γ) mRNA production from allergic rhinitis nasal mucosa (33). In tissue from nonallergic subjects, SP significantly increased only IL-6 and IL-8. This suggests that during acute allergic inflammation, SP may have a larger effect than in nonallergic rhinitis and normal mucosa. The sites of SP-induced cytokine production may include epithelial, endothelial, and inflammatory cells in these explants.

CGRP may be the mediator of vasodilation in human nasal mucosa, and is likely to be responsible for the venous sinusoid swelling that blocks nasal airflow (34). It is also likely the mediator of the flare responses after allergen skin testing and the triple response of Lewis.

In the central nervous system (CNS), trigeminal nociceptive neurons enter the pons through the sensory root and turn caudally in the trigeminal spinal tract to terminate in the pars caudalis of the nucleus of the spinal tract in the lower medulla and upper three cervical segments of the spinal cord (24). Pars caudalis interneurons cross the midline to enter the trigeminothalamic tract and terminate in the medial part of the ventral posterior thalamic nucleus. Painful and strong thermal stimuli are appreciated at the thalamic level. Tertiary neural relays to the lower third of the parietal cortical somesthetic areas provide for localization of nasal stimuli. Glossopharyngeal afferents innervate the posterior third of the tongue, upper pharynx, tonsils, eustachian tube, and middle ear, and are also of relevance to allergic rhinitis. These thermosensitive and nociceptive neurons terminate in the dorsal portion of the trigeminal spinal tract. Activation of these central registries is responsible for the sensations of itch and congestion that are the hallmarks of allergic rhinitis.

5 PARASYMPATHETIC REFLEXES

Connections between afferent trigeminal interneurons, the tractus solitarius, nucleus ambiguus, and salivatory nucleus of the seventh nerve serve to recruit parasympathetic reflexes.

Seventh nerve motor fibers synapse in the sphenopalatine ganglia and pass with sympathetic fibers through the Vidian canal to enter the nasal mucosa. These postganglionic neurons contain acetylcholine, vasoactive intestinal peptide (VIP), VIP-like peptides (e.g., peptide histidine–methionine; PHM), and nitric oxide synthase (generates nitric oxide; NO). It is possible that these are packaged in different sets of neurons. Parasympathetic reflexes are rapidly activated after allergen challenge because VIP is released within 3 min after nasal allergen provocation (35).

One of the most important functions of nociceptive nerves appears to be the activation of the central itch registries with recruitment of systemic reflexes, such as sneezing, and organ-specific parasympathetic reflexes that lead to cholinergic glandular secretion (see Fig. 6). Reflex vasodilation appears to occur, but may be of less functional significance. Suggestions of parasympathetic nerve-related cellular chemoattraction remain controversial (21,36).

Cholinergic stimulation of glandular exocytosis is probably the most important single tonically active influence regulating glandular secretion in the respiratory tract. Histamine likely induces glandular secretion by activating these nociceptive–parasympathetic reflexes. This reflex provides the rationale for the use of ipratropium bromide and other anticholinergic antagonists in allergic rhinitis (37). The M_3-muscarinic receptor is likely the most important of the five cloned muscarinic receptors in human nasal mucosa, based on functional and in situ hybridization studies (38,39). The M_2-receptors on nociceptive nerves may serve as inhibitory autoreceptors. Alkaline eosinophilic proteins (ECP), such as major basic protein (MBP), and influenza virus neuraminidase, may bind the M_2-receptor and inhibit its function. This could be one example of eosinophil-mediated neural dysfunction.

6 RECRUITMENT PHASE WITH CHEMOATTRACTION OF INFLAMMATORY CELLS

Following the immediate phase, especially if the allergic person leaves the vicinity of the allergen or has allergen provocation, there will be a diminution of symptoms after the first hour. However, the mast cell cytokines and other mediators that are released have longer durations of action than histamine, bradykinin, PGD_2, or leukotrienes. The cytokines activate endothelial and other resident cells to promote up-regulation of adhesion molecules, secondary release of chemoattractants, and adhesion of specific sets of in-

Table 3 Summary of Cytokines Relevant to Rhinitis

Chemokines					
C-X-C (α) chromosome 4	C-C (β) chromosome 17	Inflammatory cytokines	Fibrinogenic cytokines	Growth factors	Neurotrophins
IL-8	MCP-1	IL-1α,β	PDGF	GM-CSF	IL-6
PF-4	MCP-3	TNF-α	IGF	G-CSF	IL-11
NAP-2	RANTES	IL-10	FGF	M-CSF	LIF
CTAP III	MIP-1α	IL-12			CNF
(GRO-1)	IL-13				Oncostatin M
(GRO-2)	IL-15				
Lungkine					

Table 4 Nonlymphoid Sources of Cytokines

Macrophage	Epithelium	Eosinophils	Mast cells
IL-12	GM-CSF	IL-5	IL-3
IFN-α	IL-6	GM-CSF	IL-4
TNF-α	IL-8	TNF-α	IL-5
Eotaxin	Eotaxin	Eotaxin	TNF-α
			TGF-β
			IL-13
			IL-6

flammatory leukocytes (e.g., eosinophils and basophils). This "first signal" leading to enhanced adhesion is combined with the "second signal" of chemokines that act to recruit the specific and unique pattern of active inflammatory cells to the injured tissue. The chemokines and specific patterns of endothelial adhesion markers expressed during this "recruitment phase" (1) are responsible for the accumulation of eosinophils, basophils, Th2 cells, and other leukocytes that characterize the allergic late-phase response (LPR) (Table 3 and 4). Details of these cytokine-mediated effects on endothelial and inflammatory cells are discussed at length in the remainder of this book.

7 LATE PHASE-RESPONSE AND CHRONIC ALLERGIC RHINITIS

Histamine is released without a change in tryptase, suggesting release from basophils, rather than a secondary degranulation of mast cells (20,21,40,41). The role of histamine in the late-phase response (LPR) is less prominent than during the immediate phase, as evidenced by the lower level of itch and sneezing. Nasal blockage develops, but it is unclear if this is due to venous sinusoid filling, nasal secretion production, or an increase in mucosal bulk owing to leukocyte invasion of the tissue.

During prolonged, recurrent, and chronic nasal allergic inflammation, histamine may be continually released. This is indicated by the benefits of prolonged antihistamine therapy. However, the flood of cytokines and other mediators released from infiltrating eosinophils, epithelial mast cells, and Th2 lymphocytes in perennial rhinitis (see Tables 2–4) can be greater than the effects of histamine, leading to symptoms that are not amenable to antihistamine therapy.

8 EPITHELIAL CELL CHANGES IN ALLERGIC RHINITIS

The influx of inflammatory cells, and up-regulation of endothelial cell function are not the only changes in allergic rhinitis. Epithelial cells also appear to be activated because they express increased amounts of granulocyte–monocyte colony-stimulating factor (GM-CSF), IL-1α, IL-8, and IL-1-receptors; TNF-α-receptors; and class II HLA (HLA-DR) (42,43). Cytokines and ECP also up-regulate intercellular adhesion molecule (ICAM)-1 expression on nasal epithelial cells (44).

Endothelin-1 (ET1), which is expressed by epithelial and submucosal gland cells in human mucosa (45) and the enzyme that generates ET1 (endothelin-converting enzyme 1) are up-regulated in chronic rhinitis (46).

Nitric oxide is present in nasal air, and its levels in exhaled nasal air are increased during allergic rhinitis. Levels rise from 24.7 ± 2.2 ppb to 35.4 ± 2.0 ppb ($p < 0.001$) (47). The source of the NO is under active investigation, but may include endothelial cells that express constitutive type III NOS, parasympathetic neurons that express type I NOS and colocalized VIP, and macrophages, neutrophils, mast cells, arterial smooth-muscle cells, and fibroblasts that may be induced to express type II NOS (48) NO may promote vasodilation, glandular secretion, and immunomodulation, and because it is a free radical, it may have an antibacterial function.

9 GLANDULAR CHANGES

Submucosal gland area is increased in perennial allergic rhinitis (PAR) compared with normal and hypertrophic rhinitis subjects. The latter condition likely represents a form of nonallergic rhinitis, with increased turbinate size, leading to a requirement for turbinectomy. Submucosal glands represent approximately 15% of the lamina propria in normal and nonallergic subjects. However, in PAR and chronic sinusitis, gland area increases to approximately 25% (49). This is consistent with the mucous hypersecretion that has been suggested to be present in allergic airway disease.

Mucous hypersecretion is the results of increased submucosal gland mucous cell mucin exocytosis, goblet cell hyperplasia, plasma extravasation, with formation of intralumenal albumin–fibrin–mucin globules, and potentially reductions in free water or the less viscous submucosal gland serous cell products. In guinea pig and rat airways, platelet-activating factor (PAF) increases acidic mucin and MUC5 gene expression (50). This effect is potentiated by TNF-α. Epidermal growth factor (EGF) may be responsible for goblet cell hyperplasia and increased MUC5AC mRNA and protein expression (51). In lower-airway submucosal glands, MUC5B is expressed in mucous cells, whereas MUC7 is expressed only in lysozyme-producing serous cells (52). Irritants, such as acrolein, appear to increase MUC5AC mRNA, whereas, MUC5B was constitutively expressed by NCI-H292 human lung carcinoma cell line (53). IL-4 increased MUC2, MUC5, and mucous glycoconjugate expression in both NCI-H292 and mouse bronchi in vivo (54;) whereas, overexpression of IL-3 leads to rapid goblet cell proliferation and mucous hypersecretion (55).

These findings are likely applicable to human nasal mucosa given the expression of mucin genes in human nasal airways. MUC5AC mRNA levels were five- to tenfold higher than MUC1 and MUC2 in allergic rhinitis, cystic fibrosis, and normal subjects. MUC2 mRNA was similar in all subjects; whereas, MUC5A/C was significantly reduced in cystic fibrosis (56). This is in contrast with the A549 cell line in which MUC5AC was increased by neutrophil elastase, an inflammatory mediator thought to play a central role in cystic fibrosis pathophysiology (57). Conclusions drawn from human disease states, rather than in vitro cell studies, should take precedence in developing paradigms for pathogenic molecular mechanisms of mucin hyperexpression.

Treatment of mucous hypersecretion has focused on guaifenesin and related compounds. Their mechanisms of action are still debated. They may induce gastric irritation with generation of parasympathetic reflexes that increase low-viscosity serous cell exocytosis, or they may have the ability to reduce disulfide bond cross-linking of intralumenal mucins in globules (58,59). Glucocorticoids may reduce mucous hypersecretion by limiting airway inflammation, the production of mediators responsible for mucin synthesis and mucous cell hyperplasia, and normalization of epithelial histology (increase in ciliated cell expression).

10 HYPERRESPONSIVENESS

Hyperresponsiveness is a characteristic of mucosal surfaces during inflammation. Hyperresponsiveness indicates an increased mucosal response to ''nonspecific'' irritants, such as histamine, methacholine, bradykinin, hypertonic saline, cold, dry air, or other provocational agents (60,61). Persons with allergic rhinitis have increased glandular secretion when stimulated with endothelin-1, bradykinin, and histamine. Stimulation of nociceptive nerves, with recruitment of parasympathetic reflexes, is the postulated mechanism. Glandular responses to methacholine are also increased (62). In addition, VIP-immunoreactive nerve fibers may be increased in density, as has been suggested for chronic bronchitis and cholinergic nonallergic rhinitis (63,64). VIP has been proposed as an additional glandular secretagogue that participates in parasympathetic reflexes. In contrast with glandular hypersecretion, histamine-induced vascular permeability and ''exudative hyperresponsiveness'' does not appear to involve nociceptive axon responses or other neural effects (27).

The molecular mechanisms underlying the increase in nociceptive nerve sensitivity to these nocifers, the increases in the parasympathetic reflex components, and changes in mucosal mucous production, and secretory processes, still remain to be defined. When inflammatory mediators bind to their specific neurokinin-1 (NK-1), histamine H_1, muscarinic M_3, bradykinin B_2, and other seven-transmembrane receptors, conformation changes induced in the receptor lead to activation of the intracellular GTP-binding $\alpha\beta\gamma$-trimeric proteins that associate with the third intracellular loop of these receptors. This, in turn, leads to a cascade of signal transduction effects that can activate transcription factors, such as the immediate early genes c-*fos* and c-*jun* that form the activating protein-1 (AP-1) complex, and the release of active nuclear factor-κB (NF-κB) from its inhibitor (IκB). Other transduction pathways also play roles in cellular activation in atopy. These transcript factors bind to promoters of a wide range of genes in the nucleus, leading to the production of additional proinflammatory proteins, receptors, and mediators (Fig. 7). Cytokines have other transduction pathways that lead to the further up-regulation of mRNA production. In general, mRNA transcription requires continued proinflammatory mediator release and receptor binding with transcription factor activation to be maintained.

Nociceptive nerve responses and neurogenic inflammation may be up-regulated by neurotrophic cytokines, such as nerve growth factor (NGF) and IL-11 (Table 3). IL-11 may participate in the pathogenesis of viral rhinitis and asthma (65). Nasal instillation of IL-11 in mice leads 24 hr later to cholinergic bronchial reactivity, with minimal peribronchial infiltrates. Children with common colds, who have elevated IL-11 concentrations in their nasal secretions, are more likely to develop asthma. In addition, the asthmatic subset had significantly increased IL-11 lavage levels compared with those who did not develop wheezing. The role of IL-11 and similar cytokines requires further investigation in allergic rhinitis.

In contrast to this hyperresponsiveness, hyporesponsiveness can also occur. For example, in chronic sinusitis, patients have high-baseline secretion of glandular products, but have no reserve to exocytose additional materials when challenged with the glandular secretagogue methacholine (66). This suggests that the glands were acting at their maximal

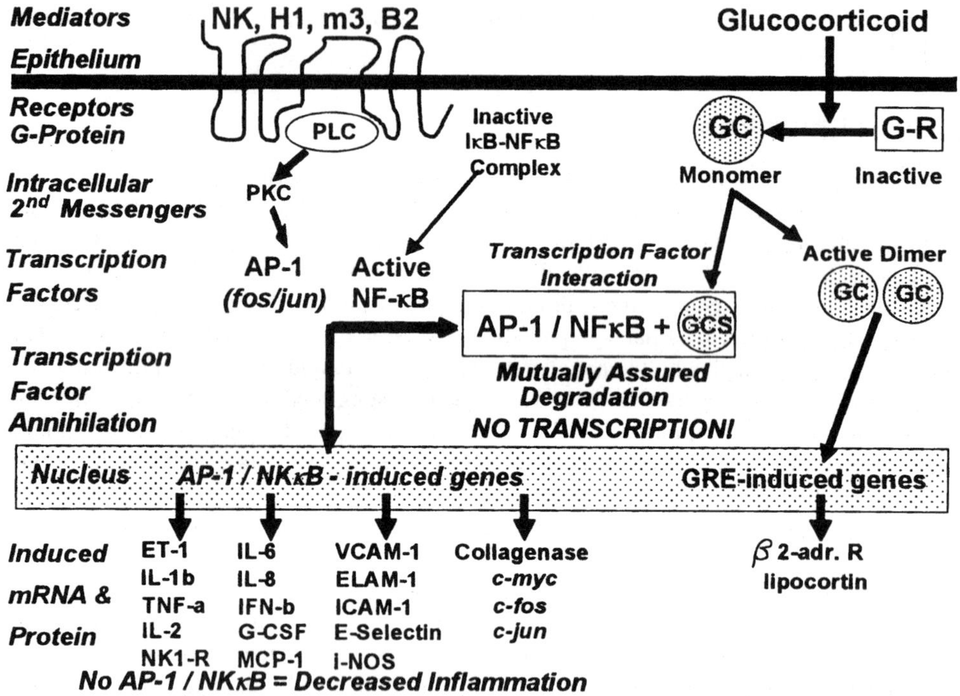

Figure 7 Hypothesis: c-*fos*/*AP-1* interactions with glucocorticoids: Activation of neurokinin (NK), histamine H_1, muscarinic M_3, bradykinin B_2, and other seven-transmembrane receptors leads to the activation of c-*fos* and c-*jun*, and the formation of *AP-1* (left). *AP-1* participates in the induction of a wide variety of proinflammatory proteins, receptors, and mediators. Glucocorticoids bind to cytoplasmic receptors, which dimerize and translocate to the nucleus to induce genes such as the β_2-adrenergic receptor (right). *AP-1* and activated glucocorticoid receptors can bind to each other, leading to their mutual proteolytic degradation, and the loss of their nuclear transcription factor effects.

rate of exocytosis because of high mucosal secretagogue levels, or that they had developed tachyphylaxis or unresponsiveness to further muscarinic challenge.

11 THERAPEUTIC MECHANISMS

Intranasal glucocorticoids remain the premier topical anti-inflammatory drugs for allergic rhinitis. They are effective at reducing basal vascular leak in allergic rhinitis and allergen-induced nasal hyperresponsiveness (44,60). Intranasal glucocorticoids reduce the densities of mucosal mast cells and eosinophils in the epithelium, which leads to a decrease in proinflammatory mediator release. Glucocorticoids also modulate c-*fos*, c-*jun*, and NF-κB activities within inflammatory and resident cells (see Fig. 7). The steroids bind to cytoplasmic glucocorticoid receptors, which dissociate from heat-shock proteins, dimerize, and translocate to the nucleus (67). There, this complex acts on glucocorticoid response elements (GRE) in promoters of genes, such as the β_2-adrenergic receptor, and increase their expression. The most critical anti-inflammatory action of steroids is mediated by the interactions between the activated glucocorticoid receptor monomers and *AP-*

1, NF-κB, and other proinflammatory gene-activating factors. These interactions lead to mutual proteolytic degradation, and the loss of all transcriptional activity for each factor. As an example, nasal steroids reduce the expression of epithelial c-*fos*-immunoreactive material in human nasal polyps in vivo (68).

The benefits of antihistamines have focused on treatment of itch and vascular permeability. These benefits are shared by both sedating and nonsedating "second-generation" antihistamines. The older drugs are less specific for the H_1 receptor and also block other receptors. The anticholinergic effects of brompheniramine and chlorpheniramine have been demonstrated. They are about 19 times less potent than atropine in a model of methacholine-induced glandular secretion from human nasal mucosal explants in vitro (69). These older antihistaminics may offer some advantages for patients with allergic rhinitis and mucous hypersecretion who are more resistant to the sedating side effects. The sedation may be related to both the antihistaminic and anticholinergic properties of these drugs in the CNS. Several other treatments may also assist in reducing the potency of histamine's effects. Following allergy immunotherapy, there is reduced histamine, bradykinin, and TAME-esterase concentrations in nasal lavage fluids collected during both the immediate and early phases after nasal allergen challenge (70).

The search for drugs to inhibit mast cell degranulation began with cromolyn, but continues now with very mixed success. Transforming growth factor-β_1 (TGF-β_1) (71) or, contrarily, antisense oligonucleotides to TGF-β_1 (72), may inhibit histamine release. Sufficiently high doses of β_2-adrenergic agonists may also be successful (29), although in isolated human lung mast cells the rank potency for inhibition of mediator release was isoproterenol > salmeterol > albuterol (salbutamol) (73). Healing "therapeutic waters" (74), herbal remedies, and prolonged use of nonsedating antihistamines (75) have been reported to reduce the release of histamine and other mediators from rat and human mast cells in several in vivo and in vitro systems. However, these reports must be viewed with deep skepticism until their claims are examined by double-blind, placebo-controlled trials in allergic rhinitis. It is anticipated that the molecular biology explosion that is engulfing medical research will lead to exciting and revolutionary new drugs, and entirely new concepts of antiallergic and anti-inflammatory therapy. For the allergic rhinitis sufferer, however, these wonder drugs may be 5–15 years away, given the current rate of development and regulatory review separating the bench from the bedside.

ACKNOWLEDGMENTS

Supported by U.S. Public Health Service Award AI42403 and Environmental Protection Agency Award R825814.

Although the research described in this chapter has been funded wholly or in part by the United States Environmental Protection Agency through grant number R825814 to James N. Baraniuk, M.D., it has not been subjected to the agency's required peer and policy review and, therefore, does not necessarily reflect the views of the Agency and no official endorsement should be inferred.

REFERENCES

1. Baraniuk JN. Pathogenesis of allergic rhinitis. J Allergy Clin Immunol 1997; 99:S763–S772.
2. Raphael GD, Meredith SD, Baraniuk JN, Druce HM, Banks SM, Kaliner MA. The pathophysi-

ology of rhinitis. II. Assessment of the sources of protein in histamine-induced nasal secretions. Am Rev Respir Dis 1989; 139:791–800.
3. Baraniuk JN, Clauw JD, Gaumond E. Rhinitis symptoms in chronic fatigue syndrome. Annl Allergy Asthma Immunol 1998; 81:359–365.
4. Baraniuk JN, Clauw D, Yuta A, Ali M, Gaumond M, Upadhyayula N, Fujita K, Shimizu T. Nasal secretion analysis in allergic rhinitis, cystic fibrosis, and nonallergic fibromyalgia/chronic fatigue syndrome subjects. Am J Rhinol 1998; 12:435–440.
5. Bonini S, Bonini O, Lambiase A, Magrini L, Rumi C, Del Prete G, Schianvone M, Rotiroti G, Onorati P, Rutella S. Vernal keratoconjunctivitis: a model of 5q cytokine gene cluster disease. Int Arch Allergy Immunol 1995; 107:95–98.
6. Mareni C, Sessarego M, Montera M, Fugazza G, Origone P, D'Amato D, Lerza R, Pistoia V, Scarra GB. Expression and genomic configuration of GM-CSF, IL-3, M-CSR receptor (C-FMS), early growth response gene-1 (EGR-1) and M-CSF genes in primary myelodysplastic syndromes. Leukemia Lymphoma 1994; 15:135–141.
7. Frazer KA, Ueda Y, Zhu Y, Gifford VR, Garofalo MR, Mohandas N, Martin CH, Pallazzolo MJ, Cheng JF, Rubin EM. Computational and biological analysis of 680 kb of DNA sequence from the human 5q31 cytokine gene cluster region. Genome Res 1997; 7:495–512.
8. Smirnov DV, Smirnova MG, Korobko VG, Frolova EI. Tandem arrangement of human genes for intereleukin-4 and interleukin-13: resemblance in their organization. Gene 1995; 155:277–281.
9. Kruskal J, Xiong M, Ferrell R, Sing CF, Turner ST, Boerwinkle E. Linkage and association of adrenergic and dopamine receptor genes in the distal portion of the long arm of chromosome 5 with systemic blood pressure variation. Hum Mol Genet 1998; 7:1379–1383.
10. Bradding P, Okayama Y, Howarth PH, Church MK, Holgate ST. Heterogeneity of human mast cells based on cytokines content. J Immunol 1995; 155:297–307.
11. Bradding P, Mediwake R, Feather IH, Madden J, Church MK, Holgate ST, Howarth PH. TNF-α is localized to nasal mucosal mast cells and is released in acute allergic rhinitis. Clin Exp Allergy 1995; 25:406–415.
12. Pawankar RU, Okuda M, Hasegawa S, Suzuki K, Yssel H, Okubo K, Okumura K, Ra C. Interleukin-13 expression in the nasal mucosal of perennial allergic rhinitis. Am J Respir Crit Care Med 1995; 152:2059–2067.
13. Juluisson S, Aldenborg F, Enerback L. Protease content of mast cells of nasal mucosa: effects of natural allergen exposure and of local corticosteroid treatment. Allergy 1995; 50:15–22.
14. Kawabori Y, Kanai N, Tosho T. Proliferative activity of mast cells in allergic nasal mucosa. Clin Exp Allergy 1995; 25:173–178.
15. Simons FE. Histamine and H1-Antagonists in Allergic Disease. New York: Marcel Dekker, 1996.
16. Terada N, Kono A, Togawa K. Biochemical properties of eosinophils and their preferential accumulation mechanism in nasal allergy. J Allergy Clin Immunol 1994; 94:629–642.
17. Naclerio RM, Baroody FM, Kagey–Sobotka A, Lichtenstein LM. Basophils and eosinophils in allergic rhinitis. J Allergy Clin Immunol 1994; 94:1303–1309.
18. Holgate ST, Bradding BM, Sampson AP. Leukotriene antagonists and synthesis inhibitors: new directions in asthma therapy. J Allergy Clin Immunol 1996; 98:1–13.
19. Sommerhof CP, Caughey GH, Finkbeiner WE, Lazarus SC, Basbaum CB, Nadel JA. Mast cell chymase: a potent secretagogue for airway gland serous cells. J Immunol 1989; 142:2450–2456.
20. Erjefalt I, Persson CG. Allergen, bradykinin, and capsaicin increase outward but not inward macromolecular permeability of guinea-pig tracheobronchial mucus. Clin Exp Allergy 1991; 21:217–224.
21. Iriyoshi N, Takeuchi K, Yuta A, Ukai K, Sakakura Y. Increased pathology of allergic rhinitis: expression of histamine H_1 receptor mRNA in allergic rhinitis. Clin Exp Allergy 1996; 26: 379–385.

22. Okayama M, Baraniuk JN, Hausfeld JN, Merida M, Kaliner MA. Characterization and autoradiographic localization of histamine H_1 receptors in human nasal turbinates. J Allergy Clin Immunol 1992; 89:1144–1150.
23. Okayama M, Yamauchi K, Sekizawa K, Okayama H, Sasaki H, Inamura N, Maeyama K, Watanabe T, Takishima T, Shirato K. Localization of histamine *N*-methyltransferase messenger RNA in human nasal mucosa. J Allergy Clin Immunol 1995; 95:96–102.
24. Baraniuk JN. Neuropeptide pharmacology. In: Townley RG, Agarwal DK, eds. Immunopharmacology of the Respiratory Tract. Clinical Allergy and Immunology 8. New York: Marcel Dekker, 1996:575–603.
25. McDonald DM. Neurogenic inflammation in the respiratory tract: actions of sensory nerve mediators on blood vessels and epithelium of the airway mucosa. Am Rev Respir Dis 1987; 136:S65–S72.
26. Stjarne P, Lacroix JS, Anggard A, Lundberg JM. Compartment analysis of vascular effects of neuropeptides and capsaicin in the pig nasal mucosa. Acta Physiol Scand 1991; 141:335–342.
27. Svensson C, Andersson M, Greiff L, Alkner U, Persson CGA. Exudative hyperresponsiveness of the airway microcirculation in seasonal allergic rhinitis. Clin Exp Allergy 1995; 25:942–950.
28. Joos GF, Germonpre PR, Pauwels RA. Neurogenic inflammation in human airways: it is important? Thorax 1995; 50:217–219.
29. Proud D, Reynolds CJ, Lichtenstein LM, Kagey–Sobotka A, Togias A. Intranasal salmeterol inhibits allergen-induced vascular permeability but not mast cell activation or cellular infiltration. Clin Exp Allergy 1998; 28:868–875.
30. Fang, S–Y, Ali M, Yuta A, Baraniuk J. Hypertonic saline nasal provocation induces substance P release: airway neurogenic inflammation redefined. Am J Respir Crit Care Med 1998; 157: A487.
31. Baraniuk JN, Ali M, Yuta A, Fang S–Y, Naranch K. Hypertonic saline nasal provocation stimulates nociceptive nerves, substance P release, and glandular mucus exocytosis in normal humans. Am J Respir Crit Care Med 1999; 160:655–662.
32. Fajac I, Braunstein G, Ickovic MR, Lacronique J, Frossard N. Selective recruitment of eosinophils by substance P after repeated allergen exposure in allergic rhinitis. Allergy 1995; 50: 970–975.
33. Okamoto Y, Shirotori K, Kudo K, Ishikawa K, Ito E, Togaw K, Saito I. Cytokine expression after the topical administration of substance P to human nasal mucosa: the role of substance P in nasal allergy. J Immunol 1993; 151:4391–4398.
34. Rinder J, Lundberg JM. Effects of hCGRP8-37 and the NK1-recptor antagonist SR140.333 on capsaicin-evoked vasodilation in the pig nasal mucosa in vivo. Allergologie 1:48, 1996.
35. Mossiman BL, White MV, Hohman RJ, Goldrich MS, Kaulbach HC, Kaliner MA. Substance P, calcitonin-gene related peptide, and vasoactive intestinal peptide increase in nasal secretions after allergen challenge in atopic patients. J Allergy Clin Immunol 1993; 92:95–104.
36. Sanico AM, Atsuta S, Togias A. Leukocyte influx after capsaicin nasal challenge is a dose dependent phenomenon. J Allergy Clin Immunol 1996; 97:A430.
37. Baraniuk NJ, Silver PB, Kaliner MA, Barnes PJ. Effects of ipratropium bromide on bradykinin nasal provocation in humans. Clin Exp Allergy 1994; 14:724–729.
38. Baraniuk JN, Kaliner MA, Barnes PJ. Localization of M_3 muscarinic receptor mRNA in human nasal mucosa. Am J Rhinol 1992; 6:145–148.
39. Mullol J, Baraniuk JN, Logun C, Merida M, Hausfeld JH, Shelhamer JH, Kaliner MA. M_1 and M_3 muscarinic antagonists inhibit human nasal glandular secretion in vitro. J Appl Physiol 1992; 73:2069–2073.
40. Gosset P, Malaquin F, Delnest Y, Wallaert B, Capron A, Joseph M, Tonnel AB. Interleukin 6 and interleukin 1β production is associated with antigen induced late nasal response. J Allergy Clin Immunol 1993; 92:878–890.

41. Togias A. Non-allergic rhinitis. In: Mygind N, Naclerio RM, eds. Allergic and Non-Allergic Rhinitis—Clinical Aspects. Philadelphia: WB Saunders, 1993:159–166.
42. Nonaka N, Nonaka R, Jordana M, Dolovich J. Am J Respir Crit Care Med 1996; 153:1675–1681.
43. Kenney JS, Baker C, Welch MR, Altman LC. Synthesis of interleukin-1α, interleukin-6, and interleukin-8 by cultured human nasal epithelial cells. J Allergy Clin Immunol 1994; 3:1060–1067.
44. Altman LC, Ayars GH, Baker C, Luchtel DL. Cytokines and eosinophil derived cationic proteins up-regulate intercellular adhesion molecule 1 on human nasal epithelial cells. J Allergy Clin Immunol 1993; 92:527–536.
45. Mullol J, Chowdoury BA, White MV, Ohkubo K, Reives RD, Baraniuk JN, Hausfield JN, Shelhamer JH, Kaliner MA. Endothelin in human nasal mucosa. Am J Respir Cell Mol Biol 1993; 8:393–402.
46. Furukawa K, Saleh D, Bayan F, Emoto N, Kaw S, Yanagisawa M, Giaid A. Coexpression of endothelin 1 and endothelin converting enzyme 1 in patients with chronic rhinitis. Am J Respir Cell Mol Biol 1996; 14:248–253.
47. Martin U, Bryden K, Devoy M, Howarth P. Increased levels of exhaled nitric oxide during nasal and oral breathing in subjects with seasonal rhinitis. J Allergy Clin Immunol 1996; 7: 768–772.
48. Fischer A, Hoffman B. Nitric oxide synthase in neurons and nerve fibres of lower airways and in vagal sensory ganglia of man. Am J Respir Crit Care Med 1996; 154:209–216.
49. Masuda S. Quantitative histochemistry of mucus-secreting cells in human nasal mucosa. Pract Otol (Kyoto) 1990; 83:1855–1863.
50. Lou YP, Takeyama K, Grattan KM, Lausier JA, Ueki IF, Agusti C, Nadel JA. Platelet-activating factor induces goblet cell hyperplasia and mucin gene expression in airways. Am J Respir Crit Care Med 1998; 157:1927–1934.
51. Takeyama K, Dabbagh K, Lee HM, Agusti C, Lausier JA, Ueki IF, Grattan KM, Nadel JA. Epidermal growth factor system regulates mucin production in airways. Proc Natl Acad Sci USA 1999; 96:3081–3086.
52. Sharma P, Dudus L, Nielsen PA, Clausen H, Yankaskas JR, Hollingsworth MA, Engelhardt JF. MUC5B and MUC7 are differentially expressed in mucous and serous cells of submucosal glands in human bronchial airways. Am J Respir Cell Mol Biol 1998; 19:30–37.
53. Borchers MT, Carty MP, Leikauf GD. Regulation of human airway mucins by acrolein and inflammatory mediators. Am J Physiol 1999; 276:L549–L555.
54. Dabbagh K, Takeyama K, Lee HM, Ueki IF, Lausier JA, Nadel JA. IL-4 induces mucin gene expression and goblet cell metaplasia in vitro and in vivo. J Immunol 1999; 162:6233–6237.
55. Wills–Karp M. Immunologic basis of antigen-induced airway hyperresponsiveness. Annu Rev Immunol 1999; 17:255–281.
56. Voynow JA, Selby DM, Rose MC. Mucin gene expression (MUC1, MUC2, and MUC5/5AC) in nasal epithelial cells of cystic fibrosis, allergic rhinitis, and normal individuals. Lung 1998; 176:345–354.
57. Voynow JA, Young LR, Wang Y, Horger T, Rose MC, Fischer BM. Neutrophil elastase increases MUC5AC mRNA and protein expression in respiratory epithelial cells. Am J Physiol 1999; 276:L835–L843.
58. Yuta A, Baraniuk JN. Therapeutic approaches to airway mucous hypersecretion. In: Rogers DF, Lethem MI, eds. Airway Mucus: Basic Mechanisms and Clinical Perspectives. Respiratory Pharmacology and Pharmacotherapy Series. Basel: Birkhauser, 1997:365–383.
59. Ziment I. Historic overview of mucoactive drugs. In: Braga PC, Allegra L, eds. Drugs in Bronchial Mucology. New York: Raven, 1989:1–34.
60. Baroody FM, Cruz AA, Lichtenstein LM, Kagey–Sobotka A, Proud D, Naclerio RM. Intranasal beclomethasone inhibits antigen induced nasal hyperresponsiveness to histamine. J Allergy Clin Immunol 1992; 90:373–376.

61. White MV. Nasal cholinergic hyperresponsiveness in atopic subjects studied out of season. J Allergy Clin Immunol 1993; 92:278–287.
62. Druce HM, Wright RH, Kossoff D, Kaliner MA. Cholinergic nasal hyperreactivity in atopic subjects. J Allergy Clin Immunol 1985; 76:445–452.
63. Kurian SS, Blank MA, Sheppard MN. Vasoactive intestinal polypeptide (VIP) in vasomotor rhinitis. Clin Biochem 1983; 11:425–426.
64. Lucchini RE, Facchini F, Turato G, Saetta M, Caramori G, Ciaccia A, Maestrelli P, Springall DR, Polak JM, Fabbri L, Mapp CE. Increased VIP-positive nerve fibers in the mucous glands of subjects with chronic bronchitis. Am J Respir Crit Care Med 1997; 156:1963–1968.
65. Einarsson O, Geba GP, Zhou Z, Landry ML, Panettiere RA Jr, Tristam D, Welliver R, Metinko A, Elias JA. Interleukin-11 in respiratory inflammation. Ann NY Acad Sci 1995; 762:31–40.
66. Jeney EV, Raphael GD, Meredith SD, Kaliner MA. Abnormal cholinergic parasympathetic responsiveness in the nasal mucosa of patients with recurrent sinusitis. J Allergy Clin Immunol 1990; 86:10–18.
67. Baraniuk JN. Glucocorticoids: bench to bedside. J Allergy Clin Immunol 1996; 97:141–182.
68. Baraniuk JN, Wong G, Ali M, Sabol M, Troost T. Glucocorticoids decrease c-*fos* expression in human nasal polyps in vivo. Thorax 1998; 53:577–582.
69. Fang S–Y, Druce HM, Baraniuk JN. Anticholinergic properties of brompheniramine, chlorpheniramine and atropine in human nasal mucosa in vitro. Am J Rhinol, 1998; 12:131–133.
70. Iliopoulos O, Proud D, Adkinson F Jr, Creticos PS, Norman PS, Kagey–Sobotka A, Lichtenstein LM. Effects of immunotherapy on the early, late, and rechallenge nasal reaction to provocation with allergen: changes in inflammatory mediators and cells. J Allergy Clin Immunol 1991; 87:855–866.
71. Bissonette EY, Encisco JA, Befus AD. TGF-beta-1 inhibits the release of histamine and tumor necrosis factor-alpha from mast cells through and autocrine pathway. Am J Respir Cell Mol Biol 1997; 16:275–283.
72. Kim HM, Lee YM. Role of TGF-beta-1 on the IgE-dependent anaphylaxis reaction. J Immunol 1999; 162:4960–4965.
73. Joly F, Charveron M, Aries MF, Bidault J, Kahhak L, Beauvais F, Gall Y. Effect of Avene spring water on the activation of rat mast cell by substance P or antigen. Skin Pharmacol Appl Skin Physiol 1998; 11:111–116.
74. Chong LK, Cooper E, Vardey CJ, Peachell PT. Salmeterol inhibition of mediator release from human lung mast cells by beta-adrenoceptor-dependent and independent mechanisms. Br J Pharmacol 1998; 123:1009–1015.
75. Jacobi HH, Skov PS, Poulsen LK, Malling MJ, Mygind N. Histamine and tryptase in nasal lavage fluid after allergen challenge: effect of 1 week of pretreatment with intranasal azelastine or systemic cetirizine. J Allergy Clin Immunol 1999; 103:768–772.

13

Nasal Polyps and Sinusitis

RAYMOND G. SLAVIN

St. Louis University School of Medicine, St. Louis, Missouri

1 NASAL POLYPS

Nasal polyps were first described more than 3000 years ago, and are the most common group of mass lesions encountered in the nose. They seem to be outgrowths of the nasal mucosa and are typically smooth, gelatinous, semitranslucent, round or pear-shaped, and pale (Fig. 1). They are located on the lateral wall of the nose, usually in the middle meatus or along the middle and superior turbinate. Most nasal polyps arise from the ethmoid sinus, with some polyps originating in the maxillary and sphenoid sinus. The ethmoid ostia are only 1–2 mm in diameter and this small area undoubtedly makes these ostia more susceptible to occlusion by mucosal edema or the growth of polypoid granulation tissue. Stammberger (1) has suggested that polyp formation occurs in contact areas between two opposing mucous membranes. Stimulation of epithelial cells induces generation and release of proinflammatory cytokines. He hypothesizes that the mechanical stimulation of surface epithelium in contact areas contributes to or even initiates the inflammatory reaction in polyps. The easy accessibility of polyps and the development of new immunohistochemical techniques has resulted in a significant increase in investigation of polyps and resultant publications in recent years.

1.1 Histopathology

The mass of a nasal polyp is made up chiefly of edema fluid, with sparse fibrous cells, a few mucous glands, and blood vessels. The surface epithelium generally reveals squamous metaplasia (Fig. 2).

The most prominent cell type in nasal polyps is the eosinophil, which is found in moderate to large numbers in polyps of 77% of patients (2). Almost all of the eosinophils

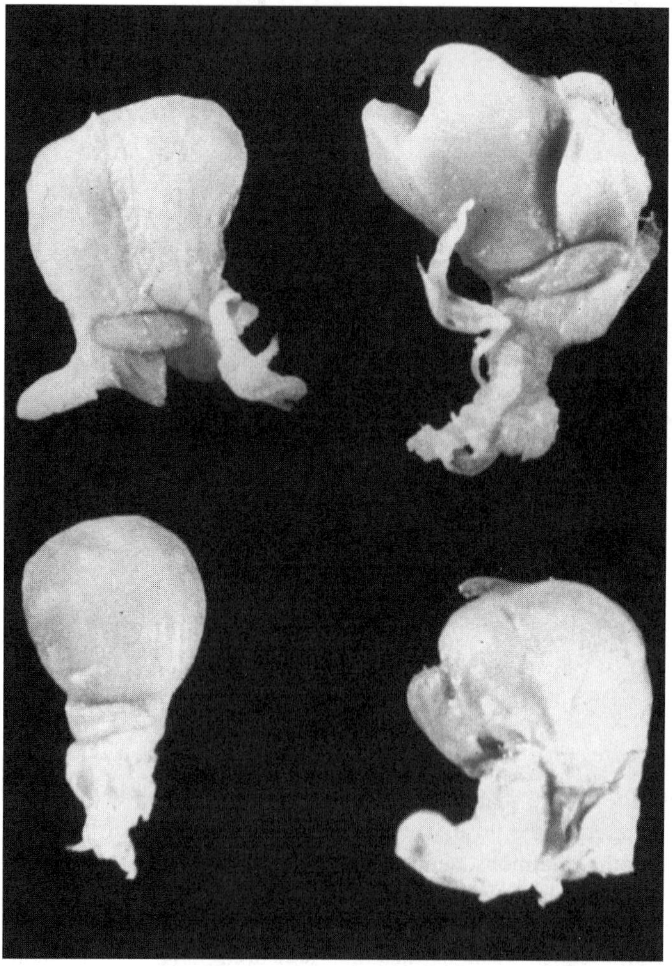

Figure 1 Four nasal polyps removed from the same individual: Upper right and lower left specimens have attached stalks. (3X). (Courtesy of Dr. Douglas R. Gnepp, Morgantown, WV.)

are $EG2^+$, indicating activation. The eosinophil is the predominant cell type in both atopic and nonatopic patients. There is a mild increase in numbers of $CD45^+$ inflammatory cells and epithelial mast cells that are tryptase-positive. The density of mast cells in the superficial layer of the mucosa is slightly higher in atopic than in nonatopic patients (3). Electron microscopic studies have shown marked and widespread mast cell degranulation, more marked than seen in allergic rhinitis (4). The total histamine content of polyps is far above other tissues and large quantities of free histamine can be measured in edema fluid (5). Although one study showed significantly more $CD8^+$ (suppressor/cytotoxic) lymphocytes than $CD4^+$ (helper/inducer) cells (6), others have claimed that $CD8^+$ cells were not increased and that $CD4^+$ T-lymphocytes were increased in nasal polyp patients with positive allergy skin tests (7).

Proliferation of stromal and epithelial elements is thought to account for the growth of nasal polyps. It has been suggested that the most prominent cell type in the nasal polyp,

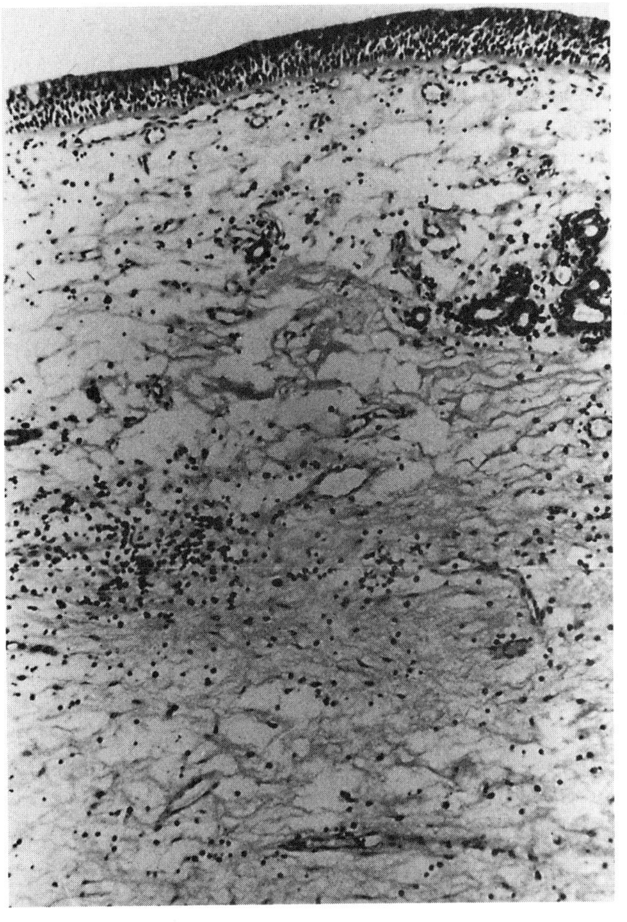

Figure 2 Photomicrograph of a nasal polyp showing spare fibrous cells, few mucous glands, and blood vessels. Surface epithelium reveals squamous metaplasia.

the eosinophil, is responsible for much of the tissue remodeling because of the release of a variety of growth factors. These growth factors, including transforming growth factor (TGF)-α and TGF-β (8), platelet-derived growth factor (PDGF) (9), epidermal growth factor (EGF), and tumor necrosis factor (TNF)-α (10), may contribute to the pathological changes seen in nasal polyps, such as thickening of epithelium and basement membrane, stromal fibrosis, angiogenesis, and epithelial and granular hyperplasia. It has been suggested that these ''hyperplastic'' features seen in the epithelium and submucosal structures of the nasal polyp, can be considered signs of airway remodeling reminiscent of those seen in chronic asthma (11).

The cellular composition of nasal polyps from cystic fibrosis (CF) and non-CF patients is considerably different (12). CF nasal polyps contain greater numbers of mast cells, endothelial cells, lymphocytes, and plasma cells. Eosinophils are rare to absent, in contrast with non-CF polyps, in which they are the predominant cell type. In CF mast cells, there are increased numbers of small granules, vacuolated granules, and lipid bodies, with evidence of 30% undergoing spontaneous degranulation.

1.2 Immunohistopathology

The predominance of eosinophils in nasal polyps seems to be due to both enhanced attraction and enhanced survival. Table 1 lists the cytokines found in nasal polyps. VLA-4–VCAM-1 interaction plays an important role in adhesion and transmigration of eosinophils, without much effect on neutrophils. Several studies have shown considerable up-regulation of VCAM-1 in microvascular endothelium of the polyp (13,14). Several cytokines that can induce VCAM-1 expression including interleukin (IL)-1, IL-3, IL-4, and TNF-α are expressed in polyp tissue (15). Another adhesion molecule, P-selectin is thought to play an important role in the initial adhesion of eosinophils to the polyp endothelium. Prolonged endothelial cell expression of P-selectin is induced by IL-3 and TNF-α.

Limited information is available on other chemoattractants, but there is some evidence that there is expression of the CC chemokines RANTES and eotaxin in nasal polyps (14). CC chemokines facilitate transendothelial migration of eosinophils and movement into the epithelium.

Other proinflammatory cytokines that are capable of recruiting and activating eosinophils are up-regulated in the epithelium and stroma of nasal polyps. These include granulocyte–macrophage colony-stimulating factor (GM-CSF), IL-6, and IL-8 (16–18). Probably the most important cytokine in the eosinophil dominated polyp is IL-5 (17). High amounts of IL-5 are found in the majority of nasal polyps, but not in normal nasal or sinus mucosa, or in antrochoanal polyps (19), which project from the antrum posteriorly into the nasopharynx. IL-5 levels are significantly higher in polyps of asthmatic subjects and in aspirin-sensitive patients than in nonasthmatics (17).

It is ironic that inflammatory cells themselves, particularly eosinophils, are rich sources of many cytokines, including those capable of inducing their own differentiation and activation in an autocrine manner. Denburg has suggested that nasal polyps can be looked on as a type of self-perpetuating inflammatory process (20).

Another reason for the preponderance of eosinophils in nasal polyps is increased survival. Ramis examined the survival of eosinophils obtained directly from nasal polyps and found a sixfold increase compared with the amount of circulating cells (21). GM-CSF, IL-3, and IL-5, which are up-regulated in nasal polyps, dramatically increase the life span of eosinophils in vitro by inhibition of programmed cell death (22). In an in vivo culture model of nasal polyp tissue, Simon et al. (23) concluded that programmed cell death, or apoptosis, was delayed in nasal polyps, compared with nasal mucosa or blood eosinophils. Tissue treatment with neutralizing concentrations of anti–IL-5, but not anti–

Table 1 Cytokines Found in Nasal Polyps

IL-1β	TNF-α
IL-3	P-selectin
IL-4	RANTES
IL-5	Eotaxin
IL-6	TGF-α and β
IL-8	PDGF
IL-13	EGF
GM-CSF	

GM-CSF or control MAb, induced eosinophil apoptosis and decreased tissue eosinophils, again pointing to IL-5 as the major support for human nasal polyp eosinophilia.

Some authors have proposed distinct mechanisms of eosinophilia in patients with and without allergy. In patients with allergy, increased expression of the Th2 cytokines IL-4, IL-5, and IL-13 mRNA is seen with very little expression of interferon (IFN)-γm RNA. In nonallergic patients, GM-CSF, IL-13, and IFN-γ are found (24). Other studies using in situ hybridization, protein measurements, immunohistochemistry, and neutralizing antibody experiments have found no significant differences between polyps from allergic and nonallergic patients (25).

There is recent evidence that inflammatory cell progenitors contribute to airway inflammation. CD34 is a cell surface, sialomucin-like glycoprotein that is expressed on hemopoietic progenitor cells and is progressively lost as cells differentiate (26). One group hypothesized that the eosinophil response in nasal polyps might be due to increased hemopoietic progenitors. They detected CD34 immunoreactive mononuclear cells and blood vessels in the lamina propria of all nasal polyps (27). They further showed that topical nasal corticosteroid treatment is associated with increased numbers of all CD34 cells, both mononuclear and endothelial. They suggest that topical corticosteroids suppress leukocyte recruitment by up-regulating CD34 expression on vascular endothelium in nasal polyps.

In another study, intranasal corticosteroids significantly reduced nasal polyp eosinophilia and $CD4^+$ T lymphocytes. The eosinophils expressing the activation marker EG_2 were more selectively reduced. In addition, P-selectin expression and the numbers of IL-4 and IL-13 $mRNA^+$ cells were reduced. In contrast, expression of endothelial VCAM-1 or the number of TNF-α or IL-1β $mRNA^+$ cells in the polyps were not affected by nasal corticosteroids. The authors suggest that these features may contribute to persistent nasal polyp disease despite intranasal steroid treatment (28).

1.3 Association of Nasal Polyps with Asthma

The association of nasal polyps with asthma has long been recognized. One large study of patients with nasal polyposis found an asthma incidence of 20%. In this same study, 32% of asthmatic patients had nasal polyps (29). In another series of 200 consecutive patients admitted for polypectomy, 30% had a history of asthma (30). Several reports have demonstrated evidence of bronchial hyperactivity in patients with nasal polyps and no history of asthma (31,32).

The pathological features of nasal polyps and asthma are strikingly similar (33). They are both expressions of airway inflammatory disease and share characteristics of fibrosis, basement membrane thickening, sloughed-off epithelium, and areas of epithelial metaplasia and eosinophils as the predominant cell type.

An association between nasal polyps and mediators of asthma has been shown (34). Polyps from patients with allergic rhinitis release histamine, leukotrienes, and eosinophil chemotactic factor of anaphylaxis when stimulated with the appropriate antigen. When polyps of patients with chronic sinusitis were passively sensitized with IgE and then challenged with antigen, there was a greater release of the leukotrienes than of histamine.

Moloney and Oliver (35) have tissue-typed patients with nasal polyps with and without asthma. They showed a significant increase in haplotype HLA-A1 and HLA-B8 in patients with both polyps and asthma. This increase indicates that tissue typing may be of some use in predicting which patients with nasal polyps are likely to develop asthma.

It may also mean that an abnormality of the immune response is associated with the pathogenesis of both nasal polyps and asthma.

A subpopulation of asthmatic patients with aspirin sensitivity has an especially high incidence of nasal polyps, on the order of 49% (36). The association of nasal polyps, bronchial asthma, and aspirin sensitivity has been well described. Vasomotor rhinitis associated with profuse rhinorrhea generally occurs first in these patients. Intense nasal congestion then follows with the subsequent development of nasal polyps; after this, bronchial asthma develops and finally, aspirin sensitivity. It has been shown that 8% of patients with nasal polyps, who were unaware of being sensitive to aspirin, were sensitive on appropriate challenge.

2 SINUSITIS

2.1 Definition and Classification

It has been suggested that the term rhinosinusitis may be more accurate than sinusitis for the following reasons: rhinitis typically precedes sinusitis; sinusitis without rhinitis is rare; the mucosa of the nose and sinuses are contiguous; and symptoms of nasal obstruction and nasal discharge are prominent in sinusitis (37).

Sinusitis is classified as acute, recurrent acute, subacute, and chronic. *Acute sinusitis* is defined as inflammation of the sinuses for less than 8 weeks in adults and less than 12 weeks in children. *Subacute sinusitis* is the development of manifestations of minimal-to-moderate signs of sinus inflammation without an overt upper respiratory infection or abrupt onset of symptoms. *Chronic sinusitis* is defined as persistent sinus inflammation for longer than 8–12 weeks. An operational definition of chronic sinusitis is persistent inflammation documented with imaging techniques at least 4 weeks after initiation of appropriate medical therapy in the absence of an intervening acute episode (38). In contrast with acute sinusitis, the role of bacterial infection in subacute and chronic sinusitis is less certain (39).

2.2 Microbiology of Sinusitis

Knowledge of the true microbiological picture in sinusitis has emerged from studies in which sinus aspirates were aseptically obtained by direct antral puncture or by sampling directly from the involved sinus during surgery.

Cultures from both adults (40) and children (41) with acute sinusitis grow predominantly aerobic organisms, with the heaviest yield being *Streptococcus pneumoniae*, *Haemophilus influenzae*, and *Moraxella* (formerly *Branhamella*) *catarrhalis*.

Although the role of viruses and bacteria in causing acute infectious sinusitis is well established, the role of microbial infection in chronic sinus disease is much less clear. Poor drainage of the chronically infected maxillary sinus reduces antral PO_2 and pH, which in turn, would be expected to encourage the growth of anaerobic bacteria by providing them with the optimal oxidation–reduction potential. It has been generally believed that anaerobic organisms played the major pathogenic role in chronic sinusitis (42), but these studies on the bacteriology of sinusitis were done before the era of endoscopic sinus surgery and the newer generation of antibiotics.

In a study of 76 adults who failed medical therapy for sinusitis and were scheduled for surgery, aerobes were isolated in 76.3% of cases and anaerobes in only 7.6% (43). Similar results have been found in children. Wald et al. studied 40 nonallergic children with chronic sinusitis. Sinus aspirates were positive in 58%, with the predominant bacteria being *S. pneumoniae*, *H. influenzae*, and *M. catarrhalis*. No anaerobes were isolated (44). In a study of chronic sinusitis in children with respiratory allergies, similar results were shown. *Moraxella catarrhalis* was the most common pathogen, with anaerobic organisms being rare (45). Maxillary antral cultures from patients with cystic fibrosis are somewhat different, with *Pseudomonas aeruginosa* being the most common followed by *H. influenzae*, *Streptococcus* species, and anaerobes (46).

The hypothesis has been offered that bacterial infection has a minor role, if any, in chronic sinusitis in many patients (39). Chronic sinusitis is relatively uncommon in children, and the data in this age-group are particularly confusing for several reasons: the variable definition of chronic sinusitis, the failure to obtain specimens aseptically, lack of quantitation of results, and concurrent use of antibiotics.

The incidence of sinusitis in acquired immunodeficiency syndrome (AIDS) patients may be as high as 68% (47). A prolonged mucociliary transit time has been reported in AIDS, and this defect with nasal obstruction is believed to represent the major mechanism for the high rate of acute and chronic sinusitis (48). The organisms causing bacterial sinusitis in human immunodeficiency virus (HIV)-infected patients are similar to those reported in the general population (49). Patients with a $CD4^+$ cell count of fewer than 150 are particularly susceptible to infection with atypical or opportunistic organisms, such as cytomegaloviruses, *Listeria monocytogenes*, *Pseudomonas*, and fungi (50).

2.2.1 The Contribution of Microbes to Inflammation

We know relatively little about how specific bacterial components trigger acute disease manifestation in the host. One direct link between the microbe to the host in disease pathogenesis would be inflammatory processes (51). Inflammatory cascades are often the first to be activated by bacteria and viruses and explain many aspects of acute disease. More specifically, the mucosal cytokine response seems to be particularly important in disease induction (52).

We know that epithelial cells respond to external stimulation and produce an array of mediators that transmit signals across the mucosal barrier. Attachment to epithelial cells is mediated by specific reactions between microbial surface ligands and host cell receptors (53). Invasion of the host cell by the bacteria or uptake of bacterial products into the cell may be required to induce a cytokine response (54). Bacteria may cross the epithelial layer and be taken up by cells such as mucosal macrophages. Release of cytokines by these infected, nonepithelial cells activates a secondary epithelial response or up-regulates the response to infection (55).

The effect of lipopolysaccharide (LPS) on epithelial cytokine responses has been well studied. LPS is an integral component of the outer membrane of gram-negative bacteria. Release of LPS in the circulation activates neutrophils, monocytes, and macrophages to release proinflammatory cytokines, such as tumor necrosis factor (TNF), IL-6, and IL-7 (53).

Concentration of IL-6 in the lumen increases following mucosal inflammation in animal models and in patients. In addition, epithelial cell lines and human mucosal biopsies secrete IL-6 following contact with bacteria in vitro (56). IL-6 is thought to enhance the maturation of mucosal B lymphocytes into IgA-producing plasma cells, and in one study of humans with mucosal inflammation, significant correlations were found between IL-6 and IgA concentration in secretions (57).

Mucosal infections trigger a broad chemokine response, including IL-8 (58,59), which is thought to play an important role in neutrophil recruitment.

The mucosal cytokine response to different pathogens is regulated by the specific immune system at the site of infection. T cells and immunoregulatory cytokines influence epithelial cell functions, including the expression of class II antigens, secretory component and intracellular adhesion molecule (ICAM) (60). Immunoregulated cytokines stimulate epithelial cell cytokine production and modify the epithelial cell cytokine response to bacteria (61). For example, IL-1 and *Escherichia coli* synergistically enhance IL-6 and IL-8 production by uroepithelial cells, whereas the combination of *E. coli* and either IL-4 or IFN-γ enhanced IL-6 production without affecting IL-8 production.

2.2.2 Acute Sinusitis

The different forms of sinusitis may be differentiated not only by clinical, but also by histological findings. In acute sinusitis (Table 2), predominantly neutrophils migrate into the inflamed tissues. A recent study investigated whether specific cytokine patterns are associated with different forms of rhinosinusitis and nasal polyps (19). Protein concentrations of nine cytokines in homogenized sinus mucosa were measured. In acute sinusitis, concentrations of proinflammatory cytokines IL-1β and IL-6 were increased compared with control mucosa, but failed to reach statistical significance. However, the concentration of IL-3 and IL-8 was significantly higher in acute sinusitis mucosa. IL-8 is known to be a potent neutrophil chemotactic protein and is constantly synthesized in the nasal mucosa (62), probably from epithelial cells to maintain neutrophils on the mucosal surfaces as important parts of nasal defense mechanisms (63). The authors state that they did not obtain mucosal samples before the fifth day of symptomatic infection and, therefore, might have missed the first events in acute inflammation, such as release of proinflammatory cytokines, including IFN-γ and IL-1β. The marked elevation of IL-3 levels would indicate the presence of activated T-lymphocytes.

2.3 Chronic Sinusitis

The histological picture of chronic sinusitis is characterized by basement membrane thickening, atypical gland formation, goblet cell hyperplasia, subepithelial edema, and mononuclear cell infiltration (64). The cellular infiltrate includes T and B lymphocytes, neutrophils, eosinophils, and macrophages. Although $CD8^+$ lymphocytes seem to predominate in adults with chronic sinusitis (65), studies in children show a predominance of $CD4^+$ cells (66).

A good deal of controversy exists relative to cytokine expression (Table 3) in chronic sinusitis. This may relate to different definition criteria of chronic sinusitis and differences in techniques. Some studies have focused on measurement of protein content of cytokines

Table 2 Cytokines Found in Acute Sinusitis

IL-1β
IL-3
IL-6
IL-8

Table 3 Cytokines Found in Chronic Sinusitis

IL-1β
IL-3
IL-4
IL-5
IL-6
IL-8
IFN-γ
TGF-β
E-selectin

and tissue, whereas other studies have looked at mRNA expression, qualitative immunohistological findings, or nasal discharge of cytokines.

In a previously cited study examining cytokine protein pattern of nine cytokines (19), only IL-3 was elevated in chronic maxillary sinusitis, compared with normals. Other investigators (67) have detected IL-1β mRNA expression in extravascular polymorphonuclear cells and in mononuclear leukocytes in chronic maxillary sinusitis mucosa together with an upregulation of ICAM-1 and E-selectin on endothelial cells.

The adherence of circulating leukocytes to the vascular endothelium is a critical step in the emigration of leukocytes through blood vessel walls to inflammatory lesions. In an elegant model using monolayers of human mucosal microvascular endothelial cells derived from the inferior turbinates, preincubation of the cells with retention fluid from the maxillary sinus of patients with chronic sinusitis induced increased neutrophil adherence (68). Recombinant IL-1β also induced adherence of neutrophils to the mucosal endothelial cells. An enzyme-linked immunosorbant assay (ELISA) detected considerable amounts of IL-1β in the chronic sinusitis retention fluids. The increased adhesion of the neutrophils by the retention fluid from chronic sinusitis patients was neutralized by incubation with anti–IL-1β antibody in a dose-dependent manner. This suggests that IL-1β in paranasal secretions induces adherence of neutrophils to vascular endothelium and subsequent infiltration of neutrophils in the paranasal sinuses, thus contributing to the persistence of chronic sinusitis.

The highly potent and selective chemoattractant for neutrophils, IL-8, has been demonstrated in chronic sinusitis in several ways. In one study, IL-8 levels measured by enzyme immunoassay was elevated in nasal discharge of chronic sinusitis patients (69). In addition, sinus mucosal specimens in chronic sinusitis, when subjected to immunohistochemical examination and in situ hybridization, showed IL-8 immunoreactivity in polymorphonuclear cells of nasal smears, in nasal gland duct cells, and in epithelial cells.

By using both a noncompetitive and a quantitative competitive reverse transcription–polymerase chain reaction (RT–PCR), sinus mucosal IL-8 gene expression was found in 55% of patients with chronic rhinosinusitis and not in control subjects (70). Furthermore, the level of IL-8 gene expression correlated well with disease severity.

In a recent report from Korea, maxillary sinus mucosa was studied in patients with chronic sinusitis who had no history of nasal allergy, asthma, or aspirin sensitivity (71). In Korea, the house dust mite is by far the most offending allergen in allergic rhinitis, and these patients were all negative by skin test and RAST to house dust mites. Use of RT-PCR and Southern blot, increased expression of IL-6, IL-8, TGF-β, IL-4, IL-5, and

IFN-γ were seen in the maxillary mucosa of patients with chronic sinusitis. The authors suggest that since TGF-β contributes to chronic inflammation and is associated with stromal fibrosis and thickening of the basement membrane (8), the increased levels seen in chronic sinusitis could explain thickening or polypoid changes of the mucosa. The increase in cytokines would result in recruitment of inflammatory cells and stimulation of secretions of other cytokines, thus resulting in chronicity of disease.

2.4 Allergic Sinusitis: Does It Exist?

Although type 1 allergy is a well-known trigger for provoking chronic inflammation, the question of whether this mechanism results in allergic inflammation in the sinuses is debatable. One group (72) evaluated tissue-specific mite IgE in the sinus mucosa and nasal turbinates of 60 mite-sensitive patients with sinusitis. Although specific mite IgE was elevated in the turbinate tissue of atopic patients, mite IgE was not found in the sinus mucosa. In a later study (73), nonatopic subjects inhaled technetium-labeled ragweed nasally. Intense reactivity was detected in the nasal cavity, but none was detected in the sinuses, suggesting that inhaled antigen does not penetrate into the sinus cavity.

Two more recent studies indicate that allergic sinusitis can be distinguished from sinusitis caused by chronic infection. In the first study (74), the number of activated eosinophils was significantly higher in patients with allergic rhinitis and chronic sinusitis than in patients with chronic suppurative sinusitis. In the second study (75), the numbers of eosinophils, activated eosinophils, and neutrophils were higher in paranasal sinus effusion from patients with allergic rhinitis and sinusitis as was the concentration of IL-5. In addition, more eosinophils and activated eosinophils infiltrated into the sinus mucosa of patients with so-called allergic sinusitis.

One group has shown increased density of cells expressing IL-4 mRNA in the sinus mucosa of allergic subjects with chronic sinusitis, but not in nonallergic subjects with chronic sinusitis. In contrast, IL-13, a cytokine with functional similarities to IL-4 was augmented in the sinus mucosa of both allergic and nonallergic patients with chronic sinusitis (76). A more recent study (77) demonstrated an increased number of cells expressing Iε the IgEε heavy-chain germline transcript and Cε the IgE heavy-chain constant region gene transcript in the sinus mucosa from allergic subjects with chronic sinusitis.

2.5 Fungal Sinusitis

Infection of the sinuses with fungi can be divided into two forms: invasive and noninvasive (78). The invasive forms, in turn, can be subdivided into acute (fulminant) invasive, granulomatous invasive, and chronic invasive. Noninvasive forms are mycetoma and allergic fungal sinusitis.

2.5.1 Invasive

Acute Invasive

Causes of this syndrome include saprophytic fungi of the order Mucorales, including *Rhizopus*, *Mucor*, and basidia. On histopathological examination, one sees hyphal invasion of blood vessels, vasculitis with thrombosis, hemorrhage, and tissue infarction. The inflammatory responses have not been well characterized. One study reports an acute neutrophilic infiltrate (79), whereas another finds a necrotizing reaction, with only minimal inflammation, thrombosis, mycotic aneurysms, and ischemic infarction (79,80).

Granulomatous Invasive

Also called indolent fungal sinusitis (81), this condition is caused by *Aspergillus flavus*. There is profuse fungal growth, with regional tissue invasion, noncaseating granulomas with giant cells and plasma cells. Central microgranulomata of eosinophils, fibrinoid necrosis, fibrosis, and vasculitis are also seen (82).

Chronic Invasive

A dense accumulation of hyphae resembling a mycetoma is seen in this syndrome. Vascular invasion by fungal elements occurs with only a sparse chronic inflammatory infiltrate (83). The condition may begin as a sinus mycetoma and becomes invasive, perhaps as a result of immunosuppression.

2.5.2 Noninvasive

Mycetoma

Also termed fungal ball, this condition is marked histopathologically by a matted, dense conglomeration of hyphae separate from, but adjacent to, the sinus mucosa. The mucosa is characterized by chronic, nongranulomatous inflammatory response of varying intensity. There is no fungal invasion of mucosa, associated blood vessels, or bone (84).

Allergic Fungal Sinusitis

Allergic fungal sinusitis (AFS) appears to represent an IgE-mediated hypersensitivity reaction to fungi resembling that occurring in the bronchi in allergic bronchopulmonary aspergillosis. Most cases have been attributed to the pigmented dematiaceous fungi, including *Bipolaris* (*Drechslera*) and *Curvularia* and the hyaline molds, such as *Aspergillus* (78). Histologically, the mucosa shows a dense inflammatory infiltrate of plasma cells, small lymphocytes, and eosinophils. Mucous glands are hypertrophied and distended with mucus. The respiratory epithelium may be desquamated and the basement membrane thickened. The involved sinus contains a brown or greenish-black material, with the consistency of peanut butter, which may obstruct sinus drainage and, along with associated polyps, lead to bacterial sinusitis. This material is referred to as ''allergic mucin'' and consists of accumulations of intact and degenerating eosinophils, Charcot–Leyden crystals, cellular debris, and sparse hyphae that are rarely visible without fungal stain, such as Fontana–Masson or methenamine-silver (78). Although hyphae are present in mucin, they are not found in the adjacent mucosa. The technique of in situ hybridization for *Aspergillus* and *Penicillium* ribosomal RNA has also been employed in diagnosing AFS (85). Allergic mucin eosinophil cationic protein levels obtained at surgery were significantly higher in patients with AFS than in patients with other forms of sinusitis. Levels appeared to correspond with disease activity. There was no significant difference in serum eosinophil cationic protein levels between the groups (86).

REFERENCES

1. Stammberger H. Examination and endoscopy of the nose and paranasal sinuses. In: Mygind N, Lildholdt T, eds. Nasal Polyposis: an Inflammatory Disease and Its Treatment. Copenhagen: Munksgaard, 1997:120–136.
2. Stoop AE, van der Heijden HA, Biewenga J, van der Baan S. Eosinophils in nasal polyps and nasal mucosa: an immunohistochemical study. J Allergy Clin Immunol 1993; 91:616–622.
3. Hamilos DL, Leung DYM, Wood R, Bean DK, Song YL, Schotman E, Hamid Q. Eosinophil

infiltration in nonallergic chronic hyperplastic sinusitis with nasal polyposis (CHS/NP) is associated with endothelial VCAM-1 upregulation and expression of TNF-α. Am J Respir Cell Mol Biol 1996; 15:443–450.

4. Drake–Lee A, Price J. Ultrastructure of mast cells in normal subjects and patients with perennial allergic rhinitis. J Laryngol Otol 1991; 105:1006–1013.
5. Drake–Lee AB, McLouhlan P. Clinical symptoms, free histamine and IgE in nasal polyps. Int Arch Allergy Appl Immunol 1982; 69:268–271.
6. Stoop AE, van der Heijden HA, Biewenga J, van der Baan S. Lymphocyte and nonlymphoid cells in human nasal polyps. J Allergy Clin Immunol 1991; 87:470–475.
7. Hamilos DL, Leung DYM, Wood R, Meyers A, Stephenns JK, Barkan J, Meng Q, Cunningham L, Bean DK, Kay AB, Hamid Q. Chronic hyperplastic sinusitis: association of tissue eosinophilia with mRNA expression of granulocyte–macrophage colony stimulating factor and IL-3. J Allergy Clin Immunol 1993; 92:39–48.
8. Elovic A, Wong DT, Weller PF, Matossian K, Galli SJ. Expression of transforming growth factors-alpha and beta 1 messenger RNA and product by eosinophils in nasal polyps. J Allergy Clin Immunol 1994; 93:864–869.
9. Ohno I, Nitta Y, Yamauchi K, Hoshi H, Honman M, Wooley K, O'Byrne P, Dolovich J, Jordana M, Tamur G, Tanno Y, Sherato K. Eosinophils as a potential source of platelet-derived growth factor B-chain (PDGF-B) in nasal polyposis and bronchial asthma. Am J Respir Cell Mol Biol 1995; 13:639–647.
10. Finotto S, Ohno I, Marshall JS, Gouldie J, Denburg JA, Dolovich J, Clark DA, Jordana M. TNF-alpha production by eosinophils in upper airways inflammation (nasal polyposis). J Immunol 1994; 153:2278–2289.
11. Jordana M, Vancheri C, Ohtoshi T, Harnish D, Gouldie J, Dolovich J, Denburg J. Hemopoietic function of the microenvironment in chronic airway inflammation. Agents Actions 1989; 28(suppl):85–95.
12. Henderson WR Jr, Chi EY. Degranulation of cystic fibrosis nasal polyp mast cells. J Pathol 1992; 166:395–404.
13. Jahnsen FL, Haraldsen G, Aanesen JP, Haye R, Brandtzaeg P. Eosinophil infiltration is related to increased expression of vascular cell adhesion molecule-1 in nasal polyps. Am J Respir Cell Mol Biol 1995; 12:624–632.
14. Beck L, Stellato C, Beall D, Schall TJ, Leopold D, Beckel CA, Baroody F, Bochner BS, Schleimer RP. Detection of chemokine RANTES and endothelial adhesion molecules in nasal polyps. J Allergy Clin Immunol 1996; 98:766–780.
15. Jahnsen FL, Haraldsen G, Haye R, Brandtzaeg P. Adhesion molecules and recruitment of eosinophils. In: Mygind N, Lildholdt T, eds. Nasal Polyposis: An Inflammatory Disease and Its Treatment. Copenhagen: Munksgaard, 1997:88–97.
16. Jordana M, Dolovich J, Ohno I, Finotto S, Denburg J. Nasal polyposis: a model for chronic inflammation. In: Busse WW, Holgate ST, eds. Asthma and Rhinitis. Boston: Blackwell Scientific, 1995:156–164.
17. Bachert C. Comparison between polyp tissue, diseased sinus mucosa and normal nasal tissue. In: Mygind N, Lildholdt T, eds. Nasal Polyposis: An Inflammatory Disease and Its Treatment. Copenhagen: Munksgaard, 1997:98–104.
18. Bachert C, Wagenman M, Hauser U, Rudack C. IL-5 synthesis is upregulated in human nasal polyp tissue. J Allergy Clin Immunol 1997; 99:837–842.
19. Rudack G, Stoll W, Bachert C. Cytokines in nasal polyposis, acute and chronic sinusitis. Am J Rhinol 1998; 12:383–388.
20. Denburg J. Nasal polyposis: cytokines and inflammatory cells. In: Mygind N, Lildholdt T, eds. Nasal Polyposis: An Inflammatory Disease and Its Treatment. Copenhagen: Munksgaard, 1997:78–87.
21. Ramis I, Finotto S, Dolovich J. Increased survival of nasal polyp eosinophils. Immunol Lett 1995; 45:219–221.

22. Bachert C, Wagenmann M, Rudack C, Hopken K, Hillebrandt M, Wang D, Van Cauwenberge P. The role of cytokines in infectious sinusitis and nasal polyposis. Allergy 1998; 53:2–13.
23. Simon HU, Yousefi S, Schranz C, Schopowal A, Bachert C, Blaser K. Direct demonstration of delayed eosinophil apoptosis as a mechanism causing tissue eosinophilia. J Immunol 1997; 158:3902–3908.
24. Hamilos DL, Leung DJ, Wood R, Cunningham L, Bean DK, Yasruel Z, Schottman E, Hamid Q. Evidence for distinct cytokine expression in allergic versus nonallergic chronic sinusitis. J Allergy Clin Immunol 1995; 96:537–544.
25. Bachert C, Wagenman M, Hauser U, Rudack C. IL-5 synthesis is upregulated in human nasal polyp tissue. J Allergy Clin Immunol 1997; 99:837–842.
26. Strauss LC, Rowley SD, LaRussa VF. Antigenic analysis of hematopoiesis V characterization of My-10 antigen expression by normal lymphohematopoietic progenitor cells. Exp Hematol 1986; 14:878–886.
27. Kim YK, Uno M, Hamilos DL, Beck L, Bochner B, Schleimer R, Denburg JA. Immunolocalization of CD34 in nasal polyposis: effect of topical corticosteroids. Am J Respir Cell Mol Biol 1999; 20:388–397.
28. Hamilos DC, Thawley SE, Kremper MA, Kamil A, Hamid Q. Effect of intranasal fluticasone on cellular infiltration, endothelial adhesion molecule expression, and proinflammatory cytokine mRNA in nasal polyp disease. J Allergy Clin Immunol 1999; 103:79–87.
29. Settipane GA. Nasal polyps. Immunol Allergy Clin North Am 1987; 7:105.
30. Drake–Lee AB, Lowe D, Swanston A, Grace A. Clinical profile and recurrence of nasal polyps. J Laryngol Otol 1984; 98:783–793.
31. Kordash TR, Gleich G, Kern EB. Evidence for increased risk of development of asthma in patients with nasal polyps [abstr]. J Allergy Clin Immunol 1978; 61:138.
32. Miles–Lawrence R, Kaplan M, Chang K. Methacholine sensitivity in nasal polyposis and the effects of polypectomy [abstr]. J Allergy Clin Immunol 1982; 69:102.
33. Chandra RK, Abol BM. Immunopathology of nasal polyps. J Laryngol Oto 1974; 88:1019–1027.
34. Kaliner M, Wasserman SI, Austen KF. Immunologic release of chemical mediators from human nasal polyps. N Engl J Med 1973; 289:277.
35. Moloney JR, Oliver RID. HLA antigens, nasal polyps, and asthma. Clin Otolaryngol 1980; 5:183–186.
36. Settipane GA, Chaffee FH, Klein DE. A critical evaluation of aspirin challenge in patients with nasal polyps [abstr]. J Allergy Clin Immunol 1982; 69:148.
37. Kaliner MA, Osguthorpe JD, Fireman P, Anon J, Georgitis J, Davis ML, Naclerio R, Kennedy D. Sinusitis: bench to bedside. J Allergy Clin Immunol 1997; 99:(S)829–848.
38. Lund VJ, Kennedy DW. Quantification for staging sinusitis. The Staging and Therapy Group. Ann Otol Rhinol Laryngol 1995; 167(suppl):17–21.
39. Wald ER. Chronic sinusitis in children. J Pediatr 1995; 127:339–347.
40. Evans FO Jr, Sydnor JB, Moore WE, Moore GP, Manwaring JL, Brill AH, Jackson RT, Hanna S, Skaar JS, Holdeman LV, Fitz–Hugh GS, Sande MA, Gwaltney JM. Sinusitis of the maxillary antrum. N Engl J Med 1975; 293:735–739.
41. Wald ER, Milmore GJ, Bowen A, Lededsma–Medina J, Salaman N, Bluestone CD. Acute maxillary sinusitis in children. N Engl J Med 1981; 304:749–754.
42. Brook I. Bacteriology of chronic maxillary sinusitis in adults. Ann Otol Rhinol Laryngol 1989; 98:426–430.
43. Ramadan HH. What is the bacteriology of chronic sinusitis in adults? Am J Otolaryngol 1995; 16:303–306.
44. Wald ER, Byers C, Guerra N, Casselbrant M, Beste D. Subacute sinusitis in children. J Pediatr 1989; 115:28–32.
45. Goldenhersh MJ, Rachelefsky GS, Dudley J, Brill J, Katz RM, Rohr AS, Spector SL, Siegel

SC, Summanen P, Baron LJ, Finegold S. The microbiology of chronic sinus disease in children with respiratory allergy. J Allergy Clin Immunol 1990; 85:1030–1039.

46. Shapiro ED, Milmore GJ, Wald ER, Rodman JB, Bowen A. Bacteriology of the maxillary sinuses I patients with cystic fibrosis. J Infect Dis 1982; 146:589–593.
47. Upadhyay S, Marks SC, Arden RL, Crane LR, Cohn AM. Bacteriology of sinusitis in human immunodeficiency virus-positive patients: implications for management. Laryngoscope 1995; 105:1058–1060.
48. Milgrim LM, Rubin JS, Small CB. Mucociliary clearance abnormalities in the HIV-infected patient: a precursor to acute sinusitis. Laryngoscope 1995; 105:1202–1208.
49. Milgrim LM, Rubin JS, Rosenstreich DLM, Small CB. Sinusitis in human immunodeficiency virus infection: typical and atypical organisms. J Otolaryngol 1994; 23:450–453.
50. Meyer RD, Gaultier CR, Yamashita JT, Babapour R, Pitchon HE, Wolfe DR. Fungal sinusitis in patients with AIDS: report of 4 cases and review of the literature. Medicine 1994; 73:69–78.
51. Hedges S, Agace W, Svanborg C. Epithelial cytokine responses and mucosal cytokine networks. Trends Microbiol 1995; 3:266–270.
52. Svanborg C, Godaly G, Hedlund M. Cytokine responses during mucosal infections: role in disease pathogenesis and host defence. Curr Opin Microbiol 1999; 2:99–105.
53. Leffler H, Svanborg–Eden C. Chemical identification of a glycosphingolipid receptor for *Escherichia coli* attaching to human urinary tract epithelial cells and agglutinating human erythrocytes. FEMS Microbiol Lett 1980; 6:127–134.
54. Eckmann L, Kagnoff MF, Fierer J. Epithelial cells secrete the chemokine interleukin-B in response to bacterial entry. Infect Immun 1993; 61:4569–4574.
55. Clerc P, Sansonetti PJ. Entry of *Shigella flaxneri* into HeLa cells: evidence for directed phagocytosis involving actin polymerization and myosin accumulation. Infect Immun 1987; 55: 2681–2688.
56. Hedges S, de Man P, Linder H, van Kooten C, Svanborg–Eden C. Interleukin-6 is secreted by epithelial cells in response to gram-negative bacterial challenge. In: Macdonald T, ed. Advances in Mucosal Immunology. International Conference of Mucosal Immunity. London: Kluwer, 1990:144–148.
57. Petersson C, Hedges S, Stenquist K, Sandberg T, Connell H, Svanborg C. Suppressed antibody and interleukin-6 responses to acute pyelonephritis in pregnancy. Kidney Int 1994; 45:571–577.
58. Agace W, Hedges S, Ceska M, Svanborg C. IL-8 and the neutrophil response to mucosal gram-negative infection. J Clin Invest 1993; 92:780–785.
59. Godaly G, Proudfoot AEI, Offord RE, Svanborg C, Agace W. Role of epithelial interleukin-8 and neutrophil IL-8 receptor A in *Escherichia coli*-induced transuroepithelial neutrophil migration. Infect Immun 1997; 65:3451–3456.
60. Kyale D, Brandzaeg P, Lov–Haug D. Up-regulation of the expression of secretory component and HLA molecules in a human colonic cell line by tumour necrosis factor-α and gamma interferon. Scand J Immunol 1988; 28:351–357.
61. Hedges S, Bjarnadotir M, Agace W, Hang L, Svanborg C. Immunoregulatory cytokines modify *Escherichia coli* induced uroepithelial cell IL-6 and IL-8 responses. Cytokine 1996; 8:686–697.
62. Bachert C, Hauser U, Prem B, Rudack C, Ganzer U. Proinflammatory cytokines in allergic rhinitis. Eur Arch Otorhinolaryngol 1995; 1(suppl):S44–S49.
63. Bazzoni F, Cassatella MA, Rossi F, Ceska M, Dewald B, Baggiolini S. Phagocytosing neutrophils produce and release high amounts of NAP-/IL-8. J Exp Med 1991; 173:771–774.
64. Georgitis JW, Matthews BL, Stone B. Chronic sinusitis: characterization of cellular influx and inflammatory mediators in sinus lavage fluid. Int Arch Allergy Immunol 1995; 106:416–421.
65. Nishimoto K, Kotaro U, Teruhiko H, et al. Lymphocyte subsets in maxillary mucosa in chronic inflammation. Acta Otolaryngol (Stockh) 1988; 106:291–298.

66. Driscoll PV, Naclerio RM, Baroody FM. CD4$^+$ lymphocyte are increased in the sinus mucosa of children with chronic sinusitis. Arch Otolaryngol Head Neck Surg 1996; 122:1071–1076.
67. Tokushige E, Itoh K, Ushikai M, et al. Localization of IL-1β mRNA and cell adhesion molecules in the maxillary sinus mucosa of patients with chronic sinusitis. Laryngoscope 1994; 104:1245–1250.
68. Itoh K, Katahira S, Matsuzoki T, Ohyama M, Fukuda K. Retention fluids of chronic sinusitis induced neutrophil adherence to microvascular endothelial cells. Acta Otolaryngol 1992; 112: 882–889.
69. Suzuki H, Takahashi Y, Wataya H, Ikeda K, Nakabayashi S, Shimomura A, Takasakaa T. Mechanism of neutrophil recruitment induced by IL-8 in chronic sinusitis. J Allergy Clin Immunol. 1996; 98:659–670.
70. Rhyoo C, Sanders SP, Leopold DA, Proud D. Sinus mucosal IL-8 gene expression in chronic rhinosinusitis. J Allergy Clin Immunol 1999; 103:395–400.
71. Min TG, Lee CH, Rhee CS, Hong SK, Kwon SH. Increased expression of IL-4, IL-5, IFN-γ, IL-6, IL-8 and TGF-β mRNAs in maxillary mucosa of patients with chronic sinusitis. Am J Rhinol 1999; 13:339–343.
72. Liu CM, Shun CT, Song HC, Lee SY, Hsu MM, How SW. Antigen-specific IgE antibody and cytogram in mucosa of the nose and sinus. Am J Rhinol 1993; 7:111–115.
73. Adkins TN, Goodgold HM, Hendershott L, Slavin RG. Does inhaled pollen enter the sinus cavities? Ann Allergy Asthma Immunol 1998; 81:181–184.
74. Ogata N, Masuyama K, Yoshida M, Samejima Y, Eura M, Ishikawa T. Preferential infiltration by activated eosinophils in allergic sinusitis. Auris Nasus Larynx 1997; 24:279–287.
75. Suzuki M, Watanabe T, Suko T, Mogi G. Comparison of sinusitis with and without allergic rhinitis: characteristics of paranasal sinus effusion and mucosa. Am J Otolaryngol 1999; 20: 143–150.
76. Al-Ghamdi K, Ghaffar O, Small P, Frankiel S, Hamid Q. IL-4 and IL-13 expression in chronic sinusitis: relationship with cellular infiltrate and effect of topical corticoseroid treatment. J Otolaryngol 1997; 26:160–166.
77. Ghaffar O, Durham SR, Al-Ghamdi K, Wright E, Small P, Frenkiel S, Gould HJ, Hamid Q. Expression of IgE heavy chain transcripts in the sinus mucosa of atopic and nonatopic patients with chronic sinusitis. Am J Respir Cell Mol Biol 1998; 18:706–711.
78. DeShazo RD, Chapin K, Swain RE. Fungal sinusitis. N Engl J Med 1997; 37:254–259.
79. Blitzer A, Lawson W, Meyers BR, Biller HF. Patient survival factors in paranasal sinus mucormycosis. Laryngoscope 1980; 90:635–648.
80. Gowing NFC, Hamlin IME. Tissue reactions to *Aspergillus* in cases of Hodgkin's disease and leukemia. J Clin Pathol 1960; 13:396–413.
81. Sandison AT, Gentles JC, Davidson CM, Branko M. Aspergilloma of paranasal sinuses and orbit in northern Sudanese. Sabouraudia 1967; 6:57–69.
82. Veress B, Malik OA, el-Tayeb AA, el-Daoud S, Mahgoub ES, el-Hassan AM. Further observations on the primary paranasal *Aspergillus* granuloma in the Sudan: a morphological study of 46 cases. Am J Trop Med Hyg 1973; 22:765–772.
83. Milroy CM, Blanshard JD, Lucas S, Michaels L. Aspergillosis of the nose and paranasal sinuses. J Clin Pathol 1989; 42:123–127.
84. Hartwick RW, Batsakis JG. Sinus aspergillosis and allergic fungal sinusitis. Ann Otol Rhinol Laryngol 1991; 100:427–430.
85. Perez–Jeffe LA, Lanza DC, Loevner LA, Kennedy DW, Montore KT. In situ hybridization for *Aspergillus* and *Penicillium* in allergic fungal sinusitis: a rapid means of speciating fungal pathogens in tissues. Laryngoscope 1997; 107:233–240.
86. Feger TA, Rupp NT, Kuhn FA, Ford JL, Dolen WK. Local and systemic eosinophil activation in allergic fungal sinusitis. Ann Allergy Asthma Immunol 1997; 79:221–225.

14

Allergic Eye Disorders

LEONARD BIELORY

UMDNJ–New Jersey Medical School, Newark, New Jersey

SERGIO BONINI

Second University of Naples and Italian National Research Council (CNR), Rome, Italy

STEFANO BONINI

University of Rome Tor Vergata, Rome, Italy

1 INTRODUCTION

Because of its localization and complete immunological repertoire, the eye is exposed to several external stimuli eliciting a wide variety of immunological and immunopathological reactions. On the other hand, in view of the wide distribution of blood and lymphatic vessels, ocular tissue also takes part in several systemic allergic reactions and diseases. Accordingly, in its broader sense, allergic eye disorders include numerous immunological and immunopathological mechanisms that are peculiar to, and dependent on, the specific functions and anatomy of the different ocular tissues: eyelids, cornea, lens, retina, uvea, and conjunctiva (1–5). This chapter will be confined to clinical conditions caused by hypersensitivity reactions of the human external eye.

The nosology of the clinical diseases resulting from conjunctival hypersensitivity is controversial (6). However, the common feature that encompasses all these clinical entities is the assumption that a common type I hypersensitivity mechanism is responsible for their pathophysiology. Accordingly, immunoglobulin E (IgE)-mediated release from mast cells and basophils has long been considered the key mechanism of allergic eye disorders and guided their diagnosis and treatment.

Recently, extensive evidence has become available for several other allergic diseases (such as asthma, rhinitis, and allergic skin diseases) indicating that their pathogenesis cannot be confined to an IgE-dependent mast cell- and basophil-mediated release, but should be extended to several other mechanisms involving other effector cells and mediators (7,8). This new and wider concept of allergy as a complex inflammatory network in which several cells and mediators take part, is also similar to the experimental findings in allergic eye diseases. Therefore, the pathogenesis of ocular allergy is more complex than previously believed. Accordingly, its nosology should possibly be revised to better distinguish among the preferential inflammatory pathways leading to inflammation and symptoms of a ''red eye.'' We hope that, this new approach will reflect a better diagnosis and treatment of the patient with allergic eye diseases.

2 INFLAMMATORY CELLS AND MEDIATORS IN ALLERGIC EYE DISEASES

2.1 Mast Cells

Mast cells that contain both tryptase and chymase have been found in increased number in allergic eye diseases (9,10). Mast cells in patients with eye allergies not only are increased in number, but also show a different distribution. In fact, in normal subjects mast cells are mainly present in the stroma, whereas in patients with allergic conjunctivitis, several intraepithelial mast cells are found. This can have relevant implication relative to the availability of mast cells to interact with allergens, other cells, and cytokines. Conjunctival mast cells can store a range of cytokines, such as interleukin (IL)-4, IL-5, IL-6 and tumor necrosis factor (TNF)-α. In seasonal allergic conjunctivitis (SAC) IL-4 appears to be secreted during the pollen season, which may have an important role in up-regulating allergic inflammation in the conjunctiva (11,12).

2.2 T Cells

T cells are present in the lymphoid tissue of the normal conjunctiva. Their number, phenotype, and distribution seem to be altered in patients with allergic eye diseases. In vernal keratoconjunctivitis (VKC), the number of $CD3^+$ cells in the subepithelium and the CD4/CD8 ratio are increased (13). In $CD3^+$ areas, there is an increased signal for IL-5, whereas there is no difference in the IL-2 mRNA. Indeed, T-cell clones from conjunctival issue of VKC patients belong mainly to the Th2 type (14). A Th2-like cytokine array (with increased levels of mRNA for IL-3, IL-4, and IL-5) was also found (15) in giant papillary conjunctivitis (GPC), whereas atopic keratoconjunctivitis (AKC) biopsies showed increased immunoreactivity for interferon (IFN)-γ and greater IL-2 mRNA expression when compared with VKC and giant papillary conjunctivitis (GPC) biopsies. Therefore, chronic allergic conjunctival diseases show signs of $CD4^+$ cell activation, but with different cytokine patterns depending on the type of disease. In SAC, the number of lymphocytes in conjunctival scrapings and tears is not significantly different from that found in normal subjects. However, it significantly increases during the late-phase allergic reaction induced by specific allergen challenge (16,17). These cells may contribute to an excessive IgE production through IL-4 and IL-13, and to influence inflammatory processes, through the modulatory effects of IL-5 on eosinophils.

2.3 Eosinophils

The eosinophil is a key effector cell in allergic eye disorders (18–20). Eosinophils represent a major diagnostic sign of VKC, having been detected in tears and conjunctival scrapings of 85% of a large series of 195 VKC patients, both in IgE- and non–IgE-mediated forms (21). In biopsies from patients with VKC, AKC, and GPC, eosinophils show an increased expression of activation antigens, such as the secreted form of eosinophil cationic protein (ECP; reacting with EG2), IL-2R intracellular adhesion molecule 1, (ICAM-1; CD54), and HLA-DR (22–24). Cytokine production varies, however, in different ocular allergic disease being greater for VKC and AKC than in GPC in which the cornea is not involved (24). In particular, whereas RANTES, transforming growth factor (TGF)-β, and TNF-α were localized to eosinophils in all disorders, in VKC, IL-4, IL-5, and IL-6; in AKC IL-4, IL-8, and granulocyte–macrophage colony-stimulating factor (GM-CSF); and in GPC, IL-5, were prominent (25).

In SAC and perennial allergic conjunctivitis (PAC), eosinophils although not present in tears and conjunctival scrapings in basal conditions are significantly increased during the late-phase allergic reaction induced by specific allergen challenge.

Interestingly enough, the involvement of eosinophils in allergic eye diseases is not confined to ocular tissues, but they are evident in peripheral blood cells. In fact, a multiparameter flow cytometry study of VKC patients showed that eosinophils were also significantly increased in the circulation (350 $\pm$ 210 vs. 190 $\pm$ 80 cells/mm^3, $p < 0.05$) and showed a more intense fluorescence signal with CD11a, CD11b, CD18, EG1, and EG2 monoclonal antibodies.

2.4 Other Cells

Macrophages expressing CD68 and dendritic cells stained with CD1a, which is prevalent on Langerhans cells, are usually increased in the tarsal conjunctiva of AKC, VKC, and GPC patients (26). Because HLA-DR is also overexpressed in VKC, AKC, and GPC, it seems that antigen presentation is up-regulated in chronic allergic eye diseases. On the contrary, little difference is observed between the allergic and the normal conjunctiva in the expression of the B-cell marker CD19 as well as in the number of natural killer (NK) cells expressing CD57 or T cells expressing the alternative T-cell receptor γδ.

Neutrophils are present in the inflamed conjunctiva of VKC patients and are significantly recruited during the early phase of allergic reactions as well as long after an allergen challenge.

Epithelial cells and fibroblasts are certainly involved in tissue damage and remodeling following allergic inflammation. Recently, increasing attention is also given to the potential role of these cells in crosstalk with other inflammatory cells and in modulating inflammatory phenomena (27). Allergic subjects with natural, persistent inflammatory conditions or after allergen challenge express ICAM-1 (28).

2.5 Mediators

Tryptase, a neutral protease stored in mast cell granules, is significantly increased in tears of VKC patients. Tryptase is not detectable in basal conditions in tears of SAC out of season, but it significantly increases during the early-phase response after effective specific allergen challenge (29,30), together with TNF-α (31), histamine, kinins, prostaglandin D (PGD), and TAME-esterase activity (32). Eosinophil products, such as ECP are present at different concentrations in tears of SAC, PAC, and VKC, and significantly increase 6 hr after effective allergen challenge (33–35). Interestingly, as observed for eosinophil activation markers, the increase of eosinophil mediators is not confined to ocular tissue, but can also be documented in the general circulation. ECP serum levels are increased in

PAC and in SAC during pollen season (36). In VKC, the increase of ECP and of eosinophil-derived neurotoxin/protein X (EDN/EPX) is even higher and is related to the number of mast cells infiltrating the conjunctiva (37).

Interleukin-5 activity was detected in tears of 4 of 13 subjects with VKC, but not in tears of controls. These data were confirmed in a larger set of patients using an immunoassay for IL-5. In fact, 6 of 32 VKC patients had measurable IL-5 in tears when compared with controls. This indicates that the positive signal for IL-5 mRNA found in conjunctival biopsies appears to be associated with detectable amounts of IL-5 protein in VKC tears. Finally, hyaluronic acid is increased in VKC tears, compared with SAC and normal tears. Therefore, the massive collagen production and collagen deposition of giant papillae in VKC is reflected by a measurable increase of this collagen marker in tear secretion. Hence many inflammatory mediators can be detected in tears (and serum) of chronic allergic eye diseases and after allergen challenge, possibly representing the communication network between a variety of inflammatory cells involved in allergic eye disease.

2.6 Neural and Nonimmune Factors

Nerve growth factor (NGF), a polypeptide produced by various cell sources including mast cells, which, through specific receptors on immune and inflammatory cells, exerts several immune functions apart from its prevalent neurotropic activity. In a recent study (38), plasma levels of NGF were significantly increased in patients with VKC and were related to the number of mast cells infiltrating the tarsal and bulbar conjunctiva. Patients with VKC also show increased plasma levels of substance P (SP) (39), a neuropeptide, the synthesis and release of which are also modulated by several factors including NGF. In fact, VKC patients with higher levels of NGF also had high levels of SP. Increased levels of NGF, however, are not confined to VKC, but also occur in other forms of allergic conjunctivitis as well as in other allergic diseases, such as asthma (40). In addition, increased expression of estrogen and progesterone receptors in conjunctival biopsies of patients with VKC has also been demonstrated (41).

Allergic inflammation is a complex phenomenon modulated by several factors. Data, briefly mentioned in the foregoing, suggest that several nonimmune factors, such as neural and endocrine factors, may have a role in influencing pathological changes and clinical expression of VKC and other allergic eye diseases.

2.7 Functional Correlates

To test the hypothesis that underlying inflammation is also responsible for an augmented responsiveness of the conjunctiva to nonspecific stimuli—as it occurs in other organs—the conjunctival responsiveness to histamine diphosphate (0.1–1.0 mg/mL) in VKC patients had been compared with that in healthy controls (42). Both VKC patients and controls reacted to histamine with a dose-dependent conjunctival redness 2–5 min after challenge. However, at low histamine doses (0.01 and 0.05 mg/mL), VKC patients had a significantly more intense reaction than controls ($p < 0.05$). Moreover, the concentration of histamine diphosphate that caused a threshold conjunctival redness (provoking concentration of histamine; PC) was significantly lower in patients with VKC than in controls ($p < 0.02$). A nonspecific conjunctival hyperreactivity to histamine has also been reported in SAC and PAC (43). The existence of a conjunctival hyperresponsiveness to histamine in VKC might be relevant for a better understanding of the pathogenesis of some clinical features of this disease, such as its variable course not related to the environmental changes of the sensitizing allergen (if any), or the hyperresponsiveness to sun, wind, dust, and other natural agents. It can also be speculated that nonspecific conjunctival hyperreactivity has a primary pathogenic role in forms of ''allergic'' conjunctivitis for which no clinical sensitization is detectable, as in many cases of VKC and contact lens conjunctivitis.

3 CLINICAL PRESENTATIONS

3.1 Allergic Conjunctivitis

Mast cell and IgE-mediated reactions are the most common hypersensitivity responses of the eye. Allergic conjunctivitis (AC) is caused by the direct exposure of the ocular mucosal surfaces to the environment. At the interface of the conjunctiva there are an estimated 50 million mast cells.

The conjunctival symptoms of itching, tearing, and burning may also include corneal symptoms of photophobia and blurring of vision. Clinical signs of AC include a milky or pale pink conjunctiva, with vascular congestion, which may progress to conjunctival swelling (chemosis). A white exudate may form during the acute state, which becomes string-like in the chronic form.

The differential diagnosis of ocular allergic disorders includes infectious causes (chlamydia, molluscum contagiosum, Parinaud's oculoglandular syndrome), chronic forms of conjunctivitis (giant papillary conjunctivitis, vernal conjunctivitis, atopic keratoconjunctivitis, superior limbic conjunctivitis, follicular conjunctivitis), and miscellaneous disorders including keratoconjunctivitis sicca, acne rosacea, and ocular cicatricial pemphigoid.

Allergic conjunctivitis is characterized histologically by infiltration of the conjunctiva with inflammatory cells, including neutrophils, eosinophils, lymphocytes, and macrophages. In contrast to asthma that has eosinophilic infiltration as a predominant feature, allergic conjunctivitis has a paucity of eosinophilic infiltration in the acute stage. However, there are numerous eosinophils in the more chronic forms. Tear fluid from these patients contains a small amount of eosinophils and histamine.

3.2 Seasonal and Perennial Allergic Conjunctivitis

Seasonal and perennial allergic conjunctivitis are the most prevalent forms of ocular allergy. Of the two, seasonal allergic conjunctivitis is more common. The importance of this condition is more due to its frequency than its severity, and it is estimated that 5–22% of the population suffers from this condition (44)

3.2.1 Seasonal Allergic Conjunctivitis

CLINICAL FEATURES. Seasonal allergic conjunctivitis (SAC) is the most common form of allergic conjunctivitis and represents half of all cases of allergic conjunctivitis. The onset of symptoms is seasonally related to specific circulating aeroallergens. Grass pollens have been noted to be associated with increased ocular symptoms noted during the spring and in some areas in the fall (''Indian summer''). The ocular symptoms are frequently associated with nasal and pharyngeal complaints. Common ocular complaints include itching, burning sensation, and watery discharge. A white exudate may form during the acute state; it becomes string-like in the chronic form. Rarely, SAC may also include corneal symptoms of photophobia and blurring of vision. The conjunctival surfaces are mildly injected with various levels of chemosis or conjunctival edema. Lid edema may sometimes occur as well as papillary hypertrophy along the tarsal conjunctival surface.

Symptoms are usually bilateral, although the degree of involvement may not be symmetrical. Affected persons usually have a history of atopy. Allergic conjunctivitis is seldom followed by permanent visual impairment.

3.2.2 Perennial Allergic Conjunctivitis

CLINICAL FEATURES. Perennial allergic conjunctivitis (PAC) is considered to be a variant of SAC that persists throughout the year, although 79% of PAC patients experience a seasonal exacerbation. Dust mites, animal dander, and feathers are the most common airborne allergens implicated in PAC. The prevalence of associated symptoms of asthma or eczema is lower than for SAC (3.5:10,000) (45). PAC is similar to SAC in age range and duration of symptoms, although SAC is subjectively more severe. When patients with PAC are compared with those who have SAC, a history of exposure to house dust was more common in PAC (42 vs. 0%), as well as the association of perennial rhinitis (75 vs. 12%).

PATHOPHYSIOLOGY. Both SAC and PAC are typical mast cell-mediated hypersensitivity reactions affecting the eye, in which the allergens react with specific IgE antibodies bound to the surface of conjunctival mast cells. The activation of mast cells leads to the release of a powerful vasoactive amine that is largely responsible for the itching, vasodilation, and edema encountered in allergic conjunctivitis.

Patients with SAC and PAC have been noted to have aeroallergen sensitivity and elevated IgE in both tears and serum. One difference between PAC and SAC includes the finding that 89% of PAC patients had specific serum IgE for house dust as compared with 43% of SAC patients. Similarly, 78% of PAC patients had tear-specific IgE for house dust, whereas none of the SAC patients had measurable IgE specific for house dust in tears. Tear samples of SAC and PAC patients also contain elevated levels of eosinophil major basic protein (MBP).

Eosinophils have been demonstrated in conjunctival scraping in 25–84% of PAC patients and in 43% of SAC patients. Various mediators from eosinophils, such as eosinophil cationic protein (ECP) have been detected in tears. However, serum levels of ECP have not been increased in children with allergic conjunctivitis (46).

3.3 Atopic Keratoconjunctivitis

Atopic keratoconjunctivitis (AKC) is a chronic inflammatory process frequently involving the lower tarsal conjunctiva. A family history of atopy, including conditions such as eczema and asthma, is common. Approximately 95% of patients with AKC also have eczema and 87% have a history of asthma. AKC typically begins in the late teens and early 20s and may persist until the fourth and fifth decades of life. The disorder presents only occasionally before the late teens. In one study evaluating pediatric atopic dermatitis patients between 1 and 10 years of age, only 21% had symptoms localized to the eyelids (47). In contrast, severe AKC was associated with complications such as blepharoconjunctivitis, and cataract, and ocular herpes simplex was observed in 40% of older patients, with the peak incidence occurring in the 30 to 50-year-old age group (48–50).

CLINICAL FEATURES. Ocular disease activity correlates with exacerbations and remissions of the dermatitis as well as with tear levels of ECP (51,52). Ocular involvement has been reported in 41 of 128 patients with atopic dermatitis: 13 had severe conjunctivitis, whereas 3 had severe keratitis (53). In another study, 85 out of 200 patients with atopic dermatitis were reported to have ocular involvement, including blepharoconjunctivitis, cataract, corneal scarring, pannus formation, keratoconus, and ocular herpes simplex (54).

The symptoms of AKC commonly include itching, burning, and tearing. These symptoms are more severe than in SAC or PAC and tend to be present throughout the year. Symptoms may worsen in the winter and summer months and may be exacerbated by exposure to animal dander, dust, and certain foods (55).

The periorbital skin, skin, and cheeks may demonstrate eczematoid changes, including erythema and thick scales. The skin of the eyelid is frequently affected by eczema that results in a single or double infraorbital crease (''Dennie–Morgan lines'') secondary to edema or thickening. The absence of the lateral eyebrow present in many older patients (''de Hertoghe's sign'') may be due to the extensive chronic eye rubbing in response to severe itching (56). Corneal scarring and neovascularization may result in blindness.

Other ocular findings include bilateral involvement of the conjunctiva in the form of fine papillary hypertrophy of the upper and lower tarsal conjunctiva, chemosis, limbal hyperemia, and limbal gelatinous hyperplasia. Cicatricial conjunctivitis with subepithelial fibrosis, fornix shortening, and symblepharon formation is observed in more severe cases. These findings are similar to the ocular manifestations of cicatricial pemphigoid (57,58).

PATHOPHYSIOLOGY. Bilateral involvement with abundant mucoid discharge is common. Secondary staphylococcal blepharitis is prevalent owing to the eyelids becoming indurated and macerated. Patients with AKC have a higher incidence of bilateral superinfection, especially with *Staphylococcus* (59,60). The corneal epithelium reveals punctate staining with fluorescein and limbal infiltration with Horner–Trantas dots. Patients with AKC are at risk for herpes simplex keratitis, which may be bilateral, severe, and recurrent (61). Keratoconus occurs in approximately 1.5–16% of patients with atopic dermatitis; conversely, eczema was reported to occur in 16% of patients with keratoconus (62–64).

Cataract as an ocular complication of atopic dermatitis was first reported in 1914 (65,66). Cataracts associated with AKC occur in 8–12% of patients in conjunction with severe forms of atopic dermatitis. Typically, they occur in young adults approximately 10 years after the onset of the atopic dermatitis (67,68). A unique feature of AKC cataracts is that they predominantly involve the anterior portion of the lens in the form of anterior subcapsular cataracts. AKC patients also develop posterior polar cataracts. Prolonged topical corticosteroid therapy may increase progression of cataract formation. There is no correlation between the severity of the atopic dermatitis, distribution of lesions, or serum IgE levels with the development of cataracts (69–72). The mechanism of corneal damage in this disorder is poorly understood, but it appears to be related to eosinophilic activation and mediator release.

3.4 Vernal Keratoconjunctivitis

Vernal keratoconjunctivitis (VKC) is a severe bilateral recurrent chronic ocular inflammatory process of the upper tarsal conjunctival surface. It has a marked seasonal incidence, classically occurring in the spring or vernal season. It occurs in children and young adults who have a history of atopy, including seasonal allergy, asthma, and eczema. Onset is usually before 10 years of age, with boys being affected twice as often as girls. After typically manifesting in prepubescent boys, its incidence becomes equally distributed among the sexes before ''burning out'' by the third decade of life. VKC may threaten sight if it involves the cornea.

CLINICAL FEATURES. Although VKC is a bilateral disease, it may affect the eyes asymmetrically. Symptoms of VKC include intense pruritus exacerbated by exposure to wind, dust, bright light, hot weather, or physical exertion associated with sweating. Symptoms include photophobia, foreign body sensation, and lacrimation. Examination of the eye in VKC reveals conjunctival hyperemia with papillary hypertrophy or ''cobblestoning'' of the upper tarsal plate. A milky-white fibrinous secretion composed of eosinophils, epithelial cells, and Charcot–Leyden crystals may be present. The mucus may be so abundant that a pseudomembrane forms on the upper lid when everted and exposed to heat (Maxwell–Lyon's sign). Transient limbal or conjunctival yellowish-white nodules lasting between 2 and 7 days (Horner–Trantas dots) may also be seen. Other signs include an extra lower eyelid crease (Dennie's line) and corneal ulcers.

Late in the course, subepithelial fibrosis may appear externally as white, linear scaring, running parallel to the lid margin (Arlt's line). Two forms of the disease, limbal and palpebral, exist and are named according to the region of the conjunctiva more extensively affected. In severe cases, an oval-shaped keratitis or ''shield ulcer'' develops superiorly on the cornea. This condition may result in severe discomfort and photophobia.

PATHOPHYSIOLOGY. Patients with VKC have demonstrated an increased responsiveness to topically applied histamine when compared with healthy controls (0.01 vs 0.05 mg/mL of histamine) (73). The effect of topically placed histamine may be due to the decreased amount of histaminases in tear fluid of VKC patients when compared with normals (74). Eosinophil cationic protein levels found in tears were directly correlated with patient symptoms and were reduced when anti-inflammatory treatment was initiated with cyclosporine or dexamethasone (75).

3.5 Giant Papillary Conjunctivitis

CLINICAL FEATURES. Giant papillary conjunctivitis (GPC), characterized by upper tarsal papillary hypertrophy or ''cobblestoning,'' is associated with continued use of contact lens and ocular prosthetics. Pruritus and tearing associated with GPC will tend to aggravate during the spring, when pollen counts are high. Signs include a white or clear exudate that often becomes thick and rope-like.

PATHOPHYSIOLOGY. GPC is associated with infiltration of basophils, eosinophils, plasma cells, and lymphocytes suggesting a mixed mast cell and lymphocyte-mediated process. The contact lens preservative thimerosal and proteinaceous deposits on the surface of the lens have been implicated as causes of GPC, but their specific role in the etiology of disease remains controversial.

Analysis of glycoprotein deposits on disposable soft contact lenses have revealed that protein deposition is more likely to occur on the tarsal surface of the lens, and protein integration is directly proportional to the lens' water content. Corneal deposits contain lysozyme, tear-specific prealbumin, and the heavy-chain components of IgG (76). In one case of lens-associated GPC, the numbers of plasma cells and mast cells were elevated (77). Tear histamine levels have not been increased (78), whereas elevations of leukotrienes (LTC_4) have been reported (79). A recent study compared normal tear fluid LTC_4 levels with tear fluid from soft contact lens wearers with and without GPC (80). The LTC_4 levels reported in that study were 210 pg/mL for control patients, 221 pg/mL for normal soft contact lens wearers, and 550 pg/mL for contact lens wearers with evidence of giant papillary conjunctivitis.

GPC may develop in both rigid and soft contact lens wearers and is estimated to affect 1–5% of rigid contact lens wearers and up to 15% of soft contact lens patients (81). Disposable contact lenses have been proposed as an alternative treatment for GPC (82,83).

4 HETEROGENEITY OF INFLAMMATION IN ALLERGIC EYE DISEASES

Allergic eye disease cannot be explained by the classic type I hypersensitivity reaction. Several cells and mediators are involved in a complex inflammatory network. However, inflammation is a heterogeneous mechanism, and it is conceivable that preferential pathophysiological inflammatory pathways play a role in the different forms of ''red eye'' and even in different patients with the same clinical diagnosis. Recently (84), it has been suggested that three major pathophysiological abnormalities—undergoing different genetic and environmental control—can be invoked to explain the heterogeneity of the spectrum of clinical phenotypes of allergic conjunctivitis:

1. An increased allergen recognition and specific IgE response
2. A Th2 cytokine profile associated with polyclonal total IgE (and IgG4) overproduction and up-regulation mast cells, basophils, and eosinophils
3. A hyperresponsiveness of target organs.

It has also been suggested that the foregoing abnormalities more or less impinge on the different forms of allergic conjunctivitis. For instance, in the typical SAC the type I hypersensitivity mechanism predominates. Because of genetic (HLA) and environmental (pollen exposure) influences, an abnormal IgE response to pollen allergens develops. Total IgE, inflammation, and target organs' hyperreactivity are usually modest out of pollen season. On the other hand, in VKC and AKC the Th2 profile (overexpression of the 5q cytokine gene cluster) is prominent, with high total IgE, mast cells, and eosinophils independently from the presence of a clinical sensitization (often to multiple allergens as the result of the polyclonal IgE activation). Finally, in GPC and other forms of nonspecific conjunctivitis, the hyperresponsiveness of the conjunctiva is the major pathophysiological abnormality, whereas specific IgE and markers of eosinophilic inflammation are absent.

Different nosological entities grouped under the umbrella term of allergic conjunctivitis are now diagnosed on the basis of clinical criteria. It is hoped that the appreciation of the pathophysiological heterogeneity of a red eye might lead to a revised classification of allergic eye diseases as well as to a more selective management based on the preferential pathogenic pathways operating in individual cases.

REFERENCES

1. Rahi AH, Garner A. Immunopathology of the Eye. Oxford: Blackwell Scientific, 1976.
2. Allansmith MR. The Eye and Immunology. St. Louis: CV Mosby, 1982.
3. Bielory L, Frohman LP. Allergic and immunologic disorders of the eye. J Allergy Clin Immunol 1992; 98:1–15.
4. Faure JP, Bloch–Michel E, Le Hoang P, Vadot E. Immunopathologie de L'Oeil. Paris: Societé Francaise d'Ophthalmologie, Masson, 1988.
5. Bonini S, Bonini S, Tomassini M. Les allergies oculaires. In: Charpin J, Vervloet D, eds. Allergologie. 3rd ed. Paris: Med Sci Flammarion, 1992:714.

6. Friedlander NH. Conjunctivitis of allergic origin: clinical presentation and differential diagnosis. Surv Ophthalmol 1993; 28(suppl 1):105–14.
7. Gleich GJ. The late phase of the immunoglobulin E-mediated reaction: a link between anaphylaxis and common allergic disease? J Allergy Clin Immunol 1982; 70:160.
8. Bonini S, Bonini S. Studies of allergic conjunctivitis. Chibret Int J 1987; 5:12.
9. Morgan SJ, Williams JH, Walls AF, Church MK, Holgate ST, McGill JI. Mast cell numbers and staining characteristics in the normal and allergic human conjunctiva. J Allergy Clin Immunol 1991; 87:111.
10. Macleod JDA, Anderson DF, Baddeley SM, Holgate ST, MaGill JI, Roche WR. Immunolocalization of cytokines to mast cells in normal and allergic conjunctiva. Clin Exp Allergy 1997; 27:1328–1334.
11. Morgan SJ, Williams JH, Walls AF, Church MK, Holgate ST, McGill JI. Mast cell numbers and staining characteristics in the normal and allergic human conjunctiva. J Allergy Clin Immunol 1991; 87:111.
12. Macleod JDA, Anderson DF, Baddeley SM, Holgate ST, MaGill JI, Roche WR. Immunolocalization of cytokines to mast cells in normal and allergic conjunctiva. Clin Exp Allergy 1997; 27:1328–34.
13. Magrini L, Metz D, Bacon A, Bonini S, Bonini S, Lightman S. Immunocytochemistry and inflammation of vernal keratoconjunctivitis. Invest Ophthalmol Vis Sci 1993; 34:857.
14. Maggi E, Biswas P, Del Prete G, Parronchi P, Macchia D, Simonelli C, Emmi L, De Carli M, Tiri A, Ricci M, Romagnani S. Accumulation of Th-2 like helper T cells in the conjunctiva of patients with vernal conjunctivitis. J Immunol 1991; 146:1169.
15. Metz D, Hingorani M, Calder VL, Buckley RJ, Lightman SL. T-cell cytokines in chronic allergic eye diseases. J Allergy Clin Immunol 1997; 100:817–824.
16. Bonini S, Bonini S, Vecchione A, Naim DM, Allansmith MR, Balsano F. Inflammatory changes in conjunctival scrapings after challenge provocation in humans. J Allergy Clin Immunol 1988; 82:462.
17. Bonini S, Bonini S, Bucci MG, Berruto A, Adriani E, Balsano F, Allansmith MR. Allergen dose response and late symptoms in a human model of ocular allergy. J Allergy Clin Immunol 1990; 86:869.
18. Abelson MB, Mediwale N, Weston JH. Conjunctival eosinophil in allergic ocular disease. Arch Ophthalmol 1983; 101:555–556.
19. Bonini S, Tomassini M, Bonini S, Capron M, Balsano F. The eosinophil has a pivotal role in allergic inflammation of the eye. Int Arch Allergy Immunol 1992; 99:354–358.
20. Trocme SD, Aldave AJ. The eye and the eosinophil. Surv Ophthalmol 1994; 39:241–252.
21. Bonini S, Bonini S, Lambiase A, Marchi S, Pasqualetti P, Zuccaro O, Rama P, Magrini L, Juhas T, Bucci MG. Vernal keratoconjunctivitis: a case series of 195 patients with long-term follow-up. Ophthalmology 2000; 107:1157–1163.
22. Bonini S, Bonini S, Lambiase A, Magrini L, Rumi C, Del Prete GF, Schiavone M, Rotiroti G, Onorati P, Rutella S. Vernal keratoconjunctivitis: a model of 5q cytokine gene cluster disease. Int Arch Allergy Immunol 1995; 107:95–98.
23. Bonini S, Bonini S. Vernal keratoconjunctivitis: a model Th2 disease. ACI Int 1998; 10:88–91.
24. Hingorani M, Calder V, Jolly G, Backley RJ, Lightman SL. Eosinophil surface antigen expression and cytokine production vary in different ocular allergic diseases. J Allergy Clin Immunol 1998; 102:821–830.
25. Rumi C, Rutella S, Puggioni PL, Lambiase A, Bonini S, Bonini S. Expression of activation markers on peripheral eosinophils in vernal keratoconjunctivitis: a flow cytometric study. Allergy 1997; 52(suppl. 37):167.
26. Metz DP, Bacon S, Holgate ST, Lightman SL. Phenotypic characterisation of T cells infiltrating the conjunctiva in chronic allergic eye disease. J Allergy Clin Immunol 1996; 98:686–696.

27. Solomon A, Shmilowich R, Shasha D, Frucht–Pery J, Pe'er J, Bonini S, Levi–Schaffer F. Conjunctival fibroblasts enhance the survival and functional activities of peripheral blood eosinophils in vitro. Invest Ophthalmol Vis Sci 2000; 41:1038–1044.
28. Ciprandi G, Buscaglia S, Pesce G, Villaggio B, Bagnasco M, Canonica GW. Allergic subjects express intercellular adhesion molecule-1 (ICAM-1 or CD54) on epithelial cells of conjunctiva after allergen challenge. J Allergy Clin Immunol 1993; 91:783–792.
29. Butrus SI, Ochsner KI, Abelson MN, Schwartz LB. The level of tryptase in human tears. An indicator of activation of conjunctival mast cells. Ophathalomlogy 1990; 97:1678.
30. Vesaluoma M, Rosenberg ME, Teppo A–M, Grönhagen–Riska C, Haahtela T, Tervo T. Tumour necrosis factor-alpha in tears of atopic patients after conjunctival allergen challenge. Clin Exp Allergy 1999; 29:537–542.
31. Proud D, Sweet J, Stein P, Settipane RA, Kagey–Sobotka A, Friedlander MH, Lichtenstein LM. Inflammatory mediator on conjunctival provocation of allergic subjects with allergen. J Allergy Clin Immunol 1991; 85:896.
32. Bonini S, Bonini S, Berruto A, Tomassini M, Carlesimo S, Bucci MG, Balsano F. Conjunctival provocation test as a model for the study of allergy and inflammation in humans. Int Arch Allergy Appl Immunol 1989; 88:144.
33. Leonardi A, Borghesan F, Faggiom D, Secchi A, Plebani M. Eosinphil cationic protein in tears of normal subjects and patients affected by vernal keratoconjunctivitis. Allergy 1995; 50:610–613.
34. Montan PG, van Hage–Hamsten M, Zetterstrom O. Sustained eosinophil cationic protein release into tears after a single high-dose conjunctival allergen challenge. Clin Exp Allergy 1996; 26:1125–1130.
35. Tomasini M, Magrini L, De Petrillo G. Serum levels of eosinophil cationic protein in allergic diseases and natural allergen exposure. J Allergy Clin Immunol 1996; 97:1350–1355.
36. Tomassini M, Magrini L, Bonini S. Increased serum levels of eosinophil cationic protein and eosinophil-derived neurotoxin (protein X) in vernal keratoconjunctivitis. Ophthalmology 1994; 101:1808–1811.
37. Rotiroti G, Magrini L, Onorati P. IL-5 in tears of vernal keratoconjunctivitis patients [abstr]. Allergy 1995; 50:180.
38. Lambiase A, Bonini S, Bonini S. Increased plasma levels of nerve growth factor in vernal keratoconjunctivitis and relationship with mast cells. Invest Ophthalmol Vis Sci 1995; 36: 2127–2132.
39. Lambiase A, Bonini S, Micera A, Tirassa P, Magrini L, Bonni S, Aloe L. Increased plasma levels of substance P and nerve growth in vernal keratoconjucntivitis. Invest Ophthalomol Vis Sci 1997; 38:2162–2164.
40. Bonini S, Lambiase A. Circulating nerve growth factor levels are increased in humans with allergic diseases and asthma. Proc Natl Acad Sci USA 1996; 93:10955–10960.
41. Bonini S, Lambiase A, Schiavone M. Estrogen and progesterone receptors in vernal keratoconjunctivitis. Ophthalmology 1995; 102:1374–1379.
42. Bonini S, Bonini S, Schiavone M, Centofanti M, Allansmith MR, Bucci MG. Conjunctival hyperresponsiveness to ocular histamine challenge in patients with vernal conjunctivitis. J Allergy Clin Immunol 1992; 89:103.
43. Ciprandi G, Buscaglia S, Pesce GP. Ocular challenge and hyperresponsiveness to histamine in patients with allergic conjunctivitis. J Allergy Clin Immunol 1993; 91:1227–1230.
44. Weeks ER. Epidemiology of hay fever and perennial allergic rhinitis. Monogr Allergy 1987; 21:1–20.
45. Dart JK, Buckley RJ, Monnickendan M, Prasad J. Perennial allergic conjunctivitis: definition, clinical characteristics and prevalence. A comparison with seasonal allergic conjunctivitis. Trans Ophthalmol Soc UK 1986; 105:513–520.
46. Sohoel P, Freng BA, Kramer J, et al. Topical levocabastine compared with orally administered

terfenadine for the prophylaxis and treatment of seasonal rhinoconjunctivitis. J Allergy Clin Immunol 1993; 92:73–81.
47. Schudel P, Wuthrich B. Klinische verlaufsbeobachtungen bei Neurodermatitis atopic dem Kleinkindersalter, eine katamnestische untersuchung anhand von 121 Fallen. Z Hautkr 1985; 60:479.
48. Garrity JA, Liesegang TJ. Ocular complications of atopic dermatitis. Can J Ophthalmol 1984; 19:21.
49. Oshinskie L, Haine C. Atopic dermatitis and its ophthalmic complications. J Am Optom Assoc 1982; 53:889.
50. Rich LF, Hanifin JM. Ocular complications of atopic dermatitis and other eczemas. Int Ophthalmol Clin 1985; 25:61.
51. Montab PG, van Hage–Hamsten M. Eosinophil cationic protein in tears in allergic conjunctivitis. Br J Ophthalmol 1996; 80:556–560.
52. Hogan MJ. Atopic keratoconjunctivitis. Am J Ophthalmol 1953; 36:937–947.
53. Karel I, Myska V, Kvicalova E. Ophthalmological changes in atopic dermatitis. Acta Dermatol Venerol 1965; 45:381–386.
54. Garrity JA, Liesegang TJ. Ocular complications of atopic dermatitis. Can J Ophthalmol 1984; 9:21–24.
55. Foster CS, Calonge M. Atopic keratoconjunctivitis. Ophthalmology 1990; 97:992–1000.
56. Rich LF, Hanifin JM. Ocular complications of atopic dermatitis and other eczemas. Int Ophthalmol Clin 1985; 25:61–76.
57. Tuft SJ, Kemeny M, Bdart JKG, Buckley RJ. Clinical features of atopic keratoconjunctivitis. Ophthalmology 1991; 98:150–158.
58. Foster CS, Calonge M. Atopic keratoconjunctivitis. Ophthalmology 1990; 97:992–1000.
59. Tuft SJ, Ramakrishnan M, Seal DV, Kemeny M, Buckley RJ. Role of *Staphylococcus aureus* in chronic allergic conjunctivitis. Ophthalmology 1992; 99:180–184.
60. Hogan MJ. Atopic keartoconjunctivitis. Trans Am Ophthalmol Soc 1952; 50:265–281.
61. Rich LF, Hanifin JM. Ocular complications of atopic dermatitis and other eczemas. Int Ophthalmol Clin 1985; 25:61–76.
62. Beetham WP. Atopic cataracts. Arch Ophthalmol 1940; 24:21–37.
63. Amemiya T, Matsuda H, Vehara M. Ocular findings in atopic dermatitis with special reference to the clinical features of the atopic cataract. Ophthalmologica 1980; 129–132.
64. Copeman PWM. Eczema and keratoconus. Br Med J 1965; 2:977.
65. Brunsting LA, Reed WB, Bair HL. Occurrence of cataracts and keratoconus with atopic dermatitis. Arch Dermatol 1955; 72:237–241.
66. Beetham W. Atopic cataracts. Arch Ophthalmol. 1940; 24:21–37.
67. Kornerup T, Lodin A. Ocular changes in 100 cases of Besnier's prurigo (atopic dermatitis). Acta Ophthalmol 1959; 37:508.
68. Uehara M, Amemiya T, Arai M. Atopic cataracts in a Japanese population. With special reference to factors possibly relevant to cataract formation. Dermatologica 1985; 170:180.
69. Tuft SJ, Kemeny M, Bdart JKG, Buckley RJ. Clinical features of atopic keratoconjunctivitis. Ophthalmology 1991; 98:150–158.
70. Garrity JA, Liesegang TJ. Ocular complications of atopic dermatitis. Can J Ophthalmol 1984; 19:21.
71. Amemiya T, Matsuda H, Uehara M. Ocular findings in atopic dermatitis with special reference to the clinical features of the atopic cataract. Ophthalmologica 1980; 180:129–132.
72. Foster CS, Calonge M. Atopic keratoconjunctivitis. Ophthalmology. 1990; 97:992–1000.
73. Abelson MB, Baird RS. Allansmith MR. Tear histamine levels in vernal conjunctivitis and other ocular inflammations. Ophthalmology 1980; 87:812–814.
74. Secchi A, Leonardi A, Abelson M. The role of eosinophil cationic protein (ECP) and histamine in vernal keratoconjunctivitis. Ocul Immunol Inflamm 1995; 3:23–28.
75. Leonardi A, Borghesan F, Faggian D, Secchi A, Plebani M. Eosinophil cationic protein in

tears of normal subjects and patients affected by vernal keratoconjunctivitis. Allergy 1995; 50:610–613.

76. Tripathi PC, Tripathi RC. Analysis of glycoprotein deposits on disposable contact lenses. Invest Ophthalmol Vis Sci 1992; 33:121–125.
77. Henriquez AS, Allansmith MR. Russell bodies in contact-lens-associated giant papillary conjunctivitis. Arch Ophthalmol 1979; 97:473–478.
78. Allansmith MR, Ross RN. Giant papillary conjunctivitis. Int Ophthalmol Clin 1988; 28:309–316.
79. Irkeç M, Orhan M. Effect of extended wear disposable contact lenses on tear LTC_4 in giant papillary conjunctivitis. Ocul Immunol Inflamm 1995; 3:107–111.
80. Irkec MT, Orhan M, Erdener E. Role of tear inflammatory mediators in contact lens-associated giant papillary conjunctivitis in soft contact lens wearers. Ocul Immunol Inflamm 1999; 7: 35–38.
81. Stenson SM. Lid, conjunctival, and corneal complications of contact lenses. In: Stenson SM, ed. Contact Lenses. Norwealk, CT: Appleton & Lange, 1987:215–217.
82. Driebe WT Jr. Disposable soft contact lenses. Surv Ophthalmol 1989; 34:44–46.
83. Coursaux G, Bloch–Michel E, Assin M. Rééquipement avec les lentilles jetables de patients porteurs de conjonctivite papillaire géante. Premiers résultats. Bull Soc Ophthalmol Fr 1989; 89:1371–1372.
84. Bonini S, Bonini S. Pathogenesis of allergic conjunctivitis. In: Denburg JA, ed. Allergy and Allergic Diseases. The New Mechanisms and Therapeutics. Totowa, NJ: Humana Press, 1998: 509–519.

15

Asthma

SAJU S. EAPEN and WILLIAM W. BUSSE

University of Wisconsin Medical School, Madison, Wisconsin

1 INTRODUCTION

Asthma is a complex clinical entity that is characterized by variable airflow obstruction, bronchial hyperresponsiveness (BHR), mucous hypersecretion, airway edema, and airway inflammation. Our understanding of the pathogenesis of asthma has undergone a major change in the last decade, with a current emphasis on airway inflammation as the principal feature of the disease. The concept of inflammation is, however, not new. Sir William Osler and Austin Flint considered asthma to be a type of bronchitis, thus implying inflammation as a component of the process. The term *inflammation* is rather nonspecific, but it better explains the chronic nature of asthma and the resulting physiology and pathophysiology, than the previous narrow view of asthma as a purely bronchospastic condition.

Bronchoscopy has provided a safe means both for challenging and sampling the airway in asthma. The use of bronchoscopy for biopsy and lavage of the asthmatic airway has overcome the limitation of autopsy material and has firmly established and begun to define the role of inflammation in the pathogenesis of asthma. New developments in immunology and molecular biology have also led to a more sophisticated analysis of the inflammatory cells and mediators. From this has emerged the knowledge that several different cell types are responsible for the airflow obstruction and hyperresponsiveness that characterize asthma. Investigations are now ongoing to determine the factors that control this process of inflammation, with interdependent and sometimes redundant roles proposed for cytokines, adhesion molecules, and neural mechanisms, in the development of inflammation in the asthmatic airway. Various stimuli, such as allergens, airborne irritants, respiratory viral infections, and occupational exposure, can provoke episodes of asthma. These stimuli act through different pathways to produce the same end result, which is an eosinophilic and lymphocytic airway inflammation. In addition, it has become recognized that a repair process occurs in asthma and may result in remodeling, thereby causing permanent changes to the airway that contribute to altered lung function. These features of injury and repair from inflammation need to be considered both for understanding the pathogenesis and mechanism of asthma, as well as to develop treatments to modify the underlying disease process. This chapter will review the role of inflammation in asthma, as well as the purported role of various cells and mediators in the progression of the disease.

2 INFLAMMATION IN ASTHMA

The concept of asthma has changed over the years from that of a ''simple'' disease caused primarily by airway smooth-muscle contraction, to a more complex persistent disease process in which there is a complex interplay between various inflammatory mediators, effector cells, and the nervous system. These rather radical changes in the concept of asthma have come about as the result of various observations made in autopsy studies of fatal cases of asthma, the use of bronchoscopy and biopsy of asthmatics with mild or even asymptomatic disease—BAL—studies, and molecular tools to more precisely define the various inflammatory mediators.

Inflammatory changes in asthma had previously been observed in autopsy specimens of patients with fatal asthma. These changes were originally thought to represent characteristic histological features of severe asthma and a terminal event. The histopathological features noted in fatal asthma included airway smooth-muscle hypertrophy, apparent basement membrane thickening, glandular hyperplasia, terminal bronchiole mucous plugging, and inflammatory cells in the lamina propria. The multicellular nature of the inflammatory infiltrate was noted even at this time. A better appreciation of the inflammatory process as being intrinsic to asthma has emerged with the availability and use of techniques such as fiber-optic bronchoscopy, lavage, and biopsy. The general consensus now is that inflammation is a characteristic feature of the disease process in asthma.

Initial bronchial biopsy studies by Beasley and associates (1) and Jeffery and coworkers (2) demonstrated characteristic features of denuded epithelium, increased collagen deposition below the basement membrane and inflammatory cell infiltrates, even in individuals with mild asthma. Some of these inflammatory cells also appeared to be activated.

Bronchoalveolar lavage (BAL) fluid analyses also provided further evidence of the inflammatory nature of asthma. Analyses of BAL fluid from moderately severe asthmatic subjects showed an increased percentage of eosinophils, mast cells, and epithelial cells, when compared with both atopic and nonatopic nonasthmatic controls. In addition, total cell counts, total lymphocytes, neutrophils, and macrophages, in contrast, were mostly unchanged (1,3,4–6). T cells were noted to be phenotypically different and expressed markers of activation, including interleukin-2 receptor (IL-2R), human leukocyte antigen (HLA)-DR and very late antigen (VLA)-1 (7,8). These T cells were also thought to belong to a T-helper cell type-2 (Th2)-like phenotype based on the cytokine mRNA and protein profile elaborated. A relation between airway function and the cellular markers of inflammation was shown by demonstrating a correlation between airway methacholine reactivity of individuals and the numbers of $CD25^+$ cells and eosinophils (9,10).

Various studies have been designed to elucidate the histology of the airways, the various cellular participants, mediators, and cytokines. These have shed light on the potential cellular products generated in response to activation of asthma and the complex interactive nature of this process, which ultimately leads to chronic airway changes. Several different models have been developed to study inflammation in asthma. Observations made from these models have been correlated with features of the natural disease or physiological markers of disease activity in asthmatic patients to ascertain pathogenic mechanisms. These approaches have resulted in an improved, but incomplete, understanding of the inflammatory process in asthma: bronchospasm, acute and chronic inflammation, persistent inflammation, and repair, and how they are initiated, interconnected, and perhaps, most importantly, self-perpetuated.

Histopathological studies have lead to the proposal that inflammation is an important aspect of asthma and contributes to the degree of bronchial hyperresponsiveness, chronic airway injury, and changes in lung function. It has also become evident that the inflammatory process in asthma involves multiple cell types and that the various cellular interactions are complex (Fig. 1), often redundant, and sometimes self-perpetuating. Increased awareness of these events has led to a better understanding of asthma pathogenesis and treatment, with greater emphasis being placed on mechanisms of inflammation and therapeutic interventions to reduce these changes.

The inflammatory response in asthma has been arbitrarily divided into three phases: acute, chronic, and injury–repair or airway remodeling. Each of these apparent continuous phases has distinct implications in relation to histopathology, physiology, therapy, and the eventual sequelae. Studies that have involved airway activation by antigen exposure

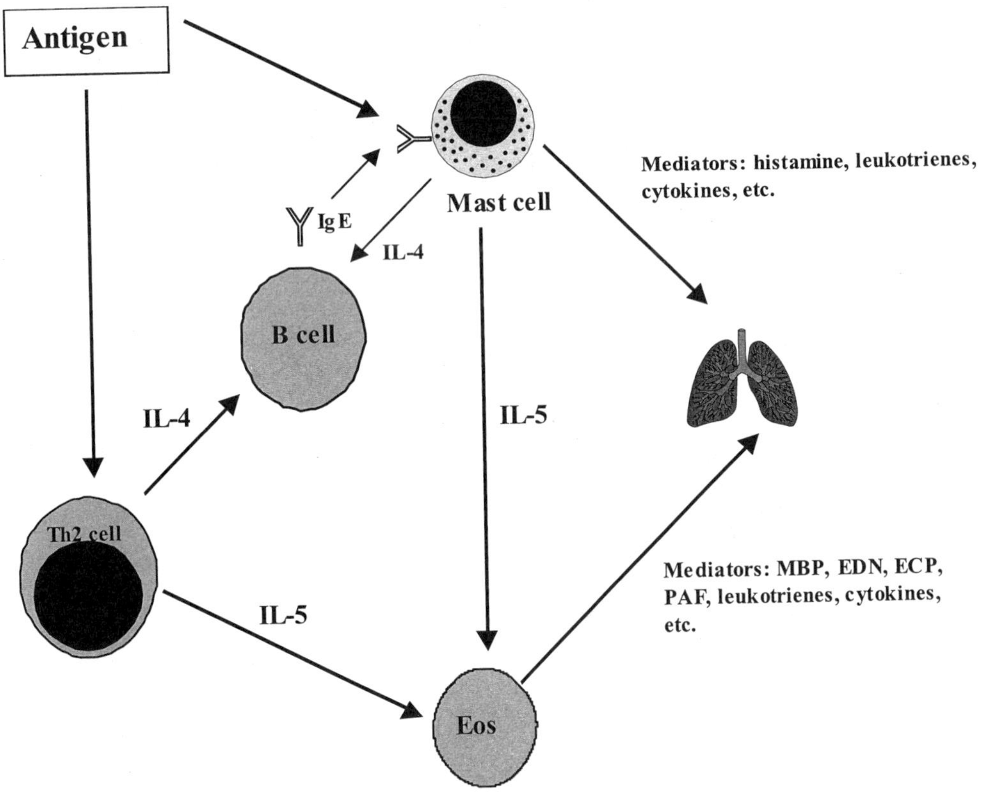

Figure 1 Inflammation in asthma: This illustration outlines the various interactions that occur in the inflammatory process in asthma.

or challenge have contributed a great deal to our understanding of the inflammatory mechanisms. It is unknown, however, whether this accurately reflects airway activation under natural circumstances. In acute inflammation, resident airway cells are apparently activated, leading to immediate-release mediators that then causes bronchospasm, edema, and a compromise in airflow. It is proposed that this acute phase of inflammation initiates a cellular recruitment to the airway, ultimately resulting in chronic persistent inflammation. Permanent injury to the airway is not generally seen at this stage, and treatment can usually resolve the acute inflammation.

As acute disease progresses into chronic inflammation, inflammatory cells are recruited into the airway, and activated. Various inflammatory mediators, including the cytokines or chemokines, are released and participate in the acute inflammatory process. The regulation of this process is poorly understood; evidence from several therapeutic intervention studies suggests that the early phase of chronic inflammation can be controlled, and changes in the airway pathology ultimately resolved.

Airway remodeling or repair and smooth-muscle hypertrophy are now thought to be components of the inflammatory disease process in asthma. Mucous hypersecretion is also a common characteristic of asthma. Loss of lung function has been noted in some patients with asthma and these changes may actually occur early in the course of the disease. Apart from airway injury, collagen products may be deposited in the airway matrix. Thus, the concept of asthma has evolved in the last decade, and it is now viewed as an inflammatory disease, rather than a purely bronchospastic process, and current investigative and therapeutic approaches focus on this.

Various stimuli can cause asthma exacerbations. Stimuli can be divided into two types: inducers and provokers (Fig. 2). Provokers usually cause a temporary increase in asthma symptoms, but do not necessarily affect underlying inflammation or responsiveness. On the other hand, inducers increase underlying inflammation, in addition to exacerbating asthma. The three major inducers are allergens, viral infections, and occupa-

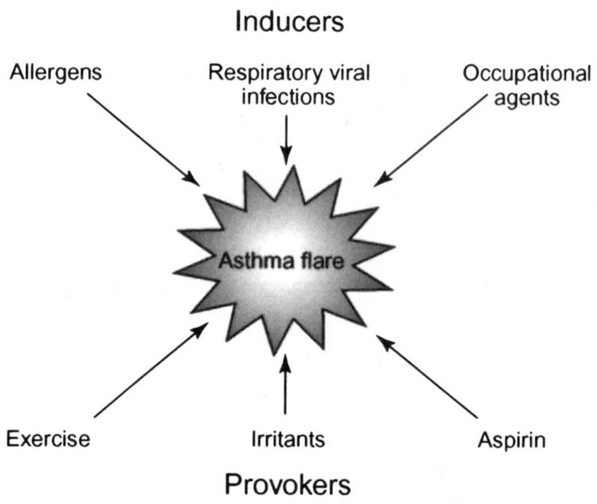

Figure 2 A range of stimuli can cause asthma exacerbations: Inducers worsen underlying disease in addition to causing an asthma exacerbation. Provokers, on the other hand, do not influence underlying inflammation and so do not affect disease severity. (From Ref. 149.)

tional exposure. It is thought that studying the interaction of the airways with these inducers can provide new insight into the underlying mechanism of asthma.

3 MODELS OF INFLAMMATION IN ASTHMA

To identify mechanisms of disease in asthma it is necessary to conduct studies in subjects with the disease and to establish animal models for experiments that cannot be performed in humans (11). Allergens, in addition to being an important precipitant of asthma, are also instrumental in the study of the mechanisms of asthma and its pathogenesis. Acute bronchospasm is usually the initial airway response to allergens and, in many individuals, it is typically followed by a late phase of airway obstruction, known as the late allergic or asthmatic response (LAR). Exposure to an allergen is usually prolonged or continuous in the natural environment, and both the immediate and late phases are likely to be a continuum. Studies of the LAR have provided evidence that acute airway inflammation is multicellular, is a part of the allergic reaction, and may play a role in the regulation of BHR. The LAR involves cell recruitment, activation, and generation of proinflammatory cytokines. It is still not entirely clear how and why this pattern of inflammation occurs in asthma or is unique to the development of persistent bronchial inflammation and eventual repair of injury. Studies on the LAR have, however, provided direction to investigate the pathogenesis of asthma.

4 THE LAR

Individuals with allergic asthma develop bronchial obstruction within minutes of exposure to inhaled antigen, with maximal airflow obstruction during the early phase of the allergic response (EAR) developing within 20–30 min (11,12). Mast cell mediators are likely responsible for this early phase of airflow obstruction. It should also be noted that these mediators also act locally on nerve endings and blood vessels to intensify the acute obstructive event by causing vasodilation and vascular leakage and by stimulating neurological events in the airway. The acute phase may subside in a relatively short time owing to a decline in short-lived mediator concentrations. In some individuals, a second phase of airflow obstruction, called the LAR, begins 4–10 hr later. The LAR is thought to be due to release of specific cytokines and chemokines along with the acute phase. These mediators then serve to attract inflammatory cells to the lung, and activate them as well as the resident airway inflammatory cells. BAL fluid obtained during the late-phase response typically contains increased numbers of eosinophils (13). The LAR has also been associated with an early eosinopenia and a late eosinophilia in the peripheral blood; the magnitude of the eosinopenia correlates with the intensity of the LAR and the degree of airway reactivity to histamine (14). They also result in the expression of specific adhesion molecules on the endothelial cell surface, which then selectively regulate cell movement into the region.

Various effector cells participate in the process of airway inflammation, including the eosinophils, lymphocytes (typically of the $CD4^+$ phenotype and having a Th2 like cytokine profile), monocytes, and neutrophils. These cells appear in the bronchial mucosa, matrix, and the lumen of the airway (15,16,17). Activation of these cells occurs by mechanisms as yet to be fully delineated and causes release of both preformed and newly synthesized factors, including toxic oxygen products, cytokines, chemokines, bronchoconstrictors, cationic proteins, and enzymes. These mediators contribute to the characteristic features of asthmatic inflammation: an increase in airway responsiveness, bronchoconstriction, epithelial cell sloughing, and edema. The initial acute inflammatory process becomes more severe and persistent. This transition may be due to persistent allergen exposure, or it may be due to the initial exposure itself and its effect on inflammatory cell function. Airway repair also begins along with the inflammatory process. Few models other than chronic asthma itself are available to study the phenomenon of persistent inflammation in asthma or the repair process (18). As our understanding of the early and late asthmatic response increases, it is becoming more apparent that some overlaps between the two responses occur. From available models, the use of antigen provocation and studies of asthma, a more complete picture of asthma, the cells, mediators, and tissues that participate in the process has emerged.

5 EOSINOPHILS

The presence of eosinophils (Fig. 3) in the sputum and blood of asthmatics was noted over 100 years ago (19). It was almost a century later that Horn and associates recognized a correlation between forced expiratory volume in 1 second (FEV_1; marker of asthma activity) and the absolute number of eosinophils in the peripheral blood of asthmatics (20). Analysis of sputum obtained from patients with acute asthmatic exacerbation also revealed clumps of desquamated airway epithelial cells, termed creola bodies, and Charcot–Leyden crystals, products of eosinophils (21).

There is now substantial evidence to suggest a pivotal role for eosinophils in the inflammatory process in asthma. The eosinophil may also be the principal effector cell responsible for tissue injury in asthma and may also have an important role in the airway response to antigen. The association between the severity of asthma and the absolute

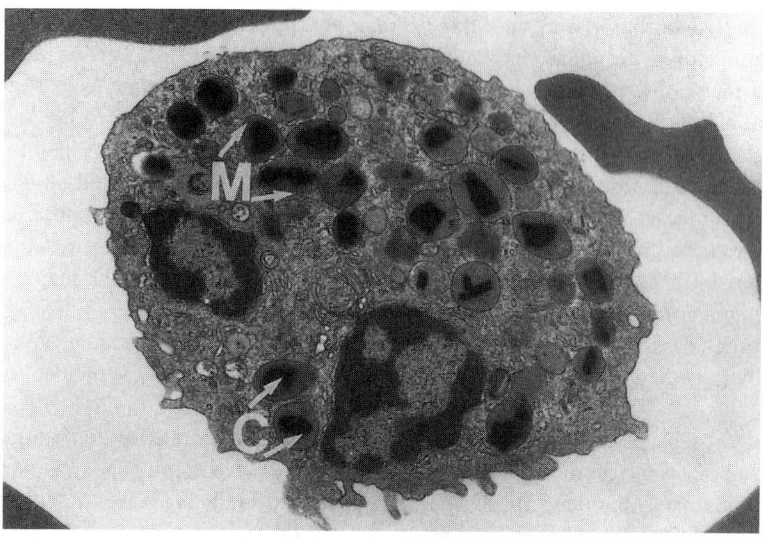

Figure 3 Electron photomicrograph of a human peripheral blood eosinophil showing intracellular granules. Original magnification × 11,500. (Courtesy of Dr. H. Kita, Mayo Clinic and Mayo Foundation, Rochester, MN.)

number of eosinophils in the peripheral blood and BAL samples was established, as determined by a graded asthma score and measurements of airflow obstruction (3). In submucosal biopsy specimens, eosinophils were observed to be degranulated, suggesting eosinophil activation in airway mucosal matrix. Also eosinophils appear in the airway lumen 24 and 48 hr after segmental airway challenge with allergen (17,22).

There is also evidence that the presence of eosinophils relates to disease activity or severity. For example, the degree of eosinophilia correlates with increases in BHR associated with antigen challenge and the appearance of sloughed airway epithelial cells (23–25). Peripheral eosinophilia also correlates with the degree of nonspecific bronchial responsiveness. This was supported by the observation by Cookson et al. of an initial peripheral eosinopenia in response to an allergen challenge, thought to be due to their rapid egress from the circulation to airway sites, followed by a subsequent eosinophilia in subjects who developed an LAR (14). Studies examining the effect of oral or inhaled corticosteroids have also demonstrated a relation between decreased numbers of eosinophils and improvement in lung function and bronchial hyperresponsiveness.

Those patients who have a dual-phase response (early and late) to an instilled airway antigen challenge show a marked increase in the number of eosinophils at 4 hr, with even higher numbers at 24 hr (26–28). The egress of eosinophils to the airway lumen is likely regulated by the action of various factors including adhesion molecules (on the cell itself and the tissues also), cytokines, and chemokines. Interleukin (IL)-18 enhances antigen-induced recruitment of eosinophils into the airways, suggesting that it may contribute to the development and exacerbation of airway inflammation in asthma (29). The eosinophil egress to the airway lumen is blocked by the action of a monoclonal antibody (MAb) targeting an adhesion molecule (α_4-integrin), which effectively prevents the development of allergen-induced airway hyperresponsiveness in primates (30). More recently, it has been shown that the nuclear factor κB (NF-κB) plays an essential role in the induction of eosinophilia in allergic airway inflammation and may be involved in the perpetuation of chronic airway inflammation (31,32). The evidence, therefore, strongly suggests that the appearance of eosinophil is causally linked and, in some cases, is correlated with the development of BHR and the severity of asthmatic responses.

Eosinophils emerge from the bone marrow as mature effector cells. The differentiating process is mediated by IL-3, IL-5, and granulocyte–macrophage colony-stimulating factor (GM-CSF). The eosinophil is then rapidly recruited into the lung tissues, mainly through the actions of T-cell cytokines and also chemokines derived from other airway tissues, including epithelium. Mature eosinophils eventually undergo apoptosis in the tissues. With persistent inflammation, increased concentrations of proinflammatory cytokines and a variety of activating factors may prolong eosinophil survival.

The eosinophil becomes activated in vivo by mechanisms that are not yet established. Circulating eosinophils are thought to vary in their metabolic state, as measured by stimulated superoxide production. Eosinophils with lower than usual density show morphological evidence of degranulation, increased oxidative metabolism, and possibly a change in the surface expression of Fcγ receptors or the integrin-common β-chain (CD18). The proportion of such lower-density eosinophils has been demonstrated in some studies to increase in subjects with asthma and also during the late-phase response to antigen. In contrast, other studies have found that eosinophil density does not accurately reflect cellular activation and surface receptor expression and that, although evidence is present for eosinophil priming in asthmatic subjects, there was no increase in the low-density eosinophil fraction (33,34).

The primary mechanism by which the eosinophils cause tissue damage is by degranulation and subsequent release of its stored granular compounds, such as major basic protein (MBP), eosinophil cationic protein (ECP), eosinophil-derived neurotoxin (EDN), and eosinophil peroxidase (EPO). In vitro, a variety of triggers enhance eosinophil degranulation, including IL-3, IL-5, and immunoglobulin complexes (35,36); however, the molecular stimuli for degranulation in vivo remain unclear. The eosinophil also synthesizes and releases certain bioactive mediators (Fig. 4) in response to stimulation. These include platelet-activating factor (PAF) that functions as a chemotactic factor and causes powerful bronchoconstriction (6,37,38) and eicosanoid derivatives of arachidonic acid, such as leukotriene-C_4 (LTC_4), which then can cause bronchoconstriction and increased airway vascular permeability (39).

Eosinophil granule proteins are present in increased concentrations in the sputum of asthmatic patients during an exacerbation of asthma (40,41). Large deposits of these granule proteins, especially MBP have been detected at sites of epithelial injury, even when intact eosinophils are scarce (42). MBP is cytotoxic to bronchial cells in animals in vivo and in human in vitro models. It has also been localized to sites of epithelial damage in the asthmatic bronchial mucosa. BAL fluid and sputum MBP levels have been correlated with the severity of asthma (43). In addition, greater levels of MBP have been detected in the BAL fluid of symptomatic asthmatic individuals than in those with an asymptomatic status, and these levels correlate with an elevated yield of eosinophils. MBP levels also correlate with the degree of BHR. MBP can also increase the airway contractility of isolated canine and guinea pig tracheal rings (44,45), and it is cytotoxic to respiratory epithelial cell cultures in vitro (46,47).

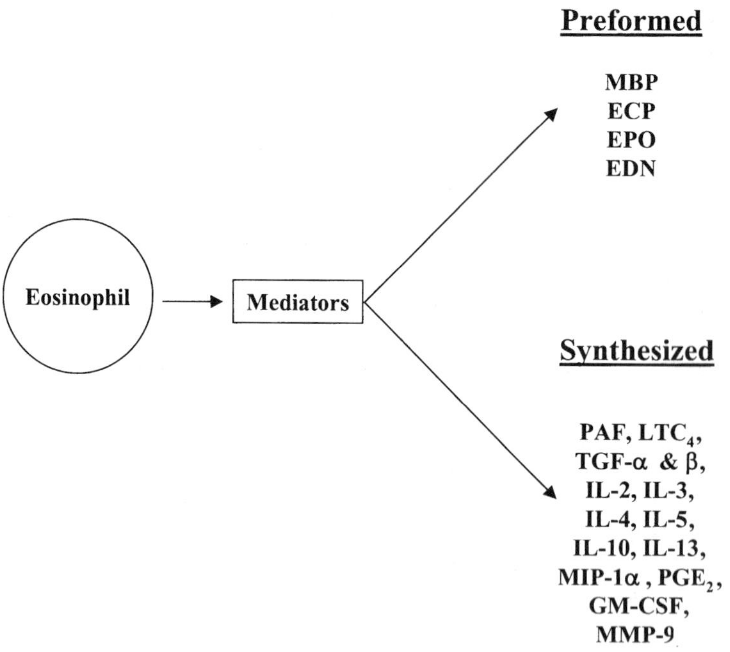

Figure 4 Examples of mediators released by the eosinophil.

Eosinophil cationic protein has been detected in the sputum during asthmatic episodes and in the serum in the setting of allergen challenge. It has also been found in the bronchial submucosa in areas of inflammation and is readily detected by the monoclonal antibodies EG1 and EG2, which are directed against the stored and secreted forms of ECP, respectively (9,48). BAL fluid from asthmatic subjects demonstrate increased levels of ECP that correlate with serum ECP levels and may also be more readily suppressed by corticosteroid therapy than are the eosinophil numbers themselves. Serum ECP levels may reflect the degree of eosinophilic airway inflammation, as well as disease activity and may be useful as an inflammatory marker in asthma (49). Other inflammatory mediators, such as EDN and EPO, have been used as indices of eosinophil activity or activation. EDN is present in increased quantities in the BAL fluid of subjects with either a single- or dual-phase response to allergen. BAL fluid EPO levels, in fact, serve as a more sensitive measure of inflammation than eosinophil numbers in primate models (50). These observations indicate that allergen recruitment of eosinophils to the airways is associated with cellular activation and release of its proinflammatory mediators.

Eosinophils are also able to generate platelet-activating factor (PAF) as well as the proinflammatory metabolites of arachidonic acid, particularly LTC_4 and LTD_4. This, along with the production of toxic superoxide anions, further enables the eosinophil to produce vasodilation, microvascular leakage, and bronchial smooth-muscle contraction. The damage to the airway epithelium caused by the eosinophil may further potentiate the inflammatory responses by neurogenic pathways. Sensory nerve endings may be exposed following the denudation of the epithelium by granule protein, and these stimulate retrograde release of potent neuropeptides, such as substance P, neurokinin A, and calcitonin gene-related peptide (CGRP). These molecules then function as spasmogens, increase vascular permeability, and lead to edema formation (51,52). Membrane-bound neutral endopeptidase, which cleaves the vasoactive mediators, has been suggested as a putative regulatory mechanism for such a system; however, studies have not detected deficiencies of this enzyme in the airways of asthmatic subjects (53).

The eosinophil appears to be the predominant effector cell in the asthmatic airway. Its presence here does not appear to be coincidental, but more likely, is the result of a coordinated effort on the part of numerous cells and their cytokines and chemokines to bring the eosinophil into the airway. The mere presence of eosinophils in the lung does not cause asthma; patients with eosinophilic pneumonia have an abundance of eosinophils, but not asthma. In addition, overexpression of IL-5 in mice causes hypereosinophilia, but does not bring about changes in lung function, such as bronchial hyperresponsiveness or airflow obstruction (54). Therefore, the airway in asthma is likely abnormal, and this abnormality results in the asthmatic response to these mediators.

Airway hyperresponsiveness failed to develop in IL-5 knockout mice when sensitized to antigen (55). However, reconstitution with IL-5 led to eosinophilia, with allergen sensitization, as airway hyperesponsiveness paralleled the appearance of eosinophilia; thus the investigators concluded that IL-5 and eosinophils are pivotal factors in the development of allergic airway disease in this model system. In contrast Corry et al. (56) also found that antigen sensitization of mice led to BHR. Treatment with anti-CD4 antibodies, or anti-IL-4 antibody, during the sensitization phase prevented the development of BHR. Administration of anti-IL-5 prevented the development of airway eosinophilia, but BHR occurred even after sensitization. These data suggest that IL-5 and eosinophils may not mediate acute BHR. Drazen et al. (57) concluded that airway hyperresponsiveness could arise through several pathways and the phenotype of asthma can be the product of multiple approaches; furthermore, as indicated, these animal models may provide examples of eosinophil-dependent and eosinophil-independent pathways to the development of BHR. The exact relation of these experiments in mice to clinical asthma is not established. With more and more evidence confirming the role of eosinophils in asthmatic inflammation, research in asthma is expanding to include the mechanisms of eosinophil recruitment and signaling, as well as their ability to cause local toxicity.

6 LYMPHOCYTES

Lymphocytes, particularly T lymphocytes, play a critical role in the initiation, regulation, and, persistence of airway inflammation in asthma. The mast cell may begin the inflammatory response immediately after antigen exposure. However, it is the lymphocyte that most likely provides the signals essential to activate and perpetuate the chronic inflammatory processes in asthma. Products from lymphocytes probably regulate endothelial cell expression of adhesion proteins and leukocyte transmigration. In addition, it is likely that lymphocytes play an important role in the initiation and regulation of the airway repair process in asthma.

Increased numbers of lymphocytes, especially T lymphocytes, have been demonstrated in the airway of asthmatics, both in autopsy as well as in bronchial biopsies (9,19). These cells are usually activated. In acute severe asthma studies, $CD4^+$ cells have demonstrated elevated levels of surface markers of T-cell activation, such as IL-2R, HLA-DR, and very late antigen (VLA-1), compared with controls. In contrast these markers were not elevated on $CD8^+$ cells. Levels of the soluble IL-2R (sIL-2R) and IFN-γ were increased in the asthmatic patients and $CD4^+$ and sIL-2R levels were inversely correlated with measures of airflow obstruction (7). However, in studies with less severe asthma, increased expression of peripheral blood T-cell activation markers has not been uniformly found (58). Increased IL-2R expression by T cells also correlates with the degree of eosinophilia. The cytokines GM-CSF, IL-3, and IL-5 were identified in both T-cell supernatants and the serum of asthmatics, and they likely contribute to prolongation of eosinophil survival (59). The expression of these activation markers thus correlates with disease severity (7) and may suggest that allergen exposure is vital in activating this process.

In another study of BAL fluid from allergic asthmatics, increased expression of IL-2R on $CD4^+$ cells correlated with the number of B cells expressing the low-affinity IgE receptor. This suggests a link between T-cell activation and increased expression of an atopic phenotype, with a similar observation being made on peripheral blood. The non-allergic asthmatics differed in displaying increased expression of IL-2R, HLA-DR, and VLA-1 on both $CD4^+$ and $CD8^+$ cells in both BAL and peripheral blood (60). BAL fluid taken 10 min after an allergen challenge demonstrated a fall in the levels of $CD3^+$, $CD4^+$, and $CD8^+$ cells, with a fall in the CD4/CD8 ratio. This may indicate the rapid egress of $CD4^+$ cells into the bronchial wall, or at least increased adhesion to the epithelium, in response to allergen exposure. No changes were noted in the markers of T-cell surface activation (61). In another study, BAL fluid was examined 48 hr after an inhalation challenge with allergen, and a rise in the proportion of $CD4^+$ cells was noted, in association with a fall in peripheral blood $CD4^+$ cells (62). The late accumulation of $CD4^+$ cells in the airway coincides with the development of bronchial hyperresponsiveness in the LAR. Thus, changes in the CD4/CD8 ratio may be implicated in determining the nature of the asthmatic response. Gonzalez et al. found greatly reduced proportions of $CD4^+$ cells and a significantly reduced CD4/CD8 ratio in BAL fluid 6 hr after allergen challenge in those patients who developed an EAR only, as compared with those who had a dual-phase response. These findings suggest that an early preponderance of $CD8^+$ cells in the airway may protect against further bronchoconstriction by down-regulation of subsequent inflammatory changes.

T lymphocytes express several inflammatory mediators. Cytokines are glycoproteins that are synthesized and released following cellular activation. T-cell–derived cytokines play a critical role in the inflammatory process in asthma. Cytokines establish the initial injury process and regulate the subsequent repair or sustained recruitment and/or activation of inflammatory cells. Cytokines, in the process of inflammation in asthma, likely function as regulators of IgE synthesis, mediators of eosinophilia and subsequent eosinophil activation, and also as activators of adhesion molecules, mediating transendothelial migration of effector cells. A characteristic pattern of cytokine expression and detection is associated with antigen exposure and asthma. The cytokine mRNA airway profile in atopic asthmatics includes IL-3, IL-4, IL-5, and GM-CSF (63). IFN-γ and IL-2 are present, but are less than or equal to normal controls (64).

Specific differences are seen in the cytokine profile in allergic and nonallergic individuals with asthma (60). Both IL-4 and IL-5 are increased in allergic asthma. In contrast, only IL-5 is increased in nonallergic asthmatics. This may explain the lack of an IgE response in the nonallergic individuals, whereas both groups manifest eosinophilia, which is regulated by IL-5. Cells other than $CD4^+$ cells produce IL-5, such as mast cells, natural killer (NK) cells, $CD8^+$ cells, and eosinophils. IL-5 appears to be one of the most important factors in the regulation of eosinophilpoiesis (65,66). It regulates eosinophil maturation from uncommitted bone marrow precursors and enhances eosinophil survival, tissue migration, and activation of mature eosinophils (65,67) Monoclonal anti-IL-5 antibodies to animals blocks airway eosinophilic response and BHR associated with antigen challenge. However, IL-5 overproduction in transgenic mice leads to eosinophilia without airway changes (68,69). Therefore, it is likely that more than one factor may be necessary for airway disease to be expressed: IL-5 and allergen, for example (57).

Chemokines are mediators that have a predominantly chemotactic function and induce cell movement (70). They are produced by several cells. Regulated on activation, normal T-cell expressed and secreted (RANTES) and eotaxin are two chemokines that act in concert with IL-5 to recruit eosinophils (71). There is now evidence that airway smooth-muscle cells also express eotaxin (72). Collins et al. (73) proposed that IL-5 increases circulating eosinophils, but has little effect on eosinophil chemotaxis. RANTES and eotaxin, in contrast, are the principal chemotactic factors for the recruitment of eosinophils to tissues. Thus, there is a cooperative effort between cytokines (IL-5) and chemokines (RANTES and eotaxin) to recruit eosinophils to the airway. Chemokine expression, in general, is increased in asthma. Epithelial cells from asthmatic patients demonstrate increased expression of monocyte chemotactic protein (MCP-1). In addition, the concentrations of macrophage inflammatory protein (MIP-1α), RANTES, and IL-8 are increased in the BAL fluid of asthmatic individuals. Thus, it is likely that chemokines play an important role, either alone or in combination with cytokines to regulate the inflammatory cell traffic to the lung. They also contribute to the complexity and redundancy of the inflammatory cascade.

Dendritic cells function as antigen-presenting cells (APCs). This further underscores the importance of the T cell early in antigen recognition and tolerance. After contact with aeroallergens, dendritic cells migrate to regional lymph nodes where they come into contact with a population of memory T cells ($CD45RO^+$). They may also be the primary

APC for the sensitization of naïve T cells ($CD45RA^+$). The regional lymph nodes probably contain most IgE-secreting plasma cells. They have also been identified as the location of IgE helper T cells and the relevant T suppressor population (74).

Subpopulations of lymphocytes, with distinct cytokine-producing profiles, have been identified (75). In mice, $CD4^+$ helper T cells are of two types, based on the differences in cytokine production (Fig. 5). Th1 cells generate IL-2, TNF-α, and IFN-γ. These cytokines are important in cell-mediated immunity against intracellular pathogens, as well as delayed-type hypersensitivity. The Th2 cells, in contrast, secrete a different cytokine profile (IL-3, IL-4, IL-5, IL-6, IL-9, and IL-13). They are involved in the regulation of IgE production and allergic inflammatory responses, as well as phagocyte-independent host defenses against parasites. IL-3 and GM-CSF are produced by both Th1 and Th2 cells. IFN-γ is thought to inhibit proliferation and cytokine production by Th2 cells and induces Th1 differentiation. In contrast, production of IL-10 by the Th2 cells inhibits Th1 cytokine production, whereas IL-4 encourages Th2 differentiation. IFN-γ thus acts as an inhibitor of allergic responses and also of IL-4–mediated IgE class switching. NK cells are also known to produce IFN-γ.

In humans, this distinction is less apparent, with most human T-cell clones producing IL-2 and some producing both IFN-γ and IL-4. However, there seems to be a generally inverse relation between the production of IFN-γ and IL-4/IL-5 (76,77). The patterns of

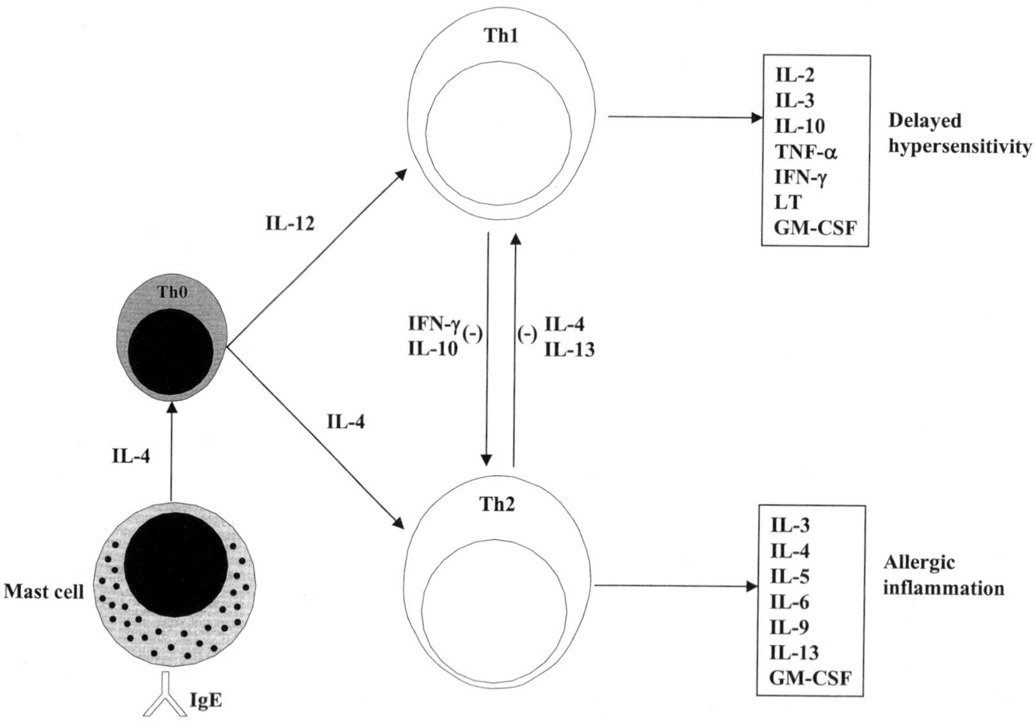

Figure 5 T helper lymphocytes in mice: T helper cells are of two types: Th1 and Th2. Th1 cells participate in delayed hypersensitivity reactions, whereas the Th2 cells are important in allergic inflammation. Th1 cytokines can inhibit Th2 activity and vice versa.

human cytokine production do not correspond precisely with that of the murine cells. IFN-γ and TNF-β remain relatively Th1-specific, and IL-4 and IL-5 are produced by the Th2 cells, and both are able to produce variable quantities of IL-2, IL-3, IL-6, IL-10, TNF-α, and GM-CSF. IFN-γ and IL-4 promote the proliferation and cytokine production of Th1 and Th2 clones, respectively; whereas IL-10 inhibits these responses in both types of clones. Peripheral blood mononuclear cell cultures from normal persons have shown that IL-4 and IFN-γ will help determine in vitro development of human $CD4^+$ cells into Th1 and Th2 like clones.

Several attempts have been made to demonstrate a Th2 involvement in atopic asthma. Bronchial biopsies from asthmatic subjects have elaborated mRNA for IL-5 in six out of ten cases, in contrast with normal controls (78). In addition, BAL fluid from allergic asthmatic subjects had increased amounts of mRNA for IL-3, IL-4, IL-5, and GM-CSF, as compared with nonatopic, nonasthmatic controls; IFN-γ levels in cells were similar in both the groups (64). A predominantly Th2 phenotype is seen in T-cell clones from atopic subjects sensitive to *Dermatophagoides pteronyssinus*. Forty percent of $CD4^+$ clones generated from endobronchial biopsies, following grass-pollen bronchoprovocation of sensitive asthmatic subjects, demonstrated Th2 cytokine release, as compared with 17% from patients with nonatopic asthma (79). Bentley et al. have shown an increase in the number of cells containing mRNA for IL-5 and GM-CSF in bronchial biopsies 24 hr after an allergen inhalation (80). Although these patterns are similar to the Th2 phenotype, they are not identical with those seen in mice, and further work is awaited. Based on these findings, allergic inflammation in asthma was proposed to represent a Th2-like cytokine profile. Although it has not been conclusively established that the Th2 subtype of T-helper cells is the explanation for airway inflammation in asthma, T lymphocytes play a major role in the allergic inflammatory process.

Several aeroallergens derived from dust mites, cockroach, *Alternaria*, and animals (especially cats), seem to be important in the development of the inflammatory process in asthma and its perpetuation (81). Early in the sensitization process, allergens are presented to the T cells, leading to the production of IgE antibodies. There is evidence that this exposure may begin prenatally (60,82), as circulating allergen-specific T cells can be detected at birth. It is also thought that, in the first year of life, these cells take up residence in the airway and begin to express a disease-related phenotype. IL-4 generation is vital to this process, for the development of Th2 subpopulations and for isotype switching of the B cells to produce IgE antibodies specific for each allergen. There is evidence that, following sensitization, the level of exposure to antigens, such as dust mites, becomes an important factor in the eventual expression of asthma (83). Further exposure to the antigen results in a rapid expansion of T-cell populations with the capacity to produce a Th2-like cytokine profile. It is proposed that a stimulus, such as an intercurrent viral infection, may enhance the expression of the disease. Airway hyperresponsiveness develops early in life, whereas allergy develops later, and it is thought that a convergence of these two factors leads to the actual expression of asthma.

It is unclear whether all asthmatic phenotypes have a similar Th2-like cytokine profile (84). An earlier study suggested that allergic asthmatic subjects had greater expression of IL-4 than patients with ''intrinsic asthma,'' with IL-5 concentrations similar in both groups (60). This differentiation on the basis of IL-4 expression has not been established. The general consensus is that both resident and acquired airway T-cell lymphocytes are essential for the initiation and perpetuation of the inflammatory response and the subsequent repair process in the airway. Thus, a possible effector function of these cells appear to be intercellular signaling through the action of specific cytokines, which may be critical for the development of an inflammatory response in asthma.

7 MAST CELLS

Several studies have attempted to define the role of mast cells (see Chap. 2) in allergic asthma and chronic airway inflammation and have indicated their involvement in both the acute and chronic phases of the inflammatory response. Mast cells in the lung are located in the airway lumen, bronchial epithelium, submucosa, and lung parenchyma. Several cytokines and growth factors derived from local cells and structures likely influence mast cell development and eventual migration to the airway lumen (85,86). The predominant mast cell subtype in the lung contains tryptase, but not chymase, referred to as the MC_T-type mast cell.

A variety of mast cell mediator inhibitors and antagonists have been demonstrated to produce modification of the response to allergen challenge. These include selective H_1-receptor antagonists, cyclooxygenase inhibitors, and cysLT1 receptor antagonists. The wealth of preformed and newly synthesized mediators, together with the presence of the high-affinity IgE receptor FCεRI to signal the presence of antigen, make this a cell type of obvious importance to allergic diseases and asthma.

In addition to granule and lipid mediators, mast cells elaborate their own specific profile of cytokines, which may play an important role in allergic inflammation. For example, the IL-4 generated by mast cells may be important in the conversion of uncommitted T cells to the Th2 phenotype and thus promote production of IL-5 (87). Thus, if large quantities of IL-4 are generated by mast cells, the response could be central to establishing a Th2-like profile in the airways and provide an appropriate environment for allergic and eosinophilic inflammation.

The increased numbers of mast cells found within BAL fluid from asthmatic subjects also supports the relevance of the mast cell to asthma (13). The proportion of mast cells and the histamine content of BAL fluid correlates with the degree of airflow obstruction and the level of hyperresponsiveness (6). A few studies have shown an increase in the number of mast cells in the epithelial layer (88,89), whereas others have not. In addition, the therapeutic effect of inhaled corticosteroids is accompanied by a reduction in epithelial and submucosal mast cell numbers, together with a reduction in eosinophils and T lymphocytes (90). However, mast cells within the airway are more likely to be in an activated state (1,48,89). Increased levels of the prostaglandin PGD_2 and the leukotriene LTC_4 have also been noted in BAL following allergen challenge early in the allergic response (26,91–93). Greater spontaneous histamine release and lavage fluid histamine levels have been found in asthma with existing airway hyperresponsiveness (6). Histamine levels in BAL fluid are elevated within minutes of an allergen challenge in asthmatic subjects and may remain elevated for a prolonged time after antigen challenge (92,94,95).

Other studies have helped define the specific role of the mast cell in the atopic asthmatic subject and determine their cellular contributions to early- and late-phase events after antigen bronchoprovocation. An increase in histamine and tryptase concentration is seen in BAL fluid following bronchoalveolar allergen challenge. Tryptase levels in the BAL fluid of atopic and nonatopic asthmatic and atopic and nonatopic controls were measured 5 min after endobronchial instillation of allergen (94). Atopic persons demonstrated higher tryptase levels, with the highest levels seen in the asthmatic group. Furthermore, the atopic asthmatic subjects also demonstrated elevated tryptase levels at baseline, which suggests a role for chronic mast cell involvement and mediator release in subjects with persistent or chronic asthma. In contrast, Sedgwick and associates examined tryptase levels 12 min and 48 hr following segmental endobronchial challenge with antigen in nonatopic asthmatic subjects (17). Tryptase levels were elevated at 12 min, but returned to baseline by 48 hr. Tryptase levels thus do not appear to increase during the late-phase response (17,95,96). Histamine levels continued to remain elevated at 48 hr after antigen challenge, suggesting that basophils, rather than mast cells, generate this mediator in a late-phase response. It is not yet clear whether these variations in tryptase levels reflect real differences between the asthmatic and nonasthmatic allergic subjects or are due to differences in study designs. The existing evidence that human mast cells elaborate cytokines, indicates that mast cells are important in the initiation and regulation of the inflammatory infiltrate following allergen exposure, with influences on accumulation and activation of T cells and eosinophils, together with the production of IgE.

8 MONOCYTES AND MACROPHAGES

Macrophages are constitutive residents of the lung and airways, and they play a major role in host defense mechanisms. Large numbers of these cells have been demonstrated in both tissue samples and BAL fluid. They are capable of releasing a variety of cytokines (IL-1, IL-6, IL-8, GM-CSF, TNF-α, and IFNs), lipid mediators (TXA_2, LTB_4, LTC_4, and PGD_2), reactive oxygen species, lysosomal enzymes, PAF, and histamine-releasing factors (HRF) (97). These mediators can contribute to airway injury in asthma. Cultured peripheral blood mononuclear cells (PBMC), from asthmatics, produce increased TNF-α, IL-1β, IL-8, and GM-CSF. Neutrophil priming activity (NPA) is another monocyte-derived factor, that increases LTB_4 and superoxide production by neutrophils. The failure of corticosteroids to inhibit NPA production appears to correspond with the presence of steroid resistance in asthmatic patients.

Macrophages also function as antigen-presenting cells that interact and then stimulate T-lymphocyte proliferation and cytokine production (98). A subpopulation of macrophages expresses low-affinity IgE receptor, in contrast with the high-affinity IgE receptor (97) found on mast cells and basophils. However, macrophages and monocytes, after activation have also been reported to express the high-affinity receptor for IgE. Such receptors are increased in atopic asthma and antigen–IgE-dependent mechanisms may culminate in the release of inflammatory mediators by these cells.

Cytokine production by Th2 cells may be down-regulated by macrophage secretion of IL-10; there is a speculation that a deficiency in IL-10 production in asthma allows Th2 cytokine generation to go "unchecked" and, thereby, perpetuate the inflammatory response. Although there is evidence that macrophages from some patients with asthma may have an increased inflammatory capacity, it is not entirely clear whether this is a consequence of asthma or a cause of this process (99).

Pulmonary alveolar macrophages (PAM) from asthmatic subjects demonstrated an increase in the generation of toxic oxygen species; when obtained following allergen challenge, PAM had higher levels of β-glucoronidase (91). PAM from such subjects also produced higher levels of TNF-α, IL-1, IL-6, and GM-CSF. Another study showed that the alveolar macrophages may be primed for the production of IL-10 and IL-12 in asthma (100). However, only one major study has identified increased numbers of macrophages in the BAL fluid 48 hr after antigen challenge (62). Furthermore, few histological studies have provided evidence for an increase in macrophages in the mucosa of extrinsic asthmatics. Thus, although macrophages release a variety of mediators and toxic substances, their precise role and specific patterns of mediator release in asthma has not been fully established, and uncertainty exists as to whether such changes are a cause or a consequence of airway inflammation.

9 BASOPHILS

Activation of basophils leads to release of both preformed (histamine and chondroitin sulfate A) and newly synthesized mediators. They also release a variety of cytokines, including IL-4, and IL-13 (101). Lipid mediators, such as LTC_4 and PAF, are also generated by the basophils. Basophils are typically scarce in both circulation and tissues, but they have been found in increased numbers both in the blood and sputum during asthma exacerbations, and an increased release of mediators from the basophils has also been noted in asthmatic individuals when compared with normal subjects (102). An increase in basophil numbers in the BAL fluid has been noted at 24 hr after antigen challenge and corresponds to the development of an LAR (103). In addition, IL-3 and GM-CSF, which are basophil chemotactic factors, have been found in BAL fluid during the LAR and their presence may be a mechanism for basophil recruitment and activation. A current view is that basophils contribute more to chronic inflammation than to an acute asthmatic episode, and they accomplish this action by the release of multiple inflammatory mediators. These actions contribute to allergic inflammation, IgE synthesis, and eosinophil recruitment.

10 NEUTROPHILS

The precise role of the neutrophil in the pathogenesis of asthma is unclear. Several mediators, such as IL-1, TNF-α, and GM-CSF, are chemoattractants for neutrophils. Neutrophils have not been consistently found in BAL fluid and lung biopsies from asthmatics (28). However, they have been found in increased numbers from lung autopsy specimens of patients who died suddenly of asthma, when compared with patients with slow-onset of status asthmaticus, in which eosinophils predominate (104). A more recent study has found bronchial neutrophilia in patients with noninfectious status asthmaticus (105). Elevated numbers of neutrophils are also found in the airway during nocturnal exacerbations of asthma (106). Another study demonstrated increased neutrophils in the sputum of subjects with severe persistent asthma. Neutrophils are also found in the BAL fluid of atopic asthmatic subjects 4 hr, but not 24 hr, after an inhaled allergen challenge (23). The foregoing data suggest that neutrophils are an early component of the inflammatory response, or they may set the stage for later events. Neutrophils contain or synthesize several molecules (myeloperoxidase, neutral serine proteases, lysozyme, myeloperoxidase, lysosomal hydrolases, superoxide metabolites, and eicosanoids, including thromboxane, LTB_4, and PAF) that can damage airway tissue or act as chemotactic factors or mediators for other inflammatory cells.

11 EPITHELIAL CELLS

In the past, the airway epithelium was thought to function primarily as a simple anatomical barrier to underlying airway tissue. Epithelium is now thought to play an active role in regulating fluid and ion transport in the airway, as well as production of mucus, and to protect airway smooth muscle. In addition, airway epithelial damage is a hallmark feature of asthma (2), which is seen even in mild clinical disease (24). The presence of epithelial cells in the creola bodies of asthmatic sputum was an early indicator of epithelial damage in asthmatic airways. The extent of epithelial injury may relate to disease severity. Eosinophil-derived granule proteins are most likely responsible for airway epithelial damage. This process begins early in allergic inflammation and subsequently results in a proliferative response and eventual remodeling. These structural changes result in altered airway epithelial function, and they may contribute to bronchial obstruction and hyperresponsiveness.

Proposed mechanisms for the cause of increased bronchial reactivity include the disruption of intercellular tight junctions, which then allows greater allergen penetration, and the exposure of nerve endings, with invoked axon reflexes. The opening of tight junctions between ciliary cells and the widening of intercellular spaces correlates with bronchial reactivity and increased number of eosinophils (107). An uncontrolled biopsy study of a small group of asthmatic subjects, with varying degrees of hyperresponsiveness (108), demonstrated epithelial damage at all airway levels. The range of epithelial changes includes complete epithelial desquamation, a residual basal cell layer, and cleavage of the basal and more superficial columnar cells. Ciliated cells demonstrated vacuolization and malalignment of the central ciliary filaments; in some biopsies, it was possible to demonstrate neural tissue in a superficial location.

Clara cell 10-kD protein (CC10), the predominant product from nonciliated cells in the epithelial lining of bronchioles (Clara cells), has immunomodulatory and anti-inflammatory activity and may play a role in controlling inflammation in the airway. Decreases of CC10-producing cells have been demonstrated in small airways of asthmatic subjects and may lead to further acceleration of inflammatory responses (109). In a fiber-optic biopsy study, three out of four symptomatic asthmatic subjects had a complete loss of surface epithelium, providing the basis for a correlation between epithelial loss and hyperresponsiveness to methacholine (2). However, another study in patients with mild asthma failed to demonstrate significant morphological changes at a light and electron microscope level, in comparison with normal controls (110). This was an important demonstration of asthma and increased hyperresponsiveness despite minimal morphological abnormalities, emphasizing that other factors, such as inflammatory cell infiltrates and the epithelial inflammatory and relaxant mediators generated were likely to be important. The artifactual epithelial damage caused by the biopsy forceps also needs to be taken into account and has been emphasized by a morphological study in normal volunteers (111). Several studies have shown an increased number of epithelial cells in BAL fluid, and this seems to correlate with hyperresponsiveness (1,43). However, this does not establish a causal relation between epithelial damage and hyperresponsiveness, as inflammation in the submucosa would be expected to affect epithelial integrity partly owing to the released products of eosinophils, such as MBP, ECP, and EPO.

Inflammatory mediators derived from the epithelial cells play an important role in the process of injury and repair. Mediators released by the epithelial cell may include lipid mediators, such as 15-hydroxyeicosatetraenoic acid (15-HETE) and PGE_2, endothelin, fibronectin, and a range of cytokines, including IL-1, IL-6, TGF-β, IL-11, and GM-CSF (112). IL-5 production has also recently been demonstrated in human airway epithelial cells (113). They also release chemokines, such as IL-8, RANTES, and MIP1-α and this probably contributes to the influx of various cells, including eosinophils, neutrophils, lymphocytes, and monocytes, to the airway. Examination of bronchial biopsies from asthmatic subjects with immunohistochemistry, polymerase chain reaction (PCR), and enzyme-linked immunosorbent assay (ELISA) on subsequent culture supernatants has established increased production of these mediators (114).

15-HETE increases production of mucus in animal models and leukotriene generation by mast cells; it can also increase the acute response to allergen challenge in asthma. Increased release of 15-HETE is seen from bronchial epithelial cells of asthmatic subjects. The cyclooxygenase products, such as PGE_2 and $PGF_{2\alpha}$, influence bronchial smooth-muscle tone, either contraction or relaxation, depending on their relative concentrations. These levels are, in turn, influenced by other factors, such as bradykinin, histamine, and PAF (115).

Endothelins (ET) have vasoconstrictor, growth-stimulating, and potent bronchoconstrictor properties. During severe asthma attacks, increased concentrations of endothelin-1 have been detected in the BAL fluid and plasma. Seventy percent of asthmatic subjects had endothelin-1 detected in the bronchial epithelium, by immunohistochemical studies, as compared with 10% of controls (116). Endothelins may also contribute to inflammatory changes by enhancing 15-lipoxygenase activity and stimulating fibroblast division. Endothelin receptor antagonists inhibit antigen-induced lung inflammation in mice; this suggests an important pathophysiological role for ET in the development of lung inflammation in asthma, and highlights the potential of ET antagonists for the treatment of the disease (117).

Neutral endopeptidase (NEP) is present in basal epithelial cells and plays an important role in degrading tachykinins. It is thought to be involved in the regulation of neurogenic aspects of inflammation (118). Induction of NEP in the bronchial epithelium by corticosteroids may reduce neurogenic inflammation.

Expression of adhesion molecules by the epithelium is implicated in the pathogenesis of asthma. An increased expression of ICAM-1 on the epithelium as well as on submucosal vessels was noted in a primate model of eosinophilic inflammation with bronchial hyperresponsiveness (30). The BAL concentration of eosinophils and the degree of hyperresponsiveness were markedly decreased by antibody to ICAM-1. Initial studies in human bronchial biopsies have shown an expression of ICAM-1 in the epithelium of both asthmatics and normal controls, whereas both ICAM-1 and E-selectin were found in the endothelium (119). ICAM-1 is the epithelial receptor for the major group of human rhinoviruses as well as for β_2-integrins on hemopoietic cells.

Nitric oxide (NO) is now thought to have a role in regulating epithelial function and mechanism of inflammation. In normal subjects, NO is constantly synthesized in small quantities and has similarities to epithelial-derived relaxing factor. NO is produced by several different cell types in the respiratory tract: airway epithelial cells, smooth-muscle cells, sensory nerves, endothelial cells, and macrophages. It is a bronchodilator and vasodilator at low levels that antagonizes endothelin and has some protective effects in the airway. In contrast, NO is found in higher levels in asthma and is due to increased inducible NO synthase (iNOS) expression (120), through the action of the cytokines IL-1, TNF-α, and INF-γ. Higher concentrations of NO react with superoxide anions in inflamed tissue to produce biological oxidants that could contribute to ongoing tissue damage and chronic asthmatic inflammation. Exhaled NO may be useful to evaluate the degree of airway inflammation in patients with mild to moderate asthma (121). Epithelial cells also express increased MHC class II antigens after allergen challenge. Furthermore, epithelial cells can express ICAM-1 that can bind neutrophils, eosinophils, and rhinoviruses.

From analyses of bronchial biopsies, interaction of eosinophils with epithelial cells appears to be an important cause of airway damage. Eosinophil exposure to IL-3, IL-5, or GM-CSF, which can be derived from multiple cellular sources, prevents apoptosis and enhances their inflammatory capacity (122). Eosinophils interact with adhesion proteins, chiefly ICAM-1, on the epithelium and then release metalloendoproteases, oxidants, and granule proteins (123). Eosinophils are a source of metalloproteinases, which can degrade both basement membrane collagen type IV and interstitial matrix molecules. This enzyme is most likely to be important in cell migration and matrix remodeling. Airway inflammation in asthma and chronic bronchitis is associated with an imbalance between metalloproteases and tissue inhibitors of metalloproteinases (TIMP) and this may have a role in the pathogenesis of remodeling and airflow obstruction (124). TIMP-1 levels were significantly higher in untreated asthmatics when compared with glucocorticoid steroid-treated subjects; this may also have important implications, as an excess of TIMP-1 could lead to airway fibrosis, a hallmark of airway remodeling (125). Inhibition of matrix metalloproteinases (MMP) prevents allergen-induced airway inflammation in a murine model of asthma (126). High levels of active elastase may also play a role in the pathogenesis of airway remodeling, probably by disruption of elastin (127).

The matrix proteoglycans are susceptible targets for the eosinophil-derived proteins. A variety of proinflammatory cytokines, including basic fibroblast growth factor, are tightly bound to the side chain of proteoglycan, and this interaction stabilizes the cytokines and localizes its activity. The interaction of the eosinophil basic proteins with proteoglycans would release these cytokines and result in further injury to the epithelium and initiation of fibroblast activity.

Basement membrane thickening was detected in early pathological studies; however, it has recently been described as ''subepithelial fibrosis.'' Deposition of collagen types II and V, tenascin, and fibronectin, which are produced by myofibroblasts (128), contribute to the thickening of the subbasement membrane in asthma. The lack of any epithelial cell-derived connective tissue types in the fibrotic layer, together with a lack of correlation with epithelial shedding, is circumstantial evidence against an epithelial origin for this collagen layer. Rather, it has been considered more likely that this may be a fibroblast reaction to cytokine secretion from nearby inflammatory cells (129). Tenascin presence in the lamina reticulosa indicates that this is a site of high matrix turnover. Furthermore, these fibroblasts also produce cytokines, such as GM-CSF, which could prolong eosinophil survival and thereby, establish a vicious cycle of injury and repair; these interactions are likely key factors in maintaining the chronic inflammatory process in asthma.

12 CELLULAR MIGRATION AND ADHESION MOLECULES IN ASTHMA

Cellular adhesion with selective diapedesis in asthma is also a complex process that involves many adhesion molecules (Fig. 6). The movement of the eosinophil to an area of inflammation in the lung is of particular importance in asthma. Initially, random contact with the endothelial cell wall may occur in a capillary vessel. The unprimed eosinophil, bearing the L-selectin surface adhesion molecule, binds to the activated endothelial surface, which expresses E-selectin, in a region of inflammation in the lung following a trigger-like antigen inhalation. This interaction results in the initial phase of eosinophil

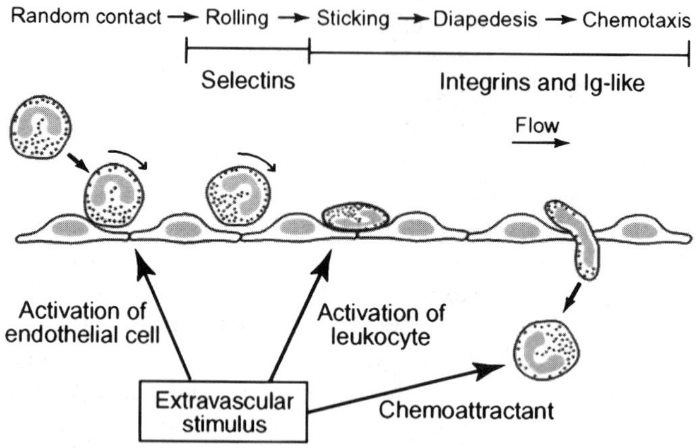

Figure 6 The sequence of events associated with recruitment of inflammatory cells to the site of inflammation. See text for details. (From Ref. 150.)

movement termed ''rolling.'' Several such interactions then occur, and the eosinophil is observed to ''skid'' along the endothelial surface.

The eosinophil is ''activated'' following exposure to a high concentration of cytokines, chemokines, and lipid mediators, likely derived from perivascular lymphocytes and sometimes the endothelial cells themselves. Endothelial production of IL-8 increases leukocyte adherence and migration (130). The activated eosinophils demonstrate increased production and affinity of the surface adhesion molecules. VLA-4 (which binds to endothelial VCAM-1), LFA-1, Mac-1, and p150, 95 (which bind to endothelial ICAM-1) are all up-regulated on the eosinophil (131). These events lead to the next phase of transendothelial migration, known as firm binding, or ''sticking,'' or ''tethering.'' Although many of the activation steps resulting in firm adhesion to the endothelium are specific to those cell types responsive to the activators produced, it is not until the next step of endothelial transmigration that cellular selectivity is accomplished. Cell-specific chemoattractants such as IL-2, IL-5, RANTES, and eotaxin, result in further selectivity for eosinophils (131). Subsequent migration of the leukocyte through the endothelial barrier requires that the firm adhesion ''loosens'' to allow movement between individual epithelial cells (132). This may be achieved either by a down-regulation (or shedding) of the receptors, or by a cyclic modulation of receptor avidity, which would result in the ''loosening'' of the firmly bound cells to allow diapedesis to take place. L-selectin is shed by eosinophils during their movement to bronchial tissue in vivo and across epithelial monolayer in vitro (133–135). RANTES stimulates transmigration across IL-1–stimulated endothelium in a fashion that is dependent on VLA-4. These cells are free to travel through the subepithelial tissue layer, once they are through the endothelial layer. In the tissue matrix, several other interactions occur between Mac-1 and fibrinogen, VLA-4 and fibronectin, and CD44 and hyaluronic acid, to help ensure continued progress toward the eosinophil's target epithelium. Eosinophil survival is enhanced by the interaction between VLA-4 and fibronectin, most likely by stimulating the autocrine production of IL-3 and GM-CSF (136). Their arrival at the airway matrix or at the epithelial junction is associated with cellular activation and the initiation of the inflammatory process in the bronchial wall.

The process of cellular adhesion and transendothelial migration permits specificity in the inflammatory response. The cytokines or chemokines and their interaction with receptors are specific; however, their presence on a variety of cells facilitates amplification of a response, as opposed to specificity. Furthermore, most cytokine functions are redundant, with several molecules capable of achieving the same end result. Therefore, it is at the venular endothelial interface that the effector cell egress to the bronchial mucosa can be limited to specific cells that can perform their effector functions leading to airway inflammation, injury, and repair.

Eosinophils bind to VCAM-1 receptors on umbilical vein endothelial cells during in vitro studies, most likely through their VLA-4 receptor (137,138). The eosinophil–endothelial cell adhesion can be inhibited by monoclonal antibodies against VLA-4 (137,139). Rats pretreated with monoclonal antibodies against VLA-4, or a combination of antibodies against LFA-1 and Mac-1, show a decrease in early- and late-phase responses to inhaled antigen (140). No overall changes in the BAL cell differential were noted, suggesting a mechanism other than cellular migration, such as a failure of these cells to be activated during the adhesion process, to account for the change in pulmonary response to antigen.

A primate model system with *Ascaris*-infected monkeys has been used to study the early- and late-phase responses to antigen (30). Allergen challenge increased airway responsiveness (as determined by methacholine challenge), eosinophil influx, and ICAM-1 expression on bronchial cells, in chronically infected animals. The airway responses, as well as the eosinophil influx, was inhibited in animals pretreated with monoclonal antibodies to ICAM-1 (30,141,142).

Various observations argue against a central role for adhesion molecules in the pathophysiology of asthma in humans. Bronchial biopsies show no significant difference in the baseline levels of ICAM-1 and E-selectin between asthmatic and nonasthmatic subjects (143). However, increased numbers of eosinophils are identified in the mucosa of asthmatic patients. Furthermore, a 6-week course of inhaled budesonide did not change expression of ICAM-1 and E-selectin, although the eosinophil numbers in the airway decreased. Such data bring into question the importance of their role in asthma. A subsequent report noted increased VCAM-1 levels in bronchial biopsies after segmental allergen challenge, but little or no change in ICAM-1 or E-selectin levels (144). Circulating forms of ICAM-1, VCAM-1, and E-selectin have been reported (145); however, their significance and precise role in asthma remains unknown. It is possible that the state of activation of these adhesion molecules, rather than their expression, determines their ultimate role in asthmatic inflammation.

Selective recruitment of eosinophils to the airway is a cardinal feature of asthma. Eosinophils, but not neutrophils, express VLA-4 ($\alpha_4\beta_1$) integrins on their cell surface. These ligands bind to VCAM-1 on endothelial cells. The particular importance of the VLA-4–VCAM-1 interaction lies in the lack of VLA-4 expression in neutrophils, thereby conferring a degree of selectivity for eosinophil and lymphocyte recruitment (146). Various animal studies have pointed to the importance of this adhesion protein interaction to the development of eosinophilic inflammation, bronchial responsiveness, and possibly, asthma. *Ascaris*-sensitive sheep treated with a monoclonal antibody to the α_4-integrin antibody demonstrated a reduced late-phase response to inhaled antigen and the development of BHR that accompanies antigen challenge (147). Treatment with antibodies against VLA-4 and VCAM-1 prevented eosinophil and T-cell infiltration of mouse trachea to an antigen challenge. In contrast, no effect on eosinophil recruitment was noted with antibodies to LFA-1 or ICAM-1 (148). This may suggest that these adhesion proteins, in addition to influencing eosinophil recruitment in the airway, also modulate their function and contribution to inflammation. In addition, these antibodies may influence T-cell recruitment to the airway and also block their interaction with endothelial adhesion proteins; this action may prevent the generation of eosinophil-attracting mediators. The evidence points overwhelmingly toward a role for the adhesion molecules in the inflammatory cell influx to the airway.

13 SUMMARY

Inflammation plays an integral role in the pathophysiology of asthma. With advances in molecular biological techniques and newer animal models, our insight into this process is advancing rapidly. A greater understanding of the interactions of the various elements of the inflammatory response and their interactions is thus evolving. This progress in our knowledge and understanding of the disease process appears to raise even more questions, but such is the nature of research. It is also known that no single abnormality of cells or mediators will suffice to explain the pathogenesis of asthma. Enhanced knowledge of molecular and cellular events in the inflammatory process would inevitably lead to newer, more specific, therapeutic agents, which would potentially be curative rather than palliative.

REFERENCES

1. Beasley R, Roche WR, Roberts JA, Holgate ST. Cellular events in the bronchi in mild asthma and after bronchial provocation. Am Rev Respir Dis 1989; 139:806–817.
2. Jeffery PK, Wardlaw AJ, Nelson FC, Collins JV, Kay AB. Bronchial biopsies in asthma. An ultrastructural quantitative study and correlation with hyperreactivity. Am Rev Respir Dis 1989; 140:1745–1753.
3. Bousquet J, Chanez P, LaCoste JY, et al. Eosinophilic inflammation in asthma. N Engl J Med 1990; 323:1033–1039.
4. Kirby JG, Hargreave FE, Gleich GJ, O'Byrne PM. Bronchoalveolar cell profiles of asthmatic and nonasthmatic subjects. Am Rev Respir Dis 1987; 136:379–383.
5. Tomioka M, Ida S, Shindoh Y, Ishihara T, Takishima T. Mast cells in bronchoalveolar lumen of patients with bronchial asthma. Am Rev Respir Dis 1984; 129:1000–1005.
6. Wardlaw DF, Dunnett S, Gleich GJ, Collins JV, Kay AB. Eosinophils and mast cells in bronchoalveolar lavage and mild asthma: relationship to bronchial hyperreactivity. Am Rev Respir Dis 1988; 137:62–69.
7. Corrigan CJ, Kay AB. CD4 T-lymphocyte activation in acute severe asthma. Relationship to disease severity and atopic status. Am Rev Respir Dis 1990; 141:970–977.
8. Walker C, Kaegi MK, Braun P, Blaser K. Activated T cells and eosinophilia in bronchoalveolar lavages from subjects with asthma correlated with disease severity. J Allergy Clin Immunol 1991; 88:935–942.
9. Azzawi M, Bradley B, Jeffery PK, et al. Identification of activated T lymphocytes and eosinophils in bronchial biopsies in stable atopic asthma. Am Rev Respir Dis 1990; 142:1407–1413.
10. Bradley BL, Azzawi M, Jacobson M, et al. Eosinophils, T-lymphocytes, mast cells, neutrophils, and macrophages in bronchial biopsy specimens from atopic subjects with asthma: comparison with biopsy specimens from atopic subjects without asthma and normal control

subjects without asthma and normal control subjects and relationship to bronchial hyperresponsiveness. J Allergy Clin Immunol 1991; 88:661–674.

11. O'Byrne PM, Dolovich J, Hargreave FE. Late asthmatic responses [review; 145 refs]. Am Rev Respir Dis 1987; 136:740–751.
12. Weersink EJ, Postma DS, Aalbers R, de Monchy JG. Early and late asthmatic reaction after allergen challenge [review; 80 refs]. Respir Med 1994; 88:103–114.
13. Djukanovic R, Roche WR, Wilson JW, et al. Mucosal inflammation in asthma. Am Rev Respir Dis 1990; 142:434–457.
14. Cookson WO, Craddock CF, Benson MK, Durham SR. Falls in peripheral eosinophil counts parallel the late asthmatic response. Am Rev Respir Dis 1989; 139:458–462.
15. Shaver JR, Zangrilli JG, Cho SK, et al. Kinetics of the development and recovery of the lung from IgE-mediated inflammation: dissociation of pulmonary eosinophilia, lung injury, and eosinophil-active cytokines. Am J Respir Crit Care Med 1997; 155:442–448.
16. Smith DL, Deshazo RD. Bronchoalveolar lavage in asthma. An update and perspective [review; 112 refs]. Am Rev Respir Dis 1993; 148:523–532.
17. Sedgwick JB, Calhoun WJ, Gleich GJ, et al. Immediate and late airway response of allergic rhinitis patients to segmental antigen challenge. Am Rev Respir Dis 1991; 144:1274–1281.
18. Roche WR. Fibroblasts and asthma [review; 37 refs]. Clin Exp Allergy 1991; 21:545–548.
19. Holloway L BRRW. The pathology of fatal asthma. In: Busse WW HS, ed. Asthma and Rhinitis. Cambridge, MA: Blackwell, 1994:109.
20. Horn BR, Robin ED, Theodore J, Van Kessel A. Total eosinophil counts in the management of bronchial asthma. N Engl J Med 1975; 292:1152–1155.
21. Naylor B. The shedding of the mucosa of the bronchial tree in asthma. Thorax 1962; 8:207.
22. Aalbers R, Kauffman HF, Vrugt B, et al. Bronchial lavage and bronchoalveolar lavage in allergen-induced single early and dual asthmatic responders. Am Rev Respir Dis 1993; 147: 76–81.
23. de Monchy JG, Kauffman HF, Venge P, et al. Bronchoalveolar eosinophilia during allergen-induced late asthmatic reactions. Am Rev Respir Dis 1985; 131:373–376.
24. Lam S, LeRiche J, Phillips D, Chan–Yeung M. Cellular and protein changes in bronchial lavage fluid after late asthmatic reaction in patients with red cedar asthma. J Allergy Clin Immunol 1987; 80:44–50.
25. Reed CE. Introduction. In: Busse WW HS, ed. Asthma and Rhinitis. Cambridge, MA: Blackwell Scientific, 1994:xxi.
26. Aalbers R, Kauffman HF, Vrugt B, et al. Bronchial lavage and bronchoalveolar lavage in allergen-induced single early and dual asthmatic responders. Am Rev of Respir Dis 1993; 147:76–81.
27. Calhoun WJ, Jarjour NN, Gleich GJ, Stevens CA, Busse WW. Increased airway inflammation with segmental versus aerosol antigen challenge. Am Rev Respir Dis 1993; 147(6 pt 1): 1465–1471.
28. Liu MC, Hubbard WC, Proud D, et al. Immediate and late inflammatory responses to ragweed antigen challenge of the peripheral airways in allergic asthmatics. Am Rev Respir Dis 1991; 144:51–58.
29. Kumano K, Nakao A, Nakajima H, et al. Interleukin-18 enhances antigen-induced eosinophil recruitment into the mouse airways. Am J Respir Crit Care Med 1999; 160:873–878.
30. Wegner CD, Gundel RH, Reilly P, Haynes N, Letts LG, Rothlein R. Intercellular adhesion molecule-1 (ICAM-1) in the pathogenesis of asthma. Science 1990; 247:456–459.
31. Yang L, Cohn L, Zhang DH, Homer R, Ray A, Ray P. Essential role of nuclear factor kappaB in the induction of eosinophilia in allergic airway inflammation. J Exp Med 1998; 188:1739–1750.
32. Hart LA, Krishnan VL, Adcock IM, Barnes PJ, Chung KF. Activation and localization of transcription factor, nuclear factor-kappaB, in asthma. Am J Respir Crit Care Med 1998; 158(5 pt+1):1585–1592.

33. Hartnell A, Moqbel R, Walsh GM, Bradley B, Kay AB. Fc gamma and CD11/CD18 receptor expression on normal density and low density human eosinophils. Immunology 1990; 69: 264–270.
34. Bruijnzeel PL, Virchow JC Jr, Rihs S, Walker C, Verhagen J. Lack of increased numbers of low-density eosinophils in the circulation of asthmatic individuals. Clin Exp Allergy 1993; 23:261–269.
35. Abu-Ghazaleh RI, Fujisawa T, Mestecky J, Kyle RA, Gleich, GJ. IgA-induced eosinophil degranulation. J Immunol 1989; 142:2393–2400.
36. Fujisawa T, Abu-Ghazaleh R, Kita H, Sanderson CJ, Gleich GJ. Regulatory effect of cytokines on eosinohil degranulation. J Immunol 1990; 144:642–646.
37. Cuss FM, Dixon CM, Barnes PJ. Effects of inhaled platelet activating factor on pulmonary function and bronchial responsiveness in man. Lancet 1986; 2:189–192.
38. Sigal CE, Valone FH, Holtzman MJ, Goetzl EJ. Preferential human eosinophil chemotactic activity of the platelet-activating factor (PAF) 1-*O*-hexadecyl-2-acetyl-*sn*-glyceryl-3-phosphocholine (AGEPC). J Clin Immunol 1987; 7:179–184.
39. Shaw RJ, Cromwell O, Kay AB. Preferential generation of leukotriene C_4 by human eosinophils. Clin Exp Immunol 1984; 56:716–722.
40. Dor PJ, Ackerman SJ, Gleich GJ. Charcot–Leyden crystal protein and eosinophil granule major basic protein in sputum of patients with respiratory diseases. Am Rev Respir Dis 1984; 130:1072–1077.
41. Frigas E, Loegering DA, Solley GO, Farrow GM, Gleich GJ. Elevated levels of eosinophil granule major basic protein in the sputum of patients with bronchial asthma. Mayo Clin Proc 1981; 56:345–353.
42. Filley WV, Holley KE, Kephart GM, Gleich GJ. Identification by immunofluorescence of eosinophil granule major basic protein in lung tissues of patients with bronchial asthma. Lancet 1982; 2:11–16.
43. Wardlaw DF, Dunnett S, Gleich GJ, Collins JV, Kay AB. Eosinophils and mast cells in bronchoalveolar lavage and mild asthma: relationship to bronchial hyperreactivity. Am Rev Respir Dis 1988; 137:62–69.
44. Brofman JD, White SR, Blake JS, Munoz NM, Gleich GJ, Leff AR. Epithelial augmentation of trachealis contraction caused by major basic protein of eosinophils. J Appl Physiol 1989; 66:1867–1873.
45. Flavahan NA, Slifman NR, Gleich GJ, Vanhoutte PM. Human eosinophil major basic protein causes hyperreactivity of respiratory smooth muscle. Role of the epithelium. Am Rev Respir Dis 1988; 138:685–688.
46. Frigas E, Loegering DA, Gleich GJ. Cytotoxic effects of the guinea pig eosinophil major basic protein on tracheal epithelium. Lab Invest 1980; 42:35–43.
47. Gleich GJ, Frigas E, Loegering DA, Wassom DL, Steimnuller D. Cytotoxic properties of the eosinophil major basic protein. J Immunol 1979; 123:2925–2927.
48. Djukanovic R, Wilson JW, Britten KM, et al. Quantitation of mast cells and eosinophils in the bronchial mucosa of symptomatic atopic asthmatics and healthy control subjects using immunohistochemistry [see comments]. Am Rev Respir Dis 1990; 142:863–871.
49. Niimi A, Amitani R, Suzuki K, Tanaka E, Murayama T, Kuze F. Serum eosinophil cationic protein as a marker of eosinophilic inflammation in asthma. Clin Exp Allergy 1998; 28:233–240.
50. Gundel RH, Wegner CD, Letts LG. Antigen-induced acute and late-phase responses in primates. Am Rev Respir Dis 1992; 146:369–373.
51. Barnes PJ. Neuropeptides and asthma [review; 88 refs]. Am Rev Respir Dis 1991; 143(3 pt 2):S28–S32.
52. McFadden ER Jr, Gilbert IA. Asthma. N Engl J Med 1992; 327:1928–1937.
53. Nadel JA, Borson DB. Modulation of neurogenic inflammation by neutral endopeptidase [review; 47 refs]. Am Rev Respir Dis 1991; 143(3 pt 2):S33–S36.

54. Lefort J, Bachelet CM, Leduc D, Vargaftig BB. Effect of antigen provocation of IL-5 transgenic mice on eosinophil mobilization and bronchial hyperresponsiveness. J Allergy Clin Immunol 1996; 97:788–799.
55. Foster PS, Hogan SP, Ramsay AJ, Matthaei KI, Young IG. IL-5 deficiency abolishes eosinophilia, airway hyperreactivity, and lung damage in a mouse asthma model. J Exp Med 1995; 183:195–201.
56. Corry DB, Folkesson HG, Warnock ML, et al. Interleukin 4, but not interleukin 5 or eosinophils, is required in a murine model of acute airway hyperreactivity. J Exp Med 1996; 183: 109–117.
57. Drazen JM, Arm JP, Austen KF. Sorting out the cytokines of asthma. J Exp Med 1996; 183: 1–5.
58. Wilson JW, Djukanovic R, Howarth PH, Holgate ST. Lymphocyte activation in bronchoalveolar lavage and peripheral blood in atopic asthma. Am Rev Respir Dis 1992; 145:958–960.
59. Walker C, Virchow J–C Jr, Bruijnzeel PLB, Blaser K. T cell subsets and their soluble products regulate eosinophilia in allergic and nonallergic asthma. J Immunol 1991; 146:1826–1835.
60. Walker C, Bode E, Boer L, Hansel TT, Blaser K, Virchow J Jr. Allergic and nonallergic asthmatics have distinct patterns of T-cell activation and cytokine production in peripheral blood and bronchoalveolar lavage. Am Rev Respir Dis 1992; 146:109–115.
61. Gratziou C, Carroll M, Walls A, Howarth PH, Holgate ST. Early changes in T lymphocytes recovered by bronchoalveolar lavage after local allergen challenge of asthmatic airways. Am Rev Respir Dis 1992; 145:1259–1264.
62. Metzger WJ, Zavala D, Richerson HB, et al. Local allergen challenge and bronchoalveolar lavage of allergic asthmatic lungs. Description of the model and local airway inflammation. Am Rev Respir Dis 1987; 135:433–440.
63. Borger P, Ten Hacken NHT, Vellenga E, Kauffman HF, Postma DS. Peripheral blood T lymphocytes from asthmatic patients are primed for enhanced expression of interleukin (IL)-4 and IL-5 mRNA: associations with lung function and serum IgE. Clin Exp Allergy 1999; 29:772–779.
64. Robinson DS, Hamid Q, Ying S, et al. Predominant T_{H2}-like bronchoalveolar T-lymphocyte population in atopic asthma. N Engl J Med 1992; 326:298–304.
65. Clutterbuck EJ, Hirst EMA, Sanderson CJ. Human interleukin-5 (IL-5) regulates the production of eosinophils in human bone marrow cultures: comparison and interaction with IL-1, IL-3, IL-6, and GM-CSF. Blood 1989; 73:1504–1512.
66. Kroegel C, Warner JA, Virchow JC Jr, Matthys H. Pulmonary immune cells in health and disease: the eosinophil leucocyte (part II) [review; 245 refs]. Eur Respir J 1994; 7:743–760.
67. Rothenberg ME, Peterson J, Stevens RL, et al. IL-5 dependent conversion of normodense human eosinophils to the hypodense phenotype uses 3T3 fibrobasts for enhanced viability, accelerated hypodensity, and sustained antibody-dependent cytotoxicity. J Immunol 1989; 143:2311–2316.
68. Dent LA, Strath M, Mellor AL, Sanderson CJ. Eosinophilia in transgenic mice expressing interleukin 5. J Exp Med 1990; 172:1425–1431.
69. Tominaga A, Takaki S, Koyama N, et al. Transgenic mice expressing a B cell growth and differentiation factor gene (interleukin 5) develop eosinophilia and autoantibody production. J Exp Med 1991; 173:429–437.
70. Alam RA. Chemokines in allergic inflammation. J Allergy Clin Immunol 1997; 99:273–277.
71. Zeibecoglou K, Macfarlane AJ, Ying S, et al. Increases in eotaxin-positive cells in induced sputum from atopic asthmatic subjects after inhalational allergen challenge. Allergy 1999; 54:730–735.
72. Ghaffar O, Hamid Q, Renzi PM, et al. Constitutive and cytokine-stimulated expression of

eotaxin by human airway smooth muscle cells. Am J Respir Crit Care Med 1999; 159:1933–1942.

73. Collins PD, Marleau S, Griffiths–Johnson DA, Jose PJ, Williams TJ. Cooperation between interleukin-5 and the chemokine eotaxin to induce eosinophil accumulation in vivo. J Exp Med 1995; 182:1169–1174.
74. Holt PG, McMenamin C, Schon–Hegrad MA, et al. Immunoregulation of asthma: control of T-lymphocyte activation in the respiratory tract [review; 86 refs.]. Eur Respir J Suppl 1991; 13:6S–15S.
75. Mosmann TR, Cherwinski H, Bond MW, Gieldin MA, Coffman RL. Two types of murine helper T cell clones: I. Definition according to profiles of lymphokine activities and secreted proteins. J Immunol 1986; 136:2348–2357.
76. Wierenga EA, Snoek M, de Groot C, et al. Evidence for compartmentalization of functional subsets of $CD2^+$ T lymphocytes in atopic patients. J Immunol 1990; 144:4651–4656.
77. Romagnani S. Th1 and Th2 subsets of $CD4^+$ T lymphocytes. Sci Am Sci Med 1994; May/June:68–77.
78. Hamid Q, Azzawi M, Ying S, et al. Expression of mRNA for interleukin-5 in mucosal bronchial biopsies from asthma. J Clin Invest 1991; 87:1541–1546.
79. Del Prete G. Human Th1 and Th2 lymphocytes: their role in the pathophysiology of atopy [review; 43 refs]. Allergy 1992; 47:450–455.
80. Bentley AM, Meng Q, Robinson DS, Hamid Q, Kay AB, Durham SR. Increases in activated T lymphocytes, eosinophils, and cytokine mRNA expression for interleukin-5 and granulocyte/macrophage colony-stimulating factor in bronchial biopsies after allergen inhalation challenge in atopic asthmatics. Am J Respir Cell Mol Biol 1993; 8:35–42.
81. Woolcock AJ PJ. Evidence for the increase in asthma worldwide. In: Chadwick DT CG, ed. The Rising Trends in Asthma. West Sussex, Engl; Wiley, 1997:122–134.
82. Warner JA, Miles EA, Jones AC, Quint DJ, Colwell BM, Warner JO. Is deficiency of interferon gamma production by allergen triggered cord blood cells a predictor of atopic eczema? [see comments]. Clin Exp Allergy 1994; 24:423–430.
83. Sporik R, Holgate ST, Platts–Mills TA, Cogswell JJ. Exposure to house-dust mite allergen (Der p I) and the development of asthma in childhood. A prospective study. N Engl J Med 1990; 323:502–507.
84. Robinson DS, Durham SR, Kay AB. Cytokines. 3. Cytokines in asthma [review; 148 refs]. Thorax 1993; 48:845–853.
85. Hultner L, Druez C, Moeller J, et al. Mast cell growth-enhancing activity (MEA) is structurally related and functionally identical to the novel mouse T cell growth factor P40/TCGFIII (interleukin 9). Eur J Immunol 1990; 20:1413–1416.
86. Moore KW, Vieira P, Fiorentino DF, et al. Homology of cytokine synthesis inhibitory factor (IL-10) to the Epstein–Barr virus gene *BCRFI* [published erratum appears in Science 1990; Oct 26; 250:494]. Science 1990; 248:1230–1234.
87. Hultner L, Druez C, Moeller J, et al. Mast cell growth-enhancing activity (MEA) is structurally related and functionally identical to the novel mouse T cell growth factor P40/TCGFIII (interleukin 9). Europe J Immunol 1990; 20:1413–1416.
88. Laitinen LA, Laitinen A, Haahtela T. Airway mucosal inflammation even in patients with newly diagnosed asthma. Am Rev Respir Dis 1993; 147:697–704.
89. Pesci A, Foresi A, Bertorelli G, Chetta A, Oliveri D. Histochemical characteristics and degranulation of mast cells in epithelium and lamina propria of bronchial biopsies from asthma and normal subjects. Am Rev Respir Dis 1993; 147:684–689.
90. Djukanovic R, Wilson JW, Britten KM, et al. Effect of an inhaled corticosteroid on airway inflammation and symptoms in asthma. Am Rev Respir Dis 1992; 145:669–674.
91. Murray JJ, Tonnel AB, Brash AR, et al. Release of prostaglandin D_2 into human airways during acute antigen challenge. N Engl J Med 1986; 315:800–804.
92. Wenzel SE, Westcott JY, Larsen GL. Bronchoalveolar lavage fluid mediator levels 5 minutes

after allergen challenge in atopic subjects with asthma: relationship to the development of late asthmatic responses. J Allergy Clin Immunol 1991; 87:540–548.
93. Wenzel SE, Larsen GL, Johnston K, Voelkel NF, Westcott, JY. Elevated levels of leukotriene C_4 in bronchoalveolar lavage fluid from atopic asthmatics after endobronchial allergen challenge. Am Rev Respir Dis 1990; 142:112–119.
94. Wenzel SE, Fowler AA III, Schwartz LB. Activation of pulmonary mast cells by bronchoalveolar allergen challenge. In vivo release of histamine and tryptase in atopic subjects with and without asthma. Am Rev Respir Dis 1988; 137:1002–1008.
95. Casale TB, Wood D, Richerson HB, et al. Elevated bronchoalveolar lavage fluid histamine levels in allergic asthmatics are associated with methacholine bronchial hyperresponsiveness. J Clin Invest 1987; 79:1197–1203.
96. Bousquet J, Chanez P, Lacoste JY, et al. Indirect evidence of bronchial inflammation assessed by titration of inflammatory mediators in BAL fluid of patients with asthma. J Allergy Clin Immunol 1991; 88:649–660.
97. Lane SJ, Sousa AR, Lee TH. The role of the macrophage in asthma [review; 90 refs]. Allergy 1994; 49:201–209.
98. Stein M, Keshav S. The versatility of macrophages [review; 55 refs]. Clin Exp Allergy 1992; 22:19–27.
99. Vachier I, Damon M, Le Doucen C, et al. Increased oxygen species generation in blood monocytes of asthmatic patients. Am Rev Respir Dis 1992; 146(5pt1):1161–1166.
100. Magnan A, van Pee D, Bongrand P, Vervloet D. Alveolar macrophage interleukin (IL)-10 and IL-12 production in atopic asthma. Allergy 1998; 53:1092–1095.
101. MacGlashan D Jr. White JM, Huang SK, et al. Secretion of IL-4 from human basophils. The relationship between IL-4 mRNA and protein in resting and stimulated basophils. J Immunol 1994; 152:3006–3016.
102. Tung R, Lichtenstein LM. In vitro histamine release from basophils of asthmatic and atopic individuals in D_2O. J Immunol 1982; 128:2067–2072.
103. Guo CB, Liu MC, Galli SJ, Bochner BS, Kagey–Sobotka A, Lichtenstein LM. Identification of IgE-bearing cells in the late-phase response to antigen in the lung as basophils. Am J Respir Cell Mol Biol 1994; 10:384–390.
104. Sur S, Crotty TB, Kephart GM, et al. Sudden-onset fatal asthma. A distinct entity with few eosinophils and relatively more neutrophils in the airway submucosa? Am Rev Respir Dis 1993; 148:713–718.
105. Lamblin C, Gosset P, Tillie–Leblond I, et al. Bronchial neutrophilia in patients with noninfectious status asthmaticus. Am J Respir Crit Care Med 1998; 157:394–402.
106. Martin RJ, Cicutto LC, Smith HR, Ballard RD, Szefler SJ. Airways inflammation in nocturnal asthma. Am Rev Respir Dis 1991; 143:351–357.
107. Ohashi Y, Motojima S, Fukuda T, Makino S. Airway hyperresponsiveness, increased intracellular spaces of bronchial epithelium, and increased infiltration of eosinophils and lymphocytes in bronchial mucosa in asthma [see comments]. Am Rev Respir Dis 1992; 145:1469–1476.
108. Laitinen LA, Heino M, Laitinen A, Kava T, Haahtela T. Damage of the airway epithelium and bronchial reactivity in patients with asthma. Am Rev Respir Dis 1985; 131:599–606.
109. Shijubo N, Itoh Y, Yamaguchi T, et al. Clara cell protein-positive epithelial cells are reduced in small airways of asthmatics. Am J Respir Crit Care Med 1999; 160:930–933.
110. Lozewicz S, Wells C, Gomez E, et al. Morphological integrity of the bronchial epithelium in mild asthma. Thorax 1990; 45:12–15.
111. Soderberg M, Hellstrom S, Sandstrom T, Lundgren R, Bergh, A. Structural characterization of bronchial mucosal biopsies from healthy volunteers: a light and electron microscopical study. Eur Respir J 1990; 3:261–266.
112. Knight DA, Stewart GA, Thompson PJ. The respiratory epithelium and airway smooth mus-

cle homeostasis: its relevance to asthma [review; 94 refs]. Clin Exp Allergy 1994; 24:698–706.

113. Salvi S, Semper A, Blomberg A, et al. Interleukin-5 production by human airway epithelial cells. Am J Respir Cell Mol Biol 1999; 20:984–991.
114. Marini M, Vittori E, Hollemborg J, Mattoli S. Expression of the potent inflammatory cytokines, granulocyte–macrophage-colony-stimulating factor and interleukin-6 and interleukin-8, in bronchial epithelial cells of patients with asthma. J Allergy Clin Immunol 1992; 89: 1001–1009.
115. Proud D. The epithelial cell as a target and effector cell in airway inflammation. In: Holgate ST, et al., eds. Asthma: Physiology, Immunopharmacology and Treatment. Fourth International Symposium. London: Academic Press, 1993.
116. Springall DR, Howarth PH, Counihan H, Djukanovic R, Holgate ST, Polak JM. Endothelin immunoreactivity of airway epithelium in asthmatic patients. Lancet 1991; 337:697–701.
117. Fujitani Y, Trifilieff A, Tsuyuki S, Coyle AJ, Bertrand, C. Endothelin receptor antagonists inhibit antigen-induced lung inflammation in mice. Am J Respir Crit Care Med 1997; 155: 1890–1894.
118. Nadel JA. Regulation of neurogenic inflammation by neutral endopeptidase [review; 59 refs]. Am Rev Respir Dis 1992; 145(2pt2):S48–S52.
119. Montefort S, Roche WR, Howarth PH, et al. Intercellular adhesion molecule-1 (ICAM-1) and endothelial leukocyte adhesion molecule-1 (ELAM-1) expression in the bronchial mucosa of normal and asthmatic subjects. Eur Respir J 1992; 5:815–823.
120. Hamid Q, Springall DR, Riveros–Moreno V, et al. Induction of nitric oxide synthase in asthma. Lancet 1993; 342:1510–1513.
121. Piacentini GL, Bodini A, Costella S, et al. Exhaled nitric oxide and sputum eosinophil markers of inflammation in asthmatic children. Eur Respir J 1999; 13:1386–1390.
122. Simon HU, Blaser K. Inhibition of programmed eosinophil death: a key pathogenic event for eosinophilia? Immunol Today 1995; 16:53–55.
123. Herbert CA, Edwards D, Boot JR, Robinson C. In vitro modulation of the eosinophil-dependent enhancement of the permeability of the bronchial mucosa. Br J Pharmacol 1991; 104: 391–398.
124. Vignola AM, Riccobono L, Mirabella A, et al. Sputum metalloproteinase-9/tissue inhibitor of metalloproteinase-1 ratio correlates with airflow obstruction in asthma and chronic bronchitis. Am J Respir Crit Care Med 1998; 158:1945–1950.
125. Mautino G, Henriquet C, Jaffuel D, Bousquet J, Capony F. Tissue inhibitor of metalloproteinase-1 levels in bronchoalveolar lavage fluid from asthmatic subjects. Am J Respir Crit Care Med 1999; 160:324–330.
126. Kumagai K, Ohno I, Okada S, et al. Inhibition of matrix metalloproteinases prevents allergen-induced airway inflammation in a murine model of asthma. J Immunol 1999; 162:4212–4219.
127. Vignola AM, Bonanno A, Mirabella A, et al. Increased levels of elastase and alpha$_1$-antitrypsin in sputum of asthmatic patients. Am J Respir Crit Care Med 1998; 157:505–511.
128. Brewster CE, Howarth PH, Djukanovic R, et al. Myofibroblasts and subepithelial fibrosis in bronchial asthma. Am J Respir Cell Mol Biol 1990; 3:507–511.
129. Roche WR, Beasley R, Williams JH, Holgate ST. Subepithelial fibrosis in the bronchi of asthmatics. Lancet 1989; 1:520–524.
130. Huber AR, Kunkel SL, Todd RF III, Weiss SJ. Regulation of transendothelial neutrophil migration by endogenous interleukin-8 [published errata appear in Science 1991 Nov 1;254: 631 and 1991 Dec 6;254:1435]. Science 1991; 254:99–102.
131. Kroegel C, Virchow JC Jr, Luttmann W, Walker C, Warner, JA. Pulmonary immune cells in health and disease: the eosinophil leucocyte (part I) [review; 322 refs]. Eur Respir J 1994; 7:519–543.
132. Ruoslahti E. Integrins [review; 40 refs]. J Clin Invest 1991; 87:1–5.

133. Georas SN, Liu MC, Newman W, Beall LD, Stealey BA, Bochner BS. Altered adhesion molecule expression and endothelial cell activation accompany the recruitment of human granulocytes to the lung after segmental antigen challenge. Am J Respir Cell Mol Biol 1992; 7:261–269.
134. Jutila MA, Rott L, Berg EL, Butcher EC. Function and regulation of the neutrophil Mel-14 antigen in vivo: comparison with LFA-1 and Mac-1. J Immunol 1989; 143:3318–3324.
135. Kishimoto TK, Jutila MA, Berg EL, Butcher EC. Neutrophil Mac-1 and MEL-14 adhesion proteins inversely regulated by chemotactic factors. Science 1989; 245:1238–1241.
136. Anwar AR, Moqbel R, Walsh GM, Kay AB, Wardlaw AJ. Adhesion to fibronectin prolongs eosinophil survival. J Exp Med 1993; 177:839–843.
137. Walsh GM, Mermod J–J, Hartnell A, Kay AB, Wardlaw AJ. Human eosinophil, but not neutrophil, adherence to IL-1-stimulated human umbilical vascular endothelial cells is alpha-4beta1 (very late antigen-4) dependent. J Immunol 1991; 146:3419–3423.
138. Weller PF, Rand TH, Goelz SE, Chi–Rosso G, Lobb RR. Human eosinophil adherence to vascular endothelium mediated by binding to vascular cell adhesion molecule 1 and endothelial leukocyte adhesion molecule 1. Proc Natl Acad Sci USA 1991; 88:7430–7433.
139. Bochner BS, Luscinskas FW, Gimbrone MA Jr, et al. Adhesion of human basophils, eosinophils, and neutrophils to interleukin 1-activated human vascular endothelial cells: contributions of endothelial cell adhesion molecules. J Exp Med 1991; 173:1553–1557.
140. Rabb HA, Olivenstein R, Issekutz TB, Renzi PM, Martin, JG. The role of the leukocyte adhesion molecules VLA-4, LFA-1, and Mac-1 in allergic airway responses in the rat. Am J Respir Crit Care Med 1994; 149:1186–1191.
141. Gundel RH, Wegner CD, Torcellini CA, Letts LG. The role of intercellular adhesion molecule-1 in chronic airway inflammation. Clin Exp Allergy 1992; 22:569–575.
142. Gundel RH, Wegner CD, Torcellini CA, et al. Endothelial leukocyte adhesion molecule-1 mediates antigen-induced acute airway inflammation and late-phase airway obstruction in monkeys. J Clin Invest 1991; 88:1407–1411.
143. Montefort S, Roche WR, Howarth PH, et al. Intercellular adhesion molecule-1 (ICAM-1) and endothelial leucocyte adhesion molecule-1 (ELAM-1) expression in the bronchial mucosa of normal and asthmatic subjects. Eur Respir J 1992; 5:815–823.
144. Lee BJ, Naclerio RM, Bochner BS, Taylor RM, Lim MC, Baroody FM. Nasal challenge with allergen upregulates the local expression of vascular endothelial adhesion molecules. J Allergy Clin Immunol 1994; 94(6pt1):1006–1016.
145. Montefort S, Lai CK, Kapahi P, et al. Circulating adhesion molecules in asthma. Am J Respir Crit Care Med 1994; 149:1149–1152.
146. Bochner BS, Luscinskas FW, Gimbrone MA, et al. Adhesion of human basophils, eosinophils and neutrophils to interleukin-1-activated human vascular endothelial cells: contributions of endothelial cell adhesion molecules. J Exp Med 1991; 173:1553–1556.
147. Abraham WM, Sielczak MW, Ahmed A, et al. alpha(4)-Integrins mediate antigen-induced late bronchial responses and prolonged airway hyperresponsiveness in sheep. J Clin Invest 1994; 93:776–787.
148. Nakajima H, Sano H, Nishimura T, Yoshida S, Iwamoto I. Role of vascular cell adhesion molecule-1/very late activation antigen-4 and intercellular adhesion molecule-1/lymphocyte function-associated antigen-1 interactions in antigen-induced eosinophil and T-cell recruitment into the tissue. J Exp Med 1994; 179:1145–1154.
149. Busse WW, Horowitz RJ, Read CE. Asthma. In: Middleton E Jr, Reed CE, Ellis EF Jr, Yunginger JW, Busso WW, eds. Allergy Principles and Practice. St Louis: Moseby, 1998: 839.
150. Carlos TM, Harlan JH. Blood 1994; 84:2068.

16

Atopic Dermatitis

PECK Y. ONG and DONALD Y. M. LEUNG

National Jewish Medical and Research Center, Denver, Colorado

1 INTRODUCTION

Atopic dermatitis (AD) is a chronically relapsing inflammatory skin disease that frequently affects children (1). In the 1930s, Sulzberger and associates first introduced the term AD in recognition of the close association of this disease with asthma and allergic rhinitis (2,3). This concept is supported by the fact that more than 50% of AD patients ultimately develop asthma or allergic rhinitis (4), and up to 85% have elevated serum IgE levels and positive immediate skin test or radioallergosorbent test (RAST) results for specific IgE directed against various food and inhalant allergens (5,6). However, the pathogenical role of allergens as the primary cause for AD has been difficult to establish, for some AD patients have no apparent sensitization to food or inhalant allergens (7), and the pathological changes of AD lesions do not resemble those of IgE-mediated immediate hypersensitivity reactions (8).

There is now increasing evidence for a cell-mediated process in AD (9). IgE^+ epidermal Langerhans cells in the skin are thought to play a central role in capturing and processing allergens to activate a cutaneous immune reaction (10). Presentation of processed allergen by IgE^+ epidermal Langerhans cells to allergen-specific T cells may result in the production of Th2 cytokines such as interleukin (IL)-4, IL-5, and IL-13, which are found in acute AD lesions (11). Th2 cytokines play crucial roles in IgE synthesis and in facilitating the migration of mononuclear cells and eosinophils to the cutaneous site of inflammation. But the roles of these cytokines in the pathogenesis of AD are not exclusive. Increased expression of interferon (IFN)-γ has recently been found in chronic AD lesions, suggesting a role for this Th1 cytokine in the chronic inflammation of AD (12). In addition to allergens, bacterial superantigens (13) and autoantigens (14) have also been implicated in the inflammation of AD. Thus, AD represents a complex disease involving a constellation of immunological triggers. An understanding of these mechanisms is important in designing strategies for the prevention and treatment of this common disease.

2 CLINICAL FEATURES

Intense pruritus and cutaneous reactivity are the hallmarks of AD. In 1891, the French dermatologist Jacquet was the first to suggest that itching is the initial event, followed by the scratching and the development of eczema. In 1936, while observing the effects of food challenge on a child with known food hypersensitivity, Engman et al. (15) showed that the development of eczema may be prevented if the skin was protected from scratching.

Table 1 Criteria for Diagnosis of Atopic Dermatitis

Major features
Pruritus
Typical distribution of dermatitis
Facial and extensor involvement in young children (< 3 years old)
Flexural involvement in older children (3 years or older) or adults
Chronic or chronically relapsing dermatitis
Personal or family history of atopy (asthma, allergic rhinitis, atopic dermatitis)
Other features
Early age of onset (< 6 years old)
Course influenced by environmental–emotional factors
Itch when sweating
Intolerance to wool and lipid solvents
Xerosis (dry skin)
White dermatographism
Recurrent conjunctivitis
Infraorbital darkening
Facial pallor or erythema
Hand–foot dermatitis
Hyperlinear palms
Keratosis pilaris
Elevated total serum IgE levels
Positive immediate skin test or RAST result
Evidence of impaired cell-mediated immunity
Frequent cutaneous infections, especially by
Staphylococcus aureus
Herpes simplex virus or other viral infections
Warts
Molluscum contagiosum
Dermatophytes
Peripheral blood eosinophilia

Source: Ref. 26.

The etiology of pruritus in AD is not well understood. It is thought that the release of inflammatory mediators as a result of immunological reactions may provoke itching. Pruritus has been induced by intracutaneous injection of histamine, leukotrienes, or proteolytic enzymes (16–18). On the other hand, Rukwied and Heyer (19) showed that the injection of acetylcholine intracutaneously in the skin of patients with AD, treated with the H_1-antagonist, cetirizine, induced significant pruritus compared with nonatopic controls. This study suggests that pruritus in AD patients may be elicited by a cholinergic, histamine-independent mechanism. AD patients also have a reduced threshold for pruritus (20). Using 48-hr Finn chamber testing with graded dilutions of sodium lauryl sulfate, Nassif et al. (21) reported that patients with active or inactive AD had significantly greater irritant skin responses than normal nonatopic controls. Children with AD also have a significantly higher rate of psychological (22) and sleep (23) disturbances than do normal controls. These disturbances may be manifested by increased anxiety and irritability (24) and lead to increased scratching and development of rash.

Table 2 Differential Diagnosis of Atopic Dermatitis

Dermatological diseases
Seborrheic dermatitis
Chronic irritant or allergic contact dermatitis
Psoriasis
Lichen simplex chronicus
Nummular eczema
Keratosis pilaris
Pityriasis rosea
Nonbullous congenital ichthyosiform erythroderma
Neoplastic diseases
Cutaneous T-cell lymphoma (mycosis fungocides, Sézary's syndrome)
Necrolytic migratory erythema associated with pancreatic tumor
Letterer–Siwe disease (Langerhans cell histiocytosis)
Immunodeficiencies
Wiskott–Aldrich syndrome
Hyper-IgE syndrome
Severe combined immunodeficiency syndrome
Infectious diseases
Human immunodeficiency virus (HIV)-associated eczema
Scabies
Candidiasis
Dermatophytosis
Tinea vesicolor
Congenital and metabolic disorders
Netherton's syndrome
Infantile-onset multiple carboxylase deficiency
Essential fatty acid deficiency
Zinc deficiency
Prolidase deficiency
Histidine deficiency
Pyridoxine (vitamin B_6) deficiency
Niacin deficiency
Phenylketonuria (PKU)

The acute lesions of AD present as pruritic, erythematous papules, with extensive serous exudate superimposed on a background of erythema (25). Subacute lesions are characterized by erythematous and excoriated papules. Repeat excoriations and trauma result in the chronic lesions of AD that are characterized by thickened plaques with increased markings (lichenification) and dry, fibrotic papules. In patients who are 2 years or older, AD lesions are most commonly localized to the antecubital and popliteal flexural areas. On the other hand, infantile AD involves the scalp, the face, especially the cheeks, and extensors surfaces of the extremities. The skin lesions of affected infants often have a shiny, erythematous appearance.

The diagnosis of AD according to Hanifin and Rajka (26) is based on the presence of a constellation of major and minor features (Table 1). Recently, a new set of diagnostic criteria for AD has been proposed by United Kingdom's Working Party (27). This set of criteria has a sensitivity of 85% and a specificity of 96%. The main features include the presence of pruritic skin and three or more of the following: history of flexural eczema, visible flexural eczema (or eczema on the cheeks, forehead, and extensor areas of extremities in a child younger than 4 years old), personal history of asthma or hay fever (or history of atopy in a first-degree relative in children younger than 4 years old), history of generalized xerosis, and onset of dermatitis before 2 years old (for patients older than 4 years old). Approximately 90% of AD patients develop the disease during the first 5 years of life (28). Thus, patients with adult-onset of AD should raise a higher index of suspicion for other diseases (Table 2).

3 IMMUNOPATHOGENESIS

3.1 Peripheral Blood Abnormalities

Atopic dermatitis is associated with several immunoregulatory abnormalities in both AD skin lesions as well as in peripheral blood (Table 3). Consistent with the high levels of serum IgE is the finding of predominant expression of Th2 cytokines by the peripheral blood mononuclear cells (PBMC) of AD patients. Enhanced expression of IL-4, IL-4

Table 3 Immunological Abnormalities in Atopic Dermatitis

Peripheral blood
Increased serum IgE levels
Eosinophilia and increased serum eosinophil granule protein levels
Increased number of $CD4^+$ and $CD8^+$ T cells secreting Th2 cytokines
Decreased number of $CD4^+$ and $CD8^+$ T cells secreting Th1 cytokines
Increased production of IL-10 and PGE_2 by monocytes
Increased expression of CD23 on mononuclear cells and B7.2 on B cells
Increased basophil spontaneous histamine release
Increased serum soluble IL-2 receptor level
Skin lesions
Increased infiltrate of $CD4^+CD45RO^+CLA^+$ T cells
Increased expression of FcεRI on Langerhans cells
Up-regulation of adhesion molecules (E-selectin, VCAM-1, ICAM-1)
Extensive deposition of eosinophil granule proteins
Predominance of IL-4, IL-13, and IL-16 in acute lesions
Predominance of IL-5, GM-CSF, and IFN-γ in chronic lesions

receptors (29), IL-5 (30), and IL-13 (31,32) has been shown in the PBMC of AD patients. Decreased expression of IFN-γ (33) and an increased ratio of IL-4/IFN-γ production (32) are also characteristics of PBMC from AD patients. Both $CD4^+$ and $CD8^+$ T cells may contribute to the increased production of IL-4 and decreased production of IFN-γ in AD (34,35). Monocytes from AD patients have elevated cAMP phosphodiesterase (36,37) and produce increased levels of IL-10 (38) and prostaglandin-E_2 (PGE_2) (39,40). Both IL-10 (41) and PGE_2 (42,43) inhibit IFN-γ production and, therefore may contribute to the decreased production of IFN-γ in AD patients. An increase in PGE_2/IL-12 production ratio by monocytes of AD patients has also been shown (40). IL-12 is a heterodimer composed of two subunits, p40 and p35 (44). It is a potent inducer of IFN-γ production (45). This increase in PGE_2/IL-12 ratio may also contribute to the increased IL-4/IFN-γ production ratio by T cells in AD.

The predominance of Th2 cytokine expression (IL-4, IL-5, and IL-13) and the decrease in Th1 cytokine expression (IFN-γ) by the PBMC of AD patients are important observations, because IL-4 and IL-13 promote IgE production by inducing IgE isotype switch in B cells (46); these cytokines, along with tumor necrosis factor (TNF) and IL-1, also induce the expression of vascular cell adhesion molecule-1 (VCAM-1) on endothelial cells to facilitate lymphocyte and eosinophil migration to the site of inflammation (47); in addition, IL-4 is involved in the differentiation and development of Th2 cells (48); IL-5 promotes the differentiation, recruitment, and survival of eosinophils (49); whereas IFN-γ mediates the type IV classic delayed type hypersensitivity reaction and inhibits the production of IgE (33). B cells of AD patients have increased expression of CD23 (low-affinity IgE receptor) (50) and B7.2 (CD86) (51), both of which promote IgE synthesis (52).

3.2 Immunopathology

Acute AD lesions are characterized by intracellular and intercellular edema of the epidermis (spongiosis), with a sparse epidermal infiltrate of T cells. In the dermis, a marked perivenular infiltrate of T cells and some monocytes–macrophages are present. Eosinophils, mast cells, and neutrophils are rarely present in acute AD lesions. In chronic AD, the epidermis is hyperplastic and hyperkeratotic with increased numbers of epidermal Langerhans cells. Cellular infiltrate in the dermis consists of predominantly macrophages and an increase in the number of eosinophils (53). Thus, different cell types in AD skin lesions contribute to skin inflammation.

3.2.1 T Cells

The majority of T cells in AD lesions are $CD4^+$ and $CD45RO^+$, suggesting a previous encounter with antigens (54,55). Most of these T cells express the skin lymphocyte-homing receptor, cutaneous lymphocyte antigen (CLA) (56), a ligand for the vascular adhesion molecule, E-selectin (57). The presence of CLA on T cells is an important factor for the development of AD. Casein-reactive T cells from patients with milk-induced eczema express significantly higher levels of CLA than *Candida albicans*-reactive T cells from the same patients or casein-reactive T cells from patients with milk-induced enterocolitis or eosinophilic gastroenteritis (58). Babi et al. (59) have shown that when the peripheral T cells of dust mite-sensitized AD and asthma patients were separated into CLA^+ and CLA^- fractions, the mite-specific T-cell proliferation response from mite-sensitized AD patients was localized to the CLA^+ fraction, whereas the mite-specific T-cell proliferation response from mite-sensitized asthma patients was localized to the CLA^- fraction. Akdis et al. (60) have shown that circulating $CLA^+CD45RO^+$ T cells from AD patients are activated Th2 cells that spontaneously released IL-4 and IL-13.

3.2.2 Epidermal Langerhans Cells

Epidermal Langerhans cells are $CD1a^+$ cells belonging to the dendritic cell lineage. These cells are effective antigen-presenting cells (APCs) and potent activators of autologous T cells (61). Normal epidermal Langerhans cells maintain an intracellular pool of the α-chain of FcεRI (high-affinity receptor for IgE) (62), but up-regulated surface expression of FcεRI has been found on epidermal Langerhans cells of AD lesions (63). FcεRI may play a critical role in facilitating the antigen-presenting function of epidermal Langerhans cells by capturing IgE-bound allergens (64). A distinct population of $CD1a^+$ cells, identified as inflammatory dendritic epidermal cells (IDEC), show especially up-regulated expression of FcεRI (65). Epidermal Langerhans cells also have increased expression of B7.2 in AD lesions and, therefore, may participate in the promotion of Th2 response and IgE production (66).

3.2.3 Eosinophils

Chronic AD lesions contain an extensive deposition of eosinophil granule proteins that include the major basic protein (MBP), the eosinophil cationic protein (ECP), the eosinophil-derived neurotoxin (EDN), and the eosinophil peroxidase (8). These proteins are deposited in AD lesions mainly through cytolytic degeneration of eosinophils (67). Eosinophil granule proteins are capable of inducing basophil and mast cell degranulation (68). In addition, MBP and ECP may cause tissue injury through their cytotoxic properties (68).

3.2.4 Mast Cells and Macrophages

Mast cells and macrophages are increased in chronic AD lesions. They are capable of producing inflammatory mediators, including leukotrienes, prostaglandins, proteases, and platelet-activating factor that contribute to the inflammation of AD. In addition, these cells are the main source of TNF-α, which can induce an up-regulation of vascular endothelial cell adhesion molecules, such E-selectin, VCAM-1, and intercellular adhesion molecules-1 (ICAM-1) in AD lesions (69). These adhesion molecules play a role in the migration of mononuclear cells and eosinophils to the cutaneous site of inflammation (70). In addition, macrophages also function as antigen-presenting cells.

3.2.5 Epidermal Keratinocytes

Granulocyte—macrophage colony-stimulating factor (GM-CSF)—plays an important role in maintaining the survival and functions of monocytes (71) and Langerhans cells (72). Enhanced production of GM-CSF by epidermal keratinocyte has been shown in AD lesions (73). Supernatants from cultured keratinocytes of AD patients induced a significantly higher proliferative response in PBMC than supernatants from control keratinocytes of nonatopic individuals, and this proliferative response could be totally abrogated by an anti-GM-CSF monoclonal antibody (MAb) (73). Supernatants from PMA-stimulated keratinocytes of AD patients, together with exogenous IL-4, also supported the maturation of monocytes into dendritic cells. Epidermal keratinocytes, when stimulated simultaneously with IFN-γ and TNF-α, produced increased levels of RANTES, which enhanced the chemotaxis of eosinophils (74). Epidermal keratinocytes are also a source of TNF-α and many other proinflammatory cytokines (75).

3.3 Cytokines and Their Receptors

By using in situ hybridization, Hamid et al. (11) found that both acute and chronic AD lesions contained significantly more cells expressing IL-4 and IL-5 mRNA than did uninvolved atopic skin and normal control skin. However, when acute AD skin lesions were compared with chronic AD lesions, the former showed an increased number of IL-4 mRNA-expressing cells and fewer IL-5 mRNA-expressing cells. In a subsequent study (76), these investigators also found that acute AD lesions contained significantly greater number of cells expressing IL-13 mRNA when compared with chronic AD lesions and normal and uninvolved atopic skin. An increase in the number of cells expressing the p40 subunit of IL-12 in chronic AD lesions compared to acute AD lesions or normal and uninvolved atopic skin was also observed. Increased IFN-γ expression has also been found in chronic AD lesions when compared with normal skin (77).

When using the atopy patch test (APT) with house dust mite allergen, a biphasic cytokine response has also been observed (12). IL-4-positive cells were increased as compared with nonlesional AD skin or normal skin during the acute phase ($<$ 24 hr) of the APT, whereas IFN-γ–positive cells predominated over IL-4–positive cells during the chronic phase, (48–72 hr) (78). $CD4^+$ T cells were the main source of IFN-γ. An influx of eosinophils that peaked at 24 hr of APT was observed. IL-4, GM-CSF, and IL-5 enhance the production of IL-12 by eosinophils in vitro (79). Thus, it was proposed that Th2 cytokines in acute AD lesions could induce eosinophils to produce IL-12, which then caused an increase in IFN-γ secretion in chronic AD lesions (79). Th2 cells may also induce dendritic cells to produce IL-12 which, in turn, stimulates IFN-γ production by Th2 cells (80). Bieber (64) has postulated that simultaneous antigen uptake and sufficient FcεRI aggregation on epidermal Langerhans cells may lead to activation of these cells and production of mediators capable of regulating a switch from Th2 to Th1 response. IFN-γ potentiates the activity and survival of eosinophils (81) and, therefore, may lead to further perpetuation of inflammation in AD.

Interestingly, because the activity of cytokines is critically dependent on the expression of their receptors, cytokine receptor expression in AD lesions (82) demonstrates that acute AD lesions contain a significantly higher number of cells expressing IL-4R-α (α-subunit of IL-4 receptor) mRNA compared with chronic AD lesions and normal and uninvolved atopic skins, whereas chronic AD lesions contained significantly more cells expressing the IL-5R-α (α-subunit of IL-5 receptor) mRNA and GM-CSFR-α (α-subunit of granulocyte–macrophage colony-stimulating factor receptor) mRNA when compared with acute AD lesions and normal and uninvolved atopic skins. The number of cells expressing IL-12R-β_2 (β_2-subunit of IL-12 receptor) mRNA was, however, not significantly higher in chronic AD lesions than acute AD lesions or normal or uninvolved atopic skins:

The mechanisms by which $CD4^+$ T cells are attracted to the cutaneous site of inflammation in AD are not fully understood. IL-16, a potent chemotactic agent for $CD4^+$ cells in vitro (83,84), is a possible chemoattractant for the influx of $CD4^+$ cells in acute AD lesions (85). IL-16 mRNA-expressing cells were significantly higher in number in acute AD lesions than in chronic AD lesions and normal and uninvolved skins. There was also a significant correlation between the number of IL-16 mRNA-expressing cells and the infiltration of $CD4^+$ cells in the uninvolved atopic skin, chronic AD lesions, and acute

AD lesions. Taken together, these studies suggest that IL-4, IL-13, and IL-16 are involved in the initiation of AD, whereas IL-5, GM-CSF, and IFN-γ play an important role in the maintenance of chronic AD.

3.4 Role of IgE

Immunoglobulin E may contribute to the pathogenesis of AD in several ways. Immediate hypersensitivity reactions involving the cross-linking of IgE molecules by allergen or microbial products on mast cells or basophils can lead to the release of histamine and inflammatory mediators (25). Food allergen challenge of patients with food allergy and AD induces the release of histamine by basophils or mast cells from these patients (86). The late-phase cutaneous reaction is characterized by an increased expression of vascular adhesion molecules (87) and a predominant Th2 cytokine profile consisting of IL-3, IL-4, IL-5, and GM-CSF (88). In addition, IL-1 and TNF-α are released in the cutaneous late-phase reaction (89). IL-1, TNF-α, and IL-4 play an important role in the induction of vascular adhesion molecule expression (70,90) and, therefore, may contribute to the recruitment to the recruitment of inflammatory cells in AD.

IgE-bound macrophages have been found in AD lesions (91). These cells may release inflammatory mediators in an IgE-dependent manner if challenged with appropriate allergens (92) or circulating IgG autoantibodies to the IgE molecules (93,94).

IgE molecules on epidermal Langerhans cells are bound to these cells predominantly by FcεRI in AD lesions (95). These IgE molecules may provide an efficient means for epidermal Langerhans cells to capture allergens before processing and presentation to allergen-specific T cells (10). IgE-bound Langerhans cells from AD lesions are 100- to 1000-fold more efficient than Langerhans cells lacking surface IgE in presenting house dust mite allergen to T cells. Thus, IgE-bound epidermal Langerhans cells may play an important role in initiating and maintaining an IgE-mediated cellular response in AD.

IgE autoantibodies against human proteins have been demonstrated by Valenta et al. (14) in a high percentage of patients with severe AD, suggesting a role for IgE autoreactivity in the pathogenesis of chronic AD. An increase in the serum level of IgE autoantibodies against the human protein, *ara* (atopy-related IgE autoantigen) NAC (nascent polypeptide-associated complex), correlates with the exacerbation of skin lesions in AD patients (96). Using serum IgE from AD patients, a cDNA coding for an IgE autoantigen, *Hom s 1*, has recently been isolated and characterized (97). *Hom s 1* was strongly expressed in human skin.

4 GENETICS AND TRIGGERING FACTORS

4.1 Genetics and Environment

The pathogenesis of AD clearly involves a genetic component. The concordance rate for monozygotic twins with AD is 77% compared with 15% for dizygotic twins with AD (98). However, the mode of inheritance for AD is unclear and does not appear to follow the classic mendelian patterns that are characteristic of single-gene diseases (99). It is likely that the interaction of multiple genes and the environment is responsible for the expression of allergic diseases, including AD (100). Major candidate genes for allergic diseases include 11q12–13 (101) and 5q31–33 (102,103). 11q12–13 contains the gene for the β-subunit of FcεRI (104), whereas 5q31–33 contains Th2 cytokine genes that regulate serum IgE levels (102) and genes that control bronchial hyperresponsiveness

(105). Linkage studies of 11q12-13 and AD have yielded conflicting results (106). However, a recent study (107), using tests of association, found a significant association of AD to polymorphisms within FcεRI-β gene. Positive linkage between AD and the T allele of the −590 C/T polymorphisms within 5q31-33 has been found in a Japanese population (108). As the T allele has been associated with higher IL-4 gene promotor activity than the C allele (109), it was postulated that predisposition to AD may be related to the genetic difference in IL-4 transcriptional activity (108). Alterations in nuclear protein interactions with IL-4 promoter elements may lead to abnormal IL-4 gene expression in AD (110). Significant association between a specific polymorphism in the mast cell chymase gene was found with AD, but not with asthma and allergic rhinitis (111). This study suggests mast cell chymase gene may have an organ-specific effect on the genetic risk of AD. However, a recent study (112) failed to confirm an association between the polymorphism in the mast chymase gene and AD. Of relevance is the finding of an association between AD and a mutation of the α-subunit of IL-4 receptor (113), which is involved in IL-4 binding and growth activation (48).

The prevalence of AD is increasing. A study by Schultz Larsen (114) showed that a cumulative incidence rate up to 7 years of age has increased from 3% for twins born between 1960 and 1964 to 12% for twins born between 1975 and 1979. Questionnaire studies of Swedish schoolchildren showed an increase in prevalence of AD from 7% in 1979 to 18% in 1991 (115). Similarly, a study of Aberdeen primary schoolchildren showed an increase in prevalence of reported eczema from 5.3% in 1964 to 12% in 1989 (116). The increase in the prevalence of AD has been attributed to various environmental factors and lifestyle changes (117). A recent worldwide study of the prevalence of AD showed significant variation in the prevalence of AD in patients of the similar ethnic backgrounds within and between countries, providing further support for the role of environmental factors in the development of AD (118).

The increase in AD prevalence parallels the increased prevalence of other allergic diseases, including asthma, throughout the world (119). It has been hypothesized that the increasing prevalence of allergic diseases may be associated with decreasing infection in early life (the ''hygiene hypothesis'') (120). In this hypothesis, a decrease in the frequency of infection, which involves delayed-type hypersensitivity, results in less IFN-γ/IL-12 production and thereby promotes Th2 cell activity and the development of allergic diseases. This hypothesis is supported by the observation that there is an inverse association between the magnitude of skin tuberculin response (Th1 response) in 1-year-old Japanese children and the eventual development of atopy (121). Interestingly, the higher socioeconomic class, which is probably least susceptible to overcrowding and infection, has a higher prevalence of AD (122).

4.2 Role of Food Allergens

The role of food allergens in the pathogenesis of AD is well documented and has been recently reviewed (123). Double-blind placebo-controlled food challenges have been documented to trigger pruritus and eczematous lesions in a subset of AD patients (124). In vitro proliferation of casein- or ovalbumin-specific T cells have been demonstrated in the peripheral blood of AD patients whose eczema is worsened by ingesting cow's milk or hen's egg, respectively (125). A prospective randomized trial of maternal and infant avoidance of cow's milk, egg, and peanut resulted in a reduction in the prevalence of AD in children with increased risk for atopy during the first 2 years (126). Food allergy is primarily a problem found in AD patients who are 5 years old or younger. Five important food allergens implicated in the pathogenesis of AD are egg, milk, peanut, soy, and wheat (123).

4.3 Role of Aeroallergens

The role of aeroallergens in the pathogenesis of AD is evidenced by a subgroup of AD patients whose skin lesions may be induced by inhalation of house dust mite allergens (127). In addition, a double-blind controlled trial has shown that avoidance of house dust mite allergens results in the improvement of skin lesions in some AD patients (128). Further support for the role of aeroallergens in the pathogenesis of AD is the derivation of aeroallergen-specific T cells from the skin lesions of AD patients (129,130). Direct skin contact with aeroallergens can also exacerbate AD as evidenced by positive alum-precipitated antigen (APT) (131,132). In addition to house dust mite, other aeroallergens that cause an exacerbation of AD include animal dander (133) and pollen (134).

4.4 Role of Microbial Agents

Recent studies have demonstrated a role for fungi and *Staphylococcus aureus* in the exacerbation of AD. The clinical improvement of AD associated with antifungal therapy (135) suggests the potential pathogenic role of fungi in AD. Specific IgEs against the yeast *Pityrosporum ovale* (136,137) and the dermatophyte *Trichophyton rubrum* (138) have been shown. In vitro stimulation of *P. ovale*-specific T cells from AD patients using anti-CD3 antibodies produced significantly higher levels of IL-4 and IL-5 compared with healthy controls (139). These findings suggest a possible role of these fungi as allergens in triggering AD exacerbation.

Most patients with AD are heavily colonized with *S. aureus*. Topical antibiotic therapy even of noninfected AD lesions has been associated with improvement of AD (140). Leung et al. (141) have shown that 57% of patients with chronic AD have serum IgE against one or more of these staphylococcal toxins: staphylococcal exterotoxin A (SEA), staphylococcal enterotoxin B (SEB), and toxic shock syndrome toxin-1 (TSST-1). Basophils from these patients released histamine only when these cells were sensitized with patients' IgE against one of these toxins (141), suggesting a potential role for them in the allergic inflammation of AD. AD patients with serum SEA/SEB-specific IgE are more likely to have severe skin disease than are AD patients without serum SEA/SEB-specific IgE (142).

In addition to their role as allergens, staphylococcal toxins, such as SEA, SEB, and TSST-1, can also act as superantigens to trigger skin inflammation in AD. Interestingly, an increased prevalence of AD has been reported in patients with Kawasaki syndrome, in which the pathogenic role of bacterial superantigens has been implicated (144). Michie and Davis (145) observed that in 68 survivors of toxic shock syndrome who had *S. aureus* producing TSST-1, 14 eventually developed chronic eczema. This was compared with gram-negative sepsis survivors who were not reported to develop eczema (145), suggesting that the development of eczema may be triggered by superantigens such as TSST-1. Indeed, direct application of SEB to the skin of healthy individuals and AD patients induced erythema and induration (146). In addition, half of AD patients experienced flaring of skin disease in the elbow flexure ipsilaterally to where SEB was applied.

TSST-1 and SEB are capable of inducing the expression of the skin-homing receptor CLA on T cells (147). This superantigen-mediated effect occured in a T-cell receptor

(TCR) Vβ-specific manner and was IL-12-dependent (147). Strickland et al. (148) have recently shown that AD patients with *S. aureus* producing TSST-1, which is known to be reactive with TCR $V\beta_2$, had selective expansion of CLA^+ T cells bearing TCR $V\beta_2$, whereas patients with *S. aureus* producing SEB, which reacts with TCR $V\beta_{17}$, had selective expansion of CLA^+ T cells bearing TCR $V\beta_{17}$. We postulate that staphylococcal superantigens stimulate accessory cells, such as epidermal Langerhans cells or macrophages, to produce IL-12, which induce the expression of CLA on T cells. These CLA^+ T cells can then recirculate to the skin where staphylococcal superantigens stimulate polyclonal expansion of these T cells with specific TCR Vβ, resulting in the elaboration of inflammatory cytokine production.

Staphylococcal superantigens may also cause inflammation in AD through other mechanisms. TSST-1, SEB, and staphylococcal exfoliative toxin-A can stimulate the release of TNF-α from activated keratinocytes. TSST-1 is also capable of enhancing the total IgE production in AD patients, possibly by up-regulating the expression of B7.2 on B cells (149). Of note, *S. aureus* strains that do not produce superantigens produce protein A and α-toxin, which are also capable of causing the release of TNF-α from activated keratinocytes (150).

5 GENERAL MANAGEMENT

5.1 Hydration and Emollient

Dryness contributes to the irritation and itching of atopic skin and should be treated with a combination of hydration therapy and effective emollients. Soaking the dry skin in lukewarm water for 15–20 min followed by trapping of the water with application of a moisturizer provides symptomatic relief for the patient. The use of a water-in-oil emollient cream (Eucerin Creme) as an adjunct to once-daily use of topical hydrocortisone 2.5% cream can be as effective as twice-daily use of the same topical corticosteroid in treating children with mild to moderate AD (151). Thus, appropriate use of an emollient may have a steroid-sparing effect.

Moisturizers are available as ointments, creams, and lotions. Creams and lotions have more of a drying effect. Ointments, on the other hand, are more occlusive and are most effective in preventing evaporation after hydration therapy. However, ointments are more likely to retain sweat and may cause further irritation and itching of the skin in selected patients. Therefore, the choice of a moisturizer should be individualized according to each patient's surrounding humidity and sweat gland function.

5.2 Irritants

Identifying and avoiding irritants is crucial as AD patients have a lowered threshold of irritant responsiveness. Potential irritants include soaps, detergents, chemicals, abrasive clothing, humidity, extremes of temperatures, and smoke. Overuse of soap, solvent, and drying agents, such as alcohol and astringents found in toiletries, should be avoided.

5.3 Allergens

In a subset of patients whose AD may be exacerbated by various food or inhalant allergens, identification of relevant allergens by careful history taking and doing selective immediate hypersensitivity skin tests is important. Negative skin tests have high-predictive value for ruling out suspected allergens, but positive skin tests must be correlated with clinical symptoms. Positive skin test to a particular food allergens should be confirmed with a double-blind, placebo-controlled food challenge, unless there is history of anaphylaxis to the food. Environmental measures, such as the use of plastic bedding encasements (152) or acaricides, (153) may have potential values in reducing the level of house dust mite allergens.

5.4 Corticosteroids

Topical corticosteroids are useful in acute flares of AD owing to their wide-spectrum anti-inflammatory actions. However, because of their side effects, which include hypothalamic–pituitary–adrenal axis suppression and skin atrophy, the least potent topical corticosteroids should be chosen to achieve the best effects. Topical corticosteroids with ointment bases can achieve more potent effects than the same corticosteroids in cream and lotion bases owing to the occlusive nature of ointment. Nonfluorinated corticosteroids with low potency should be used in areas with thinner skin such as the face, axillae, genitalia, and intertriginous regions, to avoid skin atrophy. Topical corticosteroids may be discontinued when acute flares of AD have resolved, but hydration measures should be continued.

In addition to their anti-inflammatory properties, topical corticosteroids may have an effect on bacterial colonization in AD. Several studies have found that the density of *S. aureus* on the skin could be reduced with the use of topical corticosteroids (154,155). The mechanism for reduction of *S. aureus* colonization on the skin by topical corticosteroids is unknown. It is possible that topical corticosteroids may decrease the number of attachment sites for *S. aureus* to AD lesions (13).

5.5 Infection

Superinfection by microbial agents can exacerbate AD lesions (25). The most common bacterial infections in AD lesions is *S. aureus*. Widespread, impetiginized and honey-crusted skin lesions should be treated with systemic antistaphylococcal antibiotics, such as semisynthetic penicillins or erythromycin. First-generation cephalosporins are alternative antibiotics. Topical antistaphylococcal antibiotics, such as mupirocin (Bactroban), may be effective and are particularly useful in localized infections (156). The presence of punched-out erosions and vesicles should raise suspicion for herpes simplex virus (HSV) infection. Tzanck preparation or herpes culture may be done for diagnosis. Localized HSV infection usually resolve in 1–2 weeks, but systemic acyclovir should be considered for extensive HSV infection. Antifungal medications may also be useful in selected patients.

With the increasing recognition of staphylococcal superantigens in the pathogenesis of AD, using topical antistaphylococcal antibiotics in combination with topical corticosteroids represents a rational approach in poorly controlled patients. In a double-blind, placebo-controlled crossover study (140), AD patients treated with topical corticosteroid and mupirocin showed significantly greater improvement in their skin disease compared with AD patients who received only topical corticosteroid. Thus, the combined use of topical corticosteroid–antibiotic in AD may have a steroid-sparing effect.

5.6 Antihistamines

Pruritus is the most common symptom of AD. It can cause significant distress to the patient and lead to scratching and worsening of rash. First-generation systemic antihistamines such as diphenhydramine and hydroxyzine may be effective in some patients in reducing pruritus. However, these antihistamines may cause significant drowsiness; therefore, they are best used at bedtime. Studies on the effects of second-generation nonsedating antihistamines in controlling pruritus of AD patients have produced mixed results. Terfenadine was ineffective in relieving pruritus of AD patients (157). However, a double-blind study showed that cetirizine significantly reduced pruritus and rashes in 6- to 12-year-old AD patients (158). The tricyclic antidepressant, doxepin, which has both H_1- and H_2-blocking effects, can also be effective (159).

6 EXPERIMENTAL IMMUNOMODULATORY THERAPY

A subset of patients with severe or corticosteroid-resistant AD remains a therapeutic challenge. In some of these patients, phototherapy using ultraviolet (UV)B (160), UVA1 (161), and combined UVA–UVB (162,163) have provided some therapeutic benefits, whereas in others, targeting at specific immunodysregulations using immunomodulatory therapy may offer the only effective approach.

6.1 Interferons

Because Th2 responses (i.e., production of IL-4, IL-13, and IgE) predominate the acute phase of AD and may be suppressed by IFN-γ (33), the use of recombinant(r) rIFN-γ to treat AD represents a reasonable approach. Using rIFN-γ, most published studies have shown beneficial effects of this cytokine in a subset of AD patients (164–166). Unfortunately, it is difficult to predict which subset of patients will benefit from such therapy. AD patients in one study showed persistent long-term, improvement with rIFN-γ (167).

rIFN-α has also been attempted for the treatment of AD. However, the results of various studies have been conflicting (168,169). A small study consisting of two patients showed improvement of their AD when rIFN-α and rIFN-γ were used sequentially (170).

6.2 Intravenous Immunoglobulin

High-dose intravenous immunoglobulin (IVIG) at 400 mg/kg per day for 5 days in two patients with severe AD showed significant improvement with almost complete clearing of symptoms 28 days after treatment in these patients (171). Topical IVIG applied once daily for 6 days to the skin lesions of six AD patients showed significant improvement in five out of the six patients; two of these patients showed superior improvement when compared with topical corticosteroid, and three patients had improvement equivalent to topical corticosteroid (172). The capability of IVIG in neutralizing staphylococcal toxins (173) and the increasing evidence of staphylococcal superantigens in AD inflammation may provide a theoretical basis for the beneficial effects of IVIG in AD patients. A case study showed that improvement of AD with high-dose IVIG was associated with decrease of IL-4-positive CD4 cells 2 weeks after treatment (174). In addition, IVIG may have immunomodulatory effects of autoimmune responses (175), which have also been implicated in AD.

6.3 Phosphodiesterase Inhibitors

A phosphodiesterase inhibitor, CP80,633, when applied topically, showed beneficial effects on AD patients in a double-blind, vehicle-controlled, paired comparison study (176). CP80,633 was also demonstrated to suppress AD monocyte production of PGE_2 and IL-10 (176), both of which suppress IFN-γ production (41–43).

6.4 Cyclosporin A

Cyclosporin A (CsA) is a potent immunosuppressive drug that acts primarily by suppressing cytokine gene transcription in T cells (177). CsA binds to the intracellular protein, cyclophilin, to form a complex that inhibits calcineurin, a $Ca2^+$–calmodulin-dependent protein phosphatase involved in the initiation of cytokine gene transcription (178). In an 8-week double-blind, placebo-controlled, crossover study, 33 AD patients treated with 5 mg/kg per day of oral CsA showed significant improvement in their skin disease (179). Other short-term blinded, placebo-controlled studies have confirmed the efficacy of oral CsA in the treatment of severe refractory AD (180). A long-term 48-week treatment of 100 adult patients with oral CsA resulted in significant overall improvement in disease severity, pruritus, and sleep disturbance (181). Sixty-five patients graded their AD as ''considerable improvement'' or ''no or minimal symptoms'' after the treatment; 14 patients withdrew from the study owing to adverse events (seven of which were probably treatment-related). Common side effects reported in the study include gastrointestinal symptoms, headache, musculoskeletal pains, upper respiratory tract infection, paresthesia, and skin infection. In a study of the mechanism of action for oral CsA, Campbell and Kemp (182) found significant increase in IFN-γ production and significant decrease in IL-4 production by PBMC of two children with AD treated with oral CsA over a period of 3 months. The patients also showed improvement in their skin lesions. These authors suggest that CsA may act by promoting Th1 responses and inhibiting Th2 responses in AD.

Because of concern with systemic toxicity of CsA, topical CsA has also been studied in AD patients. However, the results have not shown a consistent beneficial effect (183,184).

6.5 FK506

Tacrolimus (FK506) is a potent immunosuppressive agent that shares a similar mode of action with CsA (185). FK506 also interacts with a cyclophilin-like cytoplasmic protein, FK506-binding protein (FKBP12), to form a complex that inhibits calcineurin and decreased gene transcription for cytokines including IL-2, IL-4, or IL-5 (185). In two multicenter, well-controlled studies topical application of FK506 in ointment form (tacrolimus) resulted in clinical improvement of patients with moderate-to-severe AD (186,187). No serious side effects of tacrolimus were noted in these studies. The most common side effect was a local burning sensation at the site of application. Another study examining the pharmacokinetics of tacrolimus with similar results (188). No systemic accumulation of tacrolimus was noted in this study. The mechanism for the efficacy of tacrolimus in AD is not completely understood. It may down-regulate the expression of FcεRI on epidermal Langerhans cells (185). Tacrolimus also inhibits expression of other cytokines such as IL-1, IL-2, GM-CSF, IFN-γ, TNF-α, and IL-12 (189,190). Because recent studies suggest that both Th1 and Th2 cytokines play a role in the pathogenesis of AD. The capacity of tacrolimus to inhibit the expression of both Th1 and Th2 cytokines may account for its efficacy in AD.

6.6 SDZ ASM 981

SDZ ASM 981, an immunosuppressant that acts similar to FK506, also inhibits Th1 and Th2 cytokines (191). A randomized, double-blind, placebo-controlled study (192) has shown that twice daily topical application of 1% SDZ ASM 981 cream significantly, improved the clinical symptoms including pruritus and excoriations of AD patients. No significant adverse effects were noted in the study.

7 CONCLUSIONS

Atopic dermatitis is a complex skin disease defined by a constellation of clinical features. Currently, there is no diagnostic laboratory test, nor a curative therapy, for this disease. The search for a definitive diagnostic test and rational therapeutic solutions depends on understanding the basic mechanisms involved in the pathogenesis of this disease. Recent progress in the study of AD has revealed various immunopathogenic features of this disease. These features include (1) the presence of an up-regulated, cell-mediated immune response with IgE epidermal Langerhans cells playing a central role; (2) two defined phases of the disease process: an acute phase that is characterized by a predominance of Th2 cytokines, and a chronic phase that is associated with Th1 cytokine expression; (3) functional roles of IgE as a facilitator of allergen presentation and as autoantibodies; (4) evidence that bacterial toxins may contribute to the inflammatory process of AD by acting as allergens and superantigens. It is possible that the efficacy of IVIG can be explained by its neutralizing effects on bacterial superantigens (173). Thus, therapeutic approaches aimed at decreasing superantigenic effects may be clinically relevant.

The immunopathogenic features described in the foregoing have provided new targets for immunomodulation. For example, the use of human anti-IgE antibodies to block the binding of IgE to FcεRI (64) may down-regulate an exaggerated cell-mediated immune response in AD. By manipulating the imbalance between Th2 and Th1 cytokines, the immune abnormality of AD may be corrected. This concept has served as the basis for using rIFN-γ to down-regulate Th2 responses in the treatment of AD. The pathogenic role of IFN-γ in chronic AD is still unclear. It may play a crucial role in the perpetuation and maintenance of chronic inflammation in AD. If this is true, simultaneously decreasing both Th1 and Th2 cytokines may be important in reducing the overall inflammation of AD.

Agents such as FK 506 and SDZ ASM 981 may have multifunctional roles in modulating the inflammation of AD. These agents are capable of inhibiting multiple cytokine gene expression. They may regulate the production of both Th1 and Th2 cytokines and modulate the functions of epidermal Langerhans cells (185). Furthermore, these agents are associated with little or no systemic side effects. Understanding the disease mechanisms of AD is important, for it not only allows the manipulation of currently available therapies, but may also lead to the discovery of new therapeutic approaches.

ACKNOWLEDGMENTS

Supported in part by NIH grants AR41256 and General Clinical and Research Center grant MO1 RR00051 from the Division of Research Resources.

REFERENCES

1. Schultz Larsen F, Diepgen T, Svensson A. The occurrence of atopic dermatitis in north Europe: an international questionnaire study. J Am Acad Dermatol 1996; 34(5 pt 1):760–764.

2. Wise F, Sulzberger MB. Editorial remarks. In: Yearbook of Dermatology and Syphilogy. Chicago: Year Book Publishers, 1933:59.
3. Hill LW, Sulzberger MB. Evolution of atopic dermatitis. Arch Dermatol Syphilol 1935; 32: 451–463.
4. Roth HL, Kierland RR. The natural history of atopic dermatitis. Arch Dermatol 1964; 89: 209.
5. Jones HE, Inouye JC, McGerity JL, Lewis CW. Atopic disease and serum immunoglobulin-E. Br J Dermatol 1975; 92:17–25.
6. Sampson HA, Albergo R. Comparison of results of skin tests, RAST, and double-blind, placebo-controlled food challenges in children with atopic dermatitis. J Allergy Clin Immunol 1984; 74:26–33.
7. Guillet G, Guillet MH. Natural history of sensitizations in atopic dermatitis. A 3-year follow-up in 250 children: food allergy and high risk of respiratory symptoms. Arch Dermatol 1992; 128:187–192.
8. Ott NL, Gleich GJ, Peterson EA, Fujisawa T, Sur S, Leiferman KM. Assessment of eosinophil and neutrophil participation in atopic dermatitis: comparison with the IgE-mediated late-phase reaction. J Allergy Clin Immunol 1994; 94:120–128.
9. Leung DYM. Atopic dermatitis: the skin as a window into the pathogenesis of chronic allergic diseases. J Allergy Clin Immunol 1995; 96:302–318.
10. Mudde GC, Van Reijsen FC, Boland GJ, de Gast GC, Bruijnzeel PL, Bruijnzeel–Koomen CA. Allergen presentation by epidermal Langerhans cells from patients with atopic dermatitis is mediated by IgE. Immunology 1990; 69:335–341.
11. Hamid Q, Boguniewicz M, Leung DYM. Differential in situ cytokine gene expression in acute versus chronic atopic dermatitis. J Clin Invest 1994; 94:870–876.
12. Grewe M, Bruijnzeel–Koomen CA, Schopf E, Thepen T, Langeveld–Wildschut AG, Ruzicka T, Krutmann J. A role of Th1 and Th2 cells in the immunopathogenesis of atopic dermatitis. Immunol Today 1998; 19:359–361.
13. Leung DYM, Hauk P, Strickland I, Travers JB, Norris DA. The role of superantigens in human diseases: therapeutic implications for the treatment of skin diseases. Br J Dermatol 1998; 139(suppl 53):17–29.
14. Valenta R, Maurer D, Steiner R, Seiberler S, Sperr WR, Valent P, Spitzauer S, Kapiotis S, Smolen J, Stingl G. Immunoglobulin E response to human proteins in atopic patients. J Invest Dermatol 1996; 107:203–208.
15. Engman MF, Weiss RS, Engman ME Jr. Eczema and environment. Med Clin North Am 1936; 20:651–663.
16. Cormia FE. Experimental histamine pruritus. I. Influence of physical and psychological facts on threshold reactivity. J Invest Dermatol 1952; 19:21–34.
17. Soter NA, Lewis RA, Corey EJ, Austen KF. Local effects of synthetic leukotrienes (LTC_4, LTD_4, LTE_4, and LTB_4) in human skin. J Invest Dermatol 1983; 80:115–119.
18. Rajka G. Itch duration in the uninvolved skin of atopic dermatitis (prurigo Besnier). Acta Derm Venereol 1968; 48:320–321.
19. Rukwied R, Heyer G. Administration of acetylcholine and vasoactive intestinal polypeptide to atopic eczema patients. Exp Dermatol 1999; 8:39–45.
20. Rajka G. Atopic Dermatitis. London: W.B. Saunders Co., 1975:38.
21. Nassif A, Chan SC, Storrs FJ, Hanifin JM. Abnormal skin irritancy in atopic dermatitis and in atopy without dermatitis. Arch Dermatol 1994; 130:1402–1407.
22. Absolon CM, Cottrell D, Eldridge SM, Glover MT. Psychological disturbance in atopic eczema: the extent of the problem in school-aged children. Br J Dermatol 1997; 137:241–245.
23. Reuveni H, Chapnick G, Tal A, Tarasiuk A. Sleep fragmentation in children with atopic dermatitis. Arch Pediatr Adolesc Med 1999; 153:249–253.
24. Dahl RE, Bernhisel–Broadbent J, Scanlon–Holdford S, Sampson HA, Lupo M. Sleep disturbances in children with atopic dermatitis. Arch Pediatr Adolesc Med 1995; 149:856–860.

25. Leung DYM, Rhodes AR, Geha RS, Schneider L, Ring J. Atopic dermatitis. In: Fitzpatrick TB, Eisen AZ, Wolff K, Freeberg IM, Austen KF, eds. Dermatology in General Medicine. New York: McGraw-Hill, 1993:1543–1564.
26. Hanifin JM, Rajka G. Diagnostic features of atopic dermatitis. Acta Derm Venereol (Stockh) 1980; 92:44–47.
27. Williams HC, Burney PG, Pembroke AC, Hay RJ. The U.K. Working Party's Diagnostic Criteria for Atopic Dermatitis. III. Independent hospital validation. Br J Dermatol 1994; 131: 406–416.
28. Boguniewicz M, Leung DYM. Atopic dermatitis. In: Adkinson NF, Busse WW, Ellis EF, Middleton E, Reed CE, Yunginger JW, eds. Allergy: Principles and Practice. St Louis: Mosby, 1998:1123–1134.
29. Renz H, Jujo K, Bradley KL, Domenico J, Gelfand EW, Leung DYM. Enhanced IL-4 production and IL-4 receptor expression in atopic dermatitis and their modulation by interferon-gamma. J Invest Dermatol 1992; 99:403–408.
30. Yamamoto S, Hamasaki Y, Ishii E, Ichimaru T, Miyazaki S. Unbalanced production of interleukin-5 and interleukin-2 in children with atopic dermatitis. Ann Allergy Asthma Immunol 1997; 78:517–523.
31. Takamatsu Y, Hasegawa M, Sato S, Takehara K. IL-13 production by peripheral blood mononuclear cells from patients with atopic dermatitis. Dermatology 1998; 196:377–381.
32. Katagiri K, Itami S, Hatano Y, Takayasu S. Increased levels of IL-13 mRNA, but not IL-4 mRNA, are found in vivo in peripheral blood mononuclear cells (PBMC) of patients with atopic dermatitis (AD). Clin Exp Immunol 1997; 108:289–294.
33. Jujo K, Renz H, Abe J, Gelfand EW, Leung DYM. Decreased interferon gamma and increased interleukin-4 production in atopic dermatitis promotes IgE synthesis. J Allergy Clin Immunol 1992; 90(3 pt 1):323–331.
34. Nakazawa M, Sugi N, Kawaguchi H, Ishii N, Nakajima H, Minami M. Predominance of type 2 cytokine-producing $CD4^+$ and $CD8^+$ cells in patients with atopic dermatitis. J Allergy Clin Immunol 1997; 99:673–682.
35. Lonati A, Licenziati S, Canaris AD, Fiorentini S, Pasolini G, Marcelli M, Seidenari S, Caruso A, De Panfilis G. Reduced production of both Th1 and Tc1 lymphocyte subsets in atopic dermatitis (AD). Clin Exp Immunol 1999; 115:1–5.
36. Grewe SR, Chan SC, Hanifin JM. Elevated leukocyte cyclic AMP-phosphodiesterase in atopic disease: a possible mechanism for cyclic AMP-agonist hyporesponsiveness. J Allergy Clin Immunol 1982; 70:452–457.
37. Sawai T, Ikai K, Uehara M. Elevated cyclic adenosine monophosphate phosphodiesterase activity in peripheral blood mononuclear leucocytes from children with atopic dermatitis. Br J Dermatol 1995; 132:22–24.
38. Ohmen JD, Hanifin JM, Nickoloff BJ, et al. Overexpression of IL-10 in atopic dermatitis. Contrasting cytokine patterns with delayed-type hypersensitivity reactions. J Immunol 1995; 154:1956–1963.
39. Chan SC, Kim JW, Henderson WR Jr, Hanifin JM. Altered prostaglandin E_2 regulation of cytokine production in atopic dermatitis. J Immunol 1993; 151:3345–3352.
40. Snijders A, Van der Pouw Kraan TC, Engel M, Wormmeester J, Widjaja P, Zonneveld IM, Bos JD, Kapsenberg ML. Enhanced prostaglandin E_2 production by monocytes in atopic dermatitis (AD) is not accompanied by enhanced production of IL-6, IL-10 or IL-12. Clin Exp Immunol 1998; 111:472–476.
41. Fiorentino DF, Bond MW, Mosmann TR. Two types of mouse T helper cell. IV. Th2 clones secrete a factor that inhibits cytokine production by Th1 clones. J Exp Med 1989; 170:2081–2095.
42. Snijdewint FG, Kalinski P, Wierenga EA, Bos JD, Kapsenberg ML. Prostaglandin E_2 differentially modulates cytokine secretion profiles of human T helper lymphocytes. J Immunol 1993; 150:5321–5329.

43. Hilkens CM, Vermeulen H, van Neerven RJ, Snijdewint FG, Wierenga EA, Kapsenberg ML. Differential modulation of T helper type 1 (Th1) and T helper type 2 (Th2) cytokine secretion by prostaglandin E_2 critically depends on interleukin-2. Eur J Immunol 1995; 25:59–63.
44. Trinchieri G. Interleukin-12: a proinflammatory cytokine with immunoregulatory functions that bridge innate resistance and antigen-specific adaptive immunity. Annu Rev Immunol 1995; 13:251–276.
45. Chan SH, Perussia B, Gupta JW, Kobayashi M, Pospisil M, Young HA, Wolf SF, Young D, Clark SC, Trinchieri G. Induction of interferon gamma production by natural killer cell stimulatory factor: characterization of the responder cells and synergy with other inducers. J Exp Med 1991; 173:869–879.
46. Vercelli D, Geha RS. Regulation of IgE synthesis: from the membrane to the genes. Springer Semin Immunopathol 1993; 15:5–16.
47. Bochner BS, Klunk DA, Sterbinsky SA, Coffman RL, Schleimer RP. IL-13 selectively induces vascular cell adhesion molecule-1 expression in human endothelial cells. J Immunol 1995; 154:799–803.
48. Ryan JJ. Interleukin-4 and its receptor: essential mediators of the allergic response. J Allergy Clin Immunol 1997; 99(1 pt 1):1–5.
49. Lopez AF, Sanderson CJ, Gamble JR, Campbell HD, Young IG, Vadas MA. Recombinant human interleukin 5 is a selective activator of human eosinophil function. J Exp Med 1988; 167:219–224.
50. Bujanowski–Weber J, Brings B, Knoller I, Pfeil T, Konig W. Expression of low-affinity receptor for IgE (Fc epsilon RII, CD23) and IgE-BF (soluble CD23) release by lymphoblastoid B-cell line RPMI-8866 and human peripheral lymphocytes of normal and atopic donors. Immunology 1989; 66:505–511.
51. Jirapongsananuruk O, Hofer MF, Trumble AE, Norris DA, Leung DYM. Enhanced expression of B7.2 (CD86) in patients with atopic dermatitis: a potential role in the modulation of IgE synthesis. J Immunol 1998; 160:4622–4627.
52. Pène J. Regulatory role of cytokines and CD23 in the human IgE antibody synthesis. Int Arch Allergy Appl Immunol 1989; 90(suppl 1):32–40.
53. Leiferman KM, Gleich GJ. The role of eosinophils in atopic dermatitis. In: Leung DYM. Atopic Dermatitis: From Pathogenesis to Treatment. Austin, TX: RG Landes, 1996:145–183.
54. Leung DYM, Bhan AK, Schneeberger EE, Geha RS. Characterization of the mononuclear cell infiltrate in atopic dermatitis using monoclonal antibodies. J Allergy Clin Immunol 1983; 71(1 pt 1):47–56.
55. Bos JD, Hagenaars C, Das PK, Krieg SR, Voorn WJ, Kapsenberg ML. Predominance of ''memory'' T cells ($CD4^+$, $CDw29^+$) over ''naive'' T cells ($CD4^+$, $CD45R^+$) in both normal and diseased human skin. Arch Dermatol Res 1989; 281:24–30.
56. Picker LJ, Michie SA, Rott LS, Butcher EC. A unique phenotype of skin-associated lymphocytes in humans. Preferential expression of the HECA-452 epitope by benign and malignant T cells at cutaneous sites. Am J Pathol 1990; 136:1053–1068.
57. Picker LJ, Butcher EC. Physiological and molecular mechanisms of lymphocyte homing. Annu Rev Immunol 1992; 10:561–591.
58. Abernathy–Carver KJ, Sampson HA, Picker LJ, Leung DYM. Milk-induced eczema is associated with the expansion of T cells expressing cutaneous lymphocyte antigen. J Clin Invest 1995; 95:913–918.
59. Santamaria Babi LF, Picker LJ, Perez Soler MT, Drzimalla K, Flohr P, Blaser K, Hauser C. Circulating allergen-reactive T cells from patients with atopic dermatitis and allergic contact dermatitis express the skin-selective homing receptor, the cutaneous lymphocyte-associated antigen. J Exp Med 1995; 181:1935–1940.
60. Akdis M, Akdis CA, Weigl L, Disch R, Blaser K. Skin-homing, CLA^+ memory T cells are

activated in atopic dermatitis and regulate IgE by an IL-13-dominated cytokine pattern: IgG4 counter-regulation by CLA-memory T cells. J Immunol 1997; 159:4611–4619.

61. Taylor RS, Baadsgaard O, Hammerberg C, Cooper KD. Hyperstimulatory CD1a$^+$ CD1b$^+$ CD36$^+$ Langerhans cells are responsible for increased autologous T lymphocyte reactivity to lesional epidermal cells of patients with atopic dermatitis. J Immunol 1991; 147:3794–3802.
62. Kraft S, Wessendorf JH, Hanau D, Bieber T. Regulation of the high affinity receptor for IgE on human epidermal Langerhans cells. J Immunol 1998; 161:1000–1006.
63. Wollenberg A, Wen S, Bieber T. Langerhans cell phenotyping: a new tool for differential diagnosis of inflammatory skin diseases [letter]. Lancet 1995; 346:1626–1627.
64. Bieber T. Fc epsilon RI on human epidermal Langerhans cells: an old receptor with new structure and functions. Int Arch Allergy Immunol 1997; 113:30–34.
65. Wollenberg A, Kraft S, Hanau D, Bieber T. Immunomorphological and ultrastructural characterization of Langerhans cells and a novel, inflammatory dendritic epidermal cell (IDEC) population in lesional skin of atopic eczema. J Invest Dermatol 1996; 106:446–453.
66. Ohki O, Yokozeki H, Katayama I, Umeda T, Azuma M, Okumura K, Nishioka K. Functional CD86 (B7-2/B70) is predominantly expressed on Langerhans cells in atopic dermatitis. Br J Dermatol 1997; 136:838–845.
67. Cheng JF, Ott NL, Peterson EA, George TJ, Hukee MJ, Gleich GJ, Leiferman KM. Dermal eosinophils in atopic dermatitis undergo cytolytic degeneration. J Allergy Clin Immunol 1997; 99:683–692.
68. Gleich GJ, Adolpson CR, Leiferman KM. The eosinophils. In: Gallin JI, Goldstein IM, Snyderman R, eds. Inflammation: Basic Principles and Clinical Correlates. New York: Raven Press, 1992:663–700.
69. de Vries IJM, Langeveld–Wildschut EG, van Reijsen FC, Dubois GR, van den Hoek JA, Bihari IC, van Wichen D, de Weger RA, Knol EF, Thepen T, Bruijnzeel–Koomen CA. Adhesion molecule expression on skin endothelia in atopic dermatitis: effects of TNF-alpha and IL-4. J Allergy Clin Immunol 1998; 102:461–468.
70. Wakita H, Sakamoto T, Tokura Y, Takigawa M. E-selectin and vascular cell adhesion molecule-1 as critical adhesion molecules for infiltration of T lymphocytes and eosinophils in atopic dermatitis. J Cutan Pathol 1994; 21:33–39.
71. Bratton DL, Hamid Q, Boguniewicz M, Doherty DE, Kailey JM, Leung DYM. Granulocyte macrophage colony-stimulating factor contributes to enhanced monocyte survival in chronic atopic dermatitis. J Clin Invest 1995; 95:211–218.
72. O'Sullivan GM, Sluyter R, Boswell CM, Barnetson RS, Halliday GM. Modulation of Ia$^+$ Langerhans cell numbers in vivo by cultured epidermis derived supernatants and by GM-CSF. Exp Dermatol 1996; 5:28–37.
73. Pastore S, Fanales–Belasio E, Albanesi C, Chinni LM, Giannetti A, Girolomoni G. Granulocyte macrophage colony-stimulating factor is overproduced by keratinocytes in atopic dermatitis. Implications for sustained dendritic cell activation in the skin. J Clin Invest 1997; 99: 3009–3017.
74. Yamada H, Matsukura M, Yudate T, Chihara J, Stingl G, Tezuka T. Enhanced production of RANTES, an eosinophil chemoattractant factor, by cytokine-stimulated epidermal keratinocytes. Int Arch Allergy Immunol 1997; 114(suppl 1)28–32.
75. Pastore S, Corinti S, La Placa M, Didona B, Girolomoni G. Interferon-gamma promotes exaggerated cytokine production in keratinocytes cultured from patients with atopic dermatitis. J Allergy Clin Immunol 1998; 101(4 pt 1):538–544.
76. Hamid Q, Naseer T, Minshall EM, Song YL, Boguniewicz M, Leung DYM. In vivo expression of IL-12 and IL-13 in atopic dermatitis. J Allergy Clin Immunol 1996; 98:225–231.
77. Grewe M, Gyufko K, Schopf E, Krutmann J. Lesional expression of interferon-gamma in atopic eczema. Lancet 1994; 343:25–26.
78. Thepen T, Langeveld–Wildschut EG, Bihari IC, van Wichen DF, van Reijsen FC, Mudde

GC, Bruijnzeel–Koomen CA. Biphasic response against aeroallergen in atopic dermatitis showing a switch from an initial T_H2 response to a T_H1 response in situ: an immunocytochemical study. J Allergy Clin Immunol 1996; 97:828–837.
79. Grewe M, Czech W, Morita A, Werfel T, Klammer M, Kapp A, Ruzicka T, Schopf E, Krutmann J. Human eosinophils produce biologically active IL-12: implications for control of T cell responses. J Immunol 1998; 161:415–420.
80. Vezzio N, Sarfati M, Yang LP, Demeure CE, Delespesse G. Human Th2-like cell clones induce IL-12 production by dendritic cells and may express several cytokine profiles. Int Immunol 1996; 8:1963–1970.
81. Fujisawa T, Fukuda S, Atsuta J, Ichimi R, Kamiya H, Sakurai M. Interferon-gamma induces interleukin-3 release from peripheral blood eosinophils. Int Arch Allergy Immunol 1994; 104(suppl 1):41–43.
82. Taha RA, Leung DYM, Ghaffar O, Boguniewicz M, Hamid Q. In vivo expression of cytokine receptor mRNA in atopic dermatitis. J Allergy Clin Immunol 1998; 102:245–250.
83. Berman JS, Cruikshank WW, Center DM, Theodore AC, Beer DJ. Chemoattractant lymphokines specific for the helper/inducer T-lymphocyte subset. Cell Immunol 1985; 95:105–112.
84. Cruikshank WW, Center DM, Nisar N, Wu M, Natke B, Theodore AC, Kornfeld H. Molecular and functional analysis of a lymphocyte chemoattractant factor: association of biologic function with CD4 expression. Proc Natl Acad Sci USA 1994; 91:5109–5113.
85. Laberge S, Ghaffar O, Boguniewicz M, Center DM, Leung DYM, Hamid Q. Association of increased $CD4^+$ T-cell infiltration with increased IL-16 gene expression in atopic dermatitis. J Allergy Clin Immunol 1998; 102(4 pt 1):645–650.
86. James JM, Kagey–Sobotka A, Sampson HA. Patients with severe atopic dermatitis have activated circulating basophils. J Allergy Clin Immunol 1993; 91:1155–1162.
87. Leung DYM, Pober JS, Cotran RS. Expression of endothelial-leukocyte adhesion molecule-1 in elicited late phase allergic reactions. J Clin Invest 1991; 87:1805–1809.
88. Kay AB, Ying S, Varney V, Gaga M, Durham SR, Moqbel R, Wardlaw AJ, Hamid Q. Messenger RNA expression of the cytokine gene cluster, interleukin 3 (IL-3), IL-4, IL-5, and granulocyte/macrophage colony-stimulating factor, in allergen-induced late-phase cutaneous reactions in atopic subjects. J Exp Med 1991; 173:775–778.
89. Bochner BS, Charlesworth EN, Lichtenstein LM, Derse CP, Gillis S, Dinarello CA, Schleimer RP. Interleukin-1 is released at sites of human cutaneous allergic reactions. J Allergy Clin Immunol 1990; 86(6 pt 1):830–839.
90. Schleimer RP, Sterbinsky SA, Kaiser J, et al. IL-4 induces adherence of human eosinophils and basophils but not neutrophils to endothelium. Association with expression of VCAM-1. J Immunol 1992; 148:1086–1092.
91. Leung DYM, Schneeberger EE, Siraganian RP, Geha RS, Bhan AK. The presence of IgE on macrophages and dendritic cells infiltrating into the skin lesion of atopic dermatitis. Clin Immunol Immunopathol 1987; 42:328–337.
92. Rouzer CA, Scott WA, Hamill AL, Liu FT, Katz DH, Cohn ZA. Secretion of leukotriene C and other arachidonic acid metabolites by macrophages challenged with immunoglobulin E immune complexes. J Exp Med 1982; 156:1077–1086.
93. Quinti I, Brozek C, Wood N, Geha RS, Leung DYM. Circulating IgG autoantibodies to IgE in atopic syndromes. J Allergy Clin Immunol 1986; 77:586–594.
94. Zweiman B, Kaplan AP, Tong L, Moskovitz AR. Cytokine levels and inflammatory responses in developing late-phase allergic reactions in the skin. J Allergy Clin Immunol 1997; 100:104–109.
95. Klubal R, Osterhoff B, Wang B, Kinet JP, Maurer D, Stingl G. The high-affinity receptor for IgE is the predominant IgE-binding structure in lesional skin of atopic dermatitis patients. J Invest Dermatol 1997; 108:336–342.
96. Natter S, Seiberler S, Hufnagl P, Binder BR, Hirschl AM, Ring J, Abeck D, Schmidt T,

Valent P, Valenta R. Isolation of cDNA clones coding for IgE autoantigens with serum IgE from atopic dermatitis patients. FASEB J 1998; 12:1559–1569.

97. Valenta R, Natter S, Seiberler S, Wichlas S, Maurer D, Hess M, Pavelka M, Grote M, Ferreira F, Szepfalusi Z, Valent P, Stingl G. Molecular characterization of an autoallergen, Hom s 1, identified by serum IgE from atopic dermatitis patients. J Invest Dermatol 1998; 111:1178–1183.
98. Larsen FS, Holm NV, Henningsen K. Atopic dermatitis. A genetic–epidemiologic study in a population-based twin sample. J Am Acad Dermatol 1986; 15:487–494.
99. Sandford A, Weir T, Pare P. The genetics of asthma. Am J Respir Crit Care Med 1996; 153(6 pt 1):1749–1765.
100. Rosenwasser LJ. Genetics of asthma and atopy. Toxicol Lett 1996; 86:73–77.
101. Cookson WO, Sharp PA, Faux JA, Hopkin JM. Linkage between immunoglobulin E responses underlying asthma and rhinitis and chromosome 11q. Lancet 1989; 1:1292–1295.
102. Marsh DG, Neely JD, Breazeale DR, Ghosh B, Freidhoff LR, Ehrlich–Kautzky E, Schou C, Krishnaswamy G, Beaty TH. Linkage analysis of IL4 and other chromosome 5q31.1 markers and total serum immunoglobulin E concentrations. Science 1994; 264:1152–1156.
103. Meyers DA, Postma DS, Panhuysen CI, Xu J, Amelung PJ, Levitt RC, Bleecker ER. Evidence for a locus regulating total serum IgE levels mapping to chromosome 5. Genomics 1994; 23:464–470.
104. Sandford AJ, Shirakawa T, Moffatt MF, et al. Localisation of atopy and beta subunit of high-affinity IgE receptor (Fc epsilon RI) on chromosome 11q. Lancet 1993; 341:332–334.
105. Postma DS, Bleecker ER, Amelung PJ, Holroyd KJ, Xu J, Panhuysen CI, Meyers DA, Levitt RC. Genetic susceptibility to asthma—bronchial hyperresponsiveness coinherited with a major gene for atopy. N Engl J Med 1995; 333:894–900.
106. Folster–Holst R, Moises HW, Yang L, Fritsch W, Weissenbach J, Christophers E. Linkage between atopy and the IgE high-affinity receptor gene at 11q13 in atopic dermatitis families. Hum Genet 1998; 102:236–239.
107. Cox HE, Moffatt MF, Faux JA, Walley AJ, Coleman R, Trembath RC, Cookson WO, Harper JI. Association of atopic dermatitis to the beta subunit of the high affinity immunoglobulin E receptor. Br J Dermatol 1998; 138:182–187.
108. Kawashima T, Noguchi E, Arinami T, Yamakawa–Kobayashi K, Nakagawa H, Otsuka F, Hamaguchi H. Linkage and association of an interleukin 4 gene polymorphism with atopic dermatitis in Japanese families. J Med Genet 1998; 35:502–504.
109. Rosenwasser LJ, Klemm DJ, Dresback JK, Inamura H, Mascali JJ, Klinnert M, Borish L. Promoter polymorphisms in the chromosome 5 gene cluster in asthma and atopy. Clin Exp Allergy 1995; 25(suppl 2):74–78.
110. Chan SC, Brown MA, Willcox TM, Li SH, Stevens SR, Tara D, Hanifin JM. Abnormal IL-4 gene expression by atopic dermatitis T lymphocytes is reflected in altered nuclear protein interactions with IL-4 transcriptional regulatory element. J Invest Dermatol 1996; 106:1131–1136.
111. Mao XQ, Shirakawa T, Yoshikawa T, Yoshikawa K, Kawai M, Sasaki S, Enomoto T, Hashimoto T, Furuyama J, Hopkin JM, Morimoto K. Association between genetic variants of mast-cell chymase and eczema. Lancet 1996; 348:581–583.
112. Kawashima T, Noguchi E, Arinami T, Kobayashi K, Otsuka F, Hamaguchi H. No evidence for an association between a variant of the mast cell chymase gene and atopic dermatitis based on case–control and haplotype-relative–risk analyses. Hum Hered 1998; 48:271–274.
113. Hershey GK, Friedrich MF, Esswein LA, Thomas ML, Chatila TA. The association of atopy with a gain-of-function mutation in the alpha subunit of the interleukin-4 receptor. N Engl J Med 1997; 337:1720–1725.
114. Schultz Larsen F. Atopic dermatitis: a genetic-epidemiologic study in a population-based twin sample. J Am Acad Dermatol 1993; 28(5 pt 1):719–723.

115. Aberg N, Hesselmar B, Aberg B, Eriksson B. Increase of asthma, allergic rhinitis and eczema in Swedish schoolchildren between 1979 and 1991. Clin Exp Allergy 1995; 25:815–819.
116. Ninan TK, Russell G. Respiratory symptoms and atopy in Aberdeen schoolchildren: evidence from two surveys 25 years apart. Br Med J 1992; 304:873–875.
117. Williams HC. Atopic eczema. Br Med J 1995; 311:1241–1242.
118. Williams H, Robertson C, Stewart A, Ait–Khaled N, Anabwani G, Anderson R, Asher I, Beasley R, Bjorksten B, Burr M, Clayton T, Crane J, Ellwood P, Keil U, Lai C, Mallol J, Martinez F, Mitchell E, Montefort S, Pearce N, Shah J, Sibbald B, Strachan D, von Mutius E, Weiland SK. Worldwide variations in the prevalance of symptoms of atopic eczema in the International Study of Asthma and Allergies in Childhood. J Allergy Clin Immunol 1999; 103(1 pt 1):125–138.
119. Woolcock AJ, Peat JK. Evidence for the increase in asthma worldwide. Ciba Found Symp 1997; 206:122–134.
120. Holgate ST. The cellular and mediator basis of asthma in relation to natural history. Lancet 1997; 350(suppl 30):5–9.
121. Shirakawa T, Enomoto T, Shimazu S, Hopkin JM. The inverse association between tuberculin responses and atopic disorder. Science 1997; 275:77–79.
122. Williams HC, Strachan DP, Hay RJ. Childhood eczema: disease of the advantaged? Br Med J 1994; 308:1132–1135.
123. Sampson HA. Food sensitivity and the pathogenesis of atopic dermatitis. J R Soc Med 1997; 90(suppl 30):2–8.
124. Sampson HA, McCaskill CC. Food hypersensitivity and atopic dermatitis: evaluation of 113 patients. J Pediatr 1985; 107:669–675.
125. Reekers R, Beyer K, Niggemann B, Wahn U, Freihorst J, Kapp A, Werfel T. The role of circulating food antigen-specific lymphocytes in food allergic children with atopic dermatitis. Br J Dermatol 1996; 135:935–941.
126. Zeiger RS, Heller S, Mellon MH, Forsythe AB, O'Connor RD, Hamburger RN, Schatz M. Effect of combined maternal and infant food-allergen avoidance on development of atopy in early infancy: a randomized study [published erratum J Allergy Clin Immunol 1989 Nov; 84(5 pt 1):677]. J Allergy Clin Immunol 1989; 84:72–89.
127. Tupker RA, De Monchy JG, Coenraads PJ, Homan A, van der Meer JB. Induction of atopic dermatitis by inhalation of house dust mite. J Allergy Clin Immunol 1996; 97:1064–1070.
128. Tan BB, Weald D, Strickland I, Friedmann PS. Double-blind controlled trial of effect of housedust-mite allergen avoidance on atopic dermatitis. Lancet 1996; 347:15–18.
129. Ramb–Lindhauer C, Feldmann A, Rotte M, Neumann C. Characterization of grass pollen reactive T-cell lines derived from lesional atopic skin. Arch Dermatol Res 1991; 283:71–76.
130. van Reijsen FC, Bruijnzeel–Koomen CA, Kalthoff FS, Maggi E, Romagnani S, Westland JK, Mudde GC. Skin-derived aeroallergen-specific T-cell clones of Th2 phenotype in patients with atopic dermatitis. J Allergy Clin Immunol 1992; 90:184–193.
131. Darsow U, Vieluf D, Ring J. Evaluating the relevance of aeroallergen sensitization in atopic eczema with the atopy patch test: a randomized, double-blind multicenter study. Atopy Patch Test Study Group. J Am Acad Dermatol 1999; 40(2 pt 1):187–193.
132. Langeveld–Wildschut EG, van Marion AM, Thepen T, Mudde GC, Bruijnzeel PL, Bruijnzeel–Koomen CA. Evaluation of variables influencing the outcome of the atopy patch test. J Allergy Clin Immunol 1995; 96:66–73.
133. Szczepanski R, von Muhlendahl KE. Atopic dermatitis in a child due to cow dander [letter]. Lancet 1997; 350:114–115.
134. Darsow U, Behrendt H, Ring J. Gramineae pollen as trigger factors of atopic eczema: evaluation of diagnostic measures using the atopy patch test. Br J Dermatol 1997; 137:201–207.
135. Kolmer HL, Taketomi EA, Hazen KC, Hughs E, Wilson BB, Platts–Mills TA. Effect of

combined antibacterial and antifungal treatment in severe atopic dermatitis. J Allergy Clin Immunol 1996; 98:702–707.

136. Nordvall SL, Johansson S. IgE antibodies to *Pityrosporum orbiculare* in children with atopic diseases. Acta Paediatr Scand 1990; 79:343–348.

137. Jensen–Jarolim E, Poulsen LK, With H, Kieffer M, Ottevanger V, Stahl Skov P. Atopic dermatitis of the face, scalp, and neck: type I reaction to the yeast *Pityrosporum ovale*? J Allergy Clin Immunol 1992; 89(1 pt 1):44–51.

138. Wilson BB, Deuell B, Mills TA. Atopic dermatitis associated with dermatophyte infection and *Trichophyton* hypersensitivity. Cutis 1993; 51:191–192.

139. Tengvall Linder M, Johansson C, Bengtsson A, Holm L, Harfast B, Scheynius A. *Pityrosporum orbiculare*-reactive T-cell lines in atopic dermatitis patients and healthy individuals. Scand J Immunol 1998; 47:152–158.

140. Lever R, Hadley K, Downey D, Mackie R. Staphylococcal colonization in atopic dermatitis and the effect of topical mupirocin therapy. Br J Dermatol 1988; 119:189–198.

141. Leung DYM, Harbeck R, Bina P, Reiser RF, Yang E, Norris DA, Hanifin JM, Sampson HA. Presence of IgE antibodies to staphylococcal exotoxins on the skin of patients with atopic dermatitis. Evidence for a new group of allergens. J Clin Invest 1993; 92:1374–1380.

142. Bunikowski R, Mielke M, Skarabis H, Herz U, Bergmann RL, Wahn U, Renz H. Prevalence and role of serum IgE antibodies to the *Staphylococcus aureus*-derived superantigens SEA and SEB in children with atopic dermatitis. J Allergy Clin Immunol 1999; 103(1 pt 1):119–124.

143. Brosius CL, Newburger JW, Burns JC, Hojnowski–Diaz P, Zierler S, Leung DYM. Increased prevalence of atopic dermatitis in Kawasaki disease. Pediatr Infect Dis J 1988; 7:863–866.

144. Leung DYM, Meissner HC, Fulton DR, Murray DL, Kotzin BL, Schlievert PM. Toxic shock syndrome toxin-secreting *Staphylococcus aureus* in Kawasaki syndrome. Lancet 1993; 342: 1385–1388.

145. Michie CA, Davis T. Atopic dermatitis and staphylococcal superantigens [letter]. Lancet 1996; 347:324.

146. Strange P, Skov L, Lisby S, Nielsen PL, Baadsgaard O. Staphylococcal enterotoxin B applied on intact normal and intact atopic skin induces dermatitis. Arch Dermatol 1996;132:27–33.

147. Leung DYM, Gately M, Trumble A, Ferguson–Darnell B, Schlievert PM, Picker LJ. Bacterial superantigens induce T cell expression of the skin-selective homing receptor, the cutaneous lymphocyte-associated antigen, via stimulation of interleukin 12 production. J Exp Med 1995; 181:747–753.

148. Strickland I, Hauk PJ, Trumble AE, Picker LJ, Leung DYM. Evidence for superantigen involvement in skin homing of T cells in atopic dermatitis. J Invest Dermatol 1999; 112: 249–253.

149. Hofer MF, Harbeck RJ, Schlievert PM, Leung DYM. Staphylococcal toxins augment specific IgE responses by atopic patients exposed to allergen. J Invest Dermatol 1999; 112:171–176.

150. Ezepchuk YV, Leung DYM, Middleton MH, Bina P, Reiser R, Norris DA. Staphylococcal toxins and protein A differentially induce cytotoxicity and release of tumor necrosis factor-alpha from human keratinocytes. J Invest Dermatol 1996; 107:603–609.

151. Lucky AW, Leach AD, Laskarzewski P, Wenck H. Use of an emollient as a steroid-sparing agent in the treatment of mild to moderate atopic dermatitis in children. Pediatr Dermatol 1997; 14:321–324.

152. Nishioka K, Yasueda H, Saito H. Preventive effect of bedding encasement with microfine fibers on mite sensitization. J Allergy Clin Immunol 1998; 101(1 pt 1):28–32.

153. Cameron MM. Can house dust mite-triggered atopic dermatitis be alleviated using acaricides? Br J Dermatol 1997; 137:1–8.

154. Nilsson EJ, Henning CG, Magnusson J. Topical corticosteroids and *Staphylococcus aureus* in atopic dermatitis. J Am Acad Dermatol 1992; 27:29–34.

155. Stalder JF, Fleury M, Sourisse M, Rostin M, Pheline F, Litoux P. Local steroid therapy and bacterial skin flora in atopic dermatitis. Br J Dermatol 1994; 131:536–540.
156. Luber H, Amornsiripanitch S, Lucky AW. Mupirocin and the eradication of *Staphylococcus aureus* in atopic dermatitis. Arch Dermatol 1988; 124:853–854.
157. Berth–Jones J, Graham–Brown RA. Failure of terfenadine in relieving the pruritus of atopic dermatitis. Br J Dermatol 1989; 121:635–637.
158. La Rosa M, Ranno C, Musarra I, Guglielmo F, Corrias A, Bellanti JA. Double-blind study of cetirizine in atopic eczema in children. Ann Allergy 1994; 73:117–122.
159. Leung DYM, Hanifin JM, Charlesworth EN, Li JT, Bernstein IL, Berger WE, Blessing–Moore J, Fineman S, Lee FE, Nicklas RA, Spector SL. Disease management of atopic dermatitis: a practice parameter. Joint Task Force on Practice Parameters, representing the American Academy of Allergy, Asthma and Immunology, the American College of Allergy, Asthma and Immunology, and the Joint Council of Allergy, Asthma and Immunology. Work Group on Atopic Dermatitis. Ann Allergy Asthma Immunol 1997; 79:197–211.
160. George SA, Bilsland DJ, Johnson BE, Ferguson J. Narrow-band (TL-01) UVB air-conditioned phototherapy for chronic severe adult atopic dermatitis. Br J Dermatol 1993; 128:49–56.
161. Krutmann J, Czech W, Diepgen T, Niedner R, Kapp A, Schopf E. High-dose UVA1 therapy in the treatment of patients with atopic dermatitis. J Am Acad Dermatol 1992; 26(2 pt 1): 225–230.
162. Midelfart K, Stenvold SE, Volden G. Combined UVB and UVA phototherapy of atopic eczema. Dermatologica 1985; 171:95–98.
163. Jekler J, Larko O. Combined UVA–UVB versus UVB phototherapy for atopic dermatitis: a paired-comparison study. J Am Acad Dermatol 1990; 22:49–53.
164. Hanifin JM, Schneider LC, Leung DYM, et al. Recombinant interferon gamma therapy for atopic dermatitis. J Am Acad Dermatol 1993; 28(2 pt 1):189–197.
165. Boguniewicz M, Jaffe HS, Izu A, Sullivan MJ, York D, Geha RS, Leung DYM. Recombinant gamma interferon in treatment of patients with atopic dermatitis and elevated IgE levels. Am J Med 1990; 88:365–370.
166. Schneider LC, Baz Z, Zarcone C, Zurakowski D. Long-term therapy with recombinant interferon-gamma (rIFN-gamma) for atopic dermatitis. Ann Allergy Asthma Immunol 1998; 80: 263–268.
167. Stevens SR, Hanifin JM, Hamilton T, Tofte SJ, Cooper KD. Long-term effectiveness and safety of recombinant human interferon gamma therapy for atopic dermatitis despite unchanged serum IgE levels. Arch Dermatol 1998; 134:799–804.
168. Torrelo A, Harto A, Sendagorta E, Czarnetzki BM, Ledo A. Interferon-alpha therapy in atopic dermatitis. Acta Derm Venereol 1992; 72:370–372.
169. Paukkonen K, Fraki J, Horsmanheimo M. Interferon-alpha treatment decreases the number of blood eosinophils in patients with severe atopic dermatitis. Acta Derm Venereol 1993; 73:141–142.
170. Pung YH, Vetro SW, Bellanti JA. Use of interferons in atopic (IgE-mediated) diseases. Ann Allergy 1993; 71:234–238.
171. Kimata H. High-dose intravenous gamma-globulin treatment for hyperimmunoglobulinemia E syndrome. J Allergy Clin Immunol 1995; 95:771–774.
172. Burek–Kozlowska A, Morell A, Hunziker T. Topical immunoglobulin G in atopic dermatitis [letter]. Int Arch Allergy Immunol 1994; 104:104–106.
173. Takei S, Arora YK, Walker SM. Intravenous immunoglobulin contains specific antibodies inhibitory to activation of T cells by staphylococcal toxin superantigens [see comment]. J Clin Invest 1993; 91:602–607.
174. Jolles S, Hughes J, Rustin M. Intracellular interleukin-4 profiles during high-dose intravenous immunoglobulin treatment of therapy-resistant atopic dermatitis. J Am Acad Dermatol 1999; 40:121–123.

175. Ballow M. Mechanisms of action of intravenous immune serum globulin in autoimmune and inflammatory diseases. J Allergy Clin Immunol 1997; 100:151–157.
176. Hanifin JM, Chan SC, Cheng JB, Tofte SJ, Henderson WR Jr, Kirby DS, Weiner ES. Type 4 phosphodiesterase inhibitors have clinical and in vitro anti-inflammatory effects in atopic dermatitis. J Invest Dermatol 1996; 107:51–56.
177. Schreiber SL, Crabtree GR. The mechanism of action of cyclosporin A and FK506. Immunol Today 1992; 13:136–142.
178. Liu J, Farmer JD Jr, Lane WS, Friedman J, Weissman I, Schreiber SL. Calcineurin is a common target of cyclophilin–cyclosporin A and FKBP–FK506 complexes. Cell 1991; 66: 807–815.
179. van Joost T, Heule F, Korstanje M, van den Broek MJ, Stenveld HJ, van Vloten WA. Cyclosporin in atopic dermatitis: a multicentre placebo-controlled study. Br J Dermatol 1994; 130: 634–640.
180. Berth–Jones J, Graham–Brown RA, Marks R, Camp RD, English JS, Freeman K, Holden CA, Rogers SC, Oliwiecki S, Friedmann PS, Lewis–Jones MS, Archer CB, Adriaans B, Douglas WS, Allen BR. Long-term efficacy and safety of cyclosporin in severe adult atopic dermatitis. Br J Dermatol 1997; 136:76–81.
181. Campbell DE, Kemp AS. Cyclosporine restores cytokine imbalance in childhood atopic dermatitis. J Allergy Clin Immunol 1997; 99(6 pt 1):857–859.
182. de Prost Y, Bodemer C, Teillac D. Randomised double-blind placebo-controlled trial of local cyclosporin in atopic dermatitis. Acta Derm Venereol Suppl 1989; 144:136–138.
183. De Rie MA, Meinardi MM, Bos JD. Lack of efficacy of topical cyclosporin A in atopic dermatitis and allergic contact dermatitis. Acta Derm Venereol 1991; 71:452–454.
184. Bieber T. Topical tacrolimus (FK 506): a new milestone in the management of atopic dermatitis [editorial; comment]. J Allergy Clin Immunol 1998; 102(4 pt 1):555–557.
185. Boguniewicz M, Fiedler VC, Raimer S, Lawrence ID, Leung DYM, Hanifin JM. A randomized, vehicle-controlled trial of tacrolimus ointment for treatment of atopic dermatitis in children. Pediatric Tacrolimus Study Group. J Allergy Clin Immunol 1998; 102(4 pt 1):637–644.
186. Ruzicka T, Bieber T, Schopf E, Rubins A, Dobozy A, Bos JD, Jablonska S, Ahmed I, Thestrup–Pedersen K, Daniel F, Finzi A, Reitamo S. A short-term trial of tacrolimus ointment for atopic dermatitis. European Tacrolimus Multicenter Atopic Dermatitis Study Group. N Engl J Med 1997; 337:816–821.
187. Alaiti S, Kang S, Fiedler VC, Ellis CN, Spurlin DV, Fader D, Ulyanov G, Gadgil SD, Tanase A, Lawrence I, Scotellaro P, Raye K, Bekersky I. Tacrolimus (FK506) ointment for atopic dermatitis: a phase I study in adults and children. J Am Acad Dermatol 1998; 38:69–76.
188. Homey B, Assmann T, Vohr HW, Ulrich P, Lauerma AI, Ruzicka T, Lehmann P, Schuppe HC. Topical FK506 suppresses cytokine and costimulatory molecule expression in epidermal and local draining lymph node cells during primary skin immune responses. J Immunol 1998; 160:5331–5340.
189. Anderson J, Nagy S, Groth CG, Andersson U. Effects of FK506 and cyclosporin A on cytokine production studied in vitro at a single-cell level. Immunology 1992; 75:136–142.
190. Mrowietz U, Graeber M, Brautigam M, Thurston M, Wagenaar A, Weidinger G, Christophers E. The novel ascomycin derivative SDZ ASM 981 is effective for psoriasis when used topically under occlusion. Br J Dermatol 1998; 139:992–996.
191. Van Leent EJ, Graber M, Thurston M, Wagenaar A, Spuls PI, Bos JD. Effectiveness of the ascomycin macrolactam SDZ ASM 981 in the topical treatment of atopic dermatitis. Arch Dermatol 1998; 134:805–809.

17

Urticaria

MALCOLM WATSON GREAVES

University of London and St. John's Institute of Dermatology, St. Thomas Hospital, London, England

1 INTRODUCTION

This chapter outlines the current state of knowledge of the pathophysiology, immunopathology, and molecular basis of the urticarias. Some recent advances have had significant implications for diagnosis and therapy. These will be alluded to, but only briefly, as the remit of this book is chiefly on mechanisms, rather than management.

2 WHAT ARE THE URTICARIAS? DEFINITIONS

Urticaria describes an eruption of the skin or, very rarely, the mucous membranes. Individual lesions consist of weals: raised soft or firm lesions that range in size from a few millimeters to several centimeters. Adjacent weals have a habit of becoming confluent to form large raised red plaques. Weals may be circular (usually the smaller ones, as in cholinergic urticaria, see later discussion), or irregular, with pseudopodia (especially in acute urticaria), serpiginous, or annular. Urticarial weals classically have a pale skin-colored center owing to dermal edema causing compression-blanching of dermal postcapillary venules. The outer zone of the weal itself and the surrounding skin is usually red, the hue varying from bright red—principally in physical urticaria, such as symptomatic dermographism or cold urticaria—or dull red in chronic idiopathic urticaria. Occasionally, particularly in acute urticarial eruptions, urticarial weals may be surrounded by a white ''halo'' owing to shunting of blood through dilated arterioles in the outer portion of the weal. In true urticaria weals fade without marking the skin, apart from bruising caused by vigorous rubbing.

By definition the duration of individual weals of urticaria should be less than 24 h. In most physical urticarias individual weals last no longer than 1 hr, but in chronic idiopathic urticaria individual weals may be of up to 18-hr duration. ''Weals'' lasting longer than 24 hr raise the possibility of other causes, including urticarial vasculitis.

Itching is an almost invariable accompaniment of urticaria, although some patients complain of pain, tenderness, and stinging, rather than itching. Itching tends to be worse in the evening and at night (1). Itching leads to rubbing rather than scratching. The presence of excoriations in a patient alleged to be suffering from urticaria should raise the suspicion of an alternative or additional diagnosis.

Angioedema may accompany most forms of urticaria, including acute urticaria, where it is common, and most physical urticarias. In chronic idiopathic urticaria it occurs in 50% of cases (2). *Angioedema* is defined as the occurrence of red-or skin-colored subcutaneous or submucosal swellings caused by acute local edema. Unless very large, swellings normally last less than 24 hr. Itching is variable and angioedema of the hands or feet may be painful. In the oropharynx, respiratory obstruction can occur.

A classification of the more common forms of urticaria is listed in Table 1.

2.1 Acute Urticaria

Acute urticaria is usually arbitrarily defined as a bout of urticaria lasting less than 6 weeks. Associated angioedema is common, and itching is often severe. Systemic symptoms are common and include dyspnea, abdominal pain, and diarrhea, vomiting, faintness, and even shock in occasional patients. Attacks may be repeated (intermittent acute urticaria) over months or years.

ETIOLOGY. Classically acute urticaria is caused by an immediate hypersensitivity reaction between skin mast cell-bound IgE and specific antigen (type I allergy, Gell and Coombs classification). In such cases the offending allergen (a drug such as penicillin; an immunizing vaccine, such as antitetanus serum; a food item, such as shellfish, latex in certain fruits, peanuts, and other nuts; or insect venom) is readily identifiable by patient and family physician alike, and a specialist opinion may be sought to confirm the culprit agent by serological or (with great caution) skin-prick testing.

Besides antigen–IgE antibody reactions, other etiological factors may be important. Aspirin causes acute urticaria and angioedema by a nonimmunological mechanism, probably involving cyclooxygenase inhibition, leading idiosyncratically to redirection of arachi-

Table 1 Classification of the Urticarias

Acute
Chronic
Physical urticarias
Symptomatic dermographism
Cold urticaria
Aquagenic urticaria
Solar urticaria
Cholinergic urticaria
Aquagenic pruritus
Vibratory angioedema
Chronic ''idiopathic'' urticaria
Urticarial vasculitis

donic acid transformation through lipoxygenase pathways and formation of vasoactive leukotrienes and other lipoxygenase products.

Recent data implicates acute virus infections as a cause. Aoki et al. (3) identified a virus infection as a cause in 50 patients with urticaria of duration less than 1 week. Of these, 31 had a recent history of a respiratory or gastrointestinal infection. Viruses identified in these patients included cytomegalovirus, Coxsackie, and hepatitis B. Zuberbier (4) found no evidence of food allergy in over 100 patients with acute urticaria, although 40% had a recent history of a respiratory infection.

My own experience (unpublished) suggests that, in a hospital referral population, one or more food items can be implicated in about 40% of patients with acute urticaria. According to Zuberbier, there is no increased frequency of atopy among acute urticaria patients. How many patients with acute urticaria, especially of the intermittent variety, eventually develop chronic urticaria is unclear and needs investigating.

PATHOPHYSIOLOGY. Acute urticaria is due to release of histamine and other vasoactive mediators from skin mast cells. In acute urticaria from an allergic cause, specific antigen binds to, and cross-links membrane-bound IgE on these cells, triggering degranulation and secretion of mediators. The red flare surrounding the weals is due to the action of histamine on unmyelinated sensory ''C'' fibers leading to antidromic depolarization and release of substance P and possibly other vasodilator neuropeptides. The itch is primarily due to histamine. However, vasodilation and wealing are probably also caused by leukotrienes, prostaglandin D_2 (PG D_2), cytokines, and chemokines, including granulocyte–macrophage colony-stimulating factor (GM-CSF), interleukin (IL)-1, IL-4, IL-5, and tumor necrosis factor (TNF)-α. The cytokines also lead to local adhesion molecule expression, with consequent accumulation of activated neutrophil and eosinophil granulocytes and macrophages in lesional skin. Itching, however, is probably exclusively due to histamine acting on histamine-H_1 receptors associated with unmyelinated nociceptor C fibers (5). Rubbing relieves the itch temporarily owing to ''surround inhibition'' (6) as a result of activation of thickly myelinated A fibers that down-regulate itch through recruitment of inhibitory neuronal circuits in the substantia gelatinosa in the dorsal horns of the spinal cord gray matter.

The principal cellular and molecular participants of wealing and itching in acute and chronic urticaria are illustrated in Figure 1.

2.2 Physical Urticarias

As a group, these are characterized by positive provocation of wealing and itching caused by application of a local physical stimulus to the skin. Cholinergic urticaria, although etiologically distinct, is included under the same heading for traditional and pragmatic reasons. The most important physical urticarias are listed in Table 1. Characteristically, redness, wealing, and itching occur within seconds or 1–2 min of application of the appropriate physical stimulus to the skin. With the exception of delayed pressure urticaria, the wealing and itching of physical urticarias runs a brief time course, normally of no more than 1–2 hr before fading. After resolution, the challenged skin is usually refractory for several hours to repeated challenge at the same site, and this finding has led to utilization of tolerance treatment (''desensitization'') in cold urticaria and solar urticaria. It is common to find patients suffering from more than one physical urticaria concurrently. Common ''partners'' include cold urticaria and cholinergic urticaria, solar urticaria and heat urticaria, and dermographism and delayed pressure urticaria. Confirmation of the

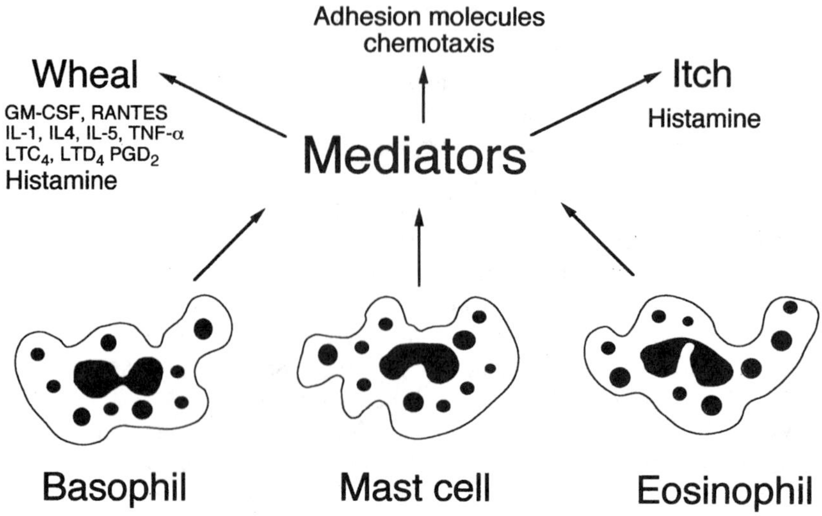

Figure 1 Mediators of urticarial wheal and itch that are derived from mast cells, basophil leukocytes, and eosinophils.

diagnosis of the urticarias depends on appropriate challenge testing, and guidelines have been published (7). Confirmation that a physical urticaria represents the patient's principal or sole problem is important for at least two reasons. First, it obviates the necessity for unnecessary laboratory investigations, allergy tests, food exclusion diets, and such, and second, it enables focused advice to be proffered on management, especially relative to occupation.

2.2.1 Symptomatic Dermographism (Syn. Factitious Urticaria)

If a blunt-pointed instrument is drawn firmly across a healthy person's skin, a transitory red line occurs, with or without mild to moderate edema. There is no itch. This physiological response, called simple dermographism, differs from symptomatic dermographism in two important aspects: a firm pressure is required to elicit the response, and there is no itching. In symptomatic dermographism even a light pressure drawn across the skin causes, within 5 min, linear redness, wealing, and itching. This reaction is best demonstrated using a spring-loaded dermographometer (8).

Although any area of skin can be affected, the mucous membranes are usually not involved. Symptomatic dermographism commonly affects young adults, although it can occur at any age. It usually runs a course of 1–2 years before clearing up spontaneously. It may occasionally present as a sequel of other pruritic disorders, including papular urticaria and scabies. Symptomatic dermographism is not associated with systemic disease.

ETIOLOGY. The etiology is unknown. Passive transfer of symptomatic dermographism has successfully been carried out using serum from affected individuals and nonhuman primates as recipients (9). This indicates the involvement of a circulating factor, although this has yet to be characterized.

PATHOPHYSIOLOGY. Skin perfusion studies (10) have demonstrated local release of histamine into the tissues of wealing skin of patients with symptomatic dermographism (10). However, the cutaneous mast cell population density is within normal limits in these patients (11,12). The brief time course of the wealing and itching (duration 30–60 min) suggests that histamine is the main mediator, and this is supported by the generally favorable symptomatic response to combined H_1 and H_2 antihistamines (8). Most, if not all, of the histamine in human skin is contained in the mast cells. The temporarily refractory state of the skin following evoked wealing is presumably due to depletion of mast cell stores of histamine.

2.2.2 Delayed Pressure Urticaria

Symptomatic dermographism and delayed pressure urticaria are frequently confused clinically. Symptomatic dermographism represents an immediate short-lived weal-and-flare response to local stroking of the skin. Delayed pressure urticaria presents as a red, swollen and indurated response occurring 2–6 hr after application of pressure perpendicular to the surface of the skin. Pain and tenderness may be more prominent than itch, especially at sites such as the palms and soles. The inflammatory response to pressure is not only delayed, but it is also prolonged, lasting 24 hr or more. It is often associated with arthralgia. Thirty-eight percent of patients with chronic idiopathic urticaria also have delayed pressure urticaria, and it is doubtful if this physical urticaria ever occurs alone (13). Systemic flu-like symptoms may accompany severe delayed pressure urticaria.

ETIOLOGY. The etiology is unknown, although histologically, this physical urticaria resembles a late-phase reaction (14).

PATHOPHYSIOLOGY. Strictly speaking, delayed pressure urticaria is not a true urticaria because the pressure-evoked swellings last longer than 24 hr. Histologically (14,15), there are large numbers of dermal eosinophils showing degranulation, together with eosinophilic granular material distributed extracellularly. There are also increased numbers of CD_4^+ dermal T lymphocytes. The population density of dermal mast cells is not increased, but there is marked up-regulation of the adhesion molecule E-selectin.

It is likely that mast cell degranulation in pressure-challenged skin is an early event followed by release of proinflammatory cytokines, including IL-1, IL-6, and possibly TNF-α (16). This leads to increased expression of adhesion molecules (E-selectin, V-CAM-1) on the microvasculature and consequently a dense inflammatory infiltrate containing lymphocytes and granulocytes, together with abundant eosinophil granule protein. There is no evidence of blood vessel damage or leukocytoclasia, which enables distinction from the superficially similar urticarial vasculitis. Our studies of tissue fluid from involved skin in delayed pressure urticaria did not show evidence of increased arachidonic acid transformation products (leukotrienes, other hydroxyeicosatetraenoic acids or prostaglandins) (17). No clues to pathogenesis emerge from observations on different drug treatments; apart from large doses of systemic corticosteroids, no drug treatments are consistently effective in this physical urticaria.

2.2.3 Cold Urticaria

Although rare, cold urticaria is one of the most intensively studied physical urticarias. The subtypes of cold urticaria are shown in Table 2. Familial cold urticaria is a rare, autosomal dominantly inherited form. Individual weals are frequently prolonged beyond 24 hr, systemic symptoms are common and, in a family I studied (18), a skin biopsy

Table 2 Cold Urticaria Subtypes

Cause	Ref.
Familial cold urticaria	18
Cold reflex urticaria	19
HIV-related cold urticaria	20
Cold-induced cholinergic urticaria	21
Delayed cold urticaria	22
Cold-dependent dermographism	23
Localized cold urticaria	24
Acquired secondary cold urticaria	(see text)
Acquired primary cold urticaria	(see text)

showed a heavy perivascular infiltrate, but no vasculitis (18). Of the remaining subtypes of cold urticaria (Table 2) only primary and secondary acquired cold urticaria will be considered in more detail here.

Primary Acquired Cold Urticaria (Essential Cold Urticaria)

Local redness, wealing, and itching occur within seconds or 1–2 min after exposure of skin to cold, which may be solid or fluid (cold air or water). The response lasts up to 1 hr and fades without leaving a mark in the skin. If exposure is widespread, systemic symptoms may ensue. Mucous membranes, including the mouth, throat, and tongue, may swell after a cold drink.

ETIOLOGY. A history of a streptococcal, mycoplasmal, or virus (e.g., Epstein–Barr or cytomegalovirus) infections (25,26) is frequent. The incidence of atopy is generally comparable with control groups (26). Passive transfer by a serum factor can be demonstrated in some patients (27–29). Arbesman et al. characterized the serum factor as having features similar to IgE (27), but a later study indicated that the immunoglobulin involved was IgM (28). Passive transfer of cold urticaria has also been demonstrated in nonhuman primate skin (29). Heterozygous deficiency of α_1-antichymotrypsin has been demonstrated in some patients (30).

PATHOPHYSIOLOGY. The histopathological appearances of biopsies of lesional skin of cold urticaria are generally unremarkable (31). The mast cell population density is within normal limits, but degranulation is usually seen. Infiltration of the dermis by inflammatory cells is minimal. Direct immunofluorescent examination was negative. Although no evidence of vasculitis is normally detectable, repeated cold challenge at the same site in five of eight patients caused vasculitic changes in the absence of circulating immunoreactants (32).

Routine examination of serum for circulating immunoreactants is, by definition, negative in primary acquired cold urticaria, although, as just discussed, passive transfer by serum may be demonstrable.

There have been several attempts to identify molecular mediators of weal and itch in cold urticaria (Table 3). Clearly, histamine, released from tissue mast cells, plays a role (33,34) and is the basis for cold tolerance treatment of cold urticaria (35). However, histamine is not the only important mediator involved. Others identified include prostaglandin D_2 (PGD_2) (36), platelet factor 4 (37), leukotriene-E_4 (LTE_4) (38), and tumor necrosis factor-α (TNF-α) (39). This probably explains the poor association between histamine

Table 3 Acquired Primary Cold Urticaria: Identified Pharmacologic Mediators

Mediator	Ref.
Histamine	34, 35, 40
Prostaglandin D_2 (PGD_2)	36, 42
Leukotriene E_4 (LTE_4)	38
Platelet factor 4	37
Eosinophil chemotactic factor of anaphylaxis (ECF-A)	33
Tumor necrosis factor-alpha (TNF-α)	39

release and wealing reported by earlier studies (34). In most of these, histamine and other mediators were recovered from the venous effluent draining a cold-immersed upper limb (34).

The molecular events linking cooling of the skin with mast cell activation are unclear, but probably involve cold-induced conformational change in either mast cell-bound IgE or the external (α-chain) portion of the high-affinity IgE receptor (FcεRI). Alternatively, in vitro experiments carried out by Kaplan (40) have raised the possibility of a cold-sensitive autoimmune mechanism, possibly involving anti-IgE autoantibodies (41).

Secondary Acquired Cold Urticaria

Secondary cold urticaria is diagnosed if a patient with cold urticaria is demonstrated to possess circulating cold-precipitating immunoreactants (cryoglobulinemia). Secondary acquired cold urticaria is much less common than the primary acquired type. A review of the literature indicates that no more than 5–10% of all acquired cold urticaria patients can be demonstrated to have circulating cold-precipitating immunoreactants (25,26).

ETIOLOGY. Underlying cryoglobulinemia can be primary (essential) or secondary. In the latter cases the cryoglobulinemia is associated with lymphoreticular malignancy (chronic lymphocytic leukemia, myelomatosis, angioimmunoblastic lymphadenopathy) or a preceding virus infection, including hepatitis B or C, glandular fever, and a range of respiratory infections especially with *Mycoplasma pneumoniae*. Allergic drug reactions are also reported to cause secondary acquired cold urticaria. This topic has been reviewed (43).

PATHOPHYSIOLOGY. In keeping with the clinical findings (cold-induced weals with a prolonged time course of 24 hr or more, often associated with purpura) a skin biopsy will reveal histological evidence of leukocytoclastic vasculitis and presence of immunoreactants deposited perivascularly on direct immunofluorescence. Systemic symptoms are common, including arthritis, Raynaud's phenomenon, and ischemic digital ulceration. Cryoglobulins may be mixed, especially in postinfection secondary acquired cold urticaria, or monoclonal, involving IgG or IgM isotypes. That these cryoglobulins play a key role in the pathogenesis of the cold-induced lesions is indicated by successful passive transfer (44). Complement activation is involved in the pathogenesis of cold-evoked lesions (44). Because mast cell degranulation can be demonstrated in lesional skin (45), mast cell-activating complement components (C5a, C3a) may be involved. Alternatively, cryoglobulins could represent IgG anti-IgE autoantibodies, which could bind to, and cross-link, mast cell receptor-bound IgE.

Other cold precipitating proteins that have been proposed to be involved include cryofibrinogens and cold agglutinins (46,47). Secondary acquired cold urticaria is well recognized to be associated with a positive syphilis serology. In these cases, a cold hemolysin is frequently involved (48).

2.2.4 Cholinergic Urticaria

Cholinergic urticaria is a common physical urticaria with a prevalence of at least 10% in the population. It has previously been comprehensively reviewed (49–51). It is common in atopic patients and in most cases is no more than a minor nuisance. Presenting as itchy papules, which may show confluence into larger weals, this urticaria is invariably associated with eccrine sweat-provoking stimuli (exercise, a hot environment, stress, or spicy or temperature-hot food or drink) and usually subsides when the patient ''cools off.'' Systemic symptoms (flushing, wheezing, and headache) are common in severely affected patients. Several rarer clinical variants have been described (Table 4). These include exercise-induced angioedema (52), persistent cholinergic erythema (53), and food- and exercise-induced cholinergic urticaria (54). The relation between exercise-induced anaphylaxis and cholinergic urticaria is more controversial, but I believe that most, if not all, of these patients have concurrent or preceding cholinergic urticaria. Cholinergic urticaria can also occur without a visible rash. These cases present with exercise, heat, or emotion-provoked pruritus (55).

ETIOLOGY. That the eruption is closely associated with stimuli (heat, exercise, emotion) that provoke eccrine sweating is widely recognized. However, production of sweat itself is probably not necessary (56). A recent report of ''sweat allergy'' in cholinergic urticaria has not been independently confirmed (57). That a serum factor is involved in the pathogenesis of cholinergic urticaria is suggested by successful passive transfer by serum to the skin of nonhuman primates in some cases (58). Patients with cholinergic urticaria have significantly lowered serum levels of a range of serine protease inhibitors (59). That this finding is of pathogenetic significance is suggested by the success of therapy by anabolic steroids (60).

PATHOPHYSIOLOGY. The pathophysiology remains to be fully elucidated. Eccrine sweat glands are activated by cholinergic sympathetic autonomic nerve pathways. That acetylcholine, released from these nerve endings, plays a role is indicated by the ability of full atropinization of the skin to suppress this urticarial response (51,61). This can be achieved readily by placing a 6% aqueous scopolamine (hyoscine) solution on the skin. Histamine release from skin has also been convincingly demonstrated (62,63), thus implicating activation of skin mast cells in the process and explaining the beneficial effect of antihistamine therapy. However, the events linking activation of cholinergic sympathe-

Table 4 Cholinergic Urticaria: Classification

Subtype	Ref.
Classic	49
With angioedema	52
Persistent cholinergic erythema	53
Food- and exercise-provoked	54
Pruritus sine urticaria	55
Exercise-induced anaphylaxis	63

tic innervation of the skin with mast cell activation are unclear. Acetylcholine is not a histamine-releasing agent, at least in humans, although it tends to produce an augmented response on intradermal injection in patients with cholinergic urticaria (61). Possibly, proteases and vasoactive peptides are involved, given the reduced plasma levels of protease inhibitors and the beneficial effects of anabolic steroids, which correct these depleted proteins (59,60). Histological examination of skin biopsy material reveals vasodilation dermal edema and mast cell degranulation, but little else (49).

2.2.5 Solar Urticaria

Solar urticaria is frequently, but usually wrongly, diagnosed in acutely sun-sensitive individuals. Most of these turn out to have an entirely different form of sun sensitivity—polymorphous light eruption. The high speed of reaction and short duration of the skin response to sun (or artificial ultraviolet) exposure (redness, wealing, and itching in sun-exposed skin) enables confirmation of the diagnosis of solar urticaria.

In children, the inborn error of metabolism, erythropoietic protoporphyria, may bring about essentially similar symptoms, although, unlike true solar urticaria, affected children usually show linear or vermiculiform facial scarring. Systemic symptoms are rare, but may occur.

ETIOLOGY. It is proposed that irradiation of the skin in susceptible patients causes a photoallergen to be produced. It has been demonstrated that intradermal injection of irradiated serum from solar urticaria patients induced wealing in exposed, but not tolerant skin of the same patients (64). They postulated that this photoallergen occupies binding sites on IgE fixed to cutaneous mast cells.

PATHOPHYSIOLOGY. Patients with solar urticaria have an action spectrum ranging from UVB (290–310 nm) through to the visible (above 400 nm) range. Examination of venous blood effluent from forearm skin irradiated with the appropriate wavelengths of UV has confirmed release of histamine, associated with mast cell degranulation (65). The good response of the itching to H_1 antihistamines in solar urticaria provides further indirect evidence of the involvement of histamine, as does the relief offered by tolerance treatment, in which repeated exposure to the appropriate wavelengths leads to depletion of histamine in the treated skin and consequent diminished reactivity to sunlight. (66).

2.2.6 Heat Urticaria

This very rare physical urticaria is a close relative of solar urticaria. Some patients with solar urticaria whose skin is sensitive to the visible wavelengths of the solar emission spectrum also respond to the adjacent infrared wavelengths and vice versa.

ETIOLOGY AND PATHOGENESIS. Contact of the skin with a warm surface or fluid causes immediate, short-lived wealing and itching. We have investigated two patients in some detail (67,68). The threshold temperature to induce wealing was 43°C in each patient (optimum 49°C), when applied for 3 min. We were unable to passively transfer heat reactivity to nonhuman primates using patients' sera. Both skin perfusion experiments and analysis of venous effluent from heat-challenge forearm skin yielded significant release of histamine and PGD_2. Histological study of skin biopsy material showed mast cell degranulation.

Other investigations have demonstrated evidence of complement activation (69). There is also a rare familial form (70) in which onset of wealing following application of heat was delayed for 2 hr. The molecular events linking heating the skin with wealing and itching are essentially unknown.

2.2.7 Aquagenic Urticaria

This is also a rare physical urticaria in which contact with water (seawater, freshwater, rain, tears, and such) causes immediate wealing and itching. All patients I have seen have been older children or young adults. Recently, it has been described in an human immunodeficiency virus (HIV)-positive patient (71).

ETIOLOGY AND PATHOGENESIS. We have previously reviewed this physical urticaria and carried out detailed observations on two patients (72). Morphologically, individual water-induced weals closely resemble those of cholinergic urticaria, and the associated pruritus is equally intense in both physical urticarias. Furthermore, development of weals in water-challenged skin can be blocked by local atropinization using topical application of 6% scopolamine aqueous solution, suggesting the involvement of acetylcholine. Both conditions are associated with elevated plasma levels of histamine during outbreaks of the physical urticaria, and in each the pruritus responds to some extent to H_1 antihistamine therapy.

How wetting the skin provokes wealing in these patients is unclear. Prior application of Vaseline to water-challenged skin prevents wealing, as does removal of the stratum corneum barrier by Scotch tape stripping, suggesting the involvement of a water-soluble stratum corneum factor. This conclusion is strengthened by the augmenting effects of application of organic solvents on water-induced wealing (72).

2.2.8 Aquagenic Pruritus

Although not strictly speaking an urticaria (there are no visible clinical signs in the skin), aquagenic pruritus needs to be mentioned here to avoid confusion. It is fairly common, but frequently misdiagnosed. It is unrelated to aquagenic urticaria or any other physical urticaria. Aquagenic pruritus, although briefly described earlier by WB Shelley, was first characterized in 1971 (73). Typically patients, usually middled-aged or elderly, suffer intense pruritus without visible signs following contact of skin with water at any temperature. Although underlying hematological disorders, especially polycythemia vera, have been identified in some patients (74), in most it is unassociated with systemic disease. Detailed investigations have confirmed the involvement of mast cell degranulation, histamine release, and increased fibrinolytic activity in this condition (73,75), which has been the subject of several recent reviews (76–79). As with aquagenic urticaria, the detailed pathophysiology is unclear.

2.2.9 Vibratory Angioedema

Vibratory angioedema is an exceptionally rare physical urticaria (I have seen only two cases) in which a vibratory stimulus (gripping the handle of a lawnmower, for example) causes local pruritus and angioedema. Other cases in the literature have had a family history (80,81).

Two reported families showed autosomal dominant inheritance (80,81). The complement C_1 esterase inhibitor level was normal. Our own case (82) had no family history, and no abnormal laboratory findings. Examination of skin biopsy material showed normal mast cell numbers, but plasma histamine levels have been reported to be elevated (83). Response to H_1-antihistamine treatment was satisfactory in our case.

2.3 Chronic Urticaria

2.3.1 Chronic Idiopathic Urticaria

Chronic ''idiopathic'' urticaria (CIU) is arbitrarily, but almost universally, defined as daily or almost daily outbreaks of urticaria for at least 6 weeks. Intermittent CIU, in which periodic prolonged remissions occur, falls under the heading of CIU, for the purposes of this discussion. CIU is accompanied by angioedema in 38–87% and delayed pressure urticaria in 50% of patients with CIU (13,84). Care must be taken to exclude urticarial vasculitis (see later) and physical urticarias (discussed earlier) before concluding that the patient's only, or main, problem is CIU. CIU affects at least 0.1% of the population and 20% of patients are still troubled by the disease after 10 years (2). Apart from the duration of the disease, the clinical features are essentially those of acute urticaria and angioedema. There is no significant association with atopy (2). The pathophysiology of angioedema and urticaria in patients with CIU is assumed to be essentially the same.

ETIOLOGY. The cutaneous mast cell is the culprit cell in CIU and its associated angioedema, although the blood-derived basophil leukocyte may also play a role (85). The problem of why this cell undergoes promiscuous activation, leading to release of histamine and other mediators (see Fig. 1) has vexed numerous investigators over many years. That the results of research up to now have been inconclusive is witnessed by the wide acceptance of the adjective *idiopathic* to describe this condition. Putative causes have included a variety of chronic infections. None of these have stood the test of time as significant etiological factors. Most recently chronic infection by *Helicobacter pylori* has been proposed by several authors, but has not been confirmed by recent controlled studies (86), and this has also been my own experience (87). Parasite infestation has never been confirmed as an underlying cause in any patient I have seen. But in regions where parasite load is high, infestation could be an important cause. This issue needs further critical study.

Most patients with CIU have been told by friends, relatives, or medical carers that their urticaria must be due to "food allergy." This can rarely be substantiated. True (type I) allergy to food items (shellfish, dairy products, nuts, fruits, or others) is nearly always well recognized by the patient and family members and presents as bouts of acute urticaria. Idiosyncratic reactions to food additives (preservatives, dyes, antioxidants, and such) does occur. However, in my experience they amount to no more than 5% of the total (88) if rigorous diagnostic criteria are used. The gold standard should be placebo-controlled challenge testing on a double-blind basis (89,90). Aspirin does exacerbate CIU nonspecifically (91), as do intercurrent virus infections. Until recently, the etiology of CIU in at least 90% of cases was either totally unknown or, at best, speculative. It has now been established, initially by my own laboratory, and subsequently by several other groups, that at least 30–45% of all chronic "idiopathic" urticaria patients have an autoimmune basis. Several earlier observations pointed toward the possible etiological role of a circulating factor in CIU. As early as 1962 Rorsman reported that some CIU patients had a lowered peripheral blood basophil count (92). That a circulating factor might also be "desensitizing" peripheral basophils was also subsequently reported by this author in 1974 (93) and subsequently confirmed (85). However, interpretation of this finding in terms of an action on basophil- (and mast cell)-bound IgE or on the receptor itself was not considered explicitly in the earlier reports.

Further indirect evidence derived from previous findings of increased frequency of organ-specific autoantibodies in CIU. Despite earlier reports (94), we have been unable to detect an increased prevalence of clinical thyroid disease in CIU (84). However, we have demonstrated increased frequency of associated autoimmune disease overall (thyroid disease, vitiligo, pernicious anemia, insulin-dependent diabetes) in autoimmune urticaria (84). We also found an increased prevalence of thyroid autoantibodies in the autoimmune chronic urticaria groups (95).

Patients with CIU do not show an increased frequency of a family history of urticaria. However, HLA class II typing showed an increased frequency of HLA-DRB1* 04 (DR4) and the associated allele HLA-DQ8 (DQB1* 0302) in CIU, in keeping with an autoimmune basis in some CIU patients (96).

Serum IgE levels are not elevated above values in control patients. Circulating non-immunoglobulin histamine-releasing factors may be important in certain patients, including cytokines and a mast cell-specific histamine-releasing factor (97–99).

That a circulating factor might be causative in CIU patients was also suggested by the demonstration of a weal-producing factor in the serum of some patients with CIU during periods of active disease (100). Further characterization of this factor proved it to be due to an IgG with a specificity for the α-chain of the high-affinity IgE receptor (FcεRIα) expressed on skin mast cells or basophil leukocytes or, less commonly, for mast cell or basophil-bound IgE itself (101,102). These antibodies were functional because they caused wealing in human skin after autologous intradermal injection, and released histamine from dermal mast cells and blood basophils of healthy donors. Confirmed independently by several other investigators, these autoantibodies were found in 30–45% of CIU patients (103–105). Their ability to cause local wealing and itching after autologous intradermal injection is the basis of the autologous serum intradermal screening test for autoimmune chronic urticaria (106). The frequency of these autoantibodies among geographically different populations of CIU patients is outlined in Table 5.

That these autoantibodies are causative in CIU in based on their functional characterization, the correlation between serum titer and disease activity in individual patients, and the induction of remission of urticaria in patients in whom the antibodies were suppressed or removed by intravenous immunoglobulin infusion (IVIG) or plasmapheresis (107,108).

Establishment of functional anti-FcεRIα and, less often, anti-IgE autoantibodies as causative factors in a subset of 30–45% of CIU patients is clearly an important step forward. However, the cause of CIU in the remaining 55–70% still has to be established. A few may be attributable to recently described cytokine-like factors alluded in the foregoing (97–99). However, it is my (unconfirmed) belief that most of these cases are actually autoimmune. The in vitro tests used Western blotting or donor basophil histamine release assays, which although acceptably specific, lack optimum sensitivity. Circumstantial evidence supporting this view derives from the finding of a positive autologous serum test (suggesting the presence of a circulating histamine-releasing factor) in some of these cases; the similarities between clinical presentation and skin histology with autoimmune chronic urticaria; and the lowered blood basophil counts, in ostensibly nonautoimmune as well as autoimmune patients (84,85,106). The etiology and pathophysiology of CIU has recently been reviewed by the author (109).

Table 5 Frequency of Functional Anti-FcεRI Autoantibodies in CIU in Recently Published Reports

Authors	Frequency (%)	Ref.
Hide et al.	30	101
Niimi et al.	30	102
Fiebiger et al.	33	103
Zweiman et al.	38	104
Tong et al.	45	105

PATHOPHYSIOLOGY. Histologically mast cell numbers are not increased in the skin in CIU, but there is evidence of mast cell degranulation. A perivascular leukocytic infiltrate is characteristic, with a predominance of $CD4^+$ over $CD8^+$ T cells. However, there is no evidence of T-cell activation (109). Other important variable histological features include eosinophils and eosinophil granule protein (110,111) and envelopment of postcapillary venules by neutrophils ("neutrophilic urticaria") without evidence of endothelial cell damage (112).

That histamine is a major mediator in CIU, especially of itching, is suggested by the favorable response to H_1-antihistamine treatment and is further supported by direct examination of tissue fluid histamine levels in involved skin (113). However, other mediators, some of which may be mast cell-derived, as illustrated in Figure 1, may also be involved, leading to adhesion molecule expression and further recruitment of inflammatory cells. Our recent studies have demonstrated moderate up-regulation of E-selectin and VCAM-1 concurrently with development of a leukocytic infiltrate (114). It is of interest that the uninvolved skin of patients with CIU shows an augmented weal-and-flare response to intradermal injection of histamine and other mediators, although this is probably a nonspecific phenomenon (115).

2.3.2 Autoimmune Chronic Urticaria

Investigation of the IgG immunoreactants in autoimmune chronic urticaria has revealed that they are predominantly of the IgG1 and IgG3 subtypes (116). No serum complement abnormalities have been demonstrated in autoimmune chronic urticaria, although complement activation may be involved in the activation of dermal mast cells by anti-FcεRI autoantibodies. The serum IgE tends to be on the low side (84). In those patients possessing anti-FcεRIα histamine-releasing autoantibodies, one-fourth these antibodies are competitive with IgE (i.e., compete with IgE for the IgE-binding site on FcεRIα), and in the remaining three-fourths, the autoantibodies are noncompetitive with IgE and, therefore, bind to a non–IgE-binding portion of the α-chain (102). However, 5% of all patients with CIU have functional autoantibodies against IgE itself (101,102). Epitope mapping has not yet been carried out.

The specificity of autoantibodies in chronic urticaria has been the subject of several studies. No evidence of anti-FcεRIα autoantibodies has been detected in healthy individuals, patients with physical urticarias, atopic eczema, asthma, or urticarial vasculitis. However, by using Western blotting, Fiebiger et al. (116) have demonstrated immunoreactive anti-FcεRIα autoantibodies in a few patients with dermatomyositis and pemphigus vulgaris. However, these antibodies, which were of the IgG isotype, were predominantly of the IgG2 and IgG4 subclasses and, furthermore, they were non–histamine-releasing and, therefore, quite distinct from the consistently histamine-releasing anti-FcεRIα autoantibodies found in chronic urticaria. As immunodetection methodology becomes more sensitive, it is likely that immunoreactive nonfunctional antibodies of these subtypes will be found in other clinical situations.

Autoimmune urticaria cannot be distinguished clinically, histologically, or immunopathologically from nonautoimmune CIU (84). Autoimmune chronic urticaria tends to run a more severe and protracted course. Basopenia is more severe (85) and histologically there tends to be more evidence of eosinophil degranulation with activated EG-2^+ eosinophils in later lesions (117). The low serum IgE concentration has already been alluded to (84). Because the IgG anti-FcεRIα and anti-IgE autoantibodies were present in only low concentrations (despite manifesting striking functional activity) they cannot be detected by routine immunopathological techniques in affected skin (Hide M, Francis DM, Greaves MW, unpublished data).

Overall these findings raise the possibility of similar pathogenetic mechanisms in both patients with autoimmune and also in apparently nonautoimmune subsets. Detection techniques that possess increased sensitivity, while retaining the present satisfactorily high level of specificity, may shed further light on this problem.

2.4 Urticarial Vasculitis

In its classic form, urticarial vasculitis was first characterized by Soter and co-workers in 1974 (118). Their cases manifested florid leukoclastic vasculitis that was histologically accompanied by systemic symptoms, including arthralgia, and serum hypocomplementemia caused by the circulating immune complexes. Nowadays criteria for diagnosis are less rigorous, and urticarial vasculitis should be suspected in any case of CIU with or without angioedema in which response to antihistamines is poor or the patient manifests atypical features. This includes prolonged duration of individual weals (>24 hr); pain or tenderness as well as, or instead of, itch; staining of the skin by purpura. Clinically weals can, and frequently do, look identical with those of classic CIU. In essence, the more frequently the clinician biopsies CIU, the more frequently he or she is going to find evidence of urticarial vasculitis. The clinical aspects of urticarial vasculitis have recently been well reviewed (119).

ETIOLOGY AND PATHOPHYSIOLOGY. Urticarial vasculitis can be an early clinical manifestation of an autoimmune connective tissue disease, especially lupus erythematosus or Sjogren's syndrome (120,121). It can also occur in association with ulcerative colitis and Crohn's disease (122), hepatitis B or C infection (123), IgM monoclonal gammopathy (Schnitzler's syndrome) (124), blood dyscrasias (125), Lyme disease (126), and serum sickness (127) (Table 6). In all these cases it is believed that in its most florid form immune complex deposition leads to local complement activation and up-regulation of endothelial adhesion molecule expression. Accumulation of activated neutrophils and eosinophils causes endothelial damage and leukocytoclasia, with fibrin deposition and diapedesis of red blood cells manifesting as purpura. Mast cell activation is variable and accounts for the unpredictable degree of itching. Indeed, itching may be absent. Local hemodynamic factors account for the propensity of urticarial vasculitis lesions to affect pressure sites (e.g., waistband).

The minimum histological criteria for diagnosis are unclear, but evidence of endothelial damage should be a sine qua non, along with leukocytoclasia and purpura. Direct immunofluorescence studies of biopsy material may show evidence of IgG and complement deposition, but these findings lack specificity. The distinguishing histological and

Table 6 Etiology of Urticarial Vasculitis

Cause	Ref.
Autoimmune connective tissue disease	120, 121
Crohn's disease and ulcerative colitis	122
Hepatitis B and C infection	123
Paraproteinemia (Schnitzler's syndrome)	124
Blood dyscrasia	125
Lyme disease	126
Serum sickness	127

immunopathological criteria between CIU and urticarial vasculitis have recently been reviewed (117,119).

Although systemic symptoms are well recognized, in most patients attending our urticaria clinic the disease seems to be clinically restricted to the skin. Occasionally, serum complement components may be depleted (118).

REFERENCES

1. Sabroe RA, Seed PT, Francis DM, Barr RM, Black AK, Greaves MW. Chronic idiopathic urticaria: comparison of the clinical features of patients with and without anti-FcεRI or anti-IgE autoantibodies. J Am Acad Dermatol 1999; 40:443–450.
2. Champion RH, Roberts SOB, Carpenter RG, Rogen JH. Urticaria and angioedema—a review of 554 patients. Br J Dermatol 1969; 81:588–597.
3. Aoki T, Kojima M, Horiko T. Acute urticaria: history and natural course of 50 cases. J Dermatol 1994; 21:73–77.
4. Zuberbier T, Ifflander J, Simmler C, Czarnetski BM. Acute urticaria—clinical aspects and therapeutic responsiveness. Acta Derm Venereol (Stockh) 1996; 76:295–297.
5. Davies MG, Greaves MW. Sensory responses of human skin to synthetic histamine analogues and histamine. Br J Clin Pharmacol 1980; 9:461–465.
6. Greaves MW, Wall PD. Pathophysiology of itching. Lancet 1996; 348:938–940.
7. Black AK, Lawlor F, Greaves MW. Consensus meeting on the definition of physical urticarias and urticarial vasculitis. Clin Exp Dermatol 1996; 21:424–426.
8. Breathnach SM, Allen R, Milford–Ward A, Greaves MW. Symptomatic dermographism: natural history, clinical features and response to therapy. Clin Exp Dermatol 1983; 8:463–476.
9. Murphy GM, Zollman PE, Greaves MW, Winkelmann RK. Symptomatic dermographism (factitious urticaria)—passive transfer experiments from human to monkey. Br J Dermatol 1987; 116:801–804.
10. Greaves MW, Sondegaard J. Urticaria pigmentosa and factitious urticaria: direct evidence for release of histamine and other smooth–muscle-contracting agents in dermographic skin. Arch Dermatol 1970; 101:418–425.
11. James MP, Eady RAJ, Black AK, Hawk JLM, Greaves MW. Physical urticaria: a microscopic and pharmacological study of mast cell involvement [abstr.]. J Invest Dermatol 1980; 74:451.
12. Lawlor F, Black AK, Murdoch RD, Greaves MW. Symptomatic dermographism, wealing, mast cells and histamine are decreased in skin following long-term application of a potent topical corticosteroid. Br J Dermatol 1989; 121:629–634.
13. Barlow RJ, Warburton F, Watson K, Black AK, Greaves MW. The diagnosis and incidence of delayed pressure urticaria in patients with chronic urticaria. J Am Acad Dermatol 1993; 24:954–958.
14. Mekori YA, Dobozin BS, Schocket AL, Kohler PF, Clark RAF. Delayed pressure urticaria histologically resembles cutaneous late-phase reactions. Arch Dermatol 1981; 127:230–235.
15. Barlow RJ, McDonald DM, Black AK, Greaves MW. Mast cells and T lymphocytes in chronic urticaria. Clin Exp Allergy 1995; 25:317–322.
16. Lawlor F, Bird C, Camp RDR, Barlow R, Barn RM, Black AK, Greaves MW. Increased interleukin-6 but reduced interleukin-1 in delayed pressure urticaria. Br J Dermatol 1993; 128:500–503.
17. Lawlor F, Barr RM, Black AK, Cromwell I, Isaacs J, Greaves MW. Arachidonic acid transformation is not stimulated in delayed pressure urticaria. Br J Dermatol 1989; 121:317–321.
18. Zip CM, Ross JB, Greaves MW, Scriver CR, Mitchell JJ, Zoar S. Familial cold urticaria. Clin Exp Dermatol 1993; 18:338–341.

19. Illig K, Paul E, Brick K, Schwennicke HP. Experimental investigations on the mechanisms of generalised type of heat and cold urticaria by means of a climate chamber. Acta Derm Venerol (Stockh) 1980; 60:373–380.
20. Lin RY, Schwarz RA. Cold urticaria and HIV infection. Br J Dermatol 1993; 129:465–467.
21. Kaplan AP, Garafolo J. Identification of a new physically-induced urticaria: cold-induced cholinergic urticaria. J Allergy Clin Immunol 1981; 68:438.
22. Sarkany I, Turk JL. Delayed hypersensitivity to cold. Proc R Soc Med 1965; 58:622.
23. Kaplan AP. Unusual cold-dependent disorders: cold-dependent dermographism and cold urticaria. J Allergy Clin Immunol 1984; 73:453–456.
24. Solomon LM, Strauss H, Leznoff A. Localised secondary cold urticaria. Acad Dermatol 1966; 94:156.
25. Neittaanmaki JJ. Cold urticaria: clinical findings in 270 patients. J Am Acad Dermatol 1985; 13:636.
26. Doeglas HMG, Rijnken WJ, Schroder FP, Schirm J. Cold urticaria and virus infections: a clinical and serological study in 39 patients. Br J Dermatol 1986; 114:311–318.
27. Houser DD, Arbesman CE, Ito K, Wicher K. Cold urticaria: immunological studies. Am J Med 1970; 49:23–33.
28. Wanderer AA, Maselli R, Ellis EF, Ishizaka KJ. Immunological characterisation of serum factors responsible for cold urticaria. Allergy 1971; 48:13–22.
29. Misch K, Black AK, Greaves MW, Almosawi T, Stanworth DR. Passive transfer of idopathic cold urticaria to monkeys. Acta Derm Venereol (Stockh) 1983; 63:163–164.
30. Wallengren LB. Heterozygous α_1-antichymotrypsin deficiency may be associated with cold urticaria. Allergy 1992; 47:456–458.
31. Lawlor F, Black AK, Breathnach AS, McKee P, Sarath Chandra P, Bhoga B, Isaacs JL, Greaves MW, Winkelmann RK. A timed study of the histopathology, direct immunofluorescence and ultrastructural findings in idiopathic cold contact urticaria over a 24 hour period. Clin Exp Dematol 1989; 14:416–420.
32. Eady RAJ, Greaves MW. Induction of cutaneous vasculitis by repeated cold challenge in cold urticaria. Lancet 1978; 1:336–337.
33. Soter NA, Wasserman SI, Austen KF. Cold urticaria: release into the circulation of histamine and eosinophil chemotactic factor of anaphylaxis during cold challenge. N Engl J Med 1976; 294:687–690.
34. Keahey TM, Greaves MW. Cold urticaria: dissociation of cold-evoked histamine release and urticaria following cold challenge. Arch Dermatol 1980; 116:174–177.
35. Bentley–Phillips CB, Black AK, Greaves MW. Induced tolerance in cold urticaria caused by cold-evoked histamine release. Lancet 1976; 2:63–66.
36. Ormerod AD, Black AK, Dawes J, Murdock RD, Koro O, Barr RM, Greaves MW. Prostaglandin D_2 and histamine release unaccompanied by evidence of platelet activation. J Allergy Clin Immunol 1988; 82:586–589.
37. Wasserman SI, Ginsberg MH. Release of platelet factor 4 into the blood after cold challenge of patients with cold urticaria. J Allergy Clin Immunol 1984; 74:275–279.
38. Malthy NH, Ind PW, Causon RC, Fuller RW, Taylor GW. Leukotriene E_4 release in cold urticaria. Clin Exp Allergy 1989; 19:33–36.
39. Tillie–Leblond I, Gosset P, Janin A, Dalenne R, Joseph M, Wallaerb B, Tonnel A–B. Tumor necrosis factor-α release during systemic reaction in cold urticaria. J Allergy Clin Immunol 1994; 93:501–509.
40. Kaplan AP, Garofalo J, Sigler R, Hauber T. Idiopathic cold urticaria in vitro demonstration of histamine release upon challenge of skin biopsies. N Engl J Med 1981; 305:1074–1077.
41. Gruber BC, Baeza MC, Marchase MJ, Aquello V, Kaplan AP. Autoantibodies in urticarial syndromes. J Invest Dermatol 1988; 90:213–217.
42. Heavey DJ, Black AK, Barrow SE, Chappell CG, Greaves MW, Dollery CT. Prostaglandin D_2 and histamine release in cold urticaria. J Allergy Clin Immunol 1986; 78:458–461.

43. Wanderer AA. Cold urticaria syndromes. Historical background, diagnostic classification, clinical and laboratory characteristics, pathogenesis and management. J Allergy Clin Immunol 1990; 85:965–981.
44. Constanzi JJ, Coltman JR, Donaldson VH. Activation of complement by a monoclonal cryoglobulin associated with cold urticaria. J Lab Clin Med 1969; 74:902–910.
45. Constanzi JJ, Coltman JR. Kappa chain cold-precipitable immunoglobulin G. Associated with cold urticaria. Clin Exp Immunol 1967; 2:167–178.
46. Kramer DW, Perilstein PK. Case report of cold sensitivity with cold haemaglutinins. Angiology 1951; 2:283–292.
47. Moroz CA, Rose B. The cryopathies. In: Samter M, ed. Immunological Diseases. 2nd ed. London: Little, Brown, 1971:459–482.
48. Harris KE, Lewis T, Vaughan JM. Haemoglobinuria and urticaria from cold occurring singly or in combinations: observations referring especially to the mechanism of urticaria with some remarks upon Raynaud's disease. Heart 1929; 14:305–336.
49. Hirschmann JV, Lawlor F, English SJC, Lowback JB, Winkelmann RK, Greaves MW. Cholinergic urticaria. Arch Dematol 1987; 123:462–467.
50. Zuberbier T, Althaus C, Chantraine–Hess H, Czarnetski BM. Prevalence of cholinegic urticaria in young adults. J Am Acad Dermatol 1994; 31:478–481.
51. Herxheimer A. The nervous pathway mediating cholinergic urticaria. Clin Sci 1956; 15:195–205.
52. Lawrence CM, Jorizzo JL, Black AK, Coutts A, Greaves MW. Cholinergic urticaria with associated angioedema. Br J Dematol 1981; 105:543–550.
53. Murphy GM, Black AK, Greaves MW. Persisting cholinergic erythema—a variant of cholinergic urticaria. Br J Dermatol 1983; 109:343–348.
54. Kivity S, Snech E, Grief J, Topilsky N, Mekori YA. The effect of food and exercise on the skin response to compound 48/80 in patients with food associated, exercise induced urticaria angioedema. J Allergy Clin Immunol 1988; 81:1155–1158.
55. Nomland R. Cholinergic urticaria and cholinergic itching. Arch Derm Syphilol 1944; 50: 247–250.
56. Kay DM, Maibach HR. Pruritus and acquired anhidrosis: two unusual cases. Arch Dematol 1969; 100:291.
57. Adachi J, Aoki T, Yamatodari A. Demonstration of sweat allergy in cholinergic urticaria. J Dermatol Sci 1994; 7:142–149.
58. Murphy GM, Greaves MW, Zollman P, Stanworth D. Cholinergic urticaria: passive transfer experiments from human to monkey. Dermatologica 1988; 177:338–340.
59. Eftekhari N, Milford Ward A, Allen R, Greaves MW. Protease inhibitor profiles in urticaria and angioedema. Br J Dermatol 1980; 103:33–39.
60. Wong E, Eftekhari N, Greaves MW, Milford Ward A. Beneficial effects of danazol on symptoms and laboratory changes of cholinergic urticaria. Br J Dermatol 1987; 116:553–556.
61. Commens CA, Greaves MW. Tests to establish the diagnosis of cholinergic urticaria. Br J Dermatol 1978; 98:47–51.
62. Soter NA, Wasserman SI, Austen KF. Release of mast cell mediators and alterations in lung function in patients with cholinergic urticaria. N Engl J Med 1980; 302:604–608.
63. Kaplan AP, Natbony SF, Tawil AP, Fructar L, Foster M. Exercise-induced anaphylaxis in a manifestation of cholinergic urticaria. J Allergy Clin Immunol 1981; 68:319–324.
64. Leeunatphong V, Holzle E, Plewig G. Solar urticaria: studies on mechanism of tolerance. Br J Dermatol 1990; 122:601–606.
65. Hawk JLM, Eady RAJ, Challoner AVJ, Black AK, Keahey TM, Greaves MW. Elevated blood histamine levels and mast cell degranulation in solar urticaria. Br J Clin Pharmacol 1980; 9:183–186.
66. Ramsay CA. Solar urticaria treatment by inducing tolerance to artificial radiation and natural light. Arch Dermatol 1997; 113:1222–1225.

67. Greaves MW, Sneddon IB, Smith AK, Stanworth DR. Heat urticaria. Br J Dermatol 1974; 90:289–292.
68. Koro O, Dover JS, Francis DM, Black AK, Kelly RW, Barr RM, Greaves MW. Release of prostaglandin D_2 and histamine in a case of localised heat urticaria and effects of treatments. Br J Dermatol 1986; 115:722–728.
69. Johansson E, Reunala T, Kostimies S, Lagerstedt A, Kauppinent K, Timoria K. Localised heat urticaria associated with a decrease in serum complement factor B (C_3 proactivator). Br J Dermatol 1984; 110:227–231.
70. Michaelsson G, Ros AM. Familial localised heat urticaria of delayed type. Acta Derm Venerol (Stockh) 1971; 51:279–283.
71. Fearfield CA, Guzzard B, Bunker CB. Aquagenic urticaria and human immunodeficiency virus infection: treatment with stanazolol. Br J Dermatol 1997; 137:620–622.
72. Sibbald RG, Black AK, Eady RAJ, James M, Greaves MW. Aquagenic urticaria: evidence of a cholinergic and histaminergic basis. Br J Dermatol 1981; 105:297–302.
73. Greaves MW, Black AK, Eady RAJ, Coutts A. Aquagenic pruritus. Br Med J 1981; 282: 2007–2010.
74. Archer CB, Camp RDR, Greaves MW. Polycythaemia vera can present with aquagenic pruritus (letter). Lancet; 1451, 1988.
75. Lotti T, Steinman HK, Greaves MW, Gabril P, Brunetti L, Panconesi E. Increased fibrinolytic activity in aquagenic pruritus. Int J Dermatol 1986; 25:508–510.
76. Steinman HK, Greaves MW. Aquagenic pruritus. J Am Acad Dermatol 1985; 13:91–96.
77. Kligman AM, Greaves MW, Steinman H. Water-induced itching without cutaneous signs. Arch Dermatol 1986; 122:183–186.
78. Greaves MW, Handfield Jones SE. Aquagenic pruritus: pharmacological findings and treatment. Eur J Dermatol 1992; 2:482–484.
79. Menage H du P, Greaves MW. Aquagenic pruritus. Semin Dermatol 1995; 14:313–316.
80. Patterson R, Melles CJ, Blankenship ML, Pruzanski JJ. Vibratory angioedema, a hereditary type of physical hypersensitivity. J Allergy Clin Immunol 1972; 50:184.
81. Epstein P, Kidd KK. Dermodistortive urticaria: an autosomal dominant dermatologic disorder. Am J Med Genet 1981; 9:307.
82. Lawlor F, Black AK, Morris A, Greaves MW. Vibratory angioedema: lesion induction, clinical features, laboratory and ultrastructural findings. Br J Dermatol 1989; 120:403–408.
83. Ting S, Reiman, BEF, Rauls DU, Mansfield LE. Non-familial vibration-induced angioedema. J Allergy Clin Immunol 1983; 71:546.
84. Sabroe RA, Seed PT, Francis DM, Barr RM, Black AK, Greaves MW. Chronic idiopathic urticaria: comparison of clinical features of patients with and without anti-FcεRI or anti-IgE autoantibodies. J Am Acad Dermatol 1999; 40:443–450.
85. Sabroe RA, Francis DM, Barr RM, Black AK, Greaves MW. Anti-FcεRI autoantibodies and basophil histamine releasability in chronic idiopathic urticaria. J Allergy Clin Immunol 1998; 102:651–658.
86. Schnyder B, Helbling A, Pichler WJ. Chronic idiopathic urticaria: natural course and association with *Helicobacter pylori* infection. Int Arch Allergy Immunol 1999; 119:60–83.
87. Burova EP, Mallet AT, Greaves MW. *Helicobacter pylori* a cause of chronic urticaria [abstr]. Br J Dermatol 1998; 139(suppl 51):43.
88. Black AK, Greaves MW, Champion RH, Pye RJ. The urticarias 1990. Br J Dermatol 1991; 124:100–108.
89. May CD. Are confusion and controversy about food hypersensitivity really necessary? J Allergy Clin Immunol 1985; 75:329–333.
90. Pastorello EA. Evaluating new tests for the diagnosis of food allergy. Allergy 1995; 50:289–291.
91. Doeglas HMG. Reactions to aspirin and food additives in patients with chronic urticaria including the physical urticarias. Br J Dermatol 1975; 93:135–144.

92. Rorsman H. Basopenia in urticaria. Acta Allergol 1962; 17:168–184.
93. Greaves MW, Plummer VM, McLaughlan P, Stanworth DR. Serum and cell-bound IgE in chronic urticaria. Clin Allergy 1974; 4:265–271.
94. Leznoff A, Sussman GL. Syndrome of idiopathic chronic urticaria and angioedema with thyroid autoimmunity—a study of 90 patients. J Allergy Clin Immunol 1989; 84:66–71.
95. O'Donnell BF, Black AK, Greaves MW. Organ- and non–organ-specific autoimmunity in chronic urticaria [abstr]. Br J Dematol 1995; 133(suppl 145):42.
96. O'Donnell BF, O'Neill CM, Francis DM, Niimi N, Barr RM, Barlow RJ, Black AK, Welsh KI, Greaves MW. Human leucocyte antigen class II associations in chronic idiopathic urticaria. Br J Dermatol 1999; 140:853–858.
97. Claveau J, Lavoie A, Brunet C, Bedford PM, Hiber J. Chronic idiopathic urticaria: possible contribution of histamine releasing factor to the pathogens. J Allergy Clin Immunol 1993; 92:132–137.
98. MacDonald SM, Rafnar T, Langdon J, Lichtenstein LM. Molecular identification of an IgE-dependent histamine releasing factor. Science 1995; 269:688–690.
99. Kermani F, Nimii N, Francis DM, Greaves MW, Barr RM. Characterisation of a novel mast cell-specific histamine releasing activity in chronic idiopathic urticaria [abstr]. J Invest Dermatol 1995; 105:452.
100. Grattan CEH, Wallington TB, Warin RP. A serological mediator in chronic idiopathic urticaria: a clinical immunological and histological evaluation. Br J Dermatol 1986; 114:583–590.
101. Hide M, Francis DM, Grattan CEH, Greaves MW. Autoantibodies against the high affinity IgE receptor as a cause for histamine release in chronic urticaria. N Engl J Med 1993; 328: 1599–1604.
102. Niimi N, Francis DM, Kermani F, et al. Dermal mast cell activation by autoantibodies against the high affinity IgE receptor in chronic urticaria. J Invest Dermatol 1996; 106:1001–1006.
103. Fiebiger E, Maurer D, Holub H, Reininger B, Hartmann G, Woisetschlager M, Stingl G. Serum IgG autoantibodies directed against the alpha-chain of FcεRI: a selective marker and pathogenetic factor for a distinct subset of chronic urticaria patients? J Clin Invest 1995; 96: 2606–2612.
104. Zweiman B, Valenzano M, Atkins PC, Tanus T, Getsy JA. Characteristics of histamine-releasing activity in the sera of patients with chronic idiopathic urticaria. J Allergy Clin Immunol 1996; 98:89–98.
105. Tong LJ, Balakrishnan G, Kochan JP, Kinet J–P, Kaplan AP. Assessment of autoimmunity in patients with chronic urticaria. J Allergy Clin Immunol 1997; 99:461–465.
106. Sabroe RA, Grattan CEH, Francis DM, Barr RM, Black AK, Greaves MW. The autologous serum skin test: a screening test for autoantibodies in chronic idiopathic urticaria. Br J Dermatol 1999; 140:446–452.
107. Grattan CEH, Francis DM, Slater NGP, Barlow RJ, Greaves MW. Plasmapheresis for severe unremitting chronic urticaria. Lancet 1992; 339:1078–1080.
108. O'Donnell BF, Barr RM, Black AK, Francis DM, Greaves MW. Intravenous immunoglobulin in chronic autoimmune urticaria. Br J Dermatol 1998; 138:101–106.
109. Greaves MW. Chronic urticaria. N Engl J Med 1995; 332:1767–1772.
110. Toyoda M, Maruyama T, Morohashi M, Bhawan J. Free eosinophil granules in urticaria: a correlation with the duration of weals. Am J Dermatopathol 1996; 18:49–57.
111. Peters MS, Schroeter ALO, Kephart GM, Gleich GJ. Localisation of eosinophil granule major basic protein in chronic urticaria. J Invest Dermatol 1983; 81:39–43.
112. Winkelmann RK, Wilson–Jones E, Smith NP, English JSC, Greaves MW. Neutrophilic urticaria. Acta Derm Venereol (Stockh) 1988; 68:129–133.
113. Kaplan AP, Horakova Z, Katz SI. Assessment of tissue fluid histamine levels in patients with urticaria. J Allergy Clin Immunol 1978; 61:350–354.
114. Barlow RJ, Ross EL, MacDonald D, Black AK, Greaves MW. Adhesion molecule expression

and the inflammatory cell infiltrate in delayed pressure urticaria. Br J Dermatol 1994; 13: 341–347.

115. Krause LB, Shuster S. Enhanced weal and flare response to histamine in chronic urticaria. Br J Clin Pharmacol 1985; 20:486–488.
116. Fiebiger E, Hammerschmid F, Stingl G, Maurer D. Anti-FcεRI autoantibodies in autoimmune-mediated disorder: identification of a structure–function relationship. J Clin Invest 1998; 101:243–251.
117. Sabroe RA, Poon E, Orchard GE, Lane D, Francis DM, Barr RM, Black MM, Black AK, Greaves MW. Cutaneous inflammatory cell infiltrate in chronic idiopathic urticaria: comparison of patients with and without anti-FcεRIα or anti-IgE autoantibodies. J Allergy Clin Immunol 1999; 103:484–493.
118. Soter NA, Austen AK, Gigli I. Urticarias and arthralgias as manifestations of necrotising angiitis (vasculitis). J Invest Dermatol 1994; 63:485–490.
119. O'Donnell BF, Black AK. Urticarial vasculitis. Int Angiol 1995; 14:1661–1674.
120. Provost T, Zone JJ, Synkowski D, Maddison PJ, Reichlin M. Unusual cutaneous manifestations of systemic lupus I: urticaria-like lesions: correlation with clinical and serological abnormalities. J Invest Dermatol 1980; 75:495–499.
121. Alexander EL, Provost T. Cutaneous manifestations of primary Sjogren's syndrome: a reflection of vasculitis and association with anti-Ro (SSA) antibodies. J Invest Dermatol 1983; 80:386–391.
122. Handfield–Jones SE, Greaves MW. Urticarial vasculitis: response to gold therapy. J R Soc Med 1991; 84:169.
123. Kuniyuki S, Katoh H. Urticarial vasculitis with papular lesions in a patient with type C hepatitis and cryoglobulinaemia. J Dermatol 1996; 23:279–283.
124. Borradori L, Rybojad M, Puissant A, Dallot A, Verola D, Morel P. Urticarial vasculitis associated with a monoclonal IgM gammopathy (Schnitzler's syndrome). Br J Dermatol 1990; 123:113–118.
125. Farrell AM, Sabroe RA, Bunker CB. Urticarial vasculitis associated with polycythaemia ruba vera. Clin Exp Dermatol 1996; 21:302–304.
126. Olson JC, Esterly NB. Urticarial vasculitis and Lyme disease. J Am Acad Dermatol 1989; 22:1114–1116.
127. Lawly TJ, Bielory L, Gascon P, Yancey KB, Young NS, Frank MM. A study of human serum sickness. J Invest Dermatol 1995; 85:129–132.

18

Anaphylaxis and Inflammation

MARK S. DYKEWICZ

St. Louis University School of Medicine, St. Louis, Missouri

1 INTRODUCTION

Anaphylaxis is an emergent, potentially fatal, systemic reaction that results from the release of biologically active mediators. Classically, anaphylaxis is triggered by antigen exposure and IgE-mediated activation of mast cells or basophils. These cells then release mediators that act on target organs. The clinical manifestations of anaphylaxis may vary, but can involve multiple sites, including the cardiovascular, respiratory and gastrointestinal systems, and skin and connective tissue. Non–IgE-mediated activation of cells or complement activation can result in a clinically indistinguishable syndrome (1). The term *anaphylactoid reaction* sometimes is used to refer to reactions that do not have an IgE-mediated basis, such as most reactions from radiographic contrast administration. However, these different initial triggering mechanisms culminate in apparently common cascades of pathophysiological processes that may include inflammation. Many of the pathological processes that occur in tissues during anaphylaxis also occur in other diseases that are limited to specific organ systems. For example, anaphylaxis can lead to inflammatory processes that are also found in the lung in asthma, in the nose in rhinitis, and in the skin and mucous membranes in urticaria and angioedema.

2 CLINICAL PRESENTATION: EARLY- AND LATE-PHASE RESPONSES

The temporal course of anaphylaxis can vary considerably. In the case of IgE-mediated anaphylaxis, clinical manifestations usually appear within minutes, but sometimes up to an hour, after exposure to a causal agent (e.g., food, drug, insect sting); the early manifestations of anaphylaxis are termed the early-phase, analogous to the early phase of allergic reactions restricted to a particular organ system. Occasionally, anaphylaxis caused by oral exposure to an allergen will have its onset somewhat later than this, a delay presumably reflecting the time required for absorption of the allergen from the gastrointestinal tract (1). Clinical manifestations of the early phase of anaphylaxis include hypotension, flushing, bronchospasm, nasal congestion and rhinorrhea, abdominal and uterine cramping, nausea, vomiting, urticaria, and angioedema. Most of these findings are thought to be caused by direct or indirect effects of mediators released by mast cells or basophils, such as histamine, leukotrienes, and tryptase, or by the activation of the complement cascade with consequent production of anaphylatoxins. During the early phase of anaphylaxis, edema and mucous production frequently occur, but cellular inflammation per se is not a prominent finding.

In many patients, anaphylaxis ends after recovery from the early phase. However, in other patients, resolution of the early phase of anaphylaxis may be followed by the return of clinical manifestations approximately 4–8 hr after the onset of early-phase, termed the late phase (2–4). There are also patients who have protracted or progressive symptoms without any diminution beyond the time period of the early phase, possibly reflecting continued mediator release (5) and uninterrupted progression from the early to late phase.

During the late phase, cellular inflammation becomes more manifest. Inflammatory findings during the late phase of anaphylaxis often mimic those that occur in late allergic responses in diseases restricted to particular organ systems, such as allergic asthma or rhinitis, or urticaria. Yet one cannot assume that late-phase responses in anaphylaxis are always mechanistically, qualitatively, and quantitatively similar. For example, animal studies suggest that there may be some differences between the required role of immunoglobulin in late-phase responses in asthma and anaphylaxis. Immunoglobulin-deficient, but sensitized, mice can develop pulmonary late-phase inflammation after allergen challenge. However, immunoglobulin-deficient sensitized mice develop neither anaphylaxis nor inflammatory responses after exposure to systemically administered allergen (6).

3 PATHOLOGY

Fatalities from anaphylaxis usually occur from respiratory obstruction or cardiovascular collapse (7–12). When death occurs from sudden cardiovascular collapse, no postmortem footprint of the preceding anaphylactic event may be present. Upper airway edema is reported in 60% of autopsy cases, and results from accumulation of transudate in the submucosa (7,8). Bronchial obstruction and lung hyperinflation are found in about half of fatalities, with obstruction resulting from bronchospasm of airway smooth muscle, submucosal edema, and secretions (7,8). Diffuse eosinophilic infiltration of the pulmonary vessels, lamina propria of the gastrointestinal tract and of the splenic sinusoids may also be present.

4 PATHOGENESIS OF INFLAMMATORY EVENTS IN ANAPHYLAXIS

4.1 Cells That May Promote Inflammation from Anaphylaxis

Many of the pathophysiological events that occur during the early phase are thought to lead to cellular inflammation that can be prominent in the late phase. Mediators released during this early phase are likely contributors to late-phase inflammation. Mast cells may play an important role in inflammation associated with anaphylaxis because preformed chemotactic factors released from mast cell secretory granules include chemoattractants for eosinophils, neutrophils, and mononuclear cells (13). Nonetheless, mast cells are not requisite for inflammation from anaphylaxis. In mouse models of systemic anaphylaxis, mast cells are not required for development of either the clinical manifestations or gastric neutrophil infiltration characteristically observed in the response (14). Basophils may also participate in the inflammatory responses of anaphylaxis, because some of the potentially proinflammatory mediators, such as cysteinyl leukotrienes (LT) produced by mast cells are also produced by basophils. However, basophils do not produce significant amounts of LTB_4, prostaglandin-(PG)D_2, platelet-activating factor (PAF), or large quantities of tryptase. Inflammation during anaphylaxis is associated with leukocyte activation (15). During anaphylaxis, neutrophils produce lysosomal enzymes that can participate in inflammatory responses (16). In addition, platelets and other cells produce platelet-activating factor, which is chemotactic for leukocytes and thus could promote cellular inflammation in anaphylaxis (17–19). From the late-phase responses seen in other allergic diseases, and limited data available from animal models of anaphylaxis, anaphylaxis upregulates cellular adhesion molecules that promote cellular inflammation and edema (20,21).

4.2 Mediators of Importance

4.2.1 Histamine

During most cases of anaphylaxis, release of histamine from secretory granules of mast cells or basophils occurs, leading to elevations in plasma or tissue histamine levels. Histamine not only plays a central role in the development of noninflammatory processes, such as bronchospasm, flushing, and hypotension, but also may contribute to other processes that promote inflammation.

Histamine stimulation of H_1- and H_2-receptors is thought to lead to mucous production of the lower and upper respiratory tract. Glycoprotein secretion from goblet cells and bronchial glands is produced by stimulation of the H_2-receptor, whereas stimulation of the H_1-receptor increases mucous viscosity (22). Throughout the body, histamine can vasodilate postcapillary venules and increase capillary permeability by creating gaps between contracted endothelial cells (23). This can lead to leakage of a plasma transudate into tissues, with consequent edema (24,25). Increased capillary permeability due to histamine could facilitate transit of cells from the circulation into tissues in response to chemotactic factors. However, there is some evidence in animal models that histamine may actually reduce cellular inflammation through receptor-mediated mechanisms, but it is unclear whether these processes are relevant in humans. In the carrageenan rat air pouch model, local administration of H_2-receptor antagonists, but not the H_1-antagonist pyrilamine, augments neutrophil infiltration at 24 hr. Because both types of histamine antagonists fail to suppress the vascular permeability response in this model, these results suggest that histamine could exert a down-regulation of neutrophil infiltration through H_2-receptors (26). Some animal data suggest that inflammation after anaphylaxis might promote histamine production. The inflammatory exudate of the postanaphylaxis phase of allergic inflammation in rats has the ability to enhance histamine production by bone marrow cells. Although the mechanisms of this process are not fully understood, it has been suggested that agents (or cells) in the inflammatory exudates stimulate de novo synthesis of histidine decarboxylase and activate protein kinase C (PKC) and tyrosine kinase (27,28).

4.2.2 Arachidonic Acid Metabolites and Platelet-Activating Factor

Several metabolites of arachidonic acid have a demonstrated importance in anaphylaxis, although only some of their actions are directly proinflammatory. These agents include leukotrienes, prostaglandins, and hydroxyeicosatetraenoic acids (HETEs). Activation of mast cells, as occurs during anaphylaxis, causes them to metabolize arachidonic acid to produce cysteinyl leukotriene (LTC_4), a smaller amount of LTB_4 and PGD_2 (17–19). LTC_4 is converted to bioactive LTD_4 and LTE_4 outside of these cells. Other cells of myeloid origin can also produce these mediators.

Cysteinyl leukotrienes, in addition to noninflammatory actions, such as playing a role in bronchospasm and hypotension, are chemotactic for eosinophils over neutrophils, whereas LTB_4 is a chemotactic factor for neutrophils over eosinophils; LTB_4 enhances neutrophil metabolic activity (13). The synthesis of these lipid mediators depends not only on the expression of the enzyme 5-lipoxygenase (5-LO), which catalyzes the first steps in the synthesis of leukotrienes, but also on expression of a nuclear membrane protein termed the 5-LO-activating protein (FLAP) (29,30). The 5-LO$^{-/-}$ mice are unable to synthesize detectable levels of leukotrienes, and have altered inflammatory responses (31,32).

Platelet-activating factor, or PAF-acether, a phospholipid derivative, is a potent aggregating agent. It is formed by platelets and also by basophils, neutrophils, monocytes, and macrophages, including alveolar macrophages. PAF is thought to contribute to manifestations of anaphylaxis because it is elevated during anaphylaxis in animal models (33), and its intravenous administration induces key manifestations of anaphylaxis, such as hypotension and bronchoconstriction in guinea pigs (34,35). In addition, it evokes eosinophil margination and diapedesis in lung parenchyma and bronchial submucosa in guinea pig models of anaphylaxis (35). PAF is felt to act largely through leukotriene-dependent mechanisms as evidenced by the finding that 5-LO$^{-/-}$ mice, who are unable to synthesize detectable levels of leukotrienes, are more resistant to lethal anaphylaxis induced by platelet-activating factor (32).

Prostaglandins may also play a role in inflammation associated with anaphylaxis (see Sec. 5).

4.2.3 β-Tryptase

β-Tryptase is strongly bound to proteoglycans in secretory granules of mast cells, and to a minimal extent, of basophils. It is released during mast cell-mediated anaphylaxis (36). As a serine protease, β-tryptase acts on protein substrates and can cleave C3 to produce C3a (37), a proinflammatory anaphylatoxin. Although this protease serves as a serum marker of systemic anaphylaxis, its role in the pathogenesis, if any, is unknown.

4.3 Proinflammatory Cascades

The complement, contact (kallikrein-kinin), clotting, and clot lysis systems all have been implicated as pathways that contribute to inflammatory responses of anaphylaxis. During activation of the complement cascade, for example, there is production of anaphylatoxins (C3a, C4a, C5a) that possess chemotactic properties and can activate a variety of cells (22,38).

4.4 Neurogenic, Glandular, and Hormonal Influences on Inflammation from Anaphylaxis

Animal studies suggest that neurogenic influences can alter inflammation associated with anaphylaxis, although it is still unclear whether this applies to humans. Bilateral decentralization of the superior cervical ganglia reduces the pulmonary inflammation that develops

4–8 hr after induction of anaphylaxis in *Nippostrongylus brasiliensis*-sensitized rats. The increase in the phagocytosis and respiratory burst of circulating neutrophils seen at 4 and 8 hr after allergen challenge in sham-operated rats is reduced significantly by decentralization. Anaphylaxis-induced pulmonary inflammation that occurs with decentralization of the superior cervical ganglia is primarily associated with down-regulation of neutrophil and macrophage functions (39).

There is evidence that glandular secretion may counteract the neurogenic inhibition of inflammation induced by anaphylaxis. In animal studies, removal of the submandibular gland (sialadenectomy) by itself does not modify the severity of pulmonary inflammation that occurs from anaphylaxis, but concurrent sialadenectomy and decentralization abolish the anti-inflammatory effect of decentralization (40). To explain this, it has been postulated that cervical sympathetic nerves tonically inhibit release of anti-inflammatory factors from submandibular glands. Both decentralization and ganglionectomy appear to increase the level of transcripts that encode immunomodulatory growth factors (nerve growth factor and epidermal growth factor) in submandibular glands, but these denervations evidently did not modify transcripts for transforming growth factor (TGF)-β_2. Accordingly, it has been proposed that systemic inflammatory events in anaphylaxis may be regulated by the central nervous system at a level superior to the superior cervical ganglia, probably through modulation of immunoregulatory factors in submandibular glands.

Insulin, in doses that do not influence the blood glucose level, potentiates anaphylactic shock in ovalbumin-sensitized mice, but moderately inhibits carrageenan-induced paw edema. Higher doses of insulin produce a dose-dependent inhibition of the inflammatory process at 2–4 hr after the onset of anaphylaxis (41). Insulin also stimulates lymphocytes to produce proinflammatory factors that can increase dextran-induced anaphylactoid reactions (42–44). These results suggest that insulin, released during anaphylaxis and other stresses, may play a complex regulatory role in hypersensitivity and inflammatory reactions, including anaphylaxis.

5 IMPLICATIONS FOR PHARMACOTHERAPY OF INFLAMMATION FROM ANAPHYLAXIS

Because glucocorticosteroids given in advance of allergen challenge reduce inflammation and late-phase responses of rhinitis, asthma, and allergic skin reactions, they are commonly administered for treatment of anaphylaxis, in part to reduce late-phase anaphylaxis responses. However, available retrospective studies (4) have not demonstrated clinical benefit from brief administration of glucocorticosteroids after anaphylaxis has begun. This might be explained because the interval between glucocorticosteroid administration and the development of the late-phase response of anaphylaxis is often too short for the anti-inflammatory effects of glucocorticosteroids to develop. This explanation would be consistent with the observation that glucocorticosteroids administered after the onset of anaphylactic shock, induced by inhalation of ovalbumin antigen in sensitized guinea pigs, can reduce bronchial inflammation that occurs 24 hr after anaphylaxis (45). In this model, bronchial inflammation is characterized by increased numbers of neutrophils, mononuclear cells, and eosinophils in the bronchoalveolar lavage (BAL) fluid. Other medications that reduce this inflammatory response include cromolyn sodium, which reduces the number of mononuclear cells and eosinophils, and theophylline, which decreases the number of eosinophils. The β-adrenergic agonist albuterol (salbutamol) actually increases neutrophil numbers, whereas the nonsteroidal anti-inflammatory agent indomethacin does not have any significant effect. Also in a guinea pig model of anaphylaxis, several different medications administered at least 1–2 hr before anaphylaxis reduce inflammatory responses; an antileukotriene agent (Sch-37224) and a PAF antagonist apafant (WEB 2086) decrease eosinophil accumulation in BAL fluid, indicating roles for 5-lipoxygenase products and PAF (46). Whether administration of these agents after the onset of anaphylaxis would have similar anti-inflammatory effects is uncertain. However, theophylline administered after allergen-induced anaphylactic shock in guinea pigs does reduce the number of eosinophils, but not the number of neutrophils in bronchoalveolar lavage (BAL) postchallenge (47).

Studies in other animal models of allergic inflammation have produced some conflicting results. Allergen challenge to the cheek pouch of immunized hamsters causes an acute inflammatory reaction that is characterized by leakage of plasma, vasodilation, and accumulation of leukocytes (48). In this model, inhibition of prostaglandin synthesis with two different nonsteroidal anti-inflammatory drugs greatly potentiates plasma leakage, leukocyte emigration, and histamine release after challenge with antigen or with compound 48/80, an agent that nonspecifically activates mast cells. The enhanced antigen-induced extravasation of plasma and leukocytes is significantly reduced by 5-LO inhibitors, but is unaffected by PAF-receptor antagonism (48). In contrast to the mast cell-dependent reactions, the inflammatory effects of the individual mediators histamine, LTB_4, and LTC_4 are not influenced by nonsteroidal anti-inflammatory drug treatment, and are markedly enhanced by both PGE_2 and PGI_2. To explain these findings, it has been suggested that vasodilating prostaglandins exert both pro- and anti-inflammatory actions in vivo. Specifically, these prostaglandins could modulate acute allergic inflammation by (1) inhibition of inflammatory mediator release, most likely unrelated to prostanoid-induced vasodilation, but caused by cAMP elevation in the mediator-secreting cells; and (2) enhancement of the target action of individual inflammatory mediators (plasma leakage and leukocyte emigration), most likely as a direct consequence of prostaglandin-induced vasodilation (48). Consequently, use of nonsteroidal anti-inflammatory drugs, which would block production of prostaglandins, might lead to either proinflammatory or anti-inflammatory effects during anaphylaxis.

Although these studies in animal models provide insight for potential therapeutic interventions in humans, it remains to be determined whether brief administration of agents with similar pharmacological effects could reduce inflammation and late-phase responses in human anaphylaxis caused by parenteral or oral allergen exposure. The unpredictable occurrence of anaphylaxis, its relatively low incidence, and its variable clinical course are barriers to performing prospective, controlled human trials to assess the efficacy of these agents.

REFERENCES

1. Bochner BS, Lichtenstein LM. Anaphylaxis. N Engl J Med 1991; 324:1785–1790.
2. Greenberg MA, Kaufman CR, Gonzales GE, et al. Late and immediate systemic–allergic reactions to inhalant immunotherapy. J Allergy Clin Immunol 1986; 77:865–870.
3. Popa VT, Lerner SA. Biphasic systemic anaphylactic reaction: three illustrative cases. Ann Allergy 1982; 53:151–155.
4. Stark BJ, Sullivan TJ. Biphasic and protracted anaphylaxis. J Allergy Clin Immunol 1986; 78:76–83.

5. Vinuya RZ, Simon MR, Schwartz LB. Elevated serum tryptase levels in a patient with protracted anaphylaxis. Ann Allergy 1994; 73:232–234.
6. Korsgren M, Erjefalt JS, Korsgren O, Sonmark B, Sundler F, Persson CG. Lack of systemic anaphylaxis and aeroallergen-induced airway plasma extravasation in allergic immunoglobulin-deficient mice. Int Arch Allergy Immunol 1999; 118:67–73.
7. Delage C, Irey NS. Anaphylactic deaths: a clinical pathologic study of 43 cases. J Forensic Sci 1972; 17:525–540.
8. Austen KF. Systemic anaphylaxis in man. JAMA 1965; 192:108–110.
9. Hunt EL. Death from allergic shock. N Engl J Med 1943; 228:502–507.
10. Lamson RW. So-called fatal anaphylaxis in man: with especial reference to diagnosis and treatment of clinical allergies. JAMA 1929; 93:1775–1778.
11. Sheppe WM. Fatal anaphylaxis in man. J Lab Clin Med 1931; 16:372–379.
12. Delage C, Mullick FG, Irey NS. Myocardial lesions in anaphylaxis. Arch Pathol Lab Med 1973; 95:185–189.
13. Horan RF, Pennoyer DS, Sheffer AL. Management of anaphylaxis. Immunol Allergy Clin North Am 1991; 11:117–141.
14. Furuta GT, Wang ZS, Wershil BK. Gastric inflammation during systemic anaphylaxis: neutrophil recruitment in stomach wall of mice does not require mast cell participation. Dig Dis Sci 1998; 43:2021–2027.
15. Wilhelms OH, Lipponer L, Seilnacht W. Chemiluminescence (CL) in blood samples reflects leukocyte activation (LA) during anaphylactoid reactions in dogs. J Biolumin Chemilumin 1990; 5:197–202.
16. Movat HZ, Uriuhara T, Taichman NS, Rowsell HC, Mustard JF. The role of PMN-leucocyte lysosomes in tissue injury, inflammation and hypersensitivity. VI. The participation of the PMN–leucocyte and the blood platelet in systemic aggregate anaphylaxis. Immunology 1968; 14:637–648.
17. An S, Goetzl EJ. Lipid mediators of hypersensitivity and inflammation. In: Middleton E Jr, Reed CE, Ellis EF, Adkinson F Jr, Yunginger J, Busse WW, eds. Allergy Principles and Practice. 5th ed. St Louis: Mosby–Year Book, 1998:168–182.
18. Church MK, Holgate ST, Robinson C, Shute JK, Walls AF, Sampson AP. Mast cell-derived mediators. In: Middleton E Jr, Reed CE, Ellis EF, Adkinson F Jr, Yunginger J, Busse WW, eds. Allergy Principles and Practice. 5th ed. St Louis: Mosby–Year Book, 1998:146–167.
19. McManus LM, Hanahan DJ, Demopoulos CA, et al. Pathobiology of the intravenous infusion of acetyl glyceryl ether phosphorylcholine (AGEPC), a synthetic platelet-activating factor (PAF), in the rabbit. J Immunol 1980; 124:2919–2924.
20. Koller ME, Berg A, Rodt SA, Westerberg E, Reed RK. alpha-Trinositol prevents increased negativity of interstitial fluid pressure in rat skin and trachea induced by dextran anaphylaxis. Eur J Pharmacol 1997; 331:259–266.
21. Withers GD, Kubes P, Ibbotson G, Scott RB. Anaphylaxis-induced mesenteric vascular permeability, granuolyte adhesion and platelet aggregation in rat. Am J Physiol 1998; 275:H272–H284.
22. Lieberman P. Anaphylaxis and anaphylactoid reactions. In: Middleton E Jr, Reed CE, Ellis EF, Adkinson F Jr, Yunginger J, Busse WW, eds. Allergy Principles and Practice. 5th ed. St Louis: Mosby–Year Book, 1998:1079–1091.
23. Majno G, Palade GE. Studies on inflammation. I. The effect of histamine and serotonin on vascular permeability: an electron microscopic study. J Biophys Biochem Cytol 1961; 11: 571–596.
24. White MV. The role of histamine in allergic diseases. J Allergy Clin Immunol 1990; 86:599–605.
25. Hoigne R. The pathogenesis of allergic inflammation. Int Z Klin Pharmakol Ther Toxikol 1971; 5:171–178.

26. Hirasawa N, Watanabe M, Mue S, Tsurufuji S, Ohuchi K. Downward regulation of neutrophil infiltration by endogenous histamine without affecting vascular permeability responses in air-pouch-type carrageenin inflammation in rats. Inflammation 1991; 15:117–126.
27. Hirasawa N, Shiraishi M, Tokuhara N, Hirano Y, Mizutani A, Mue S, Ohuchi K. Pharmacological analysis of the inflammatory exudate-induced histamine production in bone marrow cells. Immunopharmacology 1997; 36:87–94.
28. Hirasawa N, Ohuchi K, Kawarasaki K, Watanabe M, Tsurufuji S. Occurrence of histamine-production-increasing factor in the postanaphylactic phase of allergic inflammation. Int Arch Allergy Appl Immunol 1989; 88:386–393.
29. Byrum RS, Goulet JL, Griffiths RJ, Koller BH. Role of the 5-lipoxygenase-activating protein (FLAP) in murine acute inflammatory responses. J Exp Med 1997; 185:1065–1075.
30. Malo PE, Bell RL, Shaughnessy TK, Summers JB, Brooks DW, Carter GW. The 5-lipoxygenase inhibitory activity of zileuton in in vitro and in vivo models of antigen-induced airway anaphylaxis. Pulm Pharmacol 1994; 7:73–79.
31. Goulet JL, Snouwaert JN, Latour AM, Coffman TM, Koller BH. Altered inflammatory responses in leukotriene-deficient mice. Proc Natl Acad Sci USA 1994; 91:12852–12856.
32. Chen XS, Sheller JR, Johnson EN, Funk CD. Role of leukotrienes revealed by targeted disruption of the 5-lipoxygenase gene. Nature 1994; 372:179–182.
33. Watanabe M, Ohuchi K, Sugidachi A, Hirasawa N, Hayashi Y, Tsurufuji S. Platelet-activating factor in the inflammatory exudate in the anaphylactic phase of allergic inflammation in rats. Int Arch Allergy Appl Immunol 1987; 84:396–403.
34. Vargaftig BB, Chignard M, Lefort J, Benveniste J. Platelet–tissue interaction: role of platelet-activating factor (PAF-acether). Agents Actions 1980; 10:502–506.
35. Pretolani M, Lellouch–Tubiana A, Lefort J, Bachelet M, Vargaftig BB. PAF-acether and experimental anaphylaxis as a model for asthma. Int Arch Allergy Appl Immunol 1989; 88:149–153.
36. Hogan AD, Schwartz LB. Markers of mast cell degranulation. Methods 1997; 13:43–52.
37. Schwartz LB, Huff TF. Biology of mast cells. In: Middleton E Jr, Reed CE, Ellis EF, Adkinson F Jr, Yunginger J, Busse WW, eds. Allergy Principles and Practice. 5th ed. St Louis: Mosby–Year Book, 1998:261–276.
38. Silva WD, Eisele JW, Lepow IH. Complement as a mediator of inflammation. 3. Purification of the activity with anaphylatoxin properties generated by interaction of the first four components of complement and its identification as a cleavage product of C′3. J Exp Med 1967; 126:1027–1048.
39. Mathison R, Carter L, Mowat C, Bissonnette E, Davison JS, Befus AD. Temporal analysis of the anti-inflammatory effects of decentralization of the rat superior cervical ganglia. Am J Physiol 1994; 266:R1537–R1543.
40. Mathison R, Hogan A, Helmer D, Bauce L, Woolner J, Davison JS, Schultz G, Befus D. Role for the submandibular gland in modulating pulmonary inflammation following induction of systemic anaphylaxis. Brain Behav Immun 1992; 6:117–129.
41. Ottlecz A, Koltai M, Blazso G, Minker E. Contribution to the regulatory role of insulin in inflammation and anaphylaxis. Int Arch Allergy Appl Immunol 1978; 56:284–286.
42. Church MK, Miller P. Proceedings: simple models of anaphylaxis and of histamine and 5-hydroxytryptamine induced inflammation using the mouse pinna. Br J Pharmacol 1975; 55:315.
43. Koltai M, Blazso G, Minker E, Lonovics J, Ottlecz A. Anaphylactoid–inflammation-promoting factor. An insulin-induced factor derived from nonsensitized lymphocytes increases anaphylactoid inflammation in rats. Int Arch Allergy Appl Immunol 1975; 49:358–370.
44. Koltai M, Ottlecz A, Minker E, Blazso G. Sensitization by insulin of the anaphylactoid inflammation in rats. Int Arch Allergy Appl Immunol 1974; 46:261–274.
45. Tarayre JP, Aliaga M, Barbara M, Malfetes N, Vieu S, Tisne–Versailles J. Bronchial inflam-

mation and hyperreactivity after anaphylactic shock in guinea pigs actively sensitized by systemic or aerosol route. Methods Find Exp Clin Pharmacol 1991; 13:93–97.
46. Gulbenkian AR, Fernandez X, Kreutner W, Minnicozzi M, Watnick AS, Kung T, Egan RW. Anaphylactic challenge causes eosinophil accumulation in bronchoalveolar lavage fluid of guinea pigs. Modulation by betamethasone, phenidone, indomethacin, WEB 2086, and a novel antiallergy agent, SCH 37224. Am Rev Respir Dis 1990; 142:680–685.
47. Tarayre JP, Aliaga M, Barbara M, Malefetes N, Vieu S, Tisne–Versailles J. Theophyline reduces pulmonary eosinophilia after various types of active anaphylactic shock in guinea pigs. J Pharm Pharmacol 1991; 43:877–879.
48. Raud J. Intravital microscopic studies on acute mast cell-dependent inflammation. Acta Physiol Scand Suppl 1989; 578:1–58.

19

Nonanaphylactic Drug Disorders

ROLAND SOLENSKY and REBECCA S. GRUCHALLA

The University of Texas Southwestern Medical Center at Dallas, Dallas, Texas

1 INTRODUCTION

Adverse drug reactions (ADRs) are an everyday occurrence in both the inpatient and outpatient settings. An anaphylactic reaction to a medication is perhaps the most dramatic example of a drug-induced reaction. On the other hand, nonanaphylactic drug reactions are more common, and they are a greater cause of morbidity. Although some nonanaphylactic reactions, such as delayed maculopapular rashes, are not serious, others, such as toxic epidermal necrolysis, can be severe and potentially fatal. Unfortunately, the mechanisms responsible for many drug reactions remain unknown. Research in the 1960s and early 1970s resulted in major advances in the understanding of immediate-type allergic reactions to penicillin. Since this period, unlike other fields of medicine, the field of drug allergy has advanced relatively slowly. However, recent technological advances have increased interest in basic drug allergy research. Consequently, significant strides have been made in our understanding of several types of drug-induced reactions. For example, as techniques to evaluate T-cell function have improved, so has our ability to study the cellular arm of the immune system and, as a result, the importance of T cells in various allergic reactions is being recognized.

In this chapter, we will first review the classification of ADRs, as well as general concepts of drug metabolism, drug presentation to the immune system, and types of drug hypersensitivity reactions. As shown in Table 1, nonanaphylactic drug disorders encompass a wide array of reactions. Unfortunately, space limitations do not allow, in a single chapter, a comprehensive discussion of all of these disorders. Most of these disorders are assumed to be immune-mediated, but frequently the underlying immune mechanism has not been established. Because nonanaphylactic IgE-mediated drug reactions, such as urticaria, have the same underlying mechanism as anaphylactic reactions, they will not be

Table 1 Partial List of Nonanaphylactic Drug Disorders

Multisystem	Lung
Hypersensitivity syndrome	Bronchospasm
Serum sickness and serum sickness-like reactions	Pulmonary fibrosis
Drug fever	Pulmonary edema
Vasculitis	Pulmonary infiltrates with eosinophilia
Lupus erythematosus-like syndrome	Liver
Generalized lymphadenopathy	Hepatitis
Skin	Cholestasis
Maculopapular or morbilliform rashes	Kidney
Stevens–Johnson syndrome	Interstitial nephritis
Toxic epidermal necrolysis	Nephrotic syndrome
Urticaria and angioedema	Heart
Fixed drug eruptions	Myocarditis
Contact dermatitis	
Photosensitivity	
Erythema nodosum	
Bone marrow	
Hemolytic anemia	
Thrombocytopenia	
Neutropenia	
Aplastic anemia	
Eosinophilia	

included in our discussion. We refer the reader to Chapter 18 in this text, which provides a full discussion of anaphylactic reactions.

We will discuss, in detail, the following disorders: Stevens–Johnson syndrome (SJS) and toxic epidermal necrolysis (TEN), hypersensitivity syndrome (HSS), serum sickness-like reactions (SSLR), and maculopapular or morbilliform delayed cutaneous reactions. We have chosen these particular reactions because new and exciting data have emerged in recent years concerning their underlying immunopathogenesis, and our discussion will focus on the pathophysiology involved. We will discuss clinical features briefly, and we will mention diagnosis and treatment only when they help elucidate the underlying mechanisms. For a more complete review of diagnosis and treatment options, we refer the reader to several recent texts (1–3).

2 DEFINITION, INCIDENCE, AND CLASSIFICATION OF ADRs

Nonanaphylactic drug reactions, similar to all drug-induced reactions, fall under the ''umbrella'' category of ADRs. An *adverse drug reaction* (ADR) has been defined by the World Health Organization (WHO) as any noxious, unintended, and undesired effect of a drug, which occurs at doses used in humans for prevention, diagnosis, or treatment (4). Because reporting of ADRs is often incomplete and evaluation of the reactions retrospectively can be challenging, it has been difficult to determine their true incidence. Nevertheless, available studies suggest that ADRs are a significant and not uncommon problem among hospitalized patients. In a recent metanalysis of 39 studies, Lazarou et al. found that among hospitalized patients, the overall incidence of serious and nonserious ADRs

Table 2 Classification of Adverse Drug Reactions

Predictable reactions (type A)
Overdosage
Side effects
Secondary effects
Drug–drug interactions
Unpredictable reactions (type B)
Intolerance
Idiosyncratic
Allergic

was 6.7 and 8.4%, respectively (5). Furthermore, the incidence of fatal ADRs was 0.32%. Applying these findings to all hospitalized United States patients, the authors estimated that in 1994, 2,216,000 hospitalized patients had serious ADRs and that 106,000 had fatal ADRs. Although similar data for ambulatory patients is not as readily available, it is likely that ADRs also commonly occur in the outpatient setting. It is clear from such data that ADRs contribute greatly to the cost of hospital care. A recent estimate of the cost of screening, diagnosis, and therapy of ADRs in the United States was determined to be 3 billion dollars annually (6).

Although many physicians and patients commonly refer to all ADRs as being ''allergic,'' true allergic drug reactions account for only 6–10% of all observed ADRs (3). Hence, the term ''drug allergy'' should be applied only to those reactions that are known (or presumed) to be mediated by an immunological mechanism. A useful classification system for ADRs was developed by Rawlins and Thompson (7). They divided ADRs into two broad categories: predictable (also called type A) reactions, and unpredictable (or type B) reactions (Table 2). Predictable reactions are usually dose-dependent, they are related to the known pharmacological actions of the drug, and they occur in otherwise normal patients. Examples of type A reactions include acetaminophen-induced hepatic necrosis (overdose), β-agonist-associated tremor (side effect), clindamycin-associated *Clostridium difficile* pseudomembranous colitis (secondary effect), and cardiac arrhythmia resulting from the combination use of terfenadine and imidazole antifungals (drug–drug interaction).

In contrast, unpredictable reactions are usually dose-independent, they are not related to the pharmacological actions of the drug, and they occur only in susceptible individuals. Examples of type B reactions include aspirin-induced tinnitus while taking conventional dosages (intolerance), hemolytic anemia resulting from oxidant drugs given to glucose-6-phosphate dehydrogenase(G6PD)-deficient individuals (idiosyncratic reaction), and penicillin-induced anaphylaxis (allergic reaction). Although type A reactions make up approximately 80% of all ADRs, the majority of serious and life-threatening reactions are unpredictable and thus fall into the type B category (3,5).

3 CLASSIFICATION OF ALLERGIC DRUG REACTIONS

Allergic drug reactions belong to the category of type B unpredictable reactions. They are distinguished from other type B reactions in that they are mediated by an immune mechanism. Some allergic drug reactions can be classified using the Gell and Coombs

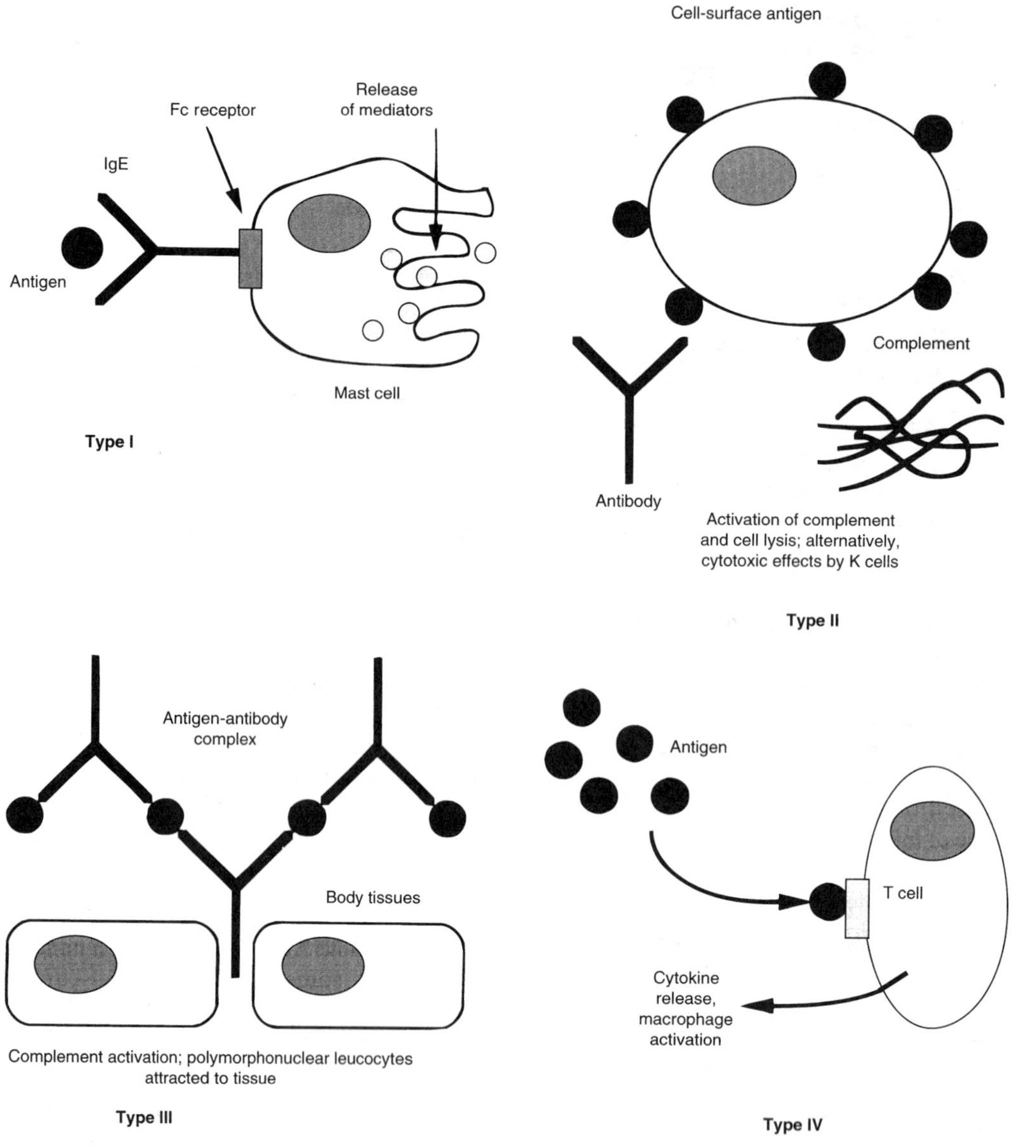

Figure 1 The Gell and Coombs classification scheme of allergic drug reactions. (From Ref. 6.)

classification scheme (8), which, although described initially for hypersensitivity reactions in general, is widely used to classify drug-induced allergic reactions. In this system, there are four types of hypersensitivity reactions (Fig. 1): immediate hypersensitivity reactions mediated by antigen-specific IgE antibodies (type I); cytotoxic antibody-mediated reactions against a cell surface (type II); immune complex deposition reactions (type III); and delayed T-cell–mediated reactions (type IV). Some drug reactions fit nicely into one of these categories. For example, treatment with penicillin has been associated with each of these four types of reactions—namely, anaphylaxis (type I), hemolytic anemia (type II), SSLR (type III), and contact dermatitis to topically applied penicillin (type IV).

Unfortunately, in many instances, it is not possible to classify drug reactions because the mechanism responsible for their elicitation is unknown. In other cases for which we have insight into the mechanism underlying drug reactions, it has become clear that some reactions cannot be classified using the traditional Gell and Coombs scheme. Several of the mechanisms to be discussed in this chapter fall in this unclassifiable category. In the future, as our understanding of basic mechanisms responsible for reactions are further elucidated, new classification schemes will need to be developed.

4 DRUG METABOLISM AND THE HAPTEN HYPOTHESIS

Some drugs, such as β-lactam antibiotics, can covalently bind to proteins (after spontaneous degradation) to cause hypersensitivity reactions without first undergoing metabolism. However, it is now well established that most drugs must be metabolized (or "bioactivated") to chemically reactive intermediates to form bonds with tissue components (9). Therefore, to understand the types of hypersensitivity reactions that drugs may produce, it is critical to understand how they are metabolized. In general, drug metabolism is considered a detoxification process, whereby drugs are converted from lipid-soluble, nonpolar compounds to more polar, hydrophilic compounds that are easily excreted. Usually metabolism takes place in two steps. The first step consists of oxidation, reduction, or hydrolysis (phase I reactions), whereas the second step is conjugation (phase II reactions). Oxidation reactions involve enzymes such as cytochrome P450, prostaglandin synthetase, and various tissue peroxidases (9). Phase II reactions are mediated by enzymes such as epoxide hydrolase, glutathione *S*-transferase (GTS), and *N*-acetyltransferase (NAT) (9).

In most instances, reactive drug intermediates are promptly detoxified (or "bioinactivated") to nonreactive products. In certain circumstances, however, reactive metabolites are able to cause injury by either direct toxicity or by immune-mediated hypersensitivity (Fig. 2) (10). Increased levels of reactive intermediates can result from increased bioactivation or from decreased detoxification, or both. In direct toxicity, chemically reactive metabolites bind to proteins or nucleic acids and cause cellular necrosis or gene mutations. Alternatively, reactive metabolites may covalently bind to macromolecules and act as haptens, leading to the initiation of an immune response. This theory is referred to as the *hapten hypothesis* (11). The immune response may be directed toward the hapten, the hapten–macromolecule complex, or toward a new antigenic determinant (neoantigen) that is created. The elicited response may be humoral, with the production of specific antibodies; cellular, with the generation of specific T lymphocytes; or both. Because they are rare, reactions of this type are not detected in early human clinical trials, nor are they generally detected by routine animal toxicology studies. In summary, the development of an ADR mediated by reactive drug metabolites is dependent on the chemical nature of the drug, the individual differences in drug metabolism, the nature of the target cellular macromolecule, and an individual's immune system genotype (12).

5 SPECIFIC DISORDERS

5.1 Stevens–Johnson Syndrome and Toxic Epidermal Necrolysis

CLINICAL FEATURES. Both SJS and TEN are mucocutaneous disorders that most clinicians believe are severity variants of the same underlying disease process. In the early 1990s, Bastuji–Garin et al. developed a commonly used classification scheme based on

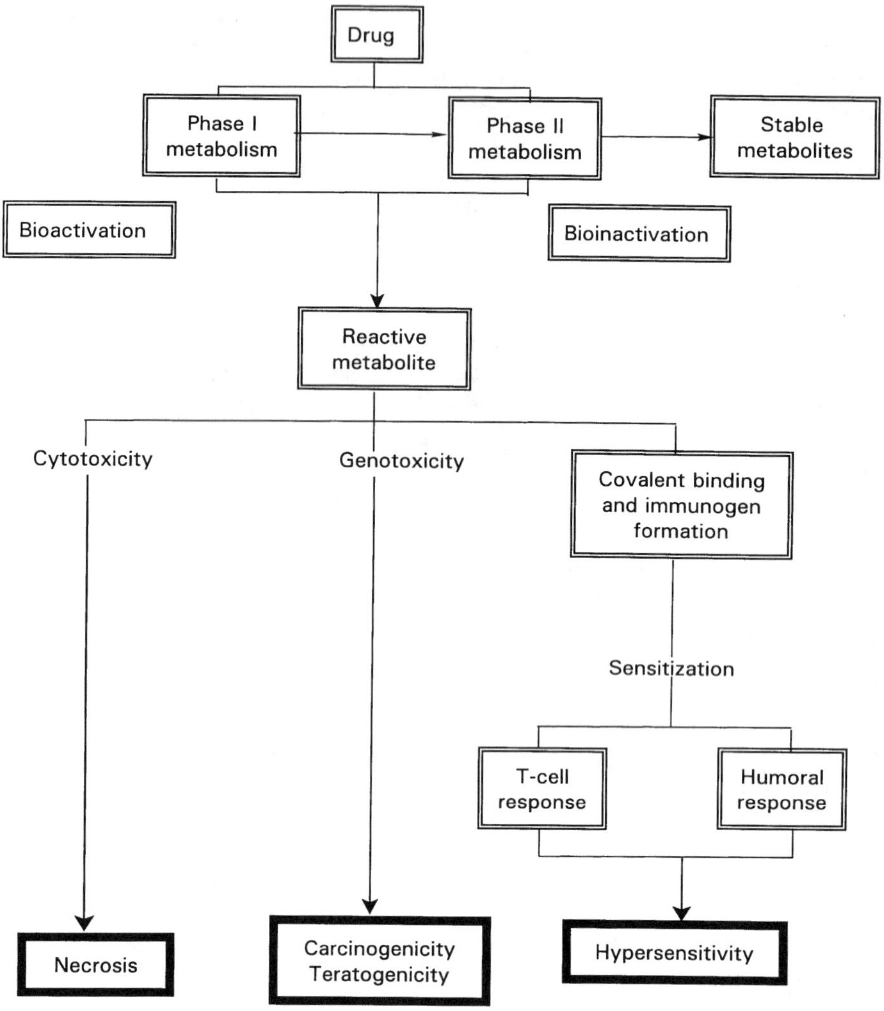

Figure 2 The role of drug-metabolizing enzymes in the bioactivation and bioinactivation of drugs. (Reprinted from Clinical Pharmacokinetics 1996; 31(3):215–230, with permission. Copyright Adis International, Inc.)

this belief (13). According to this scheme, both diseases have bullous lesions and mucosal involvement, but they differ in the extent of skin detachment: less than 10% in SJS and more than 30% in TEN. Patients with 10–30% skin detachment are classified as having "overlap SJS/TEN." Other investigators consider the two to be distinct disorders, and there continues to be no consensus on diagnostic criteria for these conditions (14). SJS and TEN are drug-induced in about 50 and 80% of patients, respectively, and the onset of symptoms is usually within 1–3 weeks after the initiation of therapy (15). More than 100 drugs have been implicated as causes of SJS and TEN (15), with the most frequent offenders being sulfonamides, aromatic anticonvulsants, β-lactam antibiotics, allopurinol, and nonsteroidal anti-inflammatory drugs (NSAIDs) (16–18).

Because there are no universally accepted definitions for SJS and TEN and some cases are classified as overlap SJS/TEN, it is difficult to discuss one disorder without the other. In the published literature, depending on the particular author's diagnostic definitions, a given patient could be classified as having either diagnosis. Hence, for this reason, and because SJS and TEN clearly share many clinical similarities, we have chosen to discuss the pathogenesis of the two disorders collectively.

PATHOGENESIS. For many years after the initial descriptions of SJS, in 1922 (19), and TEN, in 1956 (20), the pathogenesis underlying these disorders remained unknown. Research in recent years has begun to shed light on potential mechanisms by which drugs can lead to these diseases. Nevertheless, several questions remain unanswered, especially for the final pathway of tissue damage.

The initial event in the pathogenesis of SJS and TEN is thought to be an alteration in the detoxification of reactive drug metabolites that are produced by phase I metabolism (15,21). That is, susceptible individuals fail to metabolize (''detoxify'') drug intermediates normally, which subsequently lead to end-organ damage. Differences in drug metabolism predispose patients to both SJS and TEN (22,23), as well as certain other adverse drug reactions (9), some of which will be discussed later in this chapter. All of these studies utilized the ''lymphocyte toxicity assay,'' an in vitro assay developed by Spielberg (24) in which human lymphocytes are exposed to drug metabolites generated by a mouse hepatic microsomal system as a source of cytochrome P450 enzymes (Fig. 3). The level of toxicity to the cells is measured by the extent of cell death. Lymphocytes were chosen for the assay not for their immunological properties, but rather, because they are easily obtainable, and they contain detoxifying phase II enzymes that act as defenses against reactive metabolites. Therefore, it is important to realize that a positive result does not necessarily prove the causality of direct toxicity in cellular damage. Shear et al. (22) and Wolkenstein et al. (23) each have shown that when lymphocytes from patients with SJS and TEN are challenged with the culprit drug in this assay, there is a greater extent of cell death in lymphocytes from patients with SJS and TEN than in cells from normal controls when these are challenged with the culprit drug. Both investigators also found that first-degree relatives of the patients had intermediate levels of toxicity compared with patients and controls.

The issue of whether reactive drug metabolites produced by phase I metabolism cause direct cellular toxicity in SJS and TEN, or whether cell damage is mediated by the immune system remains controversial. Although it is possible that in some cases drug metabolites cause direct cellular toxicity, there are many lines of evidence that support the involvement of an immunological mechanism in these disorders. These include (1) the timing of an initial reaction (1–3 weeks after initiation of therapy) (18,25); (2) the timing of a recurrent reaction (within 48 hr of rechallenge) (18,25); (3) the linkage of SJS and TEN to particular HLA genotypes (26,27); (4) the association between TEN and graft-versus-host disease (28–30); and (5) the occurrence of Sjogren-like syndromes as sequelae in patients with TEN (16,31).

Because of these features, most experts have long suspected that SJS and TEN are immune-mediated reactions. However, direct evidence linking these disorders to particular types of allergic reactions is sparse. Efforts to demonstrate circulating cytotoxic antibodies, circulating immune complexes, complement activation, and specific cutaneous deposits have been unsuccessful, or have shown inconsistent results (32).

There is now a growing body of evidence to suggest that T lymphocytes play a critical role in the development of SJS and TEN. By using immunohistochemical staining of involved skin, several investigators have shown that the epidermal inflammatory infil-

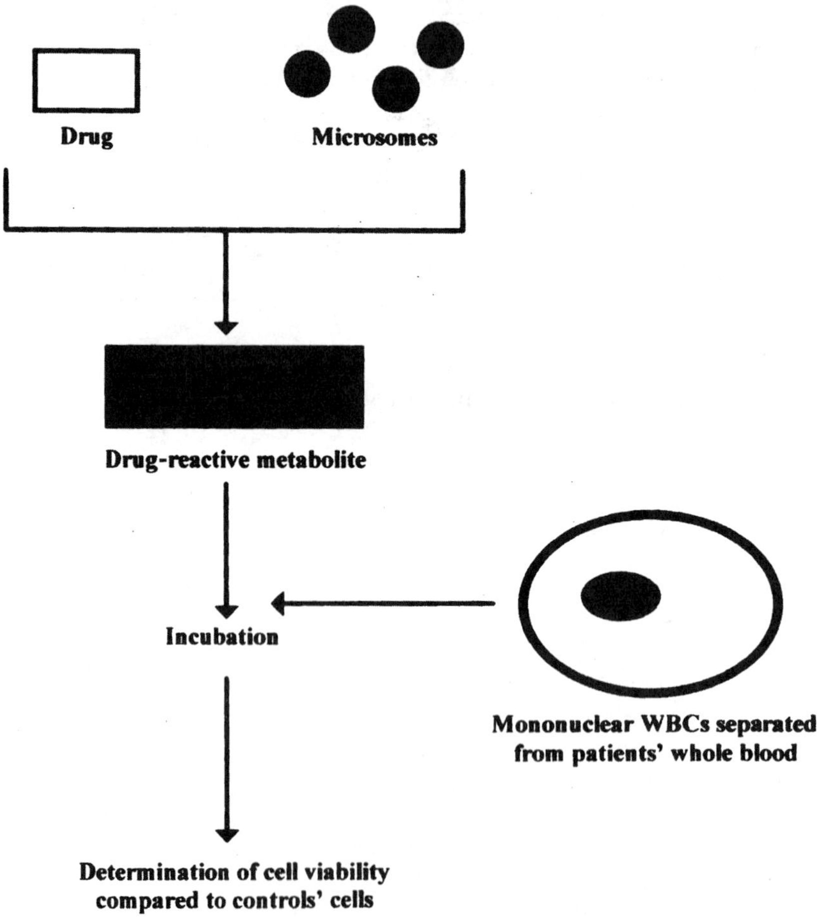

Figure 3 Lymphocyte toxicity assay using murine microsomes as a source of cytochrome P450 enzymes. (From Ref. 83.)

trate is composed primarily of $CD8^+$ T cells, whereas the dermal infiltrate is composed mostly of $CD4^+$ T cells (33–39). Similarly, analysis of blister fluid by Correia et al. revealed a predominance of $CD8^+$ lymphocytes (40). Further study of the blister lymphocytes by means of flow cytometry revealed that they, but not peripheral blood lymphocytes, were primarily $CD45RA^-$ and $CD29^+$. This finding suggests that the lymphocytes in blister fluid are antigen-primed memory T cells; they coexpress adhesion molecules, such as very late adhesion antigens (VLA), which could mediate their interaction with skin endothelium and extracellular matrix proteins. As a control, these investigators also analyzed blister fluid from burn patients. Interestingly, less than 5% of the inflammatory cells were lymphocytes, with most of the cells being neutrophils.

Although studies such as these demonstrated the presence of T lymphocytes in the skin of patients with SJS and TEN, they did not show those T cells to be specifically reactive to the suspect drug. Therefore, one could argue that the cellular infiltrate is not causal, but rather is a secondary phenomenon. Findings in more recent studies have suggested drug-specific reactivity in the T cells. In 1993, Hertl and colleagues generated epidermal $CD8^+$ T-cell clones (TCC) from the cutaneous lesions of two patients with penicillin-induced SJS (37). The TCC proliferated in response to penicillin-pulsed autologous peripheral blood mononuclear cells (PBMC), but not to allogeneic PBMC, indicating that the clones were antigen- and MHC-specific. In 1995, in a similar experiment, Hertl's group isolated dermal $CD8^+$ T-lymphocyte clones from the lesional skin of a patient with trimethoprim–sulfamethoxazole-induced TEN (39). One of the clones proliferated to sulfamethoxazole (but not trimethoprim) in a dose-dependent manner, and it was also restricted by the presence of autologous (but not allogeneic) PBMC.

From these data, it is postulated that keratinocyte damage results from $CD8^+$ T cells recognizing a given drug (or its metabolite) complexed with major histocompatibility complex (MHC) class I molecules on the surface of keratinocytes. In reality, the process is likely to be more complex, because compared with the extent of cell death that occurs, the population of T lymphocytes that is present is relatively sparse. Much of the damage is probably due to cytokines that are released, such as tumor necrosis factor-alpha (TNF-α) (41). Furthermore, it is likely that, in addition to $CD8^+$ T cells, other immune cells, such as macrophages (38,41,42), are recruited and contribute to the immune response.

Until recently, the final pathway resulting in keratinocyte death in SJS and TEN remained unknown. Cell death occurs by one of two mechanisms: apoptosis or necrosis. Apoptosis, or programmed cell death, is a genetically controlled process that provides the means for regulating the number and types of cells in tissues (43). For example, healthy skin normally contains a small percentage of apoptotic cells (44). Necrosis, on the other hand, is associated with abnormal physiological conditions, such as hypoxia and ischemia, disruption of cell membrane by complement, and exposure to toxins. Because SJS and TEN are assumed to be immunologically mediated reactions, apoptosis would be expected to play a role in the method of cell death. In 1996, Paul et al. (45) studied five patients with either TEN or overlap SJS/TEN and provided the first evidence for apoptosis as the mechanism of keratinocyte death in these diseases. Using three different methods to detect apoptotic cells, these investigators found extensive apoptosis in the epidermis of cutaneous lesions from each of the patients. The stimulus responsible for the apoptosis was not studied, although the authors hypothesized that an immune mechanism was involved.

Recently, Viard and colleagues (46) studied the potential role of Fas and Fas ligand (FasL or CD95) in TEN and provided the first clue to the mechanism responsible for enhanced keratinocyte apoptosis in this disease process. In the first part of their study, they demonstrated that (1) keratinocytes obtained by skin biopsy from patients with TEN expressed large amounts of FasL, (2) the skin section keratinocytes induced Fas-mediated cell death in Fas-sensitive target cells, and (3) this cytotoxicity was completely abrogated by incubation with FasL-blocking monoclonal antibody. In contrast, in patients with drug-induced maculopapular rashes and in healthy controls, there was no evidence of keratinocyte FasL on skin biopsy, and skin sections failed to produce cell death in target cells. In the second part of their study, they showed that physiological concentrations of intravenous immunoglobulin (IVIG) completely inhibited Fas-mediated keratinocyte apoptosis by blocking the Fas receptor. They proceeded to treat ten consecutive patients who had acute TEN with IVIG for 4 days, and reported a rapid improvement in each patient's skin disease. The authors concluded that upregulation of keratinocyte FasL expression is a critical trigger for keratinocyte destruction during TEN, and that IVIG preparations contain naturally occurring Fas-blocking antibodies, which may make it a potentially useful therapeutic agent in TEN. Clearly, the efficacy of IVIG in TEN will need to be confirmed with controlled trials in the future. From this early evidence, however, it shows promise as an antiapoptotic medication.

5.2 Hypersensitivity Syndrome

CLINICAL FEATURES. Drug-induced HSS is an uncommon, potentially fatal multiorgan disorder caused by exposure to a limited number of medications, including aromatic anticonvulsants (phenytoin, phenobarbital, and carbamazepine), sulfonamides, allopurinol, and minocycline (47). HSS usually appears 2–4 weeks after the initiation of therapy, although it may present as late as 3 months into therapy. Fever, rash, and lymphadenopathy are the first symptoms to appear, and they are also the most common. The rash, which usually begins as patchy macular erythema, may become indurated or progress to an exfoliative dermatitis. Variable numbers of patients with HSS experience or develop hepatitis, hematological abnormalities (including eosinophilia and atypical lymphocytosis), myalgias or arthralgias, renal dysfunction, and pneumonitis. Over 60% of patients have multiorgan–system involvement (excluding the hematological system) (48).

PATHOGENESIS. As in SJS and TEN, the initiating event leading to drug-induced HSS is thought to involve drug metabolism to active intermediates. Aromatic anticonvulsants are metabolized in part by cytochrome P450 to arene oxides, which are highly reactive molecules (11). Several investigators have utilized the lymphocyte toxicity assay (described earlier in Sec. 5.1) to evaluate patients who have a history of anticonvulsant-induced HSS. Following exposure to the culprit drug, the death rate of lymphocytes from these patients was significantly higher than the death rate seen in cells of controls (48–50). When hepatic microsomes were omitted from the incubation, the lymphocyte death rate was not significantly different between HSS patients and controls (48,49), proving that metabolites, rather than the parent compound, were responsible for the toxicity. In addition, the drug-induced toxicity in lymphocytes of parents of HSS patients was intermediate between that seen in lymphocytes of HSS patients and of normal controls (48,49). These data suggest that the development of HSS may be related to individual genetic polymorphism in the enzymes that metabolize these drugs. Arene oxides, for example, are detoxified by the phase II enzyme epoxide hydrolase (11). The addition of a noncompetitive inhibitor of epoxide hydrolase to the lymphocyte toxicity assay of control patients increased their lymphocyte death rate to that seen in patients with HSS (49). Therefore, it has been postulated that individuals with HSS may have an inherited deficiency of epoxide hydrolase. However, characterization of the epoxide hydrolase gene itself has failed to show any differences between patients with HSS and controls (51). It is still possible that defects occurring in the regulatory region of the gene may alter expression of the protein or, alternatively, that there is a deficiency in needed cofactors.

There is a similar body of evidence that implicates sulfonamide metabolites in the pathogenesis of sulfonamide-induced HSS. Sulfonamides are metabolized predominantly by *N*-acetylation to nonreactive metabolites, but a small amount of the drug undergoes *N*-oxidation catalyzed by cytochrome P450 enzymes to form reactive hydroxylamine and nitroso intermediates (9). In the lymphocyte toxicity assay, lymphocytes from patients who had experienced sulfonamide-induced HSS showed significantly more cell death than those of controls, and there was an intermediate level of toxicity in lymphocytes of first-degree relatives (22). Potential (and yet unproved) abnormalities in these patients include defects in phase II enzymes (such as glutathione-dependent enzymes and hydroxylase reductases) and deficiencies in certain intracellular molecules that protect against reactive metabolites (such as glutathione) (12).

Another interesting observation is that a disproportionate number of patients who experience sulfonamide HSS have a genetic polymorphism resulting in low levels of *N*-acetyltransferase (''slow acetylators''). Whereas the general population is equally divided into fast and slow acetylators, more than 90% of patients with sulfonamide HSS are slow acetylators (52). It is unclear how slow acetylation serves as a risk factor for sulfonamide HSS, but it is theorized that slow acetylators have more parent drug available for oxidative metabolism by P450 enzymes, resulting in increased production of hydroxylamines (52). It is also possible that the *N*-acetylation genetic locus simply is linked to another genetic locus that is somehow immunologically important in the generation of sulfonamide reactions (9). Clearly, as half of the population is composed of slow acetylators, yet sulfonamide reactions are rare, factors other than a metabolic defect must be present for a reaction to occur.

Although the generation of drug metabolites seems to be essential for the development of HSS, the ultimate mechanism of cellular damage is unknown. That is, the extent to which immune effects and direct toxicity play roles has not been established. For sulfamethoxazole, it appears that a nonallergic mechanism is partly operative. There is limited evidence showing that the hydroxylamine metabolite causes a direct toxic effect, leading to the suppression of T-cell proliferation, mitogen-driven immunoglobulin responses, and natural killer cell activity (53–55).

On the other hand, clinical features of HSS, such as the presence of fever, lymphadenopathy, eosinophilia, and atypical lymphocytosis, suggest an immune-mediated mechanism. Furthermore, there appears to be a period of ''sensitization'' after initiation of therapy, and when patients have been rechallenged, the onset of symptoms is within a day, if not within hours (47,56,57). According to the hapten hypothesis, one would expect that reactive metabolites would covalently bind to proteins and lead to an immune response, but until recently, confirmation of any such humoral or cellular response was lacking. Beginning in the early 1990s, Leeder and others demonstrated the presence of antimicrosomal antibodies directed against members of the cytochrome P450 family in patients with anticonvulsant HSS (58–60). Their results indicate that arene oxides may form neoantigens by binding to P450 enzymes. Analogous P450 autoantigen formation previously has been implicated in hepatotoxic reactions secondary to similarly metabolized drugs (such as halothane, tienilic acid, and dihydralazine) (61), but never in a multisystem disorder such as HSS. It is not clear how such antibodies would affect organs other than the liver, because the expression of similar antigens in other organs is not known.

Recently, convincing evidence has emerged showing the involvement of drug-specific T cells in the pathogenesis of drug-induced HSS. Mauri–Hellweg and colleagues studied patients with HSS secondary to sulfamethoxazole, phenytoin, or carbamazepine administration (62). In vitro, they demonstrated drug-induced lymphocyte proliferation of both $CD4^+$ and $CD8^+$ drug-specific T cells. The authors concluded that drug-modified peptides could be presented on either MHC class I or MHC class II molecules, because drug-modified self-proteins have access to processing pathways leading to either MHC class I or class II presentation. Analysis of cytokines produced by the drug-stimulated cell cultures revealed very high amounts of interleukin(IL)-5, which is the most important stimulus for eosinophil production, chemotaxis, and activation (63). In 1998, Choquet–Kastylevsky et al. provided further confirmation for the role of IL-5 in drug-induced HSS

(56). They prospectively followed IL-5 levels in patients with acute HSS and found that levels peaked shortly before the onset of eosinophilia, implying that the IL-5 was derived from activated lymphocytes, rather than from eosinophils.

Because HSS shares many clinical features with certain viral infections, such as infectious, mononucleosis, a role for viruses in the disorder has been postulated. Associations between viral infections and drug reactions have been described in the past, but an underlying mechanism has not been established. Two notable examples are ampicillin-induced rashes during Epstein–Barr virus mononucleosis (64,65), and the high incidence of sulfonamide-induced drug rashes in patients infected with human immunodeficiency virus (HIV) (66,67). There are no data that show a causal role for viruses in HSS, but several investigators have described patients who appeared to have a reactivation of human herpesvirus 6 (HHV-6) during acute drug-induced HSS episodes (57,68,69). An intriguing hypothesis put forth by Suzuki et al. (57) is that reactivation of HHV-6 may cause the production of autoantibodies against cytochrome P450 phase II enzymes, inhibiting their function and leading to deficient detoxification and a buildup of reactive drug intermediates. The authors pointed out that such a mechanism would be compatible with previous data showing anti-P450 antibodies in patients with HSS and in patients infected with viral hepatitis (61,70). Further research in this area will, we hope, help clarify what role, if any, viruses such as HHV-6 play in the pathogenesis of drug-induced HSS.

5.3 Serum Sickness-like Reactions

CLINICAL FEATURES. Drug-associated serum sickness-like reactions (SSLRs) are so named because they share several clinical features with serum sickness. SSLRs occur 5–10 days after the initiation of therapy and are characterized by skin rash (most commonly urticaria or erythema multiform), arthropathy, and fever. Unlike true serum sickness, lymphadenopathy is uncommon, and the presence of renal and hepatic abnormalities is rare (71). Patients with SSLRs generally recover without sequelae. SSLRs have been associated with various antibiotics (71–73). However, the second-generation cephalosporin cefaclor appears particularly prone to cause SSLRs. Soon after cefaclor was introduced into clinical practice in the United States in 1979, a cluster of SSLRs associated with its use was described (74). Subsequently, several studies have shown the incidence of cefaclor-associated SSLRs to be higher than that for other antibiotics, confirming many physicians' clinical experience (72,73, 75,76).

PATHOGENESIS. The type III hypersensitivity reaction is caused by the formation of circulating antibody–antigen complexes that are deposited in small vessels, particularly of the skin and joints, resulting in fixation of complement and tissue damage (8). Because of its similarity to serum sickness, drug-associated SSLRs have been assumed to be a type III allergic reaction, but there are no reports of circulating immune complexes, hypocomplementemia, or immunoglobulin deposition in vascular endothelium in patients with SSLRs (as there are in serum sickness) (71,76,77). It is possible that some other mechanism, such as a T-cell–mediated process, is operative in SSLRs, although the role of T cells has not been investigated. Hence, owing to a dearth of data, the underlying immunological process remains a mystery.

Because the time course and some manifestations of SSLRs are similar to sulfonamide and aromatic anticonvulsant-induced HSS, Kearns and colleagues investigated the role of drug metabolism in cefaclor-associated SSLRs (78,79). By utilizing the lymphocyte toxicity assay, they demonstrated a significantly greater extent of lymphocyte death in patients with a history of cefaclor-associated SSLRs, compared with control subjects who previously had tolerated cefaclor therapy. The level of toxicity in lymphocytes from patients who had a history of an immediate hypersensitivity reaction to cefaclor or a delayed reaction without joint involvement did not differ from those of controls. When the assay was performed in the absence of microsomes, or with microsomes that had been boiled, the extent of cell death of patients with SSLRs decreased greatly, suggesting that a metabolite, rather than the parent drug, was responsible for the observed results. Interestingly, the level of toxicity in lymphocytes of five of six mothers of SSLR patients (but only one of six fathers) was similar to that observed in the cells of the index patients. Although these data suggest a pharmacogenetic basis for the reaction, the pattern of inheritance appears to be different from that observed in patients with sulfonamide- and anticonvulsant-induced reactions, in whom intermediate levels of toxicity were found.

Less is known about the metabolism of cefaclor than about sulfonamides or aromatic anticonvulsants. The chemical nature of the reactive metabolite (or metabolites) of cefaclor has not been determined. Likewise, it is not known which phase I cytochrome P450 enzymes catalyze the conversion of cefaclor to reactive intermediates, or which phase II enzymes are possibly deficient in susceptible patients. However, the presumed cefaclor metabolic defect appears to differ from the one associated with aromatic anticonvulsants, because sera from anticonvulsant-induced HSS patients (who previously had positive lymphocyte toxicity assays with anticonvulsants) did not have positive lymphocyte toxicity assay results with cefaclor (78). Unlike sulfonamides and aromatic anticonvulsants, which show intraclass cross-reactivity in the lymphocyte toxicity assay, there is no in vitro cross-reactivity between cefaclor and other cephalosporins (including loracarbef, which differs from cefaclor only by the replacement of the sulfur at the 5 position by a methylene group) (79). Hence, it may be safe for patients who experienced cefaclor-associated SSLRs to receive other cephalosporins. Despite that metabolism of cefaclor appears to be essential for the SSLRs associated with the drug, the final mechanism of injury remains to be determined.

5.4 Maculopapular and Morbilliform Eruptions

CLINICAL FEATURES. Maculopapular or morbilliform rashes are the most common cutaneous adverse drug reactions, and they may occur with the administration of any drug. Most frequently, they are associated with the use of β-lactams, sulfonamides, anticonvulsants, allopurinol, and NSAIDs (3). These eruptions preferentially involve the trunk and extremities in a symmetrical fashion, and usually spare the face, palms, and soles. The lesions commonly appear within 10 days of the initiation of therapy, and consist of erythematous macules or papules. However, the lesions can be pleomorphic and may vary in appearance even in a single patient. The rash may be accompanied by pruritus, fever, and malaise, and occasionally, it may become confluent. The symptoms generally resolve rapidly after discontinuation of the culprit drug, in which case the patient recovers without sequelae. Rarely (and especially with continued drug administration), the rash may progress to SJS or TEN.

PATHOGENESIS. Given the variety of unrelated drugs and the heterogeneity of symptoms that are associated with drug-induced maculopapular or morbilliform rashes, it is likely that more than one mechanism is operative. Drug-specific IgE antibodies do not appear to play a role in these rashes (21,80). Likewise, no causal role for drug-specific IgG antibodies has been found (21). The delayed nature of maculopapular rashes suggests a cellular-mediated process, and this feature prompted investigation into the possible role of T cells. Indeed, results from the lymphocyte transformation test (LTT) do support their involvement. In this in vitro assay, the patient's PBMCs are cocultured with nontoxic concentrations of the suspected drug, and lymphocyte activation is determined after 5–7 days by the incorporation of radioactive thymidine. An enhanced proliferative response in the presence of the suspected drug is interpreted as a sign of drug-specific T-cell stimulation. Positive LTT results have been reported in patients who had delayed eruptions caused by a variety of drugs (81,82). Although the sensitivity, specificity, and reproducibility of the LTT are not well established, positive findings nevertheless suggest a role for T cells (81,83). Additionally, patch tests and delayed intradermal skin tests with the culprit drugs, have shown positive results in a fraction of affected patients (84–87), indicating that at least some maculopapular eruptions may be T-cell–mediated. It is possible, however, that patch testing underestimates the extent to which T cells are involved in these eruptions, because the mechanism of action may not be a simple type IV hypersensitivity mechanism. Moreover, the skin may not be able to metabolize drugs to their relevant antigenic determinants.

Research in recent years has provided further insight into the role of T cells in the pathogenesis of maculopapular rashes, and there now exist exciting data on the molecular aspects of how drugs are presented to T cells. We next will discuss these data, focusing our comments on eruptions caused by the use of penicillins and sulfonamides, as these agents have been studied most extensively.

Drugs, after covalently linking to autologous proteins (a process called haptenation), are capable of eliciting cellular immune responses (88). Namely, drug-modified serum or cell surface proteins can undergo exogenous antigen processing and can be presented by MHC class II molecules to $CD4^+$ T cells. In addition, drug-modified intracellular proteins can undergo endogenous processing and can be presented by MHC class I molecules to $CD8^+$ T cells. There is evidence for drug haptenation and for the involvement of these pathways in the pathogenesis of some penicillin- and sulfonamide-induced maculopapular or morbilliform rashes (88–98). To bind to proteins and to initiate such reactions, sulfonamides first need to be metabolized to reactive intermediates (as described earlier), whereas penicillins can covalently bind proteins after spontaneous degradation (90,91,99).

The generation of drug-specific TCC from allergic patients has led to an improved ability to study and to characterize these cells in vitro. Since the first report by Hertl et al. in 1993 (89), several groups have succeeded in isolating penicillin- and sulfonamide-specific TCC from the PBMCs of patients who experienced maculopapular or morbilliform eruptions caused by these drugs (95,100–105). Clones of both $CD4^+$ and $CD8^+$ phenotypes have been isolated, and at times, both phenotypes were present in a single patient (95,101,106). Some clones were specific for penicillin G or sulfamethoxazole, whereas others also proliferated in response to other penicillins or sulfonamides (respectively), suggesting a type of T-cell ''promiscuity'' toward its respective antigens (95,103,105).

Further analysis of penicillin- and sulfonamide-specific TCC has revealed that each bears the αβ T-cell receptor (TCR), as opposed to the γδ TCR (95,101–103,105). Various techniques have shown that drug recognition by the specific TCC occurs in an MHC-restricted manner (89,94,95,101,104). In addition to antigen recognition, the cytotoxicity of drug-specific TCC also appears to be MHC-restricted. Schnyder et al. studied the cytotoxic potential of sulfamethoxazole-specific $CD4^+$ and $CD8^+$ TCC on target cells (B lymphocytes and keratinocytes), both in the presence and absence of soluble sulfamethoxazole (106). They found that the cell lysis was MHC-restricted, and it required the presence of the soluble drug. Because cell death was abrogated by a selective inhibitor of perforin-based lysis, but not by a selective inhibitor of Fas-based apoptosis, the authors concluded that the method of cytotoxicity was perforin-mediated. Additional proof for this mechanism of cell death was provided by intense cytoplasmic immunohistochemical staining for perforin in the TCC. Keratinocytes were killed in the assay only if they were pretreated with interferon gamma (INF-γ), which up-regulates MHC class I and class II surface molecules. This mechanism may explain why patients experiencing certain viral infections, during which the expression of MHC molecules is stimulated by increased levels of INF-γ (such as HIV), are particularly predisposed to developing delayed drug-induced eruptions.

Recent research has revealed a novel mechanism of T-cell drug presentation in patients who have a history of delayed maculopapular rashes caused by the use of penicillins or sulfonamides. It has been demonstrated that these drugs are capable of binding directly, from the ''outside,'' to preformed MHC–peptide complexes that are already present on the surface of cells (107). Once this MHC–peptide–drug complex is formed, it is recognized by drug-specific T cells in an MHC-restricted manner, leading to T-cell activation. Unlike the classic antigen-processing pathways, this method of MHC binding is not dependent on the cellular-processing machinery. It has been shown in several studies that chemically fixing antigen-processing cells (APC) (thus making them unable to process antigen) before adding a penicillin or sulfonamide did not diminish their ability to activate drug-specific TCC, because the T cells were still able to proliferate, secrete cytokines, and kill autologous target cells (94,95,101,104,108). Furthermore, kinetic studies of drug-specific TCC activation were not consistent with the time required for antigen uptake, processing, and presentation on MHC molecules. After T cells have been triggered by the appropriate antigenic MHC–peptide complex, they internalize their TCRs, and the intracellular concentration of Ca^{2+} increases (109). Whereas these alterations occur after 6–12 hr with a typical processing-dependent antigen, such as tetanus toxoid, sulfonamide-specific TCC demonstrate these changes minutes after incubation with the stimulating drug (103,108), further supporting the observation that antigen processing may not always be required for antigen presentation.

Available data suggest that penicillins and sulfonamides differ in the way they bind to the cell surface MHC–peptide complex (107). For penicillins, the method of binding appears to be by covalent linkage to the peptide embedded in the groove of the MHC. Pulsing (preincubation and subsequent washing) of APC with penicillin, a process that would break noncovalent bonds, did not decrease their ability to activate drug-specific T cells, suggesting that the drug was linked covalently (94,104). The linkage of penicillin to the peptide was demonstrated in an elegant experiment by Padovan and colleagues (110). These investigators conjugated a penicilloyl group onto ''designer'' peptides containing defined anchor residues for particular MHC class II DR alleles, and they showed that these modified peptides were able to activate penicillin-specific $CD4^+$ TCC (from DR-matched patients). The peptide sequences were derived from natural peptides that are found constitutively within the groove of MHC class II molecules, and they acquired antigenic properties only after covalent modification with a penicilloyl group. Moreover, precise positioning of the hapten molecule on the peptide backbone was required for optimal T-cell recognition.

In contrast to penicillin, unmetabolized sulfonamides appear to bind to the MHC–peptide complex in an unstable, noncovalent fashion. Unlike penicillin-specific TCC, sulfonamide-specific TCC are stimulated only in the continued presence of the soluble drug.

All attempts at pulsing different APC with various concentrations of sulfonamides resulted in a complete abrogation of their ability to activate appropriate drug-specific TCC (101,103,108). Although the nature of this chemically unstable binding is unclear, it may involve hydrogen bonds or van der Waals forces that are involved in the interaction of sulfamethoxazole with its target enzymes (111). There is precedent for T-cell recognition of nonpeptide antigens; for example, the recognition of metals in contact dermatitis (112–116). In a recent review, Pichler et al. made an interesting observation that this type of drug recognition shares some features with superantigen presentation (99). They pointed out that, similar to superantigens, drugs are presented in a processing-independent manner.

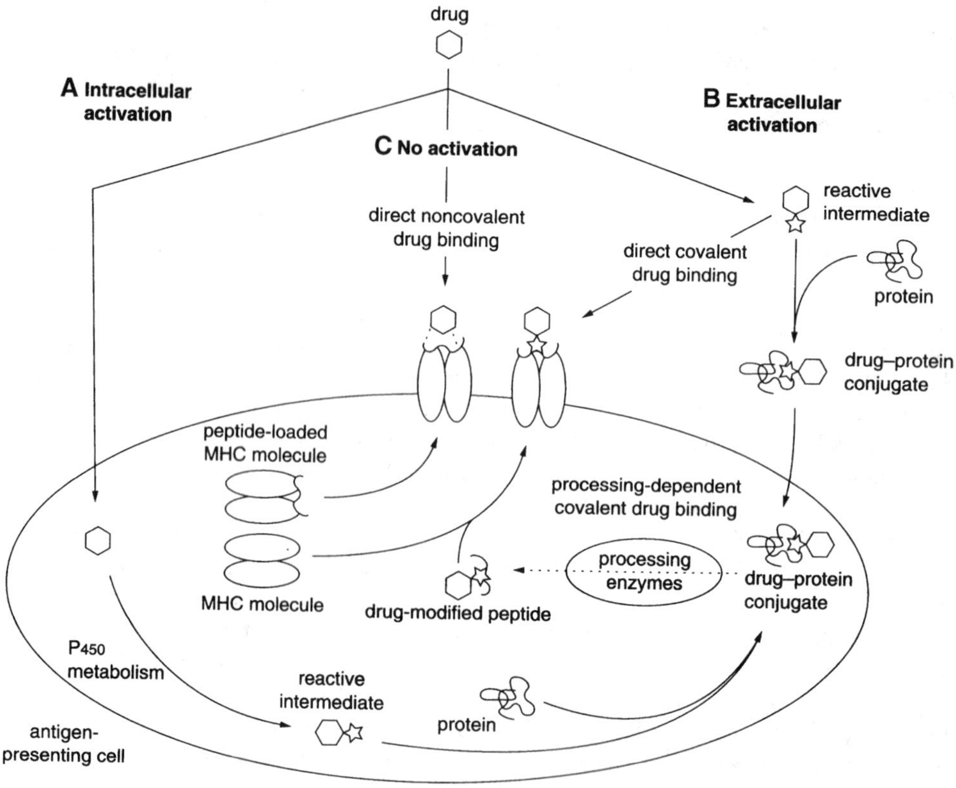

Figure 4 Possible pathways of drug presentation to T lymphocytes in maculopapular or morbilliform eruptions: (A) Drugs can undergo intra- or extrahepatic intracellular metabolism, resulting in reactive intermediates that bind covalently to proteins, are endogenously processed, and subsequently are presented in conjunction with MHC class I molecules. One example is sulfamethoxazole, which is metabolized to reactive hydroxylamine and nitroso intermediates. (B) Drugs, such as β-lactams, can undergo spontaneous degradation under physiological conditions. The reactive degradation products can either directly covalently link to the cell surface MHC–peptide complex or covalently bind to extracellular proteins. Drug-modified proteins are taken up by APC, undergo exogenous processing, and subsequently, are presented in conjunction with MHC class II molecules. (C) Drugs, such as sulfonamides, can bind directly to the cell surface MHC–peptide complex in an unstable, noncovalent manner, without first being activated. (Reprinted from TIPS, 19, Zanni et al. Involvement of T cells in drug-induced allergies, 308–310, 1998, with permission from Elsevier Science.)

In addition, they stimulate T cells of both $CD4^+$ and $CD8^+$ phenotypes, and some drug-specific TCC show an oligoclonal expansion of T cells bearing certain TCR Vβ-chains, similar to what occurs with activation by superantigens. However, drugs differ from superantigens in several ways: (1) their recognition is MHC-restricted; (2) they fail to stimulate PBMC from nonallergic donors; and (3) they result in a lesser extent of T-cell stimulation. Hence, drugs may stimulate T cells in a way that is intermediate between superantigen and peptide stimulation.

Figure 4 summarizes the possible pathways of drug presentation by APCs in T-cell–mediated delayed maculopapular or morbilliform rashes. It is likely that more than one mechanism is operative in these eruptions. The variable clinical presentations that are observed in these patients may be the result of heterogeneous T-cell responses. Importantly, these postulated modes of drug recognition are based mainly on data from experiments with activated and highly specific TCC. Therefore, the method (or methods) important for primary sensitization remain to be determined.

6 CONCLUSION

For many years, our understanding of the underlying immune mechanisms responsible for many nonanaphylactic drug disorders was limited and lagged behind the understanding of IgE-mediated reactions. The findings discussed in this chapter demonstrate that, in recent years, research has provided us with several exciting advances, and it has changed the way we think about hypersensitivity reactions. These discoveries prove that thinking ''outside'' the Gell and Coombs classification system, along with technological advances, can result in great strides in the field of drug allergy. Given the complexity of the field, work in this area will continue to require the collaboration of different groups of investigators—chemists, immunotoxicologists, pharmacologists, basic immunologists, and clinical allergists/immunologists. We hope that progress resulting from basic research will lead to the development of (1) improved predictive models for drug hypersensitivity, (2) an ability to design and manufacture drugs that are less likely to produce hypersensitivity reactions, (3) improved in vitro and in vivo tests for the diagnosis of drug hypersensitivity, and (4) superior treatment modalities of hypersensitivity reactions. Reaching some or all of these goals has the potential to greatly decrease iatrogenic morbidity and mortality from the use of medications.

REFERENCES

1. Tilles SA. Drug hypersensitivity. Immunol Allergy Clin North Am 1998; 18.
2. DeSwarte RD, Patterson R. Drug allergy. In: Patterson R, Grammer LC, Greenberger PA, eds. Allergic Diseases: Diagnosis and Management. Philadelphia: Lippincott–Raven, 1997: 317–412.
3. DeShazo RD, Kemp SF. Allergic reactions to drugs and biologic agents. JAMA 1997; 278: 1895–1906.
4. World Health Organization. International Drug Monitoring: The Role of the Hospital. Geneva, Switzerland: World Health Organization, 1966.
5. Lazarou J, Pomeranz BH, Corey PN. Incidence of adverse drug reactions in hospitalized patients: a meta-analysis of prospective studies. JAMA 1998; 279:1200–1205.
6. Rieder MJ. Immunopharmacology and adverse drug reactions. J Clin Pharmacol 1993; 33: 316–323.

7. Rawlins MD, Thompson W. Mechanisms of adverse drug reactions. In: Davies DM, ed. Textbook of Adverse Drug Reactions. New York: Oxford University Press, 1991:18–45.
8. Coombs RRA, Gell PGH. Classification of allergic reactions responsible for clinical hypersensitivity and disease. In: Gell PGH, Coombs RRA, Lachman PJ, eds. Clinical Aspects of Immunology. Oxford: Blackwell Scientific, 1975:761–781.
9. Shapiro LE, Shear NH. Mechanisms of drug reactions: the metabolic track. Semin Cutan Med Surg 1996; 15:217–227.
10. Pirmohamed M, Madden S, Park BK. Idiosyncratic drug reactions: metabolic bioactivation as a pathogenic mechanism. Clin Pharmacokinet 1996; 31:215–230.
11. Park BK, Coleman JW, Kitteringham NR. Drug disposition and drug hypersensitivity. Biochem Pharmacol 1987; 36:581–590.
12. Riley RJ, Leeder JS. In vitro analysis of metabolic predisposition to drug hypersensitivity reactions. Clin Exp Immunol 1995; 99:1–6.
13. Bastuji–Garin S, Rzany B, Stern RS, Shear NH, Naldi L, Roujeau JC. Clinical classification of cases of toxic epidermal necrolysis, Stevens–Johnson syndrome, and erythema multiforme. Arch Dermatol 1993; 129:92–96.
14. Goldstein SM, Wintroub BW, Elias PM, Wuepper KD. Toxic epidermal necrolysis: unmuddying the waters [editorial]. Arch Dermatol 1987; 123:1153–1156.
15. Roujeau JC, Stern RS. Severe adverse cutaneous reactions to drugs. N Engl J Med 1994; 331:1272–1285.
16. Revuz J, Penso D, Roujeau JC, Guillaume JC, Payne CR, Wechsler J, Touraine R. Toxic epidermal necrolysis: clinical findings and prognosis factors in 87 patients. Arch Dermatol 1987; 123:1160–1165.
17. Roujeau JC, Kelly JP, Naldi L, Rzany B, Stern RS, Anderson T, Auquier A, Bastuji–Garin S, Correia O, Locati F, Mockenhaupt M, Paoletti C, Shapiro S, Shear N, Schopf E, Kaufman DW. Medication use and the risk of Stevens–Johnson syndrome or toxic epidermal necrolysis. N Engl J Med 1995; 333:1600–1607.
18. Correia O, Chosidow O, Saiag PH, Bastuji–Garin S, Revuz J, Roujeau JC. Evolving pattern of drug-induced toxic epidermal necrolysis. Dermatology 1993; 186:32–37.
19. Stevens AM, Johnson FC. A new eruptive fever associated with stomatitis and ophthalmia: report of two cases in children. Am J Dis Child 1922; 24:526–533.
20. Lyell A. Toxic epidermal necrolysis: an eruption resembling scalding of the skin. Br J Dermatol 1956; 68:355–361.
21. Merk HF, Hertl M. Immunologic mechanisms of cutaneous drug reactions. Semin Cutan Med Surg 1996; 15:228–235.
22. Shear NH, Spielberg SP, Grant DM, Tang BK, Kalow W. Differences in metabolism of sulfonamides predisposing to idiosyncratic toxicity. Ann Intern Med 1986; 105:179–184.
23. Wolkenstein P, Charue D, Laurent P, Revuz J, Roujeau JC, Bagot M. Metabolic predisposition to cutaneous adverse drug reactions. Arch Dermatol 1995; 131:544–551.
24. Spielberg SP. Acetaminophen toxicity in human lymphocytes in vitro. J Pharmacol Exp Ther 1980; 213:395–398.
25. Guillaume JC, Roujeau JC, Revuz J, Penso D, Touraine R. The culprit drugs in 87 cases of toxic epidermal necrolysis (Lyell's syndrome). Arch Dermatol 1987; 123:1166–1170.
26. Mondino BJ, Brown SI, Rabin BS. HLA antigens in Stevens–Johnson syndrome with ocular involvement. Arch Ophthalmol 1982; 100:1453–1454.
27. Roujeau JC, Huynh TN, Bracq C, Guillaume JC, Revuz J, Touraine R. Genetic susceptibility to toxic epidermal necrolysis. Arch Dermatol 1987; 123:1171–1173.
28. Saurat JH. Cutaneous manifestations of graft-vs-host disease. Int J Dermatol 1981; 20:249–256.
29. Peck GL, Herzig GP, Elias PM. Toxic epidermal necrolysis in a patient with graft-vs-host reaction. Arch Dermatol 1972; 105:561–569.

30. Krueger GRF. Graft-vs-host disease and toxic epidermal necrolysis. Lancet 1973; 1:268–269.
31. Roujeau JC, Phlippoteau C, Koso M, Wechsler J, Andre C, Binaghi M, Revuz J, Touraine R. Sjogren-like syndrome after drug-induced toxic epidermal necrolysis. Lancet 1985; 1: 609–611.
32. Merot Y, Saurat JH. Clues to pathogenesis of toxic epidermal necrolysis [commentary]. Int J Dermatol 1985; 24:165–168.
33. Merot Y, Gravallese E, Guillen FJ, Murphy GF. Lymphocyte subsets and Langerhans' cells in toxic epidermal necrolysis. Arch Dermatol 1986; 122:455–458.
34. Miyauchi H, Hosokawa H, Akaeda T, Iba H, Asada Y. T-cell subsets in drug-induced toxic epidermal necrolysis. Arch Dermatol 1991; 127:851–855.
35. Villada G, Roujeau JC, Clerici T, Bourgault I, Revuz J. Immunopathology of toxic epidermal necrolysis. Arch Dermatol 1992; 128:50–53.
36. Heng MCY, Allen SG. Efficacy of cyclophosphamide in toxic epidermal necrolysis. J Am Acad Dermatol 1991; 25:778–786.
37. Hertl M, Bohlen H, Jugert F, Boecker C, Knaup R, Merk HF. Predominance of epidermal $CD8^+$ T lymphocytes in bullous cutaneous reactions caused by beta-lactam antibiotics. J Invest Dermatol 1993; 101:794–799.
38. Friedmann PS, Strickland I, Pirmohamed M, Park BK. Investigation of mechanisms in toxic epidermal necrolysis induced by carbamazepine. Arch Dermatol 1994; 130:598–604.
39. Hertl M, Jugert F, Merk HF. $CD8^+$ dermal T cells from a sulphamethoxazole-induced bullous exanthem proliferate in response to drug-modified liver microsomes. Br J Dermatol 1995; 132:215–220.
40. Correia O, Delgado L, Ramos JP, Resende C, Torrinha JAF. Cutaneous T-cell recruitment in toxic epidermal necrolysis. Arch Dermatol 1993; 129:466–468.
41. Paquet P, Nikkels A, Arrese JE, Vanderkelen A, Pierard GE. Macrophages and tumor necrosis factor alpha in toxic epidermal necrolysis. Arch Dermatol 1994; 130:605–608.
42. Roujeau JC, Dubertret L, Moritz S, Jouault H, Heslan M, Revuz J, Touraine R. Involvement of macrophages in the pathology of toxic epidermal necrolysis. Br J Dermatol 1985; 113: 425–430.
43. Cohen JJ, Duke RC, Fadok VA, Sellins KS. Apoptosis and programmed cell death in immunity. Annu Rev Immunol 1992; 10:267–293.
44. McCall CA, Cohen JJ. Programmed cell death in terminally differentiating keratinocytes: role of endogenous endonuclease. J Invest Dermatol 1991; 97:111–114.
45. Paul C, Wolkenstein P, Adle H, Wechsler J, Garchon HJ, Revuz J, Roujeau JC. Apoptosis as a mechanism of keratinocyte death in toxic epidermal necrolysis. Br J Dermatol 1996; 134:710–714.
46. Viard I, Wehrli P, Bullani R, Schneider P, Holler N, Salomon D, Hunziker T, Saurat JH, Tschopp J, French LE. Inhibition of toxic epidermal necrolysis by blockade of CD95 with human intravenous immunoglobulin. Science 1998; 282:490–493.
47. Morkunas AR, Miller MB. Anticonvulsant hypersensitivity syndrome. Med Toxicol 1997; 13:727–739.
48. Shear NH, Spielberg SP. Anticonvulsant hypersensitivity syndrome: in vitro assessment of risk. J Clin Invest 1988; 82:1826–1832.
49. Spielberg SP, Gordon GB, Blake DA, Goldstein DA, Herlong HF. Predisposition to phenytoin hepatotoxicity assessed in vitro. N Engl J Med 1981; 305:722–727.
50. Pirmohamed M, Graham A, Roberts P, Smith D, Chadwick D, Breckenridge AM, Park BK. Carbamazepine-hypersensitivity: assessment of clinical and in vitro chemical cross-reactivity with phenytoin and oxcarbazepine. Br J Clin Pharmacol 1991; 32:741–749.
51. Gaedigk A, Spielberg SP, Grant DM. Characterization of the microsomal epoxide hydrolase gene in patients with anticonvulsant adverse drug reactions. Pharmacogenetics 1994; 4:142–153.

52. Rieder MJ, Shear NH, Kanee A, Tang BK, Spielberg SP. Prominence of slow acetylator phenotype among patients with sulfonamide hypersensitivity reactions. Clin Pharmacol Ther 1991; 49:13–17.
53. Leeder JS, Dosch HM, Spielberg SP. Cellular toxicity of sulfamethoxazole reactive metabolites I—inhibition of intracellular esterase activity prior to cell death. Biochem Pharmacol 1991; 41:567–574.
54. Leeder JS, Nakhooda A, Spielberg SP, Dosch HM. Cellular toxicity of sulfamethoxazole reactive metabolites—inhibition of natural killer cell activity in human peripheral blood mononuclear cells. Biochem Pharmacol 1991; 41:575–579.
55. Rieder MJ, Sisson E, Bird IA, Almawi WY. Suppression of T-lymphocyte proliferation by sulphonamide hydroxylamines. Int J Immunopharmacol 1992; 14:1175–1180.
56. Choquet–Kastylevsky G, Intrator L, Chenal C, Bocquet H, Revuz J, Roujeau JC. Increased levels of interleukin 5 are associated with the generation of eosinophilia in drug-induced hypersensitivity syndrome. Br J Dermatol 1998; 139:1026–1032.
57. Suzuki Y, Inagi R, Aono T, Yamanishi K, Shiohara T. Human herpesvirus 6 infection as a risk factor for the development of severe drug-induced hypersensitivity syndrome. Arch Dermatol 1998; 134:1108–1112.
58. Riley RJ, Smith G, Wolf CR, Cook VA, Leeder JS. Human anti-endoplasmic reticulum autoantibodies produced in aromatic anticonvulsant hypersensitivity reactions recognize rodent CYP3A proteins and a similarly regulated human P450 enzyme(s). Biochem Biophys Res Commun 1993; 191:32–40.
59. Leeder JS, Riley RJ, Cook VA, Spielberg SP. Human anti-cytochrome P450 antibodies in aromatic anticonvulsant-induced hypersensitivity reactions. J Pharmacol Exp Ther 1992; 263: 360–367.
60. Leeder JS, Gaedigk A, Lu X, Cook VA. Epitope mapping studies with human anti-cytochrome P450 3A antibodies. Mol Pharmacol 1996; 49:234–243.
61. Manns MP, Obermayer–Straub P. Cytochromes P450 and uridine triphosphate-glucuronosyltransferases: model autoantigens to study drug-induced, virus-induced, and autoimmune liver disease. Hepatology 1997; 26:1054–1066.
62. Mauri–Hellweg D, Bettens F, Mauri D, Brander C, Hunziker T, Pichler WJ. Activation of drug-specific $CD4^+$ and $CD8^+$ T cells in individuals allergic to sulfonamides, phenytoin, and carbamazepine. J Immunol 1995; 155:462–472.
63. Borish L, Rosenwasser LJ. Update on cytokines. J Allergy Clin Immunol 1996; 97:719–734.
64. Pullen H, Wright N, Murdoch JMC. Hypersensitivity reactions to antibacterial drugs in infectious mononucleosis. 1967; 2:1176–1178.
65. Patel BM. Skin rash with infectious mononucleosis and ampicillin. Pediatrics 1967; 40:910–911.
66. Coopman SA, Johnson RA, Platt R, Stern RS. Cutaneous disease and drug reactions in HIV infection. N Engl J Med 1993; 328:1670–1674.
67. Koopmans PP, van der Ven A, Vree TB, van der Meer J. Pathogenesis of hypersensitivity reactions to drugs in patients with HIV infection: allergic or toxic? AIDS 1995; 9:217–222.
68. Descamps V, Bouscarat F, Laglenne S, Aslangul E, Veber B, Descamps D, Saraux JL, Grange MJ, Grossin M, Navratil E, Crickx B, Belaich B. Human herpesvirus 6 infection associated with anticonvulsant hypersensitivity syndrome and reactive haemophagocytic syndrome. Br J Dermatol 1997; 137:605–608.
69. Tohyama M, Yahata Y, Yasukawa M, Inagi R, Urano Y, Yamanishi K, Hashimoto K. Severe hypersensitivity syndrome due to sulfasalazine associated with reactivation of human herpesvirus 6. Arch Dermatol 1998; 134:1113–1117.
70. Lunel F, Abuaf N, Frangeul L, Grippon P, Perrin M, leCoz Y, Valla D, Borotto E, Yamamoto AM, Huraux JM, Opolon P, Homberg JC. Liver/kidney microsome antibody type 1 and hepatitis C virus infection. Hepatology 1992; 16:630–636.

71. Lowery N, Kearns GL, Young RA, Wheeler JG. Serum sickness-like reactions associated with cefprozil therapy. J Pediatr 1994; 1994:325–328.
72. Platt R, Dreis MW, Kennedy DL, Kuritsky JN. Serum sickness-like reactions to amoxicillin, cefaclor, cephalexin, and trimethoprim–sulfamethoxazole. J Infect Dis 1988; 158:474–477.
73. Heckbert SR, Stryker WS, Coltin KL, Manson JE, Platt R. Serum sickness in children after antibiotic exposure: estimates of occurrence and morbidity in a health maintenance organization population. Am J Epidemiol 1990; 132:336–342.
74. Murray DL, Singer DA, Singer AB, Veldman JP. Cefaclor—a cluster of adverse reactions [letter]. N Engl J Med 1980; 303:1003.
75. Stricker BHC, Tijssen JGP. Serum sickness-like reactions to cefaclor. J Clin Epidemiol 1992; 45:1177–1184.
76. Levine LR. Quantitative comparison of adverse reactions to cefaclor vs. amoxicillin in a surveillance study. Pediatr Infect Dis 1985; 4:358–361.
77. Hebert AA, Ligman EL, Levy ML. Serum sickness-like reactions from cefaclor in children. J Am Acad Dermatol 1991; 25:805–808.
78. Kearns GL, Wheeler JG, Childress SH, Letzig LG. Serum sickness-like reactions to cefaclor: role of hepatic metabolism and individual susceptibility. J Pediatr 1994; 125:805–811.
79. Kearns GL, Wheeler JG, Rieder MJ, Reid J. Serum sickness-like reaction to cefaclor: lack of in vitro cross-reactivity with loracarbef. Clin Pharmacol Ther 1998; 63:686–693.
80. Kalish RS. Drug eruptions: a review of clinical and immunological features. Adv Dermatol 1991; 6:221–237.
81. Nyfeler B, Pichler WJ. The lymphocyte transformation test for the diagnosis of drug allergy: sensitivity and specificity. Clin Exp Allergy 1997; 27:175–181.
82. Koponen M, Pichler WJ, de Weck AL. T-cell reactivity to penicillin: phenotypic analysis of in vitro activated cell subsets. J Allergy Clin Immunol 1986; 78:645–652.
83. Weiss ME, Adkinson NF. Diagnostic testing for drug hypersensitivity. Immunol Allergy Clin North Am 1998; 18:731–744.
84. Osawa J, Naito S, Aihara M, Kitamura K, Ikezawa Z, Nakajima H. Evaluation of skin test reactions in patients with non-immediate type drug eruptions. J Dermatol 1990; 17:235–239.
85. Lisi P, Lapomarda V, Stingeni L, Assalve D, Hansel K, Caraffini S, Agostinelli D. Skin tests in the diagnosis of eruptions caused by betalactams. Contact Derm 1997; 37:151–154.
86. Barbaud A, Reichert–Penetrat S, Trechot P, Jacquin–Petit MA, Ehlinger A, Noirez V, Faure GC, Schmutz JL, Bene MC. The use of skin testing in the investigation of cutaneous adverse drug reactions. Br J Dermatol 1998; 139:49–58.
87. Romano A, DiFonso M, Papa G, Pietrantonio F, Federico F, Fabrizi G, Venuti A. Evaluation of adverse cutaneous reactions to aminopenicillins with emphasis on those manifested by maculopapular rashes. Allergy 1995; 50:113–118.
88. Kalish RS. Antigen processing: the gateway to the immune response. J Am Acad Dermatol 1995; 32:640–652.
89. Hertl M, Geisel J, Boecker C, Merk HF. Selective generation of $CD8^+$ T-cell clones from the peripheral blood of patients with cutaneous reactions to beta-lactam antibiotics. Br J Dermatol 1993; 128:619–626.
90. Hertl M, Merk HF. Lymphocyte activation in cutaneous drug reactions. J Invest Dermatol 1995; 105(suppl):271–274.
91. Merk HF, Baron J, Kawakubo Y, Hertl M, Jugert F. Metabolites and allergic drug reactions. Clin Exp Allergy 1998; 28(suppl 4):21–24.
92. Gruchalla RS, Pesenko RD, Do TT, Skiest DJ. Sulfonamide-induced reactions in desensitized patients with AIDS—the role of covalent protein haptenation by sulfamethoxazole. J Allergy Clin Immunol 1998; 101:371–378.
93. Meekins CV, Sullivan TJ, Gruchalla RS. Immunochemical analysis of sulfonamide drug allergy: identification of sulfamethoxazole-substituted human serum proteins. J Allergy Clin Immunol 1994; 94:1017–1024.

94. Brander C, Mauri–Hellweg D, Bettens F, Rolli H, Goldman M, Pichler WJ. Heterogenous T cell responses to beta-lactam–modified self-structures are observed in penicillin-allergic individuals. J Immunol 1995; 155:2670–2678.
95. Padovan E, Mauri–Hellweg D, Pichler WJ, Weltzien HU. T cell recognition of penicillin G: structural features determining antigenic specificity. Eur J Immunol 1996; 26:42–48.
96. Cribb AE, Lee BL, Trepanier LA, Spielberg SP. Adverse reactions to sulphonamide and sulphonamide–trimethoprim antimicrobials: clinical syndromes and pathogenesis. Adverse Drug React Toxicol Rev 1996; 15:9–50.
97. Rieder MJ, Uetrecht J, Shear NH, Cannon M, Miller M, Spielberg SP. Diagnosis of sulfonamide hypersensitivity reactions by in-vitro ''rechallenge'' with hydroxylamine metabolites. Ann Intern Med 1989; 110:286–289.
98. Naisbitt DJ, Hough SJ, Gill HJ, Pirmohamed M, Kitteringham NR, Park BK. Cellular disposition of sulphamethoxazole and its metabolites: implications for hypersensitivity. Br J Pharmacol 1999; 126:1393–1407.
99. Pichler WJ, Schnyder B, Zanni MP, Hari Y, von Greyerz S. Role of T cells in drug allergies. Allergy 1998; 53:225–232.
100. Kalish RS, LaPorte A, Wood JA, Johnson KL. Sulfonamide-reactive lymphocytes detected at very low frequency in the peripheral blood of patients with drug-induced eruptions. J Allergy Clin Immunol 1994; 94:465–472.
101. Schnyder B, Mauri–Hellweg D, Zanni M, Bettens F, Pichler WJ. Direct, MHC-dependent presentation of the drug sulfamethoxazole to human alpha-beta T cell clones. J Clin Invest 1997; 100:136–141.
102. Zanni MP, von Greyerz S, Schnyder B, Mauri–Hellweg D, Brander C, Kalbermatten C, Pichler WJ. T cell reactions in patients showing adverse immune reactions to drugs. Inflamm Res 1996; 45(suppl 2):79–84.
103. von Greyerz S, Zanni MP, Frutig K, Schnyder B, Burkhart C, Pichler WJ. Interaction of sulfonamide derivatives with the TCR of sulfamethoxazole-specific human $\alpha\beta^+$ T cell clones. J Immunol 1999; 162:595–602.
104. Horton H, Weston SD, Hewitt CRA. Allergy to antibiotics: T-cell recognition of amoxicillin is HLA-DR restricted and does not require antigen processing. Allergy 1998; 53:83–88.
105. Mauri–Hellweg D, Zanni M, Frei E, Bettens F, Brander C, Mauri D, Padovan E, Weltzien HU, Pichler WJ. Cross-reactivity of T cell lines and clones to beta-lactam antibiotics. J Immunol 1996; 157:1071–1079.
106. Schnyder B, Frutig K, Mauri–Hellweg D, Limat A, Yawalkar N, Pichler WJ. T-cell–mediated cytotoxicity against keratinocytes in sulfamethoxazole-induced skin reaction. Clin Exp Allergy 1998; 28:1412–1417.
107. von Greyerz S, Burkhart C, Pichler WJ. Molecular basis of drug recognition by specific T-cell receptors. Int Arch Allergy Immunol 1999; 119:173–180.
108. Zanni MP, von Greyerz S, Schnyder B, Brander KA, Frutig K, Hari Y, Valitutti S, Pichler WJ. HLA-restricted, processing- and metabolism-independent pathway of drug recognition by human $\alpha\beta$ T lymphocytes. J Clin Invest 1998; 102:1591–1598.
109. Valitutti S, Muller S, Cella M, Padovan E, Lanzavecchia A. Serial triggering of many T-cell receptors by a few peptide-MHC complexes. Nature 1995; 375:148–151.
110. Padovan E, Bauer T, Tongio MM, Kalbacher H, Weltzien HU. Penicilloyl peptides are recognized as T cell antigenic determinants in penicillin allergy. Eur J Immunol 1997; 27:1303–1307.
111. Zanni MP, Schnyder B, von Greyerz S, Pichler WJ. Involvement of T cells in drug-induced allergies. Trends Pharmacol Sci 1998; 19:308–310.
112. Moulon C, Vollmer J, Weltzien HU. Characterization of processing requirements and metal cross-reactivities in T cell clones from patients with allergic contact dermatitis to nickel. Eur J Immunol 1995; 25:3308–3315.
113. Kapsenberg ML, Wierenga EA, Stiekema FEM, Tiggelman AMBC, Bos JD. Th1 lymphokine

production profiles of nickel-specific CD4+ T-lymphocyte clones from nickel contact-allergic and non-allergic individuals. J Invest Dermatol 1992; 98:59–63.
114. Sinigaglia F, Scheidegger D, Garotta G, Scheper R, Pletscher M, Lanzavecchia A. Isolation and characterization of Ni-specific T-cell clones from patients with Ni-contact dermatitis. J Immunol 1985; 135:3929–3932.
115. Lofstrom A, Wigzell H. Antigen specific human T-cell lines specific for cobalt chloride. Acta Derm Venereol (Stockh) 1986; 66:200–206.
116. Porcelli SSA, Morita CT, Modlin RL. T cell recognition of non-peptide antigens. Curr Opin Immunol 1996; 8:510–516.

20

Vasculitis

NABIH I. ABDOU

University of Missouri School of Medicine and St. Luke's Hospital, Kansas City, Missouri

1 INTRODUCTION

1.1 Definition

Inflammation in allergic–immune diseases could present itself as vasculitis with predominant inflammatory response of the blood vessels. The classic pathological features of vasculitis include endothelial thickening (proliferation), necrosis of the vessel wall, and perivascular cell infiltrate. The consequences of these blood vessels inflammatory changes are: (1) weakening of vessel wall resulting in aneurysmal dilation in some vasculitides, (2) slowing or pooling of blood in vessel lumen with subsequent thrombosis and ischemia of affected tissues, and (3) swelling and induration of an affected area caused by perivascular infiltrates that release certain cytokines and chemokines that magnify the inflammatory response.

1.2 Heterogeneity

Vasculitic syndromes are heterogenous and their immunopathological–clinical presentations depend on the type of vessel, target organ(s) affected, predominant cell infiltrates, severity of disease, and associated immune–allergic diseases. Moreover, genetic–ethnic background, patient gender, and age could influence vasculitis manifestations and severity. Vasculitis could be a localized or systemic, mild or life-threatening, and primary or secondary to immune, autoimmune, infectious, or malignant process.

2 CLASSIFICATION

The American College of Rheumatology, in 1990, established criteria for classification of vasculitis (1). This was followed by an international consensus conference on nomenclature of vasculitis (2). Both of these reports are helpful guidelines for classification and for establishing criteria for several forms of vasculitis. It is important that both the classification and nomenclature are based on the type of vessel affected, the histopathological features on biopsy or autopsy, or more importantly, the clinical parameters and modes of presentation.

2.1 Classification Based on Vessel Type and Size

Classification by vessel type and size is mainly pathological based on results of biopsy or clinical syndrome. A mild, self-limited form of vasculitis could present as venulitis and is usually due to a drug reaction or viral infection. An example would be certain cases of allergic drug reaction with superficial mild vasculitis. On the other hand extensive vasculitis could involve large arteries, such as in giant cell arteritis; Takayasu's arteritis, or temporal arteritis. A classic example of medium-sized arteritis is polyarteritis nodosa.

2.2 Classification Based on Histopathological Features

Histopathological classifications are based on the type of cell infiltrate: polymorphonuclear, lymphocytic, or eosinophilic. The presence of necrosis, giant cells, or alterations in internal elastic lamina of the vessel wall will be an added feature to classify the vasculitis syndrome. Presence of immune deposits (complement components, immunoglobulins, antibody, and antigen) as detected by immunofluorescence, electron microscopy, or by molecular biological techniques [polymerase chain reaction (PCR), or in situ hybridization] will shed light on immune–allergic pathogenesis of vasculitis. Importantly, vasculitis is a dynamic state, and immune deposits could be a transient phenomenon and even if detected could be the result of an inflammatory insult and not the cause of the disease.

2.3 Classification Based on Clinical Presentation

Certain vasculitides have characteristic features that will facilitate their diagnosis or could narrow the differential diagnosis. Examples are the predominant temporal artery involvement in giant cell arteritis, upper and lower respiratory tract involvement of granulomatous necrotizing vasculitis of Wegener's granulomatosis, and mucosal (buccal, genital) involvement in Behçet's syndrome. In the clinical presentation of vasculitis, it is important to note whether it is primary or secondary or associated with another collagen vascular disease (e.g., systemic lupus erythematosus, rheumatoid arthritis, or Sjögren's syndrome).

3 INFLAMMATORY MECHANISMS

3.1 Immune Complexes

Although immune complexes are the most extensively studied mechanism in animal models of vasculitis, the direct proof of their role in human primary vasculitis is still weak. In animal models of serum sickness, repeated injections of heterologous proteins result in antigen–antibody complexes that could result in vasculitis if the ratio of antigen/antibody is in slight antigen excess (3). This will result in complement fixation. There are several optimal factors required to induce tissue injury, which include the size (intermediate or small) (4) and net charge (cationic or positive) of immune complexes (5), nature of antibody response (isotype and IgG subclass), and the functional status of the reticuloendothelial system (RES) (6). The latter predominantly depends on the status of IgG receptor (FcγR3A). A dysfunctional RES with abnormal receptors will result in poor clearance of immune deposits, with subsequent tissue localization and injury of the vessels (7). Immune complex deposits will result in complement activation of the classic cascade, release of anaphylatoxins C3a and C5a, which will facilitate recruitment of inflammatory cells, clotting factors, and vasoactive factors, such as cytokines, adhesion molecules, histamine, and platelet-activating factor (8).

3.2 Inflammatory Cells

3.2.1 Neutrophils and Monocytes

Important cell types in immune complex vasculitis are neutrophils and monocytes. They are attracted to and bind to immune complexes by their C5a, C3b, and IgG receptors (8). The recruited neutrophils and monocytes will release toxic oxygen radicles (H_2O_2, O_2^-) and proteases (cathepsin G, elastase). The released enzymes will damage the elastic layer of the vessel wall by digesting elastin (9). Metalloproteases are also released by the recruited inflammatory cells and result in further vessel wall damage by digesting collagen and proteoglycans, and disruption of the basement membrane (10). Procollagenase in neutrophils at the inflammatory sites are converted to collagenases by plasma enzymes, such as plasmin and kallikrein (11). The resultant collagenases will digest type I and III collagen. This is followed by further degradation by gelatinases. These enzymatic steps will result in degradation of vessel wall elastin and basement membrane collagen (type IV).

3.2.2 Lymphocytes

Lymphocytes' role in pathogenesis of vasculitis has been suggested in giant cell arteritis and Takayasu's arteritis (12). CD4 T lymphocytes were the predominant cell phenotype in temporal artery biopsies. A small number of these CD4 T cells showed up-regulation of interleukin(IL)-2R expression, indicating in vivo activation (13). Those activated T cells produce interferon (INF)-γ and are clonally expanded. These findings would point to a localized antigen-driven immune response. The nature of this antigen remains to be seen (14,15).

3.3 Autoantibodies

3.3.1 Antineutrophil Cytoplasmic Antibodies

Two types of antineutrophil cytoplasmic antibodies (ANCA) have been described, based on the pattern of immunofluorescence of alcohol-fixed neutrophils. Cytoplasmic ANCA (C-ANCA) gives coarse granular fluorescence of cytoplasm. Proteinase-3 (PR-3) is the predominant target antigen in the neutrophil that gives the C-ANCA pattern. PR-3 is a 95-kDa neutral serine protease and has also been detected in mast cell granules, a subset of monocytes, and on human endothelial cells (16). Perinuclear ANCA (P-ANCA) is directed predominantly against myeloperoxidase and less often against lactoferrin and elastase (16,17).

C-ANCA has been predominantly associated with Wegener's granulomatosis, and P-ANCA, although less specific, has been associated with crescentic glomerulonephritis and some other forms of systemic necrotizing vasculitis, such as Churg–Strauss vasculitis and polyarteritis nodosa.

The role of ANCA in the vasculitis disease process is under intensive investigation. Tumor necrosis factor-alpha (TNF-α) up-regulates cell adhesion molecules, translocates PR-3 and myeloperoxidase to the cell surface and makes the enzymes accessible to circulating ANCA (18–20). The activated neutrophils can then induce endothelial injury and migrate to the vessel wall and thus magnify their tissue damage (19,20). Another plausible mechanism is the up-regulation of PR-3 on the endothelial cell surface, and thereby allowing ANCA to recruit activated neutrophils and induce cell damage by antibody-dependent cell cytotoxicity (19). The precise role of ANCA in vasculitis still awaits documentation by human in vivo studies, such as demonstration of ANCA at the site of granulomatous vasculitis. The specificity, sensitivity, and diagnostic value of ANCA in vasculitis syndromes have been critically reviewed (17). The current consensus is that clinical correlations are essential for the diagnosis of vasculitides with positive ANCA. Diagnosis and follow-up of patients with vasculitis should not be dependent on only the status of an ANCA blood test (17).

3.3.2 Antiendothelial Antibodies

Antiendothelial antibodies have been demonstrated in sera of patients with vasculitis, including Wegener's granulomatosis, microscopic polyarteritis, and vasculitis associated with rheumatoid arthritis (21). Antiendothelial antibodies could induce vessel wall injury by recruiting cytotoxic cells or neutrophils to vessel walls or by fixing complement and initiating the complement cascade.

3.4 Cytokines and Chemokines

There are no conclusive studies detailing the role of certain cytokines or chemokines in vasculitis. Endothelial cells on stimulation secrete IL-8, interferons, and colony stimulating factors. Neutrophils secrete IL-8 and TNF-α, and monocytes secrete IL-1, TNF-α, IL-6, and IL-8. Monocytes also secrete β-chemokines, including monocyte chemotactic protein and macrophage inflammatory peptides. The role these cytokines and chemokines play in human vasculitis awaits future studies (21,22).

3.5 Adhesion Molecules

A limited number of studies have focused on the role of adhesion molecules' expression in human vasculitis (21). In most studies up-regulation of adhesion molecules was important for initiation and progression of vasculitis. These adhesion molecules were intercellular adhesion molecule (ICAM-1) on endothelial cells and polymorphonuclear leukocytes, and vascular cell adhesion molecules (VCAM-1) on endothelial cells. Infiltrating leukocytes generally carry the β_1-integrins VLA-4 and LFA-1. These data would indicate that adhesive mechanisms could be playing a role in the immunopathology of vasculitis. However, the exact role needs to await further studies detailing the stage of the vasculitic lesion, early versus late disease, and quantitative data on adhesion molecules. In the future, use of knockout or transgenic animals with various mutations in adhesion molecules will enhance the knowledge of their role in vasculitis.

3.6 Infectious Agents and Superantigens

Infectious causes of vasculitis are now under extensive investigation. In hepatitis B infection a serum sickness-like syndrome is noted, and circulating immune complexes made up of hepatitis B surface antigen and IgG antibody were detected and may cause glomerulonephritis (23).

There are several animal models for infection-mediated vasculitis. The use of PCR and the availability of probes of conserved sequences for various infectious agents that could amplify microbial nucleic acid sequences have opened a new chapter and renewed the interest in a possible infectious agent in the pathogenesis of vasculitis (24). In animal models with interferon-γ(INF-γ)-deficient and IFN-γ receptor-deficient mice, Dal Canto and Virgin were able to induce arteritis-like lesion by herpesvirus (25). The arteritis was first detected in media of arteries, was regulated by INF-γ, and was dependent on B and T cells (25).

Streptococcal-derived superantigens could possibly play a role in a variety of human vasculitides (26). Superantigen could activate and expand autoreactive T cells and result in vessel wall damage. In patients with Kawasaki disease, Wegener's granulomatosis, and infection-related vasculitis, superantigen-producing microorganisms were detected. Skewing of T-cell repertoire in which T-cell receptor (TCR) Vβ expansions were shown on T cells at the time when microbial superantigen was detected, provide evidence for the role of superantigen in the expansion of the T-cell clone, with possible involvement in the pathophysiology of vasculitis (26).

Hepatitis C virus has been suggested to play a primary role in the induction of type II mixed cryoglobulinemia (27). Clonal expression of intrahepatic B lymphocytes from hepatitis C virus-infected patients was detected and preferentially involved rheumatoid factor-producing cells (28). With in situ hybridization, hepatitis C virus was detected in skin biopsy specimens of patients with cutaneous vasculitis and type II cryoglobulinemia (29). The role of hepatitis C virus in other primary vasculitides is unlikely (30).

Modern technology could permit identification of infectious agents in vasculitides of unknown cause. Broad-range rDNA PCR, using evolutionary-conserved sequences as probes for PCR primers, could be very useful in future studies (24).

3.7 Vascular Endothelium

Vascular endothelium secretes several cytokines and expresses several adhesion molecules or their ligands (21). Endothelial cells play an important regulatory function, mediated in part by various mediators, such as prostaglandins, adenosine nucleotide, and platelet-activating factor. They carry major histocompatibility complex (MHC) molecules, which are ligands for CD8 and CD4 T cells. MHC-I could serve as a target for cell-mediated cytotoxicity, and MHC-II could present antigen to CD4 T cells in an MHC-restricted fashion (21).

In an animal model of Shwartzman's hemorrhagic vasculitis, binding of leukocyte integrins (CD18) to ICAM-1 on endothelial cells plays a critical role in the expression of vasculitis (31). The hemorrhagic vasculitis could be inhibited by administration of antibodies to either CD18 or ICAM-1.

3.8 Genetic Factors

Except for giant cell arteritis (GCA), there are no data on the predominance or influence of genetic factors in human vasculitis. In GCA overrepresentation of HLA-DR4 haplotype was found. This association was mapped to HLA-DR B1 locus (32). In the study of Weynad et al., a sequence polymorphism within the hypervariable region of two of the HLA-DR B1 gene-spanning amino acid positions 28–31 was identified in patients with GCA

(32). This finding would suggest that antigen selection and presentation is operative in the pathogenesis of GCA. Both CD4 and CD8 T lymphocytes have selected usage of T-cell antigen receptor V and J gene segments, indicative of oligoclonal expansion. Certain V_b–J_b combinations are favored, thus, again indicating the recognition of a disease-related antigen (33).

4 PATHOLOGICAL–CLINICAL VASCULITIS SYNDROMES

4.1 Hypersensitivity Angiitis

The entity hypersensitivity angiitis has also been labeled as hypersensitivity vasculitis or allergic vasculitis. It includes a heterogeneous, large group of disorders, all associated with superficial cutaneous vasculitis. The vessel involved is usually a small vessel, such as postcapillary venules, venules, and arterioles. The disease usually follows an exogenous insulting agent, such as microbial or viral infection. The disease is usually of abrupt onset and associated with superficial necrotizing vasculitic lesions with palpable purpura (34). The necrotizing lesions could ulcerate and could be associated with transient arthralgias, myalgias, and nephritis (35).

A biopsy of the cutaneous lesions usually shows leukocytoclastic vasculitis of the arterioles and postcapillary venules, with endothelial thickening, fragmentation, and necrosis of the vessel wall (karyorrhexis), neutrophil infiltrates, nuclear fragments, mild perivascular hemorrhage, and fibrinoid deposits in the vessel wall. Usually, a few eosinophils and lymphocytes are mixed with the neutrophils (35).

The disease onset is usually abrupt and generally the cutaneous vasculitic lesions are of the same age, and in many instances, the disease spontaneously resolves after the exogenous insult goes away or is treated. However, in a few patients, the disease becomes chronic, and this could be a signal for other types of vasculitis or other collagen vascular autoimmune diseases.

Several other vasculitides could present as hypersensitivity angiitis; namely serum sickness, Schönlein–Henoch purpura, cryoglobulinemia, small vessel vasculitis associated with connective tissue diseases, and in rare cases this could be the manifestation of a neoplasm, particularly B-cell lymphoma or Hodgkin's disease (36).

The immunopathology of hypersensitivity angiitis is most likely an immune complex-type response and in several cases immunoglobulin or complement components could be detected in early vasculitic lesions. The nature of the antigen has not been clearly identified in many instances.

4.2 Schönlein–Henoch Purpura

Schönlein–Henoch purpura is occasionally labeled as anaphylactoid purpura, associated with cutaneous vasculitis, and frequently, palpable purpura could be detected (37). The disease is associated with abdominal pain and in certain groups of patients with glomerulonephritis and arthralgias. Most of the patients are children younger than 7 years of age; however, recently adults have been described with Schönlein–Henoch purpura. The disease is usually self-limited and lasts 10 days to 2 weeks, but in a few patients it could progress to persistent nephritis (37).

The etiology of the disease is unknown, but a drug reaction or prior streptococcal infection has been noted.

The pathology of the disease is that of leukocytoclastic angiitis. Characteristically

IgA deposits and the alternative complement pathway components can be detected in the biopsy. Serum IgA levels are usually elevated (37).

4.3 Urticarial Vasculitis

The true nature of this entity has been questioned, but in some patients with urticaria the rash persists beyond 24 hr, leaves a residual pigmentation, and is usually associated with a burning sensation. When these features are seen in urticarial patients a skin biopsy usually demonstrates evidence of edema, with leukocytoclastic vasculitis characteristics and immunoglobulin and complement deposits. Some patients with urticarial vasculitis have systemic manifestations, with arthralgias and myalgias, with elevated erythrocyte sedimentation rate and a drop of serum complement levels (38). In certain cases circulating immune complexes have been detected (38).

4.4 Churg–Strauss Vasculitis

Churg–Strauss vasculitis has also been labeled as allergic angiitis and granulomatosis. It could be considered as a variant of Wegener's granulomatosis or polyarteritis nodosa (39). The target organs in Churg–Strauss syndrome are usually the lung and gastrointestinal tract, but not the kidneys, with predominant involvement of the pulmonary vessels and associated with bronchospasm and eosinophilia. High-titer P-ANCA has been detected in some patients. The vasculitis is of the necrotizing type and, in certain patients, could be associated with granuloma formation (40). The insult on the vessels could be a result of eosinophilic cationic protein deposition, which has been demonstrated in the granulomas of Churg–Strauss syndrome (41). No etiological factors have been detected, including infectious agents or allergens.

4.5 Polyarteritis Nodosa

Polyarteritis nodosa is a small and medium-sized arterial vessel disease, systemic in nature, and may be due to immune complex deposition in the vessel wall. The immunopathology of the disease is that of fibrinoid necrosis, with perivascular infiltrates of neutrophils and, occasionally, aneurysmal dilation (42). In about one-third or fewer of the patients, there is associated hepatitis B infection that could be demonstrated by immunofluorescence in the vessel wall (43). A report by one group, using more sensitive techniques for hepatitis B, such as monoclonal antibodies and molecular probes for viral DNA in affected patients' blood lymphocytes or tissue biopsies, showed the incidence of hepatitis B to be much higher, approaching 75% (44). The causal relation between hepatitis B antigen or antibody and polyarteritis nodosa immunopathology needs to be documented by other groups. Other infectious agents have been implicated in the pathogenesis of polyarteritis nodosa; namely, cytomegalovirus, human immune deficiency virus 1 (HIV), and parvovirus.

Polyarteritis nodosa is a systemic disease, and any organ system could be affected. Patients with polyarteritis nodosa could present with several manifestations, depending on the target organ, whether it is CNS disease, peripheral nerves, abdominal, or cardiac involvement (45). In certain individuals, polyarteritis nodosa could present without necrotizing skin manifestations, and in these cases, arteriogram of internal vessels (mesenteric, renal, cerebral) for demonstrating aneurysmal dilation would be very helpful to support the diagnosis.

Polyarteritis nodosa is one of the vasculitides in which immune mechanism is highly suspected, particularly immune complex pathogenesis, and viral antigens need to be looked at in these patients as well as evidence of complement activation (46).

4.6 Microscopic Polyangiitis

Microscopic polyangiitis affects small arterioles and possibly venules and is very similar to polyarteritis nodosa immunopathology. Most patients with polyangiitis have a positive P-ANCA blood test. This entity has been labeled as minipolyarteritis or pauci-immune polyarteritis (47).

4.7 Wegener's Granulomatosis

The characteristic immunopathological features of Wegener's granulomatosis (WG) is that of necrotizing granulomatous vasculitis, involving predominantly the upper and lower respiratory tracts, and in about one-fourth of the patients it could affect the kidneys. Monocytes, not neutrophils, play an important role in the vasculitis process.

The importance of recognizing WG is that it could be misdiagnosed early on as infectious sinusitis or allergic rhinosinusitis. The presence of nasal mucosal ulcerations, with hearing loss and granulomatous pulmonary involvement should suggest the WG diagnosis.

The classic biopsy of WG is that of necrotizing granulomas with giant cell formation. In our experience nasal or sinus biopsies have not been diagnostic for Wegener's owing to extensive necrosis of the tissues at the time of biopsy. Biopsy of early, fresh lesions will help in demonstrating the classic WG features before onset of extensive late necrosis.

Serology is very helpful in the diagnosis of WG. As stated in the previous section the demonstration of C-ANCA occurs in more than 80% of patients with WG and is almost specific for the disease, particularly if the C-ANCA is confirmed by the presence of serum PR-3 antibodies by enzyme-linked immunosorbent assay (ELISA). There are recent reports that some Wegener's patients could have positive P-ANCA (48).

There is work in progress to shed light on the immune mechanisms contributing to the vasculitis in WG. Cytokines, such as TNF-α, up-regulate endothelial cell and neutrophil adhesion molecules, resulting in adherence of circulating inflammatory cells to endothelial wall, followed by immigration of the inflammatory cells to the tissues. Several enzymes from the neutrophils and monocytes are then released in the tissues, resulting in the inflammatory response and granuloma formation (18–20).

The inciting agent or agents that lead to the immunopathology of WG are unknown. Epidemiological studies have failed to show any environmental factors, the disease is not inherited, and there is no familial aggregation in the disease (49).

4.8 Giant Cell Arteritis

These groups of arteritides include temporal arteritis and cranial arteritis. The disease also is associated with polymyalgia rheumatica in about 50% of the patients.

The immunopathology of the disease is under extensive investigation. It is not due to immune complexes in the vessel wall, but it is a T-cell–mediated phenomenon. CD4 helper cells were seen in the temporal artery biopsies. The CD4 cells produce IL-2 and IFN-γ, which must be playing a role in pathogenesis. Work in progress is dissecting the cell infiltrates in temporal arteritis and detecting the cytokines released (15). This work has shown that the main cytokines are IL-1, IL-6, and IFN-γ. Recent work has also demonstrated the clonality of the T-lymphocyte infiltrates, and the selected usage of T-cell antigen receptor V and J gene segments indicate a possible putative disease-related antigen. The latter has not yet been identified (15).

4.9 Takayasu's Arteritis

This form of arteritis predominantly involves the aorta, carotid, subclavian, and vertebral arteries, and in some cases, could affect the pulmonary circulation. There are isolated reports of involvement of the abdominal aorta (50,51). The vasculitis is predominantly a giant cell arteritis and, histologically, could be similar to giant cell arteritis of temporal arteritis.

The precipitating factors and the pathogenesis of Takayasu's arteritis are unknown. Genetic studies in Japanese patients showed predominance of HLA antigen BW52. The significance of this finding is still unclear (50).

4.10 Mixed Cryoglobulinemia

Type II mixed cryoglobulinemia in which there is a monoclonal rheumatoid factor, usually IgM, associated with polyclonal IgG is seen predominantly in lymphoproliferative disorders and collagen vascular diseases and in several patients with hepatitis C viral infections. Hepatitis C was detected in the cryoglobulin precipitates and in skin biopsies of vasculitis lesions (27–29).

In other types of cryoglobulinemia, namely types I and III, hepatitis C could not be demonstrated. Type I cryoglobulinemia is associated with B-cell malignancies and monoclonal immunoglobulin is detected in the cryoprecipitates. In type III cryoglobulinemia there are polyclonal IgM or IgA immunoglobulins and polyclonal IgG complex, and the disease is associated with collagen vascular diseases and is usually immune complex-mediated (52).

4.11 Vasculitis of the Central Nervous System

Several forms of vasculitis could affect the central nervous system (CNS), or the latter could be affected by vasculitis without any other organ involvement, which is known as isolated CNS vasculitis. In the latter condition the brain is predominantly involved and the disease is manifested by focal signs, seizures, dementia, headaches, intellectual dysfunction, or cranial nerve involvement. In rare cases, the spinal cord could be involved and the disease manifested as transverse myelitis.

The immunopathology of the disease is predominantly granulomatous vasculitis, and there are cases that have been described to be associated with herpes zoster, human T lymphotropic virus type III, and HIV. To confirm the diagnosis a cerebral angiogram or meningeal or brain biopsy is required (53).

5 DISORDERS MIMICKING VASCULITIS

5.1 Atherosclerosis

There is renewed interest in the immunopathology or pathogenesis of atherosclerosis and whether vasculitis with an inflammatory or immunological mechanism is contributing to the pathology of the disease. This subject has recently been reviewed (54). There is evidence from biopsy studies that inflammatory cells could infiltrate the vessel wall at the sites of arteriosclerotic lesions. In animal models that are given a high-cholesterol diet, monocytes adhere to the endothelium, migrate to the vessel wall, and transform into foam cells. Similar lesions were found in human disease. The lipid lesion in atherosclerotic area is characterized by the presence of T lymphocytes. Moreover, adhesion molecules, cytokines, and chemokines were expressed at the atherosclerotic plaque (54).

Apolipoprotein E gene knockout mice developed profound atherosclerosis. The latter markedly decreases if the B and T lymphocytes are eliminated by generating crossbreeds with deficient B and T lymphocytes. These animal data indicate that inflammatory–immune mechanisms could play a role in the induction of atherosclerotic plaques (54).

5.2 Atrial Myxoma

Microemboli of myxomatous tissue could result in distant infarctions. Myxomatous tissue could invade the vessel wall and simulate vasculitis with microaneurysmal formation. Several patients with left atrial myxoma could have constitutional symptoms with fever, elevated erythrocyte sedimentation rate, and hypergammaglobulinemia, simulating vasculitis.

5.3 Antiphospholipid Syndrome

Antiphospholipid syndrome (APS) could manifest itself by arterial or venous thrombosis, recurrent fetal loss, and thrombocytopenia. Circulating lupus anticoagulant with anticardiolipin antibody is usually detected in sera of APS patients. In primary APS there is vasculopathy with thrombosis of the vessels, but it is very rarely associated with any inflammatory infiltrates. However, in patients with APS with another collagen vascular disease, such as systemic lupus erythematosus, vasculopathy could be associated with an inflammatory component of the vessel wall owing to the collagen vascular disease and not to the antiphospholipid antibody (55).

5.4 Cholesterol Atheroembolism

Atheromatous plaques could embolize to the extremities, kidneys, or the CNS and could mimic vasculitis. Distinction could be made by visualization of cholesterol crystals in biopsies of the involved tissue. Occasionally, patients with cholesterol atheroemboli could have an elevated sedimentation rate, eosinophilia, leukocytosis, thrombocytopenia, and hypocomplementemia. All these laboratory features could simulate systemic vasculitis.

6 SUMMARY

Progress has been made in the classification, characterization, and identification of vasculitis; a heterogeneous disease with various vessel sizes and types of involvement. Understanding pathogenetic mechanisms and the kinetics of the inflammatory–immune response is still in its infancy. With the availability of new tools for diagnosis and the use of molecular biological techniques at the cellular, tissue, and fluid phase levels will open the doors for new understanding of the etiology and mechanism(s) of this group of diseases.

REFERENCES

1. Hunder GG, Arend WP, Bloch DA, Calabrese LH, Fauci AS, Fries JF, Leavitt RY, Lie JT, Lightfoot RW Jr, Masi AT, McShane DJ, Michel BA, Mills JA, Stevens MB, Wallace SL, Zvaifler NJ. American College of Rheumatology 1990 criteria for the classification of vasculitis. Arthritis Rheum 1990; 33:1065–1067.
2. Jennette JC, Falk RJ, Andrassy K, Bacon PA, Churg J, Gross WL, Hagen EC, Hoffman GS, Hunder GG, Kallenburg CG, McCluskey RT, Sinico RA, Rees AJ, vanEs LA, Waldherr R, Wiik A. Nomenclature of systemic vasculitides: proposal of an international consensus conference. Arthritis Rheum 1994; 37:187–194.
3. Wilson CB, Dixon FJ. Quantitation of acute and chronic serum sickness in the rabbit. J Exp Med 1971; 134(suppl):7S–8S.
4. Theofilopoulos AN, Dixon FJ. The biology and detection of immune complexes. Adv Immunol 1980; 28:89–220.
5. Gauthier VJ, Mannik M, Striker CE. Effect of cationized antibodies in preformed immune complexes on deposition and persistence in renal glomeruli. J Exp Med 1982; 156:766–777.
6. Clarkson SB, Kimberly RP, Valinsky JE, Witmer MD, Bussel JB, Nachman RL, Unkeless JC. Blockade of clearance of immune complexes by an anti Fc gamma receptor monoclonal antibody. J Exp Med 1986; 164:479–489.
7. Frank MM, Hamburger MI, Lawley TJ, Kimberly RP, Plotz PH. Defective reticuloendothelial system Fc-receptor function in systemic lupus erythematosus. N Engl J Med 1979; 300:518–523.
8. Fernandez HN, Henson PM, Otani A, Hugli TE. Chemotactic response to human C3a and C5a anaphylatoxins. I. Evaluation of C3a and C5a leukotaxis in vitro and under stimulated in vivo conditions. J Immunol 1978; 120:109–115.
9. Klebanolt SJ. Oxygen metabolites from phagocytes. In: Gallin JI, Goldstein I, Synderman R, eds. Inflammation: Basic Principles and Clinical Correlates. 2nd ed. New York: Raven Press, 1992:541–588.
10. Keiser H, Greenwald RA, Reinstein G, Janoff A. Degradation of cartilage proteoglycan by human leukocyte granule neutral proteases—a model of joint injury. II. Degradation of isolated bovine nasal cartilage proteoglycan. J Clin Invest 1976; 57:625–632.
11. Katsuda S, Okada Y, Okada Y. Matrix metalloproteinase-9 (92-kd gelatinase/type IV collagenase equals gelatinase B) can degrade arterial elastin. Am J Pathol 1994; 145:1208–1218.
12. Cid MC, Campo E, Ercilla G, Palacin A, Vilaseca J, Villalta J, Ingelmo M. Immunohistochemical analysis of lymphoid and macrophage cell subsets and their immunologic activation markers in temporal arteritis. Arthritis Rheum 1989; 32:884–893.
13. Weyand CM, Hicok KC, Hunder GG. Tissue cytokine patterns in patients with polymyalgia rheumatica and giant cell arteritis. Ann Intern Med 1994; 121:484–494.
14. Weyand CM, Schonberger J, Oppitz U, Hunder GG, Hicok KC, Goronzy JJ. Distinct vascular lesions in giant cell arteritis share identical T cell clonotypes. J Exp Med 1994; 179:951–960.
15. Weyand CM, Goronzy JJ. Giant cell arteritis as an antigen-driven disease. Rheum Dis Clin N Am 1995; 21:1027–1039.
16. Hagen EC, Ballieux BE, vanEs LA, Daha MR, van der Woude FJ. Antineutrophil cytoplasmic antibodies: a review of the antigen involved, the assays and the clinical and possible pathogenetic consequences. Blood 1993; 81:1996–2002.
17. Rao JK, Weinberger M, Oddone EZ, Allen NB, Landsman P, Feussner JR. The role of antineutrophil cytoplasmic antibody (c-ANCA) testing in the diagnosis of Wegener granulomatosis. A literature review and meta-analysis. Ann Int Med 1995; 123:925–932.
18. Falk RJ, Terell RS, Charles LA, Jennette JC. Antineutrophil cytoplasmic autoantibodies induce neutrophils to degranulate and produce oxygen radicals in vitro. Proc Natl Acad Sci USA 1990; 87:4115–4119.

19. Keogan MT, Esnault VLM, Green AJ, Lockwood CM, Brown DL. Activation of normal neutrophils by anti-neutrophil cytoplasm antibodies. Clin Exp Immunol 1992; 90:228–234.
20. Roshan B, Wenger J, Evans M, Abdou NI. C-ANCA in Wegener's granulomatosis sera upregulates ICAM-1 and superoxide production in presence of TNF by normal neutrophils [abstr]. Arthritis Rheum 1996; 39:S40.
21. Kevil CG, Bullard DC. Roles of leukocyte/endothelial cell adhesion molecules in the pathogenesis of vasculitis. Am J Med 1999; 106:677–687.
22. Cassatella MA, Bazzoni F, Ceska M, Ferro I, Baggiolini M, Berton G. IL8 production by human polymorphonuclear leukocytes. The chemoattractant formyl-methionyl-leucyl-phenylalanine induces the gene expression and release of IL-8 through a pertussis toxin-sensitive pathway. J Immunol 1992; 148:3216–3220.
23. Combes B, Shorey J, Berrera A, Stastny P, Eigenbrodt EH, Hull AR, Carte NW. Glomerulonephritis with deposition of Australia antigen–antibody complexes in glomerular basement membrane. Lancet 1971; 2:234–237.
24. Nikkari S, Relman DA. Molecular approaches for identification of infectious agents in Wegener's granulomatosis and other vasculitides. Curr Opin Rheumatol 1999; 11:11–16.
25. Dal Canto AJ, Virgin HW IV. Animal models of infection-mediated vasculitis. Curr Opin Rheumatol 1999; 11:17–23.
26. Cohen Tervaert JW, Popa ER, Bos NA. The role of superantigens in vasculitis. Curr Opin Rheumatol 1999; 11:24–33.
27. Agnello V, Chung RT, Kaplan LM. A role for hepatitis C virus infection in type II cryoglobulinemia. N Engl J Med 1992; 327:1490–1495.
28. Sansonno D, DeVita S, Iacogelli AR, Cornacchiulo V, Boiocchi M, Dammacco F. Clonal analysis of intrahepatic B cell from HCV-infected patients with and without mixed cryoglobulinemia. J Immunol 1998; 160:3594–3601.
29. Agnello V, Abel G. Localization of hepatitis C virus in cutaneous vasculitic lesions in patients with type II cryoglobulinemia. Arthritis Rheum 1997; 40:2007–2015.
30. Servant A, Bogard M, Delaugerre C, Cohen P, Deny P, Guillevin L. GB virus C in systemic medium- and small-vessel necrotizing vasculitides. Br J Rheumatol 1998; 37:1292–1294.
31. Argenbright LW, Barton RW. Interactions of leukocyte integrins with intercellular adhesion molecule 1 in the production of inflammatory vascular injury in vivo. J Clin Invest 1992; 89: 259–272.
32. Weyand CM, Hicok KC, Hunder GG, Goronzy JJ. The HLA-DRB1 locus as a genetic component in giant cell arteritis. Mapping of a disease-linked sequence motif to the antigen binding site of the HLA-DR molecule. J Clin Invest 1992; 90:2355–2361.
33. Grunwald J, Andersson R, Rydberg L, Gigliotti D, Schaufelberger C, Hansson GK, Wigzell H. $CD4^+$ and $CD8^+$ T cell expansions using selected TCR V and J gene segments at the onset of giant cell arteritis. Arthritis Rheum 1994; 37:1221–1227.
34. Fauci AS, Haynes B, Katz P. The spectrum of vasculitis: clinical, pathologic, immunologic and therapeutic considerations. Ann Intern Med 1978; 89:660–676.
35. Winkelmann RK, Ditto WB. Cutaneous and visceral syndromes of necrotizing or ''allergic'' angiitis: a study of 38 cases. Medicine 1964; 43:59–89.
36. Green JM, Longley S, Edwards NL, Elfenbein GJ, Panush RS. Vasculitis associated with malignancy. Experience with 13 patients and literature review. Medicine 1988; 67:220–230.
37. Dillon MJ, Ansell BM. Vasculitis in children and adolescents. Rheum Disease Clin North Am 1995; 21:1115–1136.
38. Soter NA, Austen KF, Gigli I. Urticaria and arthralgias as a manifestation of necrotizing angiitis (vasculitis). J Invest Dermatol 1974; 63:485–490.
39. Lanham JG, Elkon KB, Pusey CD, Hughes GR. Systemic vasculitis with asthma and eosinophilia: a clinical approach to the Churg–Strauss syndrome. Medicine 1984; 63:65–81.
40. Masi AT, Hunder GG, Lie JT, Michel BA, Bloch DA, Arend WP, Calabrese LH, Edworthy SM, Fauci AS, Leavitt RY, Lightfoot RW Jr, McShane DJ, Mills JA, Stevens MB, Wallace

SL, Zvaifler NJ. The American College of Rheumatology 1990 criteria for the classification of the Churg–Strauss syndrome (allergic granulomatosis and angiitis). Arthritis Rheum 1990; 33:1094–1100.

41. Tai PC, Holt ME, Denny P, Gibbs AR, Williams BD, Spry CJ. Deposition of eosinophil cationic protein in granulomas in allergic granulomatosis and vasculitis: the Churg–Strauss syndrome. Br Med J Clin Res Ed 1984; 289:400–402.
42. Zeek PM. Periarteritis nodosa and other forms of necrotizing angiitis. N Engl J Med 1953; 18:764–772.
43. Sergent JS, Luckshin MD, Christian CL, Gocke DJ. Vasculitis with hepatitis B antigenemia: long-term observation in nine patients. Medicine 1976; 55:1–18.
44. Christian CL. Hepatitis B virus (HBV) and systemic vasculitis. Clin Exp Immunol 1991; 9: 1–2.
45. Holsinger DR, Osmundson PJ, Edwards JE. The heart in periarteritis nodosa. Circulation 1962; 25:610–618.
46. Sundy JS, Haynes BF. Pathogenic mechanisms of vessel damage in vasculitis syndromes. Rheum Disease Clin North Am 1995; 21:861–881.
47. Guillevin L, Lhote F. Distinguishing polyarteritis nodosa from microscopic polyangiitis and implications for treatment. Curr Opin Rheumatol 1995; 7:20–24.
48. Bajema IM, Hagen EC. Evolving concepts about the role of antineutrophil cytoplasm autoantibodies in systemic vasculitis. Curr Opin Rheumatol 1999; 11:34–40.
49. Hoffman GS, Drucker Y, Cotch MF, Locker GA, Easley K, Kwoh K. Wegener's granulomatosis: patient-reported effects of disease on health, function and income. Arthritis Rheum 1998; 41:2257–2262.
50. Kerr GS, Hallahan CW, Giordano J, Leavitt RY, Fauci AS, Rottem M, Hoffman GS. Takayasu arteritis. Ann Intern Med 1994; 120:919–929.
51. Gardner JD, Lee KR, Abdou NI. Takayasu arteritis. Reversal of pulse deficit after early treatment with corticosteroids. J Rheumatol 1984; 11:92–93.
52. Cohen SJ, Pittelkow MR, Su WP. Cutaneous manifestations of cryoglobulinemia: clinical and histopathologic study of seventy-two patients. J Am Acad Dermatol 1991; 25:21–27.
53. Calabrese LH, Duna GF. Evaluation and treatment of central nervous system vasculitis. Curr Opin Rheumatol 1995; 7:37–44.
54. Juvonen T, Juvonen J, Savolainen MJ. Is vasculitis a significant component of atherosclerosis? Curr Opin Rheumatol 1999; 11:3–10.
55. Englert HJ, Loizou S, Derue GG, Walport MJ, Hughes GR. Clinical and immunological features of livedo reticularis in lupus: a case–control study. Am J Med 1989; 87:408–410.

21

Allergic Bronchopulmonary Aspergillosis, Allergic Fungal Sinusitis, and Hypersensitivity Pneumonitis

PAUL A. GREENBERGER

Northwestern University Medical School, Chicago, Illinois

1 INTRODUCTION

1.1 General

Allergic bronchopulmonary aspergillosis (ABPA) is a hypersensitivity disease associated with saprophytic growth, typically of hyphae of *Aspergillus fumigatus* (Af), that results in a marked inflammatory response including sputum plugs or "glue" that is not expectorated by the patient. A chest physician may spend 30 min during bronchoscopy of a patient with asthma and undiagnosed ABPA and be unable to remove mucus. In contrast, accumulation of mucus in patients with cystic fibrosis may be removed during bronchoscopy without such difficulty. ABPA occurs in patients with intermittent or persistent asthma (1,2), patients with cystic fibrosis (3–8), and patients with neutrophil disorders, such as the hyperimmunoglobulin E syndrome (HIE) or chronic granulomatous disease (CGD) (9). Allergic fungal sinusitis (AFS) often occurs in patients with a history of nasal polyposis and chronic sinusitis in whom, on histological examination of mucoid material obtained from the sinuses, there are eosinophils, septate hyphae, and recovery of Af or other fungi from the sinus secretions (10–15). Fungal balls of the sinuses have been found, and material is inspissated in sinuses, making removal very difficult by pharmacological means, such as administration of prednisone and topical nasal corticosteroids. Invasive aspergillosis is rare, unless immunodeficiency (e.g., neutropenia) is present.

Hypersensitivity pneumonitis (HP) has been typically described in the context of acute or chronic disease (16). Also, nonacute early disease, with a normal chest x-ray

(CXR) film has been reported (17). Alternatively, years of antigen exposure may result in pulmonary fibrosis, bronchiolitis obliterans, and death (18,19). Exposure to antigenic material may be brief, such as when a large, intermittent exposure to fungi occurs while overturning moldy, wood chips or contaminated hay, or more subtle (e.g., when a person is subjected to birds at their workplace or at home). Similarly, moldy rugs serving as floor coverings are associated with summer-type HP in Japan (20).

1.2 *Aspergillus*-Related Conditions

Immediate cutaneous reactivity to *Aspergillus* species indicates the presence of *Aspergillus*-specific IgE antibodies and occurs in approximately 25–28% of patients with asthma (2,21). It is unknown whether *Aspergillus*-sensitized patients with asthma have an altered natural history, as compared with patients with asthma and sensitization to other fungal allergens. ABPA occurs in about 1–2% of patients with persistent asthma and may result in bronchiectasis before the diagnosis is made. Prednisone is the drug of choice for ABPA because it clears chest infiltrates, as evidenced by improved CXR, reverses peripheral blood eosinophilia, and resolves sputum plugs without having fungicidal activity (2). Patients with allergic fungal sinusitis are atopic and immunocompetent. In one series of 67 patients, all patients had nasal polyps and a history of seasonal or perennial allergic rhinitis, with at least two positive immediate skin tests to common allergens. Forty-three (64%) had asthma and 9 (13%) had aspirin or nonsteroidal anti-inflammatory drug (NSAID) hypersensitivity. Fifty (75%) patients reported a history of nasal casts (rubber consistency and green in color) being self-extracted or expelled (13).

Initially, it was thought that *Aspergillus* infections would be frequent in patients with human immunodeficiency virus (HIV) infection, but the number of cases of invasive aspergillosis is fewer than predicted (22). This finding emphasizes that immunity against invasive aspergillosis requires intact innate immunity, particularly neutrophil and monocyte–macrophage function, in contrast to cellular (lymphocytes) and humoral (antibody) immunity. *Aspergillus* species may be recovered from sputum of HIV-infected patients, but such patients do not have *Aspergillus*-related disease (23). In one series of 975 patients with acquired immune deficiency syndrome (AIDS), 45 (4%) had *Aspergillus* species recovered either from sputum or bronchoscopy specimens (23). Five of the 45 subsequently died from invasive aspergillosis, but many of the other colonized patients who died did not have autopsy evidence of invasive disease (23).

In non-AIDS–immunosuppressed patients, *Aspergillus* infections may occur primarily in association with 2 weeks or more of severe neutropenia ($<$ 500 granulocytes per cubic millimeter) (24). High-dose corticosteroids, alcoholism, and malignancies may magnify the risks in neutropenic patients. *Aspergillus* infections may result in sepsis, postlung-transplantation pneumonia or incision-site infections (25), pseudomembranous tracheobronchitis (26), or not be detected until autopsy.

2 ALLERGIC BRONCHOPULMONARY ASPERGILLOSIS

2.1 Classification and Stages of ABPA

ABPA may result in central bronchiectasis (ABPA-CB) which is detectable on standard chest roentgenograms or computerized tomography (CT). Thin-section scanning during CT examinations shows bronchial wall widening in the proximal two-thirds of lung fields without extension to the periphery (27). In the absence of central bronchiectasis, ABPA is considered to be present and is designated as ABPA-seropositive (ABPA-S) in contrast with ABPA-CB (2,28). ABPA-S may be a less aggressive condition, as most patients are under surveillance and treatment, so it does not evolve to ABPA-CB (28).

2.1.1 ABPA-Central Bronchiectasis

ABPA-central bronchiectasis (CB) can be classified into any of five different stages. Early diagnosis and appropriate treatment can help avoid progression to end-stage fibrocavitary lung disease from ABPA. The classic presentation, which is stage I (acute), is when there are new, upper or middle lobe chest roentgenographic infiltrates, that may or may not cavitate, associated with an elevated total serum IgE concentration and peripheral blood eosinophilia (29). Criteria for diagnosis include 1) asthma; 2) chest roentgenographic infiltrates; 3) immediate cutaneous reactivity to *A. fumigatus* or *Aspergillus* sp; 4) total serum IgE concentration higher than 1000 ng/mL (or $>$ 400 IU/mL); 5) precipitating antibodies in gel to *A. fumigatus*; 6) central (proximal) bronchiectasis; 7) peripheral blood eosinophilia ($>$ 1000 cells per cubic millimeter); and 8) elevated serum IgE and IgG antibodies to Af or the specific *Aspergillus* sp. involved. An additional finding in some patients is the expectoration of sputum plugs (tenacious, golden brown) from which Af can be cultured. The minimal essential criteria for the diagnosis of ABPA-CB are 1) asthma; 2) immediate cutaneous reactivity to Af or *Aspergillus* sp.; 3) total serum IgE concentration higher than 1000 ng/mL; and 4) central bronchiectasis without distal bronchiectasis. The diagnosis would be secured by demonstration of increased serum IgE and IgG antibodies to Af. These minimal four or five essential criteria should be of use, as the primary eight criteria may be affected by prednisone, which clears chest roentgenographic infiltrates and causes disappearance of peripheral blood eosinophilia, sometimes associated with declines in precipitating antibodies to Af or in the total serum IgE concentration.

Stage II (remission) is present after prednisone treatment has cleared the infiltrates observed in the CXR, and the prednisone has been tapered and discontinued for 6 months or more. In stage II, the patient receives treatment for asthma, but the CXR is clear of infiltrates, but may show some minor scarring from previous infiltrates. The total serum IgE concentration will have declined sharply, as reported in three patients in whom stage I (acute) levels of 10,350, 8,500, and 7,360 ng/mL declined to levels in stage II of 1,314, 1,800, and 1,143 ng/mL, respectively (29). It is not necessary to continue treating the patient with prednisone to try to reduce the total serum IgE concentration to less than 1000 ng/mL.

Stage III (exacerbation) resembles stage I (acute) when there is a new chest roentgenographic infiltrate unexplained by other causes, with a 100% increase in the total serum IgE concentration over the patient's baseline. Peripheral blood eosinophilia may not be present if the patient is receiving moderate doses of an inhaled corticosteroid or a recent course of prednisone for asthma. Some exacerbations are clinically subtle, identified only by a mild cough, a decline in the forced vital capacity (FVC) and forced 1-sec expiratory volume (FEV_1), or an increase in the total serum IgE concentration. Prednisone should clear the infiltrates as in stage I disease. Other patients will be diagnosed as stage III ABPA because of a more florid presentation (e.g., pneumonia or chest roentgenographic infiltrates), and bronchoscopy examinations may reveal tenacious inspissated mucus that grows Af, or an unsuspected homogeneous infiltrate(s) in the upper lobe(s) that necessitates evaluation.

Stage IV (corticosteroid-dependent asthma) is defined when it becomes apparent that the patient either continues to have chest roentgenographic infiltrates when prednisone is tapered, or if the asthma becomes of such severity that it is prednisone-dependent despite avoidance measures and pharmacotherapy (30). The initial total serum IgE concentration at original diagnosis of ABPA in one study of such patients ranged from 514 to 48,000 ng/mL, and after a mean of 10.2 years of treatment from 208 to 4250 ng/mL (30). Patients in stage IV may have exacerbations (new chest roentgenographic infiltrates, with a 100% rise in the total serum IgE concentration), especially if the dose of prednisone is less than 30 mg on alternate days.

Patients with stage V (fibrotic) ABPA have persistent fibrotic lesions on chest roentgenograms and moderate to very severe obstruction or restrictive pulmonary function changes (31). New radiographic infiltrates more likely are from disease of bronchiectatic airways, such as hemoptysis, *Pseudomonas aeruginosa* pneumonia, *Staphylococcus aureus* pneumonia, or atypical mycobacteria. In a series of 17 patients identified as stage V ABPA, initial total serum IgE concentrations (mostly before emergence of stage V status) ranged from 360 to 25,000 ng/mL (31). The 5 patients whose mean FEV_1 was 0.77 L after prednisone and other pharmacotherapy, all subsequently died of respiratory failure (31). The 11 stage V patients whose mean FEV_1 was 1.2 L after initial intensive treatment did not die of ABPA-associated respiratory failure.

2.1.2 ABPA-Seropositive

Some patients with asthma can have a diagnosis of ABPA without evidence for central bronchiectasis on high-resolution (thin section) CT examinations (28). The patients fulfill other diagnostic criteria, including a history of or current CXR infiltrates. Twenty-eight such patients, designated as ABPA-S, were identified over a 12-year period (28). Most patients were in stage II (remission), and all had persistent asthma. Some 11 patients were examined longitudinally for a total of 63 patient-years, but only four exacerbations (stage III) were recorded, suggesting a less aggressive form of ABPA. Patients who received surveillance with clinical examinations, prospective monitoring of the total serum IgE concentrations to identify latent exacerbations, and prednisone for diagnosed infiltrates, did not have progression of their disease to the end-stage–fibrotic stage. Thus, by definition and follow-up, ABPA-S patients can be classified into stages I–IV, but not V (fibrotic).

Differences in the serological findings between ABPA-S and ABPA-CB patients were not striking. For example, at the initial diagnosis, the mean total serum IgE concentration in the ABPA-S group was 6,663 ng/mL versus 11,880 ng/mL in ABPA-CB ($p > 0.05$) (28). Serum IgE-Af levels also were comparable with high indices in both groups (4.1 vs. 4.8, respectively, with > 2.0 being consistent with ABPA) (28). There was a reduced amount of serum IgG-Af in ABPA-S compared with ABPA-CB (3.6 vs. 7.8, respectively, with >2.0 consistent with ABPA) (28).

2.2 Clinical Characteristics

Patients with ABPA are highly ''atopic'' in the sense that there are several allergic diagnoses that are present, in addition to asthma and ABPA (32). For example, in a series of 38 ABPA-CB patients, 31 of 38 had a diagnosis of allergic rhinitis made before and 36 of 38 asthma before ABPA was recognized. One patient had just exercise-induced asthma. Typically, the diagnosis of asthma was known for 10 years before ABPA was identified or became manifested. Only three patients reported symptoms of asthma after nonimmunological stimuli, such as cold air, infection, and exercise, as opposed to allergens such as mold. Immediate cutaneous reactivity was common, with ABPA patients reacting to nine of ten inhalant allergens and nine of ten fungi (32). However, when compared with ''mold-sensitive asthma'' controls, who had immediate cutaneous reactivity to *Aspergillus* sp., no differences were present, as in numbers of allergen-specific positive skin tests. ABPA patients were much more likely to have histories of food and drug allergies than the control allergic asthma patients.

2.3 Natural History

ABPA-CB need not progress to end-stage fibrotic disease. With screening of asthma patients, greater clinical suspicion of patients with ''pulmonary eosinophilia,'' and use of assays for IgE-Af and IgG-Af, there has been earlier diagnosis and treatment. As stated, if patients present with extensive bronchiectasis and are in stage V with FEV_1 less than 0.8 L after maximal therapy, the prognosis is poor (31). However, for new patients who present with pulmonary infiltrates on CXR and are in stage I or III, prednisone treatment improves respiratory status and halts progression to stage V. Similarly, many of the corticosteroid-dependent asthma (stage IV) patients do not develop new areas of bronchiectasis or fibrosis. A retrospective analysis showed that many patients with stage III or IV ABPA, who had a delay in diagnosis or ineffective treatment, developed stage V (fibrotic) disease and become disabled or died of end-stage bronchiectasis (31,33).

3 PATHOLOGIC FINDINGS OF ALLERGIC BRONCHOPULMONARY ASPERGILLOSIS

3.1 Bronchiectasis

Gross pathological features of ABPA lung include bronchiectasis of any lobe, inspissated mucus, and ''semihardened masses'' along with green–yellow or green purulent material (34). Bronchopneumonias have been identified, along with pleural thickening and adhesions to the lung. Alternatively, lungs may be contracted from pulmonary fibrosis without any evidence of infections.

3.2 Histological Findings

Mucoid impactions of bronchi associated with septate hyphae and eosinophils in mucin are commonly found, as is bronchocentric granulomatosis. This latter finding involves replacement of the bronchiolar wall with granulomatous inflammation consisting of ''palisading'' histiocytes surrounded by lymphocytes, plasma cells, and eosinophils (34). The infiltrate may erode adjacent bronchial cartilage. The bronchial lumen can contain sloughed epithelial cells, necrotic eosinophils, Charcot–Leyden crystals, fungal hyphae, and neutrophils.

Some areas of lung have inflammatory cell infiltrates of the pulmonary arteries, but without necrosis. There is no evidence for invasion of fungi into blood vessels. Other histological findings include bronchiolitis consisting of lymphocytes and plasma cells admixed with eosinophils. Bronchiolitis obliterans can be present, which is a result of the inflammation that occurs in the distal lung. In contrast, bronchiectasis is proximal. Areas of eosinophilic pneumonia are found in distal lung parenchyma, whereas eosinophils and macrophages are present in the alveolar spaces with interstitial infiltration by eosinophils, lymphocytes, and macrophages (34). Some areas of lung have an ''exudative bronchiolitis,'' characterized by the necrotic debris of eosinophils and neutrophils in the bronchiolar lumen (34). This occurs in areas distal to bronchocentric granulomatosis.

In summary, histological findings include those of asthma, and usually mucoid impactions or bronchocentric granulomatosis, or both. Eosinophils are the dominant cell type in all active lesions. ABPA may yield multiple histological diagnoses in the same patient, such as eosinophilic pneumonia, mucoid impaction, bronchocentric granulomatosis, and even bronchiolitis obliterans.

4 IMMUNOLOGICAL ABNORMALITIES

4.1 Humoral

4.1.1 Total Serum IgE

Humoral abnormalities include sharp elevations of total serum IgE that may not normalize despite prednisone-induced remission of CXR infiltrates and peripheral blood eosinophilia. In an early series of 15 patients, the presenting total serum IgE concentrations ranged from 6,100 to 64,600 ng/mL (35). However, some patients at presentation will have lower IgE concentrations, 1,000–2,000 ng/mL. Prednisone administration results in a sharp decline in the total serum IgE concentration of at least 35% by 6 weeks (36). If a patient is in stage II (remission) or Stage V (fibrotic), the total serum IgE may approach the upper limits of normal for nonatopic persons or 300 ng/mL. Similarly, after prednisone administration in stage IV (corticosteroid-dependent asthma), the total serum IgE concentration may be less than 1000 ng/mL.

Most of the total serum IgE is not directed to epitopes of Af (37), because removal of Af-binding IgE from ABPA sera does not cause a substantial decline in the total IgE concentration. These findings were in contrast to serum from patients with ragweed-induced allergic rhinitis, for which much of the total serum IgE was removed by incubation with ragweed. There are immunostimulating (38) and immunomodulating (39) peptides of Af that may account for the high total IgE levels in ABPA.

4.1.2 Serum Isotypic Antibodies to *Aspergillus fumigatus*

The demonstration of sharply elevated levels of serum IgE–Af, IgG–Af, and IgA–Af in ABPA sera has resulted in sensitive and specific serological diagnostic aids for ABPA (40–42). There is a differentiation between the changes in total serum IgE and serum IgE–Af, the latter not correlating well with pulmonary exacerbations of ABPA. Thus, elevation of the isotypic antibodies to Af may be present when the total serum IgE concentration is not increased in stage IV (corticosteroid-dependent asthma) ABPA.

With immunoblotting, there is remarkable heterogeneity of isotypic antibody binding to Af. ABPA exacerbations are associated with a sharp rise in total serum IgE, but not with a specific antigen-binding pattern of IgE, IgG, and IgA (43). When exacerbation sera were compared with preexacerbation and posttreatment sera, various patterns of intensified binding to Af were found. For example, in a patient whose total IgE increased from 4,272 to 14,694 ng/mL during an exacerbation, a predominant IgG-binding pattern was present with six intensified bands from 24- to 90-kDa molecular weights. Few bands were present with IgE and IgA and IgA1 immunoblots, and there was little difference in blots using exacerbation sera. The clinical correlations between isotypic antibody patterns and exacerbations still have not been clarified, and these experiments suggest that varying patterns of immune response occur during ABPA exacerbations.

4.1.3 Precipitating Antibodies

Most patients with acute (stage I) or exacerbation (stage III) ABPA have precipitating antibodies to Af. Their absence should not be used as evidence against the diagnosis of ABPA, as prednisone administration can lead to disappearance of precipitating antibodies. A more common reason for negative results is poorly reactive fungal extracts and failure to concentrate sera before testing.

4.1.4 Bronchoalveolar Compartment Antibodies

Eight patients with ABPA-CB underwent bronchoalveolar lavage (BAL) safely and had cells and antibodies analyzed (44). There was a predominance of macrophages (62%), with fewer epithelial cells (12%), lymphocytes (16%), eosinophils (6%), and PMNs (4%). These cell counts were found despite that seven of eight patients were receiving alternate-day or daily prednisone and inhaled corticosteroids. Antibodies were standardized based on albumin concentration in lavage fluid or serum. Surprisingly, the standardized ratio of total IgE in BAL fluid/total IgE in serum was 0.93, whereas for IgE–Af and IgA–Af the BAL fluid/serum ratios were very high (44). The BAL fluid/serum ratio for IgE–Af was 48 and for IgA–Af was 96. There was no evidence for local bronchoalveolar compartment production of IgG–Af in that the BAL fluid/serum ratio was 0.94. These results were consistent with bronchoalveolar compartment synthesis of IgE–Af and IgA–Af, but not total IgE or IgG–Af. The data support the concept that other locations (such as bone marrow, pharnygeal lymphoid tissue, or gut-associated lymphoid tissue) are the sites of total IgE synthesis. These findings emphasize the need for caution in interpreting in vitro results from cell culture experiments in which IgE is measured, so as not to imply that IgE–Af may be affected similarly.

4.2 Cellular

4.2.1 Basophil Hyperreleasability

Incubation of peripheral blood basophils from patients with ABPA with Af or anti-IgE caused greater release of histamine in vitro than similarly treated basophils from asthma patients with immediate cutaneous reactivity to *Aspergillus* (45). Furthermore, release of histamine was higher with basophils from ABPA patients in stages IV and V than from patients in stages I, II, and III. Other fungi (including *Penicillium, Fusarium*, Dematiaceae, and *Chaetomium*) also resulted in greater histamine release from cells from ABPA patients compared with cells from asthmatic controls. Extrapolation of these observations to mast cells in the bronchial lumen or mucosa suggests such fungi may activate mast cells in the lungs and thereby contribute to the advanced, destructive stages as well as the bronchospasm seen in ABPA.

4.2.2 T-Lymphocyte Activation

There is a growing body of literature consistent with $CD4^+$ T-lymphocyte activation in ABPA. Supporting data include elevations of sIL-2R (46). Most T-cell clones from ABPA patients (38,39,47,48,50) are of the $CD4^+$ Th2 phenotype, but Th1 phenotypes also have been produced, depending on the stimulating Af peptides (50). With at least 18 Af allergens being recognized by the World Health Organization (WHO) and the International Union of Immunological Societies (IUIS), there are many opportunities to identify specific Af allergens that stimulate or down-regulate IgE production or $CD4^+$ lymphocyte clones, bind to antibodies, or act as growth factors for eosinophils. To establish the clinical significance of each factor in ABPA remains a challenge.

4.2.3 Fluorescence-Activated Cell Sorter (FACS) Analysis

Activation of peripheral blood lymphocytes has shown at least two response patterns in ABPA (51). One pattern shows increased numbers of $CD19^+$ $CD23^+$ B cells, whereas the other shows increased numbers of $CD3^+$ $CD4^+$ T cells. The number of activated B cells in the former case is extremely high in that most of the $CD19^+$ cells were also $CD23^+$. The presence of an ABPA exacerbation did not dramatically change the phenotypic patterns when serial studies were done, suggesting other factors contribute to ABPA exacerbations. Clinical and serological differences could not explain the B-cell ''exacerbations'' from the T-cell ''exacerbations.''

5 RADIOLOGIC FINDINGS

5.1 Plain Chest Roentgenograms

The chest roentgenogram findings include 1) homogeneous, smooth margin infiltrates usually of upper lobes (including posterior segments that mimic *Mycobacterium tuberculosis* infection); 2) air–fluid levels in infiltrates; 3) pulmonary fibrosis with scarring in limited areas, to an involvement in all lobes; 4) bronchial wall thickening called ''tramlines'' (also seen in asthma and congestive heart failure); 5) parallel line shadows, where the bronchus extends distally—evidence for bronchiectasis; 6) ring shadows—1- to 2-cm

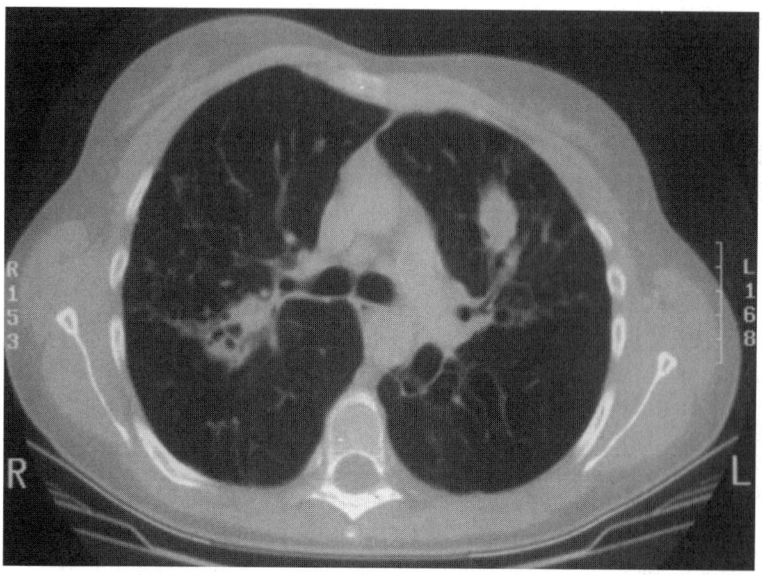

Figure 1 A 29-year-old woman, with pneumonia 6 years previously, presented with clubbing, nasal polyps, and bilateral fibrosis on PA and lateral CXRs. A CT scan just below the level of the carina demonstrated a cavitary mass in the right lung field, an infiltrate in the left anterior lung field, and cystic areas of bronchiectasis in the left lower lobe (bottom of figure). A sweat test was normal.

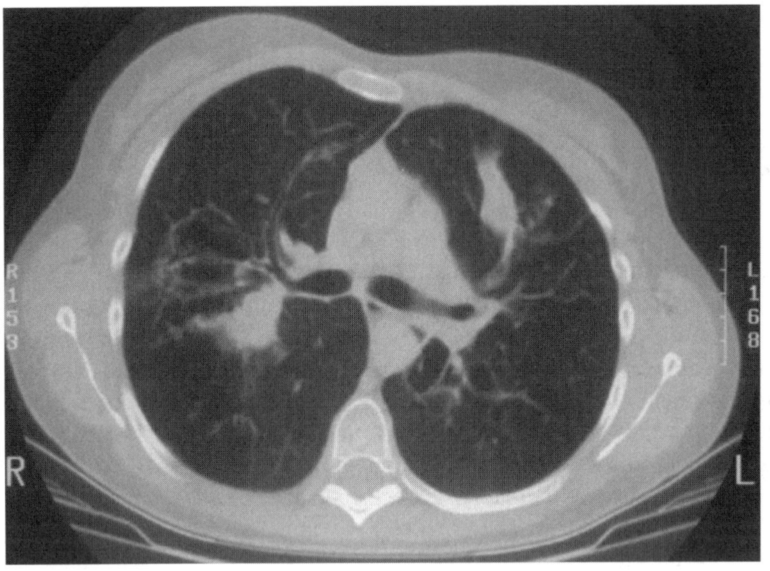

Figure 2 Same patient as in Figure 1: The CT scan section is below the previous cut. Bronchiectasis can be seen in the right midlung along with bilateral infiltrates. There are cystic areas in both lung fields representing areas of bronchiectasis and bronchial wall widening.

rings representing bronchiectatic bronchi when viewed in the coronal perspective on a posteroanterior film; and 7) blebs, bullae, cavities, pneumothorax, and volume loss (52).

5.2 Computerized Tomography

With use of thin sections (1.5-mm collimation) with cuts taken every 10–20 mm from the aortic knob to the diaphragm, infiltrates representing consolidation or cavitation not visible on the CXR can be appreciated (27,53). Bronchiectasis is present when dilated bronchi are viewed tangentially (axial) so that a bronchus appears longitudinally. Central bronchiectasis refers to the inner two-thirds of the CT field. Bronchiectasis may be cylindrical, varicose, or cystic (27).

Examples of infiltrates and bronchiectasis in a patient with ABPA-CB who had only known of one or two episodes of ''pneumonia'' are presented in Figures 1 and 2.

6 MANAGEMENT

6.1 Avoidance Measures

Obvious sources of moisture in a home favor fungal growth and should be corrected. For example, wet wood inside of walls because of a leaky roof may provide for growth of fungi, such as Af for several years thereafter. Basements and crawl spaces that flood should be improved to remove and prevent mold. Patients with ABPA should avoid working and sleeping in presumably moldy basements. Some patients have been helped by moving from homes with crawl spaces that had flooded.

6.2 Medications

6.2.1 Oral Corticosteroids

The most effective treatment for ABPA exacerbations is prednisone (28,29,54–56), even for patients in stage IV (corticosteroid-dependent asthma) (30) and stage V (fibrotic) (31). At the time of CXR infiltrates and total serum IgE elevations, an empiric course of prednisone at a moderate oral dosage of 0.5 mg/kg, given daily, is usually sufficient to result in complete or nearly complete resolution of the acute CXR infiltrates. Scarring may remain in some patients. After the initial 2 weeks of prednisone, the dose is administered on alternate days for 2 months, and then it is tapered and discontinued. The total serum IgE concentration can be measured after 4–6 weeks, when at least a 33% decline is expected (36). Often the decline is much greater. Concurrently, there are reductions in symptoms of asthma, improvements in spirometric values, and resolution of peripheral blood eosinophilia. Production and expectoration of mucous plugs should cease. The patient's asthma or cystic fibrosis may be more aggressive after the diagnosis of ABPA. In such cases, inhaled corticosteroids, bronchodilators, nedocromil, and leukotriene antagonists may be inadequate to control symptoms. These patients develop corticosteroid-dependent asthma, stage IV ABPA (30). They may or may not have subsequent ABPA exacerbations. Clinical suspicion should remain high and total serum IgE concentrations obtained, especially when flares of asthma occur. In the presence of wheezing, bronchial breath sounds can be absent.

Patients with ABPA-S appear to have a less aggressive form of ABPA (28). During 63 patient-years of serial total serum IgE measurements, just four ABPA exacerbations occurred. No patient was a chronic sputum producer, although in two of the four exacerbations, Af was present in expectorated sputum.

The physician managing a patient with ABPA needs to make the patient aware that recurrent, often silent infiltrates, which can be detected in a CXR, may cause additional bronchiectasis and worsen respiratory status. Also, alternate-day prednisone avoids nearly all of the serious side effects seen with high-dose daily prednisone. If ABPA enters stages II (remission) or III (recurrent exacerbation), prednisone will not be required on a regular basis.

6.2.2 Antifungal Agents

Although different antifungal agents continue to be evaluated in patients with ABPA, prednisone has remained the drug of choice since 1973 (56). For example, in 11 patients who received inhaled pimaricin or nystatin, CXR infiltrates occurred in all patients from 1 month to 2 years later. Thus, a single course of antifungal therapy did not prevent "recurrent consolidations" (56). In that same study, cromolyn sodium was administered to one group of patients and prednisone in an average dose of 10.5 mg daily to another group. New exacerbations occurred in 60% of the former and 20% of the latter (56). A limitation of this 1973 study was that total serum IgE assays were not available.

The administration of itraconazole as adjunctive therapy in addition to prednisone has been described in ABPA (55,57–59) and cystic fibrosis (60). In a study of 14 ABPA patients, for which a 2-year retrospective period was used as a control, the administration of itraconazole 200 mg/day for 12 months resulted in 7 of 14 patients discontinuing oral corticosteroids (58). The number of ABPA exacerbations decreased from 2.0 to 0.9/yr with a reduction of prednisone from 22 to 6.5 mg/day. The authors stated that there had been no change in the prednisone dosage in the 2-year control period. These results should be considered as evidence for adjunctive use of itraconazole in ABPA. However, itraconazole is a potent inhibitor of cytochrome 3A4 (P-450), which in turn, would decrease the clearance of prednisone and inhaled corticosteroids. Thus, itraconazole could be a steroid-enhancing agent, and this effect, rather than its antifungal activity, might account for its apparent success in the treatment in ABPA. In addition, at Northwestern University, only 10% of 29 Af isolates from inpatients were susceptible to itraconazole (and 15% to ketoconazole), compared with 97% with amphotericin B. Antifungal drug resistance may not be as high in outpatient sputum samples from patients with ABPA, but widespread use of itraconazole likely will result in resistant strains. Should a patient be treated with prednisone and continue to expectorate Af in sputum, itraconazole could be considered. Nevertheless, many ABPA patients stop producing sputum after prednisone is initiated and who do not have sputum in-between exacerbations. Because of its high cost, adverse drug interactions, and low fungicidal activity against many strains of Af, itraconazole use should remain adjunctive in ABPA if it is used at all.

6.3 Coexisting Conditions

Allergic bronchopulmonary aspergillosis may occur in patients with asthma that is intermittent to persistent and mild to severe, with cystic fibrosis, and occasionally, with allergic fungal sinusitis. ABPA should be suspected in patients with cystic fibrosis when wheezing episodes become more pronounced even though prior serological tests for ABPA may have been negative. What processes result in conversion of asthma or cystic fibrosis without ABPA into ABPA is uncertain, but may involve activation of antigen-presenting cells, T cells; or B cells by Af allergens. It remains unclear why the patients generate such thick mucus that contains eosinophils and Af hyphae. On a fundamental level, why do Af hyphae colonize bronchial mucus in patients with ABPA? There are many questions remaining to be answered about initial steps in development of ABPA, but from a clinical perspective, nearly all the patients are broadly atopic.

6.4 Screening for ABPA in Patients with Asthma

6.4.1 In Asthma and Cystic Fibrosis

A high index of suspicion is required in managing patients with asthma and some patients with cystic fibrosis in that unrecognized and untreated ABPA can be indolent and result in bronchiectasis and bronchiolitis obliterans. Although the incidence of ABPA is 1–2% in patients with persistent asthma (2), the irreversible consequences of untreated ABPA require that physicians identify cases as early as possible. Patients with asthma should be tested for immediate cutaneous reactivity to Af and have total IgE levels measured (sensitive albeit nonspecific tests). Follow-up of patients testing positive with a highly specific set of serological assays (serum precipitins to Af, serum IgE–Af and IgG–Af) will improve diagnostic specificity. Negative results exclude ABPA (2,21,41).

6.4.2 Allergic Bronchopulmonary Mycoses

Allergic bronchopulmonary mycosis (ABPM) may present clinically similar to ABPA, but with negative Af serologies (61). The presence of CXR infiltrates, peripheral blood eosinophilia, an elevated total serum IgE concentration, and the recovery of other fungi from sputum can lead to this diagnosis. End-stage ABPM cases are very rare (62), suggesting that there may be differences in immune and inflammatory responses resulting in areas of bronchiectasis or pulmonary fibrosis in ABPA as opposed to ABPM. There may be differences in intrinsic properties of the fungi themselves. For example, proteases (63) and ribotoxins (which could inhibit protein synthesis) (64) have been identified from strains of Af that bind to serum IgE–Af and IgG–Af and may contribute to localized areas of inflammation and bronchial wall destruction. In contrast, the proteins produced by the fungi that cause ABPM may be less toxic or less immunogenic.

7 ALLERGIC FUNGAL SINUSITIS

7.1 Description and Histology

Patients with allergic fungal sinusitis (AFS) have a history of chronic sinusitis, nasal polyps, recurrences of purulent sinusitis despite medical and surgical interventions, and sinus radiography demonstrates opacified sinuses (10–15). Differential weighting of magnetic resonance imaging (MRI) examinations can provide support for AFS on the T1-weighted image when signal intensity is decreased. The T2-weighted image shows sinuses without signal in areas of allergic mucin. Some patients produce nasal casts or thick, viscous (peanut butter consistency) mucus that should be examined for fungi and eosinophils. Histological examination of sinus mucus confirms the diagnosis when eosinophils and fungal hyphae are observed (10,13). Silver methenamine staining of the allergic mucin should be performed to show the fungal hyphae. The density of hyphae is less than one sees in mycetoma (13). In some cases, fungi will not be revealed by the silver stain, but will be recovered in cultures. After hematoxylin and eosin (H&E) staining, eosinophils and Charcot–Leyden crystals will be visible in the ''allergic'' mucin. Fungal invasion into the sinus mucosa and mycetoma is not present. Similar to findings in patients with asthma, the epithelium of the mucosa of the sinuses is denuded and the subepithelium is infiltrated with lymphocytes and eosinophils. Non-Af fungi causing AFS include *Bipolaris spicifera* [especially in the southwestern United States (13)], *Alternaria*, and *Pullularia* (65).

To secure the diagnosis of AFS, histological examination and cultures of mucus should be performed in atopic, immunocompetent patients with nasal polyps, opacified sinuses, and difficult-to-manage sinusitis. In the future, advanced MRI and CT scans may permit a diagnosis without need for surgical specimens and cultures.

7.2 Immunological Findings

Immediate cutaneous reactivity to the incriminated fungus and serum precipitating antibodies are present in AFS, usually without peripheral blood eosinophilia, and without markedly elevated total serum IgE and serum antifungal IgE and IgG levels (10,13). Some confusion may exist when a patient with AFS also has ABPA or ABPM (66), peripheral blood eosinophilia, or a modestly elevated total serum IgE concentration. Serum IgA–Af antibodies are not helpful in distinguishing AFS from chronic sinusitis. There is no serological diagnostic test to confirm AFS.

7.3 Treatment

7.3.1 Medications

Once the diagnosis of AFS is made, prednisone, in a regimen similar to ABPA, should be initiated, but a good response is less certain than for ABPA. In AFS the thick inspissated mucus is located in a closed space, unlike the more open bronchi in ABPA. If the prednisone trial is not successful, surgical intervention may be necessary to establish effective sinus drainage and to debulk sinus debris. Sinus debridement also may need to be considered. Sinus irrigations by the patient are recommended. Unfortunately, topical intranasal corticosteroids and antifungal agents have not been helpful. Some authors believe that fungal allergen immunotherapy has a role (65,67), but efficacy remains unproved.

7.3.2 Surgery

The surgical goal in AFS is to establish effective sinus drainage. Patients often will have had one or more sinus surgical procedures before the diagnosis of AFS is made. Removal of inferior turbinates and creation of larger ostia does not always prevent recurrences. Once adequate sinus marsupialization is performed, polyps removed, and drainage established with removal of the allergic mucin, prednisone therapy may reduce the frequency of recurrence. Physicians should be alert for acute bacterial sinusitis. If polyps recur, intranasal corticosteroids should be administered after prednisone is discontinued. Some patients appear to be cured of their AFS after several surgical procedures combined with prednisone treatment.

7.3.3 Controversies

Naturally, some patients will seek out therapy with antifungal agents in an attempt to avoid prednisone use or additional surgical procedures. The current state of knowledge is that such an approach will fail, and it is not a suitable alternative for ''prednisone phobia'' patients. With education that prednisone treatment is not lifelong for AFS, such patients may be more compliant. Prednisone has been used successfully for as short a time as 1 month postoperatively, but it is followed by a topical intranasal corticosteroid (11).

8 HYPERSENSITIVITY PNEUMONITIS

8.1 Clinical

Hypersensitivity pneumonitis (HP) presents as acute, subacute, or chronic disease. The diagnosis requires a high level of clinical suspicion in some settings because the antigen may be unknown or new, and the severity of symptoms may be mild if the inhaled dose of antigen is low. Many of the names given to HP refer to the occupation or hobby of the affected subject. Much experience has been obtained in studies of avian HP; aerosol challenges with avian antigens result in acute (hours after exposure), subacute, and chronic disease (68).

8.1.1 Acute HP

The acute response may occur 4–6 hr after challenge and the temporal relation to the antigen may not be appreciated by the patient. Acute symptoms can include chest tightness, dyspnea, cough, fever, chills, and myalgias (68). If a CXR is obtained, nodular infiltrates will usually be present, and pulmonary function tests (PFTs) show a restrictive pattern. Examination of the chest may reveal rales. Rarely, severe arterial hypoxemia or respiratory failure occurs.

8.1.2 Subacute HP

Subacute HP is insidious. Dyspnea, fatigue, and nonproductive cough, possibly with hypoxemia and fever, occur over weeks or months (69). For example, an 11-year-old child with exposure to nine cockatiels and two doves in the home, after 4 months of respiratory symptoms, presented with a Po_2 of 49 mmHg on room air (69). The CXR did not show infiltrates, but a high-resolution CT of the lung demonstrated a groundglass pattern. PFTs revealed a diffusing capacity for CO of just 24% of predicted, an FVC of 29%, and an FEV_1 of 28%, consistent with severe restriction (69). Subacute and acute presentations may overlap, but fever is less likely to occur in subacute cases of HP. Although the CXR often shows infiltrates, patients fail to improve with antibacterial agents.

8.1.3 Chronic HP

Chronic HP also may be insidious and results in pulmonary fibrosis to the point of honeycombing on CXR, dyspnea, and eventually respiratory failure (18,19). Pulmonary function tests show a restrictive pattern with varying degrees of obstruction, sometimes resembling asthma (19). In contrast with acute and subacute forms of HP, there is little to no meaningful response to oral corticosteroids. Furthermore, avoidance of the antigen does not result in improvement in respiratory status.

8.2 Immunology

8.2.1 Precipitating Antibodies

Precipitating antibodies to the antigen(s) involved are present and provide supportive evidence for the diagnosis. Sera should be concentrated before being combined with suspected antigens. Delays in the diagnosis of HP are common because of poorly reactive antigens. For avian hypersensitivity pneumonitis an extract from fresh bird excreta should be prepared and tested with sera from the affected individual when standard laboratory tests are reported as negative, but the index of suspicion is high. However, subjects often will have precipitins to antigens without having HP, suggesting sensitization, but not clinical disease. Thus, a diagnosis of HP requires both an appropriate clinical presentation and consistent laboratory test results.

8.2.2 Bronchoalveolar Lavage

Findings from BAL include a substantial increase in $CD8^+$ lymphocytes, up to 60–80% in both symptomatic and nonsymptomatic (exposed) individuals (70). Lymphocytes are activated as demonstrated by being $CD25^+$ (IL-2 receptor) or Ia^+, but show minimal suppressor activity in vitro. Symptomatic subjects with summer-type HP in Japan have increases in BAL sICAM, likely triggered by the pivotal cytokines, TNF-α, IFN-γ, or IL-1β (71). BAL lymphocytes and macrophages express increased levels of ICAM-1 compared with controls. The concentrations of BAL sICAM correlated well ($r = 0.71$) with the alveolar–arterial oxygen difference (71). These findings suggest that antigen inhalation in HP activates lymphocytes and alveolar macrophages to express ICAM-1 and shed this adhesion molecule into the bronchoalveolar compartment and into the peripheral blood (71).

Unexpectedly, mitogen responsiveness of BAL lymphocytes is reduced in HP when phytohemagglutinin (PHA) and concanavalin A (Con A) are used (72). Moreover, addition of alveolar macrophages, serving as accessory cells, to separated $CD4^+$ or $CD8^+$ lymphocytes increase lymphocyte responsiveness to normal. Thus, despite lymphocytic alveolitis, lymphocyte responsiveness to various agonists may be reduced, possibly accounting for some of the clinical and pathological findings of HP.

Incubation of an alveolar epithelial tumor cell line with *Saccharopolyspora rectivirfula*, the thermophilic bacteria formerly known as *Micropolyspora faeni*, caused IL-6 and IL-8 to be produced (73). Of interest, *S. rectivirfula* caused increased expression of NF–

κB, which activates transcription of the IL-8 gene. In these experiments, IL-10 and dexamethasone inhibited production of IL-8, a potent chemotactic factor for PMNs and an agonist for angiogenesis. The relevance of these results to HP is uncertain, because neutrophils are not abundant in the BAL fluid. As an example of the heightened activation state of macrophages in HP, BAL macrophages spontaneously secreted high levels of TNF-α and IL-1, which were suppressed by oral prednisone, 20 mg daily (74). Natural killer (NK) cell activity was also high at baseline, but paradoxically increased with prednisone administration (74).

To investigate why lymphocytic alveolitis occurs, BAL samples from 18 patients with HP were compared with nonsmokers for expression of costimulatory molecules (70). The absolute number of cells recovered was tenfold higher in BAL samples from patients with HP than in those from controls, with the percentage of lymphocytes being 64 in HP compared with 13 in controls (70). The percentages of BAL alveolar macrophages stained, respectively, with anti-CD80 (B7-1) and anti-CD86 (B7-2) were 35 and 62 in HP samples, compared with 7 and 24 in controls (70). Thus, costimulatory molecules on alveolar macrophages are up-regulated in HP compared with controls. The high levels of CD80 and CD86 expression are important because such alveolar macrophages may be more effective at presenting antigen to T cells. There were no differences between the percentages of HP and control T cells staining positive for CD28 and CTLA-4, receptors for CD80 and CD86.

8.3 Pathological Findings

8.3.1 Fatal Cases

Advanced pulmonary fibrosis (honeycomb lung) is a characteristic of fatal cases of HP (18,19,75). Cystic areas are seen on gross examination. Microscopically, HP involves the interstitium, terminal bronchioles, and alveoli. Histological examination can demonstrate lymphocyte and plasma cell interstitial and peribronchiolar infiltrates without vasculitis or infectious organisms (18). The alveoli can be replaced by fibrous connective tissue (19). Bronchiolitis obliterans may be present, but organizing pneumonias are not seen. Granulomas usually are absent (18,19,75), but were present in a dairy farmer who died 1 day after bagging moldy grain (75).

8.3.2 Nonfatal Cases

Biopsies of lung tissue in an acute form of avian HP reveals ''foamy'' histiocytes in alveolar septa surrounded by infiltrates comprised of lymphocytes and plasma cells (76). The histological pattern is consistent with interstitial pneumonitis. In chronic pigeon-breeder's disease, instead of histiocytes, one finds noncaseating granulomas, with giant cells in interstitial spaces and in alveoli. The bronchiole lumen is obstructed with inflammatory cells, and peribronchiolar smooth-muscle hypertrophy occurs to a greater extent than pulmonary fibrosis (77). The combination of inflammation surrounding bronchioles and fibrosis of alveoli explain the arterial hypoxemia that occurs in HP, even when the CXR does not show an infiltrate.

8.4 Treatment

8.4.1 Avoidance

Without exception primary treatment requires avoidance of the culprit antigens. Because the offending antigenic material may be related to workplace exposures or hobbies (birds), there may be reluctance to comply. Especially in the case of avian hypersensitivity pneumonitis, the birds in the home may function as dear companions. Some bird-fanciers have become depressed or suicidal when birds were removed from the home environment.

8.4.2 Pharmacological Therapy

Prednisone can be administered for short periods to resolve CXR infiltrates, raise arterial oxygen, and improve overall respiratory status. Dosages for adults of 40–60 mg daily taken as a single morning dose for 1–2 weeks can be effective in the acute and subacute states of HP. It is hoped that the antigenic exposure can be reduced or eliminated during that time period so that prednisone can be discontinued. In patients with chronic forms of HP in whom end-stage pulmonary fibrosis has occurred, home oxygen may be needed. Prednisone given on alternate days or in low daily doses may be useful as a maintenance medication in patients who resemble corticosteroid-dependent asthmatics (19). If HP progresses to pulmonary-based disability and cyanosis, a lung transplant may be indicated. However, even successful transplantation still requires the patient to comply with medications and environmental control. Clearly, one hopes to avoid having patients progress to end-stage fibrosis from HP by early diagnosis and intervention.

ACKNOWLEDGMENTS

Supported by USPHS AI 42349 and the Ernest S. Bazley Grant to Northwestern Memorial Hospital and Northwestern University.

REFERENCES

1. Ricketti AJ, Greenberger PA, Patterson R. Varying presentations of allergic bronchopulmonary aspergillosis. Int Arch Allergy Appl Immunol 1984; 73:283–285.
2. Greenberger PA, Patterson R. Allergic bronchopulmonary aspergillosis and the evaluation of the patient with asthma. J Allergy Clin Immunol 1988; 81:646–650.
3. Mearns M, Young W, Batten J. Transient pulmonary infiltrates in cystic fibrosis due to allergic aspergillosis. Thorax 1965; 20:385–392.
4. Becker JW, Burke W, McDonald G, Greenberger PA, Henderson WR, Aiken ML. Prevalence of allergic bronchopulmonary aspergillosis and atopy in adult patients with cystic fibrosis. Chest 1996; 109:1536–1540.
5. Laufer P, Fink JN, Bruns WT, Unger GF, Kalbfleisch JH, Greenberger PA, Patterson R. Allergic bronchopulmonary aspergillosis in cystic fibrosis. J Allergy Clin Immunol 1984; 73:44–48.
6. Nikolaizik WH, Moser M, Crameri R, Little S, Warner JO, Blaser K, Schoni MH. Identification of allergic bronchopulmonary aspergillosis in cystic fibrosis patients by recombinant *Aspergillus fumigatus* I/a-specific serology. Am J Respir Crit Care Med 1995; 152:634–639.
7. Geller DE, Kaplowitz H, Light MJ, Colin AA. Allergic bronchopulmonary aspergillosis in cystic fibrosis: reported prevalence, regional distribution, and patient characteristics. Chest 1999; 116:639–646.
8. Hutcheson PS, Knutsen AP, Rejent AJ, Slavin RG. A 12-year longitudinal study of *Aspergillus* sensitivity in patients with cystic fibrosis. Chest 1996; 110:363–366.
9. Eppinger TM, Greenberger PA, White DA, Brown AE, Cunningham–Rundles C. Sensitization to *Aspergillus* species in the congenital neutrophil disorders chronic granulomatous disease and hyper-IgE syndrome. J Allergy Clin Immunol 1999; 104:1265–1272.
10. Katzenstein A–LA, Sale SR, Greenberger PA. Allergic *Aspergillus* sinusitis: a newly recognized form of sinusitis. J Allergy Clin Immunol 1983; 72:89–93.

11. Marple BF, Mabry RL. Comprehensive management of allergic fungal sinusitis. Am J Rhinol 1998; 12:263–268.
12. Schwartz HJ. Allergic fungal sinusitis: experience in an ambulatory allergy practice. Ann Allergy Asthma Immunol 1996; 77:500–502.
13. Schubert MS, Goetz DW. Evaluation and treatment of allergic fungal sinusitis. I. Demographics and diagnosis. J Allergy Clin Immunol 1998; 102:387–394.
14. Schubert MS, Goetz DW. Evaluation and treatment of allergic fungal sinusitis. II. Treatment and follow-up. J Allergy Clin Immunol 1998; 102:395–402.
15. deShazo RD, Chapin K, Swain RE. Fungal sinusitis. N Engl J Med 1997; 337:254–259.
16. Schuyler M. The diagnosis of hypersensitivity pneumonitis. Chest 1997; 111:534–536.
17. Saltoun CA, Harris KE, Mathisen TL, Patterson R. Hypersensitivity pneumonitis resulting from community exposure to Canada goose droppings: when an external environmental antigen becomes an indoor environmental antigen. Ann Allergy Asthma Immunol 2000; 84:84–86.
18. Nakagawa–Yoshida K, Ando M, Etches RI, Dosman JA. Fatal cases of farmer's lung in a Canadian family: probable new antigens, *Penicillium brevicompactum* and *P. olivicolor*. Chest 1997; 111:245–248.
19. Greenberger PA, Pien LC, Patterson R, Robinson P, Roberts M. End-stage lung and ultimately fatal disease in a bird fancier. Am J Med 1989; 86:119–122.
20. Yoshizawa Y, Ohtani Y, Hayakawa H, Sato A, Suga M, Ando M. Chronic hypersensitivity pneumonitis in Japan: a nationwide epidemiologic survey. J Allergy Clin Immunol 1999; 103: 315–320.
21. Schwartz HJ, Greenberger PA. The prevalence of allergic bronchopulmonary aspergillosis in patients with asthma, determined by serologic and radiologic criteria in patients at risk. J Lab Clin Med 1991; 117:138–142.
22. American Thoracic Society. Fungal infection in HIV-infected persons. Am J Respir Crit Care Med 1995; 152:816–822.
23. Pursell KJ, Telzak EE, Armstrong D. *Aspergillus* species colonization and invasive disease in patients with AIDS. Clin Infect Dis 1992; 14:141–148.
24. Gerson SL, Talbot GH, Hurwitz S, Strom BL, Lusk EJ, Cassileth PA. Prolonged granulocytopenia: the major risk factor for invasive pulmonary aspergillosis in patients with acute leukemia. Ann Intern Med 1984; 100:345–351.
25. Tomee JFC, Mannes GPM, van der Bij W, van der Werf TS, de Boer WJ, Koeter GH, Kauffman HF. Serodiagnosis and monitoring of *Aspergillus* infections after lung transplantation. Ann Intern Med 1996; 125:197–201.
26. Kramer MR, Denning DW, Marshall SE, Ross DJ, Berry G, Lewiston NJ, Stevens DA, Theodore J. Ulcerative tracheobronchitis after lung transplantation: a new form of invasive aspergillosis. Am Rev Respir Dis 1991; 144:552–556.
27. Neeld DA, Goodman LR, Gurney JW, Greenberger PA, Fink JN. Computerized tomography in the evaluation of allergic bronchopulmonary aspergillosis. Am Rev Respir Dis 1990; 142: 1200–1205.
28. Greenberger PA, Miller TP, Roberts M, Smith LL. Allergic bronchopulmonary aspergillosis in patients with and without evidence of bronchiectasis. Ann Allergy 1993; 70:333–338.
29. Patterson R, Greenberger PA, Radin RC. Allergic bronchopulmonary aspergillosis: staging as an aid to management. Ann Intern Med 1982; 96:286–291.
30. Patterson R, Greenberger PA, Lee TA, Liotta JL, O'Neill EA, Roberts M, Sommers H. Prolonged evaluation of patients with corticosteroid-dependent asthma stage of allergic bronchopulmonary aspergillosis. J Allergy Clin Immunol 1987; 80:663–668.
31. Lee TM, Greenberger PA, Patterson R, Roberts M, Liotta JL. Stage V (fibrotic) allergic bronchopulmonary aspergillosis. Arch Intern Med 1987; 147:319–323.
32. Ricketti AJ, Greenberger PA, Patterson R. Immediate-type reactions in patients with allergic bronchopulmonary aspergillosis. J Allergy Clin Immunol 1983; 71:541–545.

33. Greenberger PA, Patterson R, Ghory AC, Arkins JA, Walsh T, Graves T, Saker J. Late sequelae of allergic bronchopulmonary aspergillosis. J Allergy Clin Immunol 1980; 66:327–335.
34. Bosken CH, Myers JL, Greenberger PA, Katzenstein A–LA. Pathologic findings of allergic bronchopulmonary aspergillosis. Am J Surg Pathol 1988; 12:216–222.
35. Rosenberg M, Patterson R, Mintzer R, Cooper BJ, Roberts M, Harris KE. Clinical and immunologic criteria for the diagnosis of allergic bronchopulmonary aspergillosis. Ann Intern Med 1977; 86:405–414.
36. Ricketti AJ, Greenberger PA, Patterson R. Serum IgE as an important aid in management of allergic bronchopulmonary aspergillosis. J Allergy Clin Immunol 1984; 74:68–71.
37. Patterson R, Rosenberg M, Roberts M. Evidence that *Aspergillus fumigatus* growing in the airway of man can be a potent stimulus of specific and nonspecific IgE formation. Am J Med 1979; 63:257–262.
38. Kurup VP, Banerjee B, Murali PS, Greenberger PA, Krishnan M, Hari V, Fink JN. Immunodominant peptide epitopes of allergen, Asp f I from the fungus *Aspergillus fumigatus*. Peptides 1998; 19:1469–1477.
39. Murali PS, Kurup VP, Bansal NK, Fink JN, Greenberger PA. IgE down regulation and cytokine induction by *Aspergillus* antigens in human allergic bronchopulmonary aspergillosis. J Lab Clin Med 1998; 131:228–235.
40. Greenberger PA, Liotta JL, Roberts M. The effects of age on isotypic antibody responses to *Aspergillus fumigatus*: implications regarding in vitro measurements. J Lab Clin Med 1989; 114:278–284.
41. Krasnick J, Greenberger PA, Roberts M, Patterson R. Allergic bronchopulmonary aspergillosis: serologic update for 1995. J Lab Clin Immunol 1995; 46:137–142.
42. Apter AJ, Greenberger PA, Liotta JL, Roberts M. Fluctuations of serum IgA and its subclasses in allergic bronchopulmonary aspergillosis. J Allergy Clin Immunol 1989; 84:367–372.
43. Bernstein JA, Zeiss CR, Greenberger PA, Patterson R, Marhoul JF, Smith LL. Immunoblot analysis of sera from patients with allergic bronchopulmonary aspergillosis: correlation with disease activity. J Allergy Clin Immunol 1990; 86:532–539.
44. Greenberger PA, Smith LJ, Hsu CCS, Roberts M, Liotta JL. Analysis of bronchoalveolar lavage in allergic bronchopulmonary aspergillosis: divergent responses of antigen-specific antibodies and total IgE. J Allergy Clin Immunol 1988; 82:164–170.
45. Ricketti AJ, Greenberger PA, Pruzansky JJ, Patterson R. Hyperreactivity of mediator-releasing cells from patients with allergic bronchopulmonary aspergillosis as evidenced by basophil histamine release. J Allergy Clin Immunol 1983; 72:386–392.
46. Brown JE, Greenberger PA, Yarnold PR. Soluble serum interleukin 2 receptors in patients with asthma and allergic bronchopulmonary aspergillosis. Ann Allergy Asthma Immunol 1995; 74:484–488.
47. Chauhan B, Knutsen AP, Hutcheson PS, Slavin RG, Bellone CJ. T cell subsets, epitope mapping, and HLA-restriction in patients with allergic bronchopulmonary aspergillosis. J Clin Invest 1996; 97:2324–2331.
48. Chauhan B, Santiago L, Kirschman DA, Hauptfeld V, Knutsen AP, Hutcheson PS, Woulfe SL, Slavin RG, Schwartz HJ, Bellone CJ. The association of HLA-DR alleles and T cell activation with allergic bronchopulmonary aspergillosis. J Immunol 1997; 159:4072–4076.
49. Kurup VP, Grunig G, Knutsen AP, Murali PS. Cytokines in allergic bronchopulmonary aspergillosis. Res Immunol 1998; 149:466–477.
50. Kurup VP, Hari V, Guo J, Murali PS, Resnick A, Krishnan M, Fink JN. *Aspergillus fumigatus* peptides differentially express Th1 and Th2 cytokines. Peptides 1996; 17:183–190.
51. Greenberger PA, Grammer LC, Goulsby C. Lymphocyte activation during and after exacerbations of allergic bronchopulmonary aspergillosis. Clin Res 1994; 42:385A.
52. Mendelson EB, Fisher MR, Mintzer RA, Halwig JM, Greenberger PA. Roentgenographic and clinical staging of allergic bronchopulmonary aspergillosis. Chest 1985; 87:334–349.

53. Shah A, Pant CS, Bhagat R, Panchal N. CT in childhood allergic bronchopulmonary aspergillosis. Pediatr Radiol 1992; 22:227–228.
54. Wang JLF, Patterson R, Roberts M, Ghory AC. The management of allergic bronchopulmonary aspergillosis. Am Rev Respir Dis 1979; 120:87–92.
55. Leon EE, Craig TJ. Antifungals in the treatment of allergic bronchopulmonary aspergillosis. Ann Allergy Asthma Immunol 1999; 82:511–517.
56. Safirstein BH, D'Souza MF, Simon G, Tai EH–C, Pepys J. Five-year follow-up of allergic bronchopulmonary aspergillosis. Am Rev Respir Dis 1973; 108:450–459.
57. Denning DW, Van Wye JE, Lewiston NJ, Stevens DA, Adjunctive therapy of allergic bronchopulmonary aspergillosis with itraconazole. Chest 1991; 100:813–819.
58. Salez F, Brichet A, Desurmont S, Grosbois J–M, Wallaert B, Tonnel A–B. Effects of itraconazole therapy in allergic bronchopulmonary aspergillosis. Chest 1999; 116:1665–1668.
59. Stevens DA, Schwartz HJ, Lee JV, Moskovitz BL, Jerome DC, Catanzaro A, Bamberger DM, Weinmann AJ, Tuazon CU, Judson MA, Platts–Mills TAE, DeGraff AC. A randomized trial of itraconazole in allergic bronchopulmonary aspergillosis. N Engl J Med 2000; 342:756–762.
60. Nepomuceno IB, Esrig S, Moss RB. Allergic bronchopulmonary aspergillosis in cystic fibrosis: role of atopy and response to itraconazole. Chest 1999; 115:364–370.
61. Miller MA, Greenberger PA, Amerian R, Toogood JH, Noskin GA, Roberts M, Patterson R. Allergic bronchopulmonary mycosis caused by *Pseudallescheria boydii*. Am Rev Respir Dis 1993; 148:810–812.
62. Pinson P, Van Der Straeten M. Fibrotic stage of allergic bronchopulmonary candidiasis. Chest 1991; 100:565–567.
63. Piechura JE, Kurup VP, Daft LJ. Isolation and immunochemical characterization of fractions from membranes of *Aspergillus fumigatus* with protease activity. Can J Microbiol 1990; 36: 33–41.
64. Kurup VP, Kumar A, Kenealy WR, Greenberger PA. *Aspergillus* ribotoxins react with IgE and IgG antibodies of patients with allergic bronchopulmonary aspergillosis. J Lab Clin Med 1994; 123:749–756.
65. Marple BF, Mabry RL. What we now know about allergic fungal sinusitis. J Respir Dis 2000; 21:23–31.
66. Bhagat R, Shah A, Jaggi OP, Khan ZU. Concomitant allergic bronchopulmonary aspergillosis and allergic *Aspergillus* sinusitis with an operated aspergilloma. J Allergy Clin Immunol 1993; 91:1094–1096.
67. Folker RJ, Marple BF, Mabry RL, Mabry CS. Treatment of allergic fungal sinusitis: a comparison trial of postoperative immunotherapy with specific fungal antigens. Laryngoscope 1998; 108:1623–1627.
68. Fink JN. Hypersensitivity pneumonitis. In: Patterson R, Grammer LC, Greenberger PA, eds. Allergic Diseases: Diagnosis and Management. Philadelphia: Lippincott–Raven, 1997:543–553.
69. McClellan JS, Albers GM, Noyes BE, Sotelo C, Petterchak JA, Knutsen AP. B-lymphocyte aggregates in alveoli from a child with hypersensitivity pneumonitis (bird breeders lung). Ann Allergy Asthma Immunol 1999; 83:357–360.
70. Israel–Assayag E, Dakhama A, Lavigne S, Laviolette M, Cormier Y. Expression of costimulatory molecules on alveolar macrophages in hypersensitivity pneumonitis. Am J Respir Crit Care Med 1999; 159:1830–1834.
71. Shijubo N, Imai K, Shigehara K, Hirasawa M, Tsujisaki M, Hinoda Y, Abe S. Soluble intercellular adhesion molecule-1 (ICAM-1) in sera and bronchoalveolar lavage (BAL) fluids of extrinsic alveolitis. Clin Exp Immunol 1995; 102:91–97.
72. Yamasaki H, Kinoshita T, Ohmura T, Ando M, Soda K, Sakata T, Araki S, Onoue K. Lowered responsiveness of bronchoalveolar lavage T lymphocytes. Am J Respir Cell Mol Biol 1991; 4:417–425.

73. Gudmundsson G, Hunninghad GW. Respiratory epithelial cells release interleukin-8 in response to a chemophilic bacteria that causes hypersensitivity pneumonitis. Exp Lung Res 1999; 25:217–228.
74. Denis M, Bedard M, Laviolette M, Cormier Y. A study of monokine release and natural killer activity in the bronchoalveolar lavage of subjects with farmer's lung. Am Rev Respir Dis 1993; 147:934–939.
75. Kokkarinen J, Tukiainen H, Terho EO. Mortality due to farmer's lung in Finland. Chest 1994; 106:509–512.
76. Fink JN, Sosman AJ, Barboriak JJ, Schleuter DP, Holmes RA. Pigeon breeder's disease: a clinical study of hypersensitivity pneumonitis. Ann Intern Med 1968; 68:1205–1219.
77. Perez–Padilla R, Gaxiola M, Salas J, Mejia M, Ramos C, Selman M. Bronchiolitis in chronic pigeon breeders disease: morphologic evidence of a spectrum of small airway lesions in hypersensitivity pneumonitis induced by avian antigens. Chest 1996; 110:371–377.

22

Pharmacological Approaches

PEDRO C. AVILA, JEFFREY L. KISHIYAMA, and DANIEL C. ADELMAN

University of California at San Francisco, San Francisco, California

1 INTRODUCTION

The etiology of the rise in prevalence of allergic diseases is unknown, but recent evidence suggests changes in lifestyle may play a role. The increase in incidence of allergic disease has been most noticeable as developing nations undergo the transformation from rural communities to industrialized societies with western lifestyles (1). Epidemiological studies have identified some factors associated with ''western lifestyles'' and an increased prevalence of atopy. These factors include, but are not limited to, the following:

1. Increased home insulation and decreased ventilation which increases exposure to indoor allergens such as dust mites, cat dander, and cockroach antigen (2,3).
2. Decreased childhood exposure to infections (e.g., measles, hepatitis A, tuberculosis, and lactobacillus) owing to more hygienic habits and vaccinations. Some investigators hypothesize that exposure to common childhood infections preferentially induces T-helper 1 (Th1) immunological response patterns, which reciprocally inhibit development of atopy (Th2-responses) on later exposure to environmental antigens (4–8).
3. Air pollution, particularly exposure to diesel exhaust particles that may act as an adjuvant for allergic inflammation (9).

Until the environmental factors responsible for the increase in prevalence and morbidity of atopic diseases are elucidated, primary prevention in children born with genetic predisposition for atopy is unlikely to be accomplished and a reliance on pharmacological management will remain. The current armamentarium of drugs (Table 1) to treat allergic diseases is sufficiently diverse to allow physicians to adequately manage most patients suffering from allergic diseases. Among the most efficacious and widely used drugs are

Table 1 Medications Available for Treatment of Allergic Diseases

Class	Drug
Topical corticosteroids	Beclomethasone dipropionate Budesonide Flunisolide Fluticasone propionate Mometasone Triamcinolone acetonide
Antihistamines	
First-generation	Brompheniramine Clemastine Chlorpheniramine Cyproheptadine Diphenhydramine Hydroxyzine Phenothiazine
Second-generation	Azelastine Cetirizine Ebastine Fexofenadine Levocabastine Loratidine Terfenadine[a]
Decongestants	
Topical	Ephedrine Oxymetazoline
Systemic	Pseudoephedrine Phenylpropanolamine
Nonsteroidal anti-inflammatory drugs[b]	Colchicine Indomethacin
β_2-Agonists	
Short-acting	Albuterol Pirbuterol Terbutaline Levalbuterol Metaproterenol
Long-acting	Salmeterol Formoterol[a]
Mast cell stabilizers	Cromolyn sodium Nedocromil sodium Olopatadine Ketotifen[a]
Methylxantines	Aminophylline Theophyline
Anticholinergic agents	Ipratropium bromide[b]
Leukotriene antagonists	Montelukast Pranlukast[a] Zafirlukast Zileuton
Immunosuppressants[b]	Cyclosporin A[b] Methotrexate[b]
Desensitization	Allergen immunotherapy Aspirin

[a] Not available in the United States.
[b] Not approved by the U.S. Food and Drug Administration for treatment of allergic diseases.

corticosteroids, which inhibit many aspects of atopic inflammation and are very effective in the treatment of allergic diseases. Although partially ameliorated through the development and utilization of topical preparations, the long-term toxicity of corticosteroids remains a major problem. Consideration of drug safety, in the context of a worldwide increase in prevalence of allergic diseases (10,11), has fostered considerable interest and research into the development of novel and efficacious therapeutics.

2 INFLAMMATORY PROCESSES IN ATOPIC DISEASE

The mechanisms of allergic inflammation are extremely complex and involve several different cell types and chemical mediators. More detailed characterization of immunopathogenetic mechanisms and elucidation of inflammatory cascades has contributed toward the development of better treatments for allergic disease. Ongoing trials with investigational therapies often have the dual objectives of developing potential therapeutics and providing insight toward the underlying immunopathogenesis of disease. A brief description of the allergic inflammatory cascade is provided in Figure 1. Mast cell activation occurs after allergen exposure, causing the release of histamine and generation of newly formed mediators and leukotrienes, which cause vasodilation, increased vascular permeability, chemoattraction of leukocytes, and bronchoconstriction. Whereas this early allergic response can cause symptoms in affected individuals, it also sets the stage for the development of late-phase allergic reactions and the development of chronic inflammation with persistent allergen exposure. Chronic inflammation is characterized by morphological tissue changes and infiltration by sensitized and activated leukocytes. In affected tissues, allergens are processed by antigen-presenting cells (APCs), including macrophages, dendritic cells, and B lymphocytes, and presented to T helper lymphocytes in the context of major histocompatibility complex (MHC) (Fig. 2).

A current paradigm of T-helper cell function is useful when considering the role of sensitized T cells in the pathogenesis of inflammation. Naive or resting $CD4^+$ T lymphocytes can mature and develop down one of two dichotomous pathways to become a T-helper type-1 (Th1) or T-helper type-2 (Th2) lymphocyte (12,13). The phenotype of these functional T cells is determined by examination of their cytokine production and profile. Th1 cells preferentially synthesize interleukin (IL)-2 and interferon (IFN)-γ, which contribute to cell-mediated immune responses. Th2 cells produce IL-4, IL-5, IL-9, and IL-13, which promote humoral immunity and IgE-mediated hypersensitivity.

There has been an increased appreciation that allergic diseases are characterized by chronic inflammatory tissue changes, associated with antigen-specific, activated T lymphocytes demonstrating T helper 2 (Th2) phenotype (see Fig. 1) (11,14,15). Th2 responses promote allergic inflammation through the promotion of IgE-mediated reactions and eosinophilia. In mice, passive transfer of antigen-specific, sensitized Th2 cells is sufficient to generate an asthma phenotype in nonallergic animals subsequently exposed to inhaled allergen (16–18). The Th2 cells are thought to orchestrate the tissue inflammation (see Fig. 2) (16,19) by releasing not only IL-4 and IL-13, which induces B cell immunoglobulin isotype switch from IgM to IgE, but also through the generation of IL-3, IL-5, and granulocyte–monocyte colony-stimulating factor (GM-CSF). IL-5 recruits, activates, and prolongs the survival of eosinophils (15) and IL-3; GM-CSF contributes to mast cell differentiation.

Production and synthesis of Th2 cytokines may not be exclusive to T cells, however, as numerous other cells (as described in Chapters 2–11) secrete proinflammatory media-

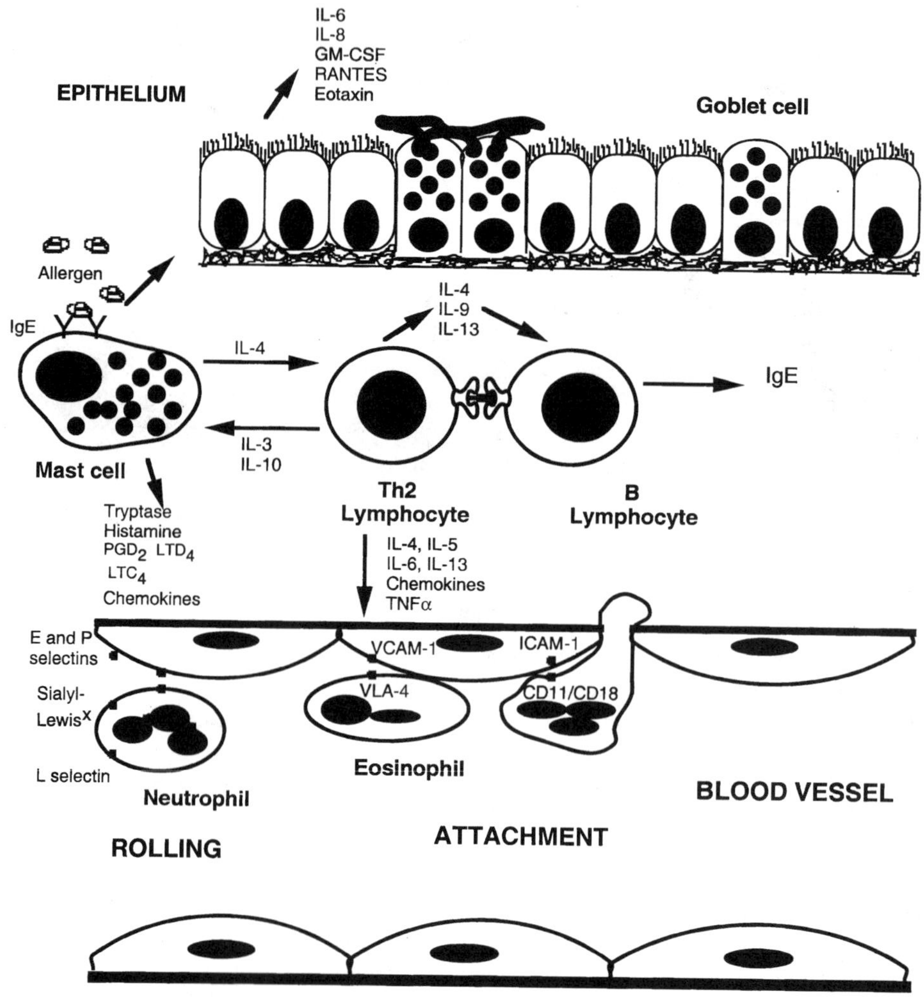

Figure 1 Allergic inflammation: Mast cells are activated by the allergen binding to surface IgE, which causes release of granular contents and production of lipid mediators, cytokines, and chemokines. Those mediators cause vasodilation, increase permeability in blood vessels, and cause the early allergic response. They also attract inflammatory cells, such as eosinophils and neutrophils, that characterize the late allergic response. The eosinophils and neutrophils in the bloodstream first slow down by rolling over the activated endothelium, a process mediated by selectins. Then, eosinophils and neutrophils attach tightly to the endothelium through integrins and traverse the vessel wall toward the inflamed tissue, guided by chemokines. T lymphocytes are the most important cells driving the allergic inflammation. T lymphocytes are activated by antigen-presenting cells (e.g., B lymphocytes and dendritic cells) and release cytokines and chemokines that affect all cells involved in the allergic inflammation. B lymphocytes are activated by allergen, by cell contact and interaction with T lymphocytes (CD40–CD40 ligand interaction), and by IL-4 and IL-13, which promote B-cell proliferation and differentiation to plasma cells and production of IgE. Epithelial cells also produce cytokines and chemokines that further enhance airway inflammation. Abbreviations: Th2, T helper 2; IL, interleukin; RANTES, regulated on activation, normal T-cell expressed and secreted; GM–CSF, granulocyte–monocyte colony-stimulating factor; PG, prostaglandin; LT, leukotriene; TNF-α, tumor necrosis factor-alpha; VCAM-1, vascular cell adhesion molecule 1; ICAM-1, intercellular adhesion molecule 1; VLA-4, very late antigen 4; LTD_4, leukotriene D_4; LTC_4, leukotriene C_4.

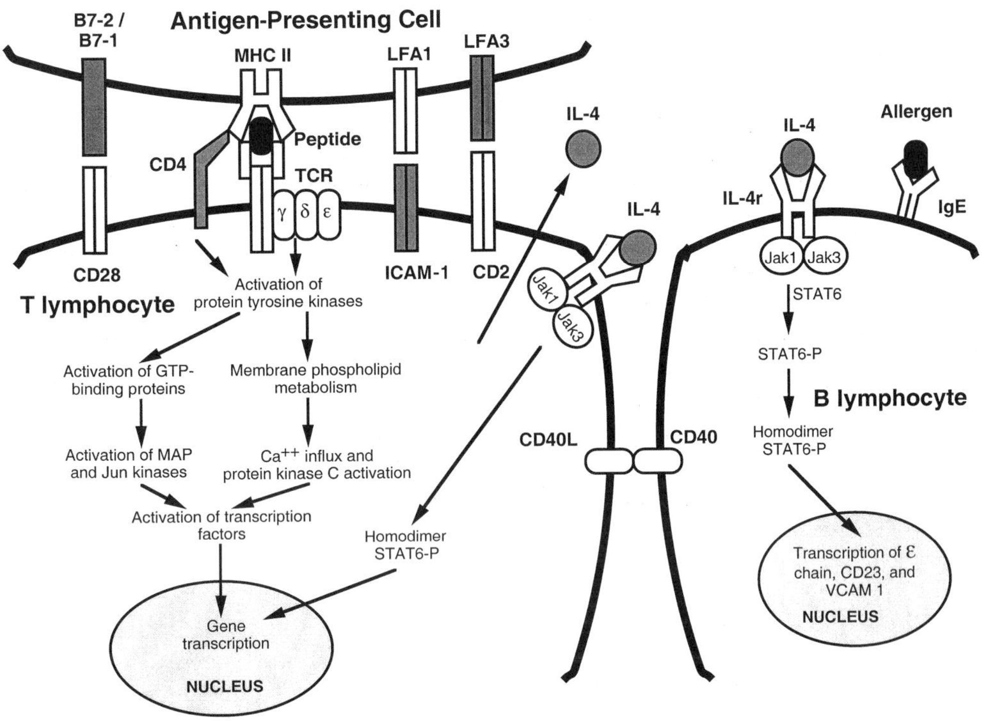

Figure 2 Activation of lymphocytes: T cells interact with antigen-presenting cells through several molecules that provide adhesion and stimulation signals. Peptide from the allergen is presented in the major histocompatibility complex class II (MHC II), which interacts with the T-cell receptor (TCR) and CD4. This interaction activates protein tyrosine kinases (PTKs such as Lck, Fyn) in the intracytoplasmic tails of TCR and CD4 which, in turn, activate other PTKs such as Zap-70. Zap-70 then activates guanosine triphosphate (GTP)-binding proteins such as RAS and phospholipase C. RAS activates mitogen-activated protein kinases, and phospholipase C initiates membrane phospholipid catabolism. These processes lead to activation of transcription factors and gene expression. Interleukin 4 (IL-4) is secreted by T-helper cells and binds to the IL-4 receptor (IL-4r) to activate PTKs in its intracytoplasmic tails (Jak1 and Jak3), which phosphorylate signal transducer and activator of transcription 6 (STAT6). Phosphorylated STAT6 (STAT6-P) forms dimers that are translocated into the nucleus and causes transcription of many genes related to allergic inflammation, such as epsilon (ε) chain of IgE, VCAM-1, and low-affinity Fc receptor for IgE (CD23). Interaction between B7-2 (or B7-1) and CD28 provides essential costimulatory signal for T-cell activation, and adhesion molecules maintain APC and T-cell attachment. B lymphocytes are activated by cell interaction with T cells through CD40 and CD40 ligand (CD40L), IL-4, and binding of allergen to surface IgE. For abbreviations see Figure 1. LFA, lymphocyte-function associated antigen.

tors and actively contribute to allergic inflammation, including neurons (20), epithelial cells (21), fibroblasts (22–25), smooth muscle (26–28), and endothelial cells (29–31). Furthermore, T cells, together with epithelial cells, macrophages, and other cell types, release chemokines (that play an important role in chemoattraction of lymphocytes, monocytes, eosinophils, and neutrophils) into the site of allergic inflammation (32). Additionally, although the inflammation of allergic diseases is more of a Th2 type, some markers of Th1 response can also be found in tissues affected by allergic inflammation (see Fig. 1).

3 AVAILABLE PHARMACOLOGICAL APPROACHES FOR ALLERGIC DISEASES

3.1 Topical and Systemic Corticosteroids

Corticosteroids are presently the mainstay for treatment of chronic allergic inflammatory diseases because of their inhibitory effects on the cells involved in inflammation as well as their ability to block the generation of mediators such as proinflammatory cytokines, chemokines, adhesion molecules, and lipid mediators (33). This broad anti-inflammatory action is reflected by their marked effectiveness in clinical trials (33,34), so that now they are the gold standard treatment for chronic allergic inflammatory disorders. However, even topically applied corticosteroids can cause several adverse effects that concern clinicians, particularly pediatricians, and have encouraged the search for new anti-inflammatory agents with more attractive side effect profiles.

Topical corticosteroids are the most effective drugs in the long-term treatment of asthma in children and adults. Clinical studies have shown that topical corticosteroids markedly reduce local inflammation, improve lung function, and that early intervention improves pulmonary physiological and clinical outcomes. Topical corticosteroids are also cost-effective and improve quality of life (33). In comparative studies, topical corticosteroids are more effective than any other medication for the long-term treatment of asthma and should be considered the first-line treatment for chronic disease management (33).

Several inhaled topical corticosteroids are available for the treatment of allergic airways disease (Table 2). Although many clinical trials have compared the different formulations, a definite conclusion cannot be reached on their comparability because of vari-

Table 2 Comparison of Inhaled Corticosteroids

Parameter	BDP/BMP	BUD	FLUN	FLUT	TAA
Bioavailability after oral dose	<20%	11%	21%	<1%	10%
Bioavailability after inhaled dose	20%	25%	39%	20%	21.5%
Hydrosolubility (μg/mL)	0.1/10	14	100	0.04	40
GR binding[a]	0.4/13.5	9.4	1.8	18–22	2.3–3.6
Clearance (L/min)	3.8	0.9–1.5	1.0	0.9	0.8–1.2
Half-life (hr)	15	1.5–2.8	1.6	3.1–14	1.5
Glucocorticoid receptor complex half-life (hr)	NA/7.5	5.1	3.5	10.5	3.9
Volume distribution (L/kg)	NA	4.3	1.8	3.5	1.4
Dissolution time in bronchial fluid	>5 hr	6 min	<2 min	>6 hr	NA
Relative glucocorticoid receptor affinity	NA/3.3	2.5	0.45	5.0	0.5
Relative clinical equivalence estimations (μg)[b]	1.5	1.5	3.0	1.0	3.0

BDP/BMP, beclomethasone dipropionate/beclomethasone monopropionate. BDP is metabolized into BMP, an active metabolite; BUD, budesonide; FLUN, flunisolide; FLUT, fluticasone propionate; TAA, Triamcinolone acetate; NA, not available.

[a] Glucocorticoid receptor (GR) binding is relative to dexamethasone; the higher the number the higher is the affinity of the corticosteroid for the GR.

[b] Clinical equivalence in micrograms among the different corticosteroids (e.g., 1 μg FLUT = 3 μg TAA) is based on estimations from limited clinical data available.

Source: Refs. 126–128.

ability in delivery devices, lack of control for confounding factors, and flat dose–response curves seen in studies of early inhaled corticosteroid preparations. Newer-generation preparations, fluticasone propionate and budesonide, have a better risk/benefit ratio than older inhaled preparations because of their high first-pass metabolism by the liver, which reduces the risk of systemic side effects (35). Mometasone, a recently developed topical corticosteroid, seems to have similar characteristics and is under investigation for the treatment of asthma. When the topical corticosteroids are compared on a microgram-to-microgram basis, flunisolide and triamcinolone are felt to be the weakest inhaled corticosteroids, followed by beclomethasone dipropionate, budesonide, and fluticasone in ascending order of potency (35,36) (see Table 2). The frequency of adverse effects to topical corticosteroids therapy is directly proportional to the total daily dose administered and duration of treatment. Side effects are myriad and can include oral candidiasis (5%), dysphonia (up to 58%), alterations in bone metabolism, suppression of the hypothalamic–pituitary–adrenal axis, cataract formation, glaucoma, growth suppression in children, and dermal thinning with easy bruisability in older female patients (33).

Oral or systemic corticosteroids, including prednisone, prednisolone, methylprednisolone, and hydrocortisone, are very effective treatment for exacerbations of asthma and more rarely, very severe allergic rhinoconjunctivitis or atopic dermatitis. They are usually given for 7–10 days for acute exacerbations, but occasionally some patients with severe refractory disease require prolonged treatment. Long-term use of systemic corticosteroids is associated with increased risk for adverse effects, such as systemic hypertension, glucose intolerance, osteoporosis, cataracts, immunosuppression, and growth suppression in children (33).

At a molecular level, a corticosteroid molecule (CS) binds to a cytoplasmic glucocorticoid receptor (GR), forming a homodimeric complex (CS–GR). This CS–GR complex is transported into the nucleus where it binds to regions on the DNA called glucocorticoid response elements (GRE). The GRE are located 5′ upstream from promoter regions, and the interaction between CS–GR and GRE results in activation of promoter genes and increased gene expression. Binding of CS–GR to negative GRE (nGRE) may inactivate the promoter regions and decrease gene expression.

Corticosteroids also increases expression of IκB, an inhibitor of cytoplasmatic nuclear factor κB (NF-κB). Inhibition of NF-κB decreases cytokine (IL-1, IL-2, and IL-6; tumor necrosis factor-alpha [TNFα]), chemokines (IL-8, RANTES, monocytic chemotactic protein [MCP-1]), inducible NO synthase (iNOS), and adhesion molecules (ICAM-1 and VCAM-1) gene transcription. The complex CS–GR also binds and inhibits transcription factors such as activator protein 1 (AP-1) and transcription factor–CREB by binding to cyclic-AMP responsive elements (CREB) on genes. Corticosteroids can modulate transcription of 10–100 genes in a single cell, including suppression of many relevant gene products: IL-1, IL-2, IL-3, IL-4, IL-5, IL-6, IL-8, IL-11, IL-12, IL-13, TNFα, GM-CSF, RANTES, MIP-1α, MCP-1, MCP-3, MCP-4, eotaxin, stem cell factor (SCF, stimulates mast cells), iNOS, cyclooxygenase-2, inducible PLA_2, endothelin-1, ICAM-1, VCAM-1, and E-selectin.

Corticosteroids can also stimulate production of several gene products, including β_2-adrenergic receptors, IκB, IL-1 receptor antagonist, and neutral endopeptidase. In the airway, glucocorticoid receptors are mainly localized in epithelial cells, endothelial cells and, to a lesser extent, in smooth muscle and leukocytes (33,37). The inhibitory effect of corticosteroids on transcription factors appears to mediate most of the anti-inflammatory action (transrepression), whereas the binding of CS–GR to DNA is responsible for tran-

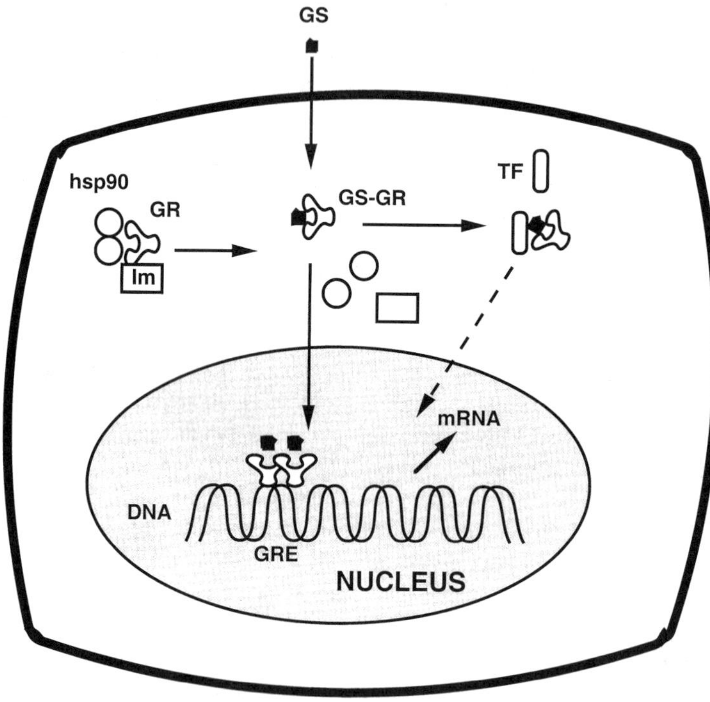

Figure 3 Mechanism of action of corticosteroids: Glucocorticoids (GS) bind to their receptor in the cytoplasm (GR) to form a complex (GS–GR). Normally, GRs are bound to heat-shock protein 90 (hsp 90), immunophylin (Im), and other inhibitory proteins, which keep GR inactive. GS–GR migrates into the nucleus where it forms dimers that bind to glucocorticoid responsive elements (GRE) on the DNA. There are positive GREs, which, once bound to GS–GR, cause increased gene transcriptions (e.g., lipocortin, β_2-adrenoceptor), and negative GREs, which cause decreased gene transcription (e.g., inducible nitric oxide synthase, cyclooxygenase 2). GS–GR also bind to transcriptor factors (TF) and inactivate them as is the case for nuclear factor κB (NF-κB), transcriptor factor activator protein (AP-1), transcriptor factor AMP responsive element (CREB), and STAT5 and STAT6. The interaction of GS–GR with transcription factors can lead to inhibition or stimulation of their action, so that corticosteroids affect transcription of 10–100 genes.

scription of genes (transactivation) responsible for many of the systemic side effects of corticosteroids (33,38,39). Developing new corticosteroids or small molecules that selectively inhibit transcription factors without causing transactivation may lead to drugs with anti-inflammatory properties comparable with the ones from current corticosteroids, but without systemic adverse effects (Fig. 3) (33,37,40).

3.2 Antihistamines

Histamine is produced and stored in cytoplasmic granules of mast cells and basophils and released after activation through surface IgE cross-linked by allergens. It binds to histamine receptors 1, 2, and 3 (H_{1r}, H_{2r}, and H_{3r}), which are G protein-coupled receptors. H_{1r} is the principal mediator or histamine effects in allergic diseases and is localized on the surface of smooth muscles in blood vessels, airways, and gastrointestinal tract. Biochemical signaling, after histamine–H_{1r} interaction, occurs via cytoplasmic inositol triphosphate and diacylglycerol. Clinically, activation of H_{1r} results in pruritus, sneezing, local pain, increased vascular permeability, hypotension, tachycardia, headache, flushing, bronchospasm, cough, and stimulation of endothelial cell nitric oxide production, further increasing vascular permeability and vasodilation. In the central nervous system (CNS), H_{1r} is involved in the control of vigilance and sleep (41).

The H_2 receptors are located in the gastric mucosa, heart, uterus, and CNS. Binding of histamine to H_{2r} leads to activation of adenylate cyclase and formation of cAMP. As a result, histamine causes gastric acid secretion, vasodilation, bronchospasm, mucous secretion in the airway, hypotension, tachycardia, headache, flushing, and proliferation of lymphocytes. H_{3r} plays a role in neurotransmission in the CNS, airways, and gastrointestinal tract. The mechanisms of H_{3r} activation are not well established.

There are several antihistamines that block H_{1r}. They are classified in seven categories:

1. Alkylamines (e.g., brompheniramine, chlorpheniramine)
2. Piperazines (e.g., hydroxyzine, meclizine, cetirizine)
3. Piperidines (e.g., cyproheptidine, astemizole, ebastine, levocabastine, loratadine, fexofenadine, terfenadine)
4. Ethanolamines (e.g., clemastine, diphenhydramine)
5. Ethylenediamines (e.g., antazoline)
6. Phenothiazines (e.g., promethazine)
7. Others (e.g., azelastine)

Their side effects are drug-specific, and can include depressive and stimulatory CNS symptoms, neuropsychiatric disorders, QTc prolongation, dry mouth, urinary retention, and altered taste. However, the second-generation antihistamines have a much safer adverse effect profile than first-generation antihistamines.

Second-generation antihistamines, such as loratadine, fexofenadine, and cetirizine, block H_{1r}, have long half-lives and are less sedative. The decreased sedative side effects are a consequence of their lipophobic structures, which decrease their ability to cross the blood–brain barrier. Tolerance to the CNS side effects has been reported in some studies, whereas tachyphylaxis owing to prolonged use up to 12 weeks, does not occur (41). Antihistamines do not inhibit late-phase response to allergen challenge, but decrease mucous production, sneezing, and pruritus.

Comparative studies have shown similar efficacy of H_{1r} antihistamines, topical cromolyn, and nedocromil in allergic rhinoconjunctivitis (41). Antihistamines are also effective for urticaria and skin pruritus in atopic dermatitis (41), but they are of limited benefit for asthma (42–44). The H_{2r} antihistamines have a limited role in the treatment of allergic diseases, but may benefit patients with chronic urticaria, anaphylaxis, and asthma associated with gastroesophageal reflux (41).

3.3 Adrenergic Agonists and Decongestants

Activation of alpha(α)$_1$- and α_2-adrenergic receptors (AR), which are G protein-coupled receptors, causes vasoconstriction and reduction of mucosal edema in allergic respiratory and ocular diseases. Decongestants stimulate α_1-AR, which activates the phosphoinositol pathway leading to intracellular influx of calcium, contraction of smooth muscle, decrease in plasma transudation, and reduction of edema. Activation of α_2-AR results in formation of cyclic-adenosine monophosphate (cAMP) and release of intracellular calcium, but it is not clear that decongestants stimulate α_2-AR (45). Use of systemic and topical decongestants can improve nasal and conjunctival vascular congestion. Prolonged regular use of topical decongestants can, however, cause unremitting nasal vascular congestion, soreness, and mucosal edema, which is called rhinitis medicamentosa. This disorder is attributed to down-regulation of expression of α-AR resulting in tachyphylaxis to decongestants. Thus, it is advisable to use topical decongestants for no longer than 2–3 days. Similar problems can occur with prolonged use of ocular α-AR agonists, which may give rise to conjunctivitis medicamentosa. Systemic decongestants do not cause those local adverse effects, but are weakly effective and may cause CNS stimulation.

3.4 β_2-Adrenergic Agonists: Short- and Long-Acting

The short-acting β_2-adrenergic receptor agonists are the most effective and fast-acting bronchodilators; therefore, they are the first choice for the treatment of acute exacerbations of asthma. The selectivity of albuterol, terbutaline, and pirbuterol for the β_2-AR allows more bronchodilation, with less tachycardia and tremors than nonselective β-AR bronchodilators, such as metaproterenol and fenoterol. Selective β_2-agonists have rapid onset of action (minutes) and their bronchodilatory effects last for 4–6 hr. They are available in inhaled, subcutaneous, and oral formulations. Those different formulations provide the same degree of bronchodilation, but the oral and subcutaneous formulations cause more side effects and have longer duration of action (46). Inhaled administration by metered-dose inhaler with a spacer is more efficacious than by jet nebulizer, although the use of jet nebulizer is easier and simpler.

Comparative studies with other drugs show that β_2-agonists produce more bronchodilation than ipratropium bromide and theophylline (46). Regular use of bronchodilator does not cause deleterious side effects (47), but is as effective when used on an as-needed basis. Although long-term regular use of β_2-agonists can be associated with loss of protection to methacholine and exercise challenges, significant tachyphylaxis to the bronchodilatory response does not occur (46).

A newly approved short-acting β_2-agonist, levalbuterol, is a pure preparation of the right isomer of albuterol (*R*-albuterol). Synthetic drugs are typically produced as racemic mixtures containing equal amounts of right and left isomers, but usually only one of the isomers is biologically active. Levalbuterol contains only the pure and biologically active *R*-albuterol. In one clinical trial, levalbuterol produced greater and longer bronchodilation than double the amount of the racemic mixture (comparable amounts of *R*-albuterol), suggesting that the presence of the *L*-albuterol in the racemic mixture jeopardizes the action of *R*-albuterol to a small extent (48).

There are two long-acting β_2-agonists (46), salmeterol and formoterol (not available in the United States), that may be used for the extended treatment of asthma, but not for acute symptom relief owing to their slow-onset action. Both salmeterol and formoterol have long lipophylic side chains that interact with the cell membrane and allow the bronchodilator to stimulate the β_2-AR for a prolonged time. The effects of either long-acting β_2-agonist are detected for up to 24 hr after a single dose, which allows twice-daily dosing. Formoterol has a faster onset of action than salmeterol. They are both effective in asthma for nocturnal and daytime symptoms and exercise-induced bronchoconstriction. Regular use for up to 1 year does not cause tachyphylaxis to the bronchodilatory effect or to the response to short-acting β_2-agonists in most patients, but may be associated with partial loss of protection to methacholine challenges (46). Many clinicians use long-acting β_2-

agonists to improve symptom control in asthmatic subjects already taking inhaled corticosteroids. This approach was more efficacious than doubling the dose of inhaled corticosteroid (46). Regular use of long-acting β_2-agonists without an anti-inflammatory drug is not advisable, because ongoing worsening of airway inflammation may be masked by bronchodilation and temporary symptom control (49,50).

In addition to their bronchodilatory effects, β_2-agonists inhibit mediator release from mast cells, basophils, and eosinophils; increase mucociliary clearance; and decrease vascular permeability (46). Side effects can include tremor, palpitations, increased QTc interval, paradoxical bronchoconstriction and, in high doses, hypokalemia and hypomagnesemia. Another side effect is tachyphylaxis occurring over a period of days or weeks. Although most studies have failed to show the development of clinical tachyphylaxis with regular use of β_2-agonists, a few have demonstrated a decreased duration of action with preserved peak response (46), necessitating increased frequency of dosing.

3.5 Anticholinergic Agents

Ipratropium bromide, a quaternary ammonium derivative, is a short-acting bronchodilator that is poorly absorbed from the respiratory and gastrointestinal tract. It binds to M_2 and M_3 muscarinic receptors on airway smooth muscle, decreasing the acetylcholine-induced bronchospasm. It also binds to M_2 receptors on the postganglionic parasympathetic nerves, inhibiting the release of acetylcholine, and to M_3 receptors in the mucous glands, decreasing secretion (51). Some studies have shown inhaled ipratropium to produce further mild bronchodilation after treatment when given after short-acting β_2-agonists in asthmatic patients with acute exacerbations, particularly children. Nasal ipratropium decreases production of mucus in allergic rhinitis and common colds. It appears to be very safe, rarely causing adverse effects (e.g., mucosal dryness) (51).

3.6 Mast Cell Stabilizers

Cromolyn sodium and *nedocromil* sodium are purported to be mast cell stabilizers and clear rapidly from the lungs following inhalation. Cromolyn has a half-life of 81 min, and both medications are metabolized by the liver and eliminated mostly in the feces. Both agents inhibit calcium influx after mast cell activation, suppressing release of histamine and prostaglandin-D_2 (PGD_2) after allergen challenge. These medications also possess anti-inflammatory activity, block activation of eosinophils, inhibit immunoglobulin isotype switching from IgM to IgE, decrease chemotaxis of eosinophils and neutrophils, and decrease synthesis of tumor necrosis factor-alpha (TNF-α) from rat mast cells. Nedocromil modestly decreases interleukin (IL)-6 release from macrophages, expression of adhesion molecules in the endothelial and epithelial cells, and accumulation of eosinophils in the bronchial submucosa in asthmatic subjects (52–55).

Clinical trials demonstrate that both agents taken shortly before bronchial challenges modestly decrease early and late asthmatic responses after provocation with allergen, and reduce airway obstruction in response to exercise and cold air challenges. They also decrease symptoms and provide a small improvement in airway function when used for the long-term treatment of asthma (52). Topical ocular cromolyn sodium is also effective in allergic conjunctivitis, vernal keratoconjunctivitis, and allergic rhinitis. Topical nasal nedocromil also is effective for allergic rhinitis, although it is not currently available in the United States.

The greatest advantage of cromolyn and nedocromil is the near absence of significant adverse effects, despite their overall modest clinical efficacy. Although both medications are indicated for the prolonged treatment of patients with mild and moderate asthma, they are less effective than inhaled corticosteroids and do not decrease airway inflammation to a significant extent, as do topical corticosteroids. Cromolyn is more effective in children than in adults and is most effective when taken four times a day. Nedocromil is effective in children and adults and is taken twice to four times a day. Some patients may complain about the unpleasant taste of nedocromil.

Olopatadine is an antihistamine and mast cell stabilizer, which can be used twice a day, and is the most effective topical treatment for allergic conjunctivitis (56). *Ketotifen* is also an antihistamine and mast cell stabilizer used for the topical treatment of allergic conjunctivitis (56). In some countries, but not in the United States, ketotifen is available in an oral formulation for the treatment of asthma. It has mild anti-inflammatory effects, decreasing the number of mucosal T cells and eosinophils (57), but it is of only modest benefit for the treatment of asthma. In a comparison trial, ketotifen was less efficacious than inhaled cromolyn for the treatment of asthma (58).

3.7 Theophylline and Methylxanthines

Theophylline was initially used in the 1930s as a bronchodilator in asthmatic patients who did not respond to adrenergic agonists. Over time, several clinical benefits and multiple mechanisms of action have been observed. Bronchoprotection, anti-inflammatory, and immunomodulatory actions can occur at serum levels of more than 5 μg/mL. When used as monotherapy, therapeutic levels for theophylline was 10–20 μg/mL, but used adjunctively, lower levels are preferred and are associated with decreased complication rates. Theophylline protects against bronchoconstriction induced by methacholine, histamine, allergens, sulfur dioxide, distilled water, and adenosine. Theophylline has been reported to modestly attenuate certain aspects of allergen-induced airway inflammation, such as early- and late-allergenic challenges (to the same degree as cromolyn), release of leukotrienes from mast cells, airway influx, and activation of several cells including T cells, eosinophils, and neutrophils (59,60). Furthermore, theophylline decreases fatigue of diaphragmatic muscles, increases mucociliary clearance, increases respiratory drive, and decreases microvascular fluid leakage into the airways (60).

The exact mechanism of action is not completely elucidated, but theophylline seems to inhibit phosphodiesterases (PDE), thereby decreasing the hydrolysis and increasing intracellular levels of cyclic nucleotides. Inhibition of PDE types III and IV mediates the airway smooth-muscle relaxation effects of theophylline, whereas inhibition of PDE IV mediates the anti-inflammatory effects, such as inhibition of T cells, eosinophils, mast cells, and macrophages (60).

Theophylline is completely absorbed when given orally, and sustained-release preparations allow dosing at 12 or 24 hr. Its half-life varies among individuals from 3.5 hr in children to 9 hr in adults. It is metabolized in the liver and excreted mostly in the bile (61). Many drugs, as well as liver and cardiopulmonary conditions, interfere with the metabolism of theophylline, requiring dose adjustment (61). Side effects are numerous; correlate directly with serum levels; and include headache, dizziness, agitation, seizures, nausea, vomiting, worsening gastroesophageal reflux, palpitation, hypotension, precordial pain, tachyarrhythmias, and sudden death (61).

Because of its modest efficacy and toxicity, theophylline has been relegated to a third or fourth choice for the treatment of asthma. Clinical benefits are seen with therapeutic levels of 5–10 μg/mL, which cause fewer side effects than levels of 10–20 μg/mL. In chronic asthma, theophylline has a role in relieving nocturnal symptoms, if inhaled corticosteroids and long-acting bronchodilators have failed, and as a corticosteroid-sparing drug (60,62). In acute asthma, theophylline may provide further bronchodilation and other beneficial effects if symptoms are refractory to short-acting β-agonists, systemic corticosteroids, and ipratropium bromide (60,61).

3.8 Leukotriene Antagonists

Two classes of leukotriene antagonists are available for oral treatment of asthmatic patients: leukotriene receptor antagonists (montelukast, zafirlukast, and pranlukast—the latter is not available in the United States), and leukotriene synthesis inhibitors (zileuton). The leukotriene receptor antagonists bind competitively to the cysteine leukotriene 1 ($CysLT_1$) receptor, a seven–transmembrane-spanning receptor, the ligands of which are cysteinyl leukotrienes LTC_4, LTD_4, and LTE_4. Those leukotrienes mediate airway smooth-muscle contraction, chemotaxis, and increased vascular permeability (63). The only currently available leukotriene synthesis inhibitor is zileuton, which inhibits 5-lipoxygenase and decreases formation of the cysteinyl leukotrienes and of LTB_4, a potent neutrophil chemoattractant. In a given cell type, the synthesis of leukotrienes is biased toward either the production of cysteinyl leukotrienes or the production of LTB_4. Alveolar macrophages, eosinophils, and mast cells produce cysteinyl leukotrienes, whereas neutrophils produce LTB_4 (63).

Clinical trials have shown that leukotriene antagonists can decrease the airway response to several stimuli, such as cold air, exercise, sulfur dioxide, and allergen (63,64). Zileuton is administered four times daily, but has been associated with hepatotoxicity (drug-induced hepatitis), thus requiring monitoring of liver function (64). The $CysLT_1$ receptor inhibitors do not demonstrate the same degree of hepatotoxicity and, therefore, do not require monitoring of liver function. Moreover, they have a more convenient dosing schedule (once to twice daily) and are at least as effective as zileuton in controlling asthma (63). Clinical trials have demonstrated their effectiveness in asthmatic patients with mild to moderate disease. Patients with severe asthma may also benefit, although these drugs have not been well studied in this group. Leukotriene antagonists are the drugs of choice to treat patients with aspirin-induced asthma. Another approach in selected aspirin-sensitive patients is a cautious attempt at aspirin desensitization (65,66).

Comparisons of leukotriene antagonists with other drugs have shown that montelukast is less effective than beclomethasone for chronic asthma treatment (67), and more effective than salmeterol for exercise-induced asthma (68). Zileuton is more effective than theophylline for chronic asthma treatment (69). In a preliminary study, zafirlukast was not beneficial in seasonal allergic rhinitis (70), and leukotriene antagonists have not been properly studied in atopic dermatitis.

3.9 Methotrexate

Methotrexate is an alkylating agent that interferes with folate metabolism leading to accumulation of intracellular adenosine and immunosuppression. It leads to profound suppression of cell-mediated immunity and host defense, and it can be associated with gastrointestinal side effects, lung toxicity, liver toxicity, and an increased risk for development of malignancy. Because of its steroid-sparing effects in autoimmune and rheumatic diseases, it has been used in steroid-dependent asthmatics with inconsistent success.

Two recent metanalyses reviewed the relevant studies of methotrexate in steroid-dependent asthmatics (71,72). Data from 12 studies and 250 patients show that methotrexate 15 mg/week decreases prednisone dose by 3.3–4.4 mg (or 18–24% reduction), without changing pulmonary function. It was associated with gastrointestinal adverse effects, elevated liver enzymes, and opportunistic infections. Therefore, its use in asthma has to be considered individually after careful assessment of risks and benefits.

3.10 Cyclosporin and Tacrolimus

Both cyclosporin A (CSA) and tacrolimus (FK 506) inhibit the signal transduction in lymphocytes in a similar manner and cause selective inhibition of T cells. They have produced marked advances in the field of transplantation.

The mechanism of action of these two drugs involves inhibition of the transcription factor NF-AT. After T-cell activation, a complex composed of the cytoplasmic and nuclear subunits of NF-AT translocates to the nucleus and binds response elements in the DNA, activating gene transcription (73). Cyclosporin and tacrolimus enter the T cell where they bind to cytoplasmic proteins called cyclophilin, and FK 506-binding protein (FKBP), respectively. The complex drug–cytosolic protein blocks the action of the calcineurin–calmodulin complexes, thereby preventing activation of the cytoplasmic NF-AT. As a result, CSA and tacrolimus can block transcription of IL-2 and other cytokine genes (73).

The half-life of CSA is 6 hr and of tacrolimus is 11–21 hr. The oral bioavailabilities are 20–30% and 6–56%, for CSA and FK 506, respectively, and both drugs are metabolized in the liver with 94% or more excreted in the bile (74). Side effects of CSA include nephrotoxicity (75% of patients), hypertension, hepatotoxicity, neurotoxicity, hirsutism, gingival hyperplasia, and gastrointestinal toxicity. Tacrolimus has a similar side effect profile, including nephrotoxicity, neurotoxicity, gastrointestinal toxicity, hypertension, hyperkalemia, hypomagnesemia, and hyperglycemia (74). Neither drug is FDA-approved for the treatment of allergic diseases.

Cyclosporin has been used for the treatment of steroid-dependent asthmatics with less than clearcut results. Two trials from a group of investigators, involving a total of 72 patients, have shown that low-dose CSA (5 mg/kg per day) improved peak flow by 12% forced expirator volume in 1 sec (FEV_1) by 17.6%, reduced exacerbations requiring systemic steroids by 48%, and reduced daily dose of prednisolone by 4 mg (37%) compared with placebo (75,76). There were no severe side effects. Another trial, however, found no beneficial effects of CSA in a cohort of 34 steroid-dependent asthmatics (77). Side effects were hypertension, nephrotoxicity, and hepatotoxicity. Thus, similar to methotrexate, CSA is not very effective for patients with oral steroid-dependent asthma and causes several adverse effects. Therefore, CSA treatment in asthma has to be carefully considered and discussed with individual patients.

Tacrolimus ointment has been studied in refractory atopic dermatitis and shows very promising results and little toxicity even after a few months of treatment. However, this preparation is not yet commercially available, and there is still some concern about its toxicity with long-term topical use (78–81).

3.11 Nonsteroidal Anti-inflammatory Drugs

Because thromboxanes and prostaglandins are involved in the pathogenesis of airway inflammation in asthma, several small studies have suggested a potential benefit for nonsteroidal anti-inflammatory drugs (NSAIDs) in asthma. Problems with this approach relate to complications seen in aspirin-sensitive subjects and adverse effects associated with prolonged use. A well-controlled trial of colchicine in moderate asthmatics, however, showed negligible benefits (82).

3.12 Intravenous Immunoglobulin

Based on well-controlled studies, the FDA currently approves the use of intravenous immunoglobulin G (IVIG) for six conditions:

1. Primary immunodeficiencies (IgG deficiency)
2. Immune-mediated thrombocytopenia
3. Kawasaki syndrome
4. Recent bone marrow transplantation in patients older than 20 years of age
5. Chronic B-cell–lymphocytic leukemia
6. Pediatric human immunodeficiency virus type 1 (HIV-1) infection

Except for immune thrombocytopenic purpura and Kawasaki syndrome, in which IVIG modulates immune dysregulation, all other indicated uses of IVIG are for antibody replacement in immune-deficient patients. When used for antibody replacement, IVIG is given monthly at 400 mg/kg, whereas immunomodulatory doses are much higher, up to 1–2 g/kg per day. Because of its purported immunomodulatory effects, IVIG has recently been studied in more than 50 other inflammatory, autoimmune, and allergic diseases. Proposed mechanisms of action include Fc receptor blockade, idiotype–anti-idiotype antibody interactions, inhibition of B-cell function, induction of T-cell suppressor activity, inhibition of cytokine production, inhibition of complement uptake and activation on target cells (e.g., endothelium), neutralization of toxins, and enhancement of natural killer cell activity (83–85). It is possible that other molecules present in the IVIG preparations (e.g., soluble HLA class I and II antigens, CD4 and CD8 molecules) may play a role in some of these observed actions (83–85). Considering the potential application of IVIG to allergic diseases, in vitro studies have shown that high doses of IVIG can inhibit IgE production by B cells, decrease IL-2 and IL-4 production by T cells, act synergistically with dexamethasone to suppress T-cell proliferation, and improve glucocorticoid affinity for its receptor (84).

Two open-label trials of IVIG in severe asthma have suggested a steroid-sparing effect, but three randomized, double-blind, placebo-controlled studies have not confirmed clinical efficacy. Niggemann et al. studied IVIG 1 g/kg daily for 2 days then monthly for 2 months in 31 children and adolescents with moderate to severe asthma who were receiving inhaled corticosteroids. Compared with placebo, IVIG resulted in no significant improvement in symptom control, pulmonary function, inhaled corticosteroid dose, and total serum IgE (86). In a randomized, controlled study of 40 oral corticosteroid-dependent asthmatics with a mean steroid-requirement of 16 mg/day, Kishiyama et al. assessed the efficacy of IVIG 1 g/kg, 2 g/kg, or placebo for 6 months. There were no significant differences among the groups in terms of reduction in oral corticosteroid dose (about 33–39% for all groups), symptoms, and pulmonary function tests (87). Interestingly, the large placebo effect in this trial, might have been mistaken for clinical benefits from therapy, if there had been no control group. Three patients receiving 2 g/kg monthly were hospitalized with aseptic meningitis, and subgroups analysis failed to find a subgroup that might have benefited from IVIG (87). In a third controlled trial of IVIG treatment in asthma, Salmun et al. (88) assessed the steroid-sparing effect of IVIG, 400 mg/kg every 3 weeks for 9 months (after a 2 g/kg loading dose), in 38 children and adults with steroid-dependent asthma. A post hoc analysis showed that among the subjects who had taken 2000 mg or more of prednisone in the previous year, those who receive IVIG had a significantly larger reduction in the prednisone dose compared with placebo (73 vs. 33%; $p = 0.04$). However, there were no significant differences between those two subgroups relative to other outcome variables, including symptoms, pulmonary function, and other medications consumption, and missed days of work or school.

The half-life of IVIG (IgG) is 21 days and it is mostly metabolized by the reticuloendothelial (monocyte–phagocytic) system. It may cause several adverse effects, which occur in 1–10% of the patients, particularly with high doses or fast administration. Its adverse effects include headache, nausea, vomiting, fever, myalgias, light-headedness, aseptic meningitis, anaphylaxis (particularly in IgA-deficient patients who receive IVIG with high IgA contend), anaphylactoid reactions, tachycardia, and acute renal failure (mainly in those receiving IVIG preparations that contain sucrose as the stabilizing sugar to prevent IgG aggregation) (85,89). In 1993–1994, IVIG therapy caused an epidemic of hepatitis C in immunodeficient patients (90), but the current IVIG preparations undergo pasteurization or solvent–detergent treatment to kill potential viral contaminants. The use of IVIG will likely be restricted to the appropriate indications at this time, which do not include allergic diseases, owing to the high expense, toxicity, and shortage of the product in the United States since 1997 (91).

4 PHARMACOLOGICAL APPROACHES IN DEVELOPMENT FOR ALLERGIC DISEASES

As the immunopathological basis of atopic disorders is becoming better characterized, novel therapies are being developed to treat allergic inflammation and disease with more selective and targeted approaches. Improved efficacy, with a reduction in side effects and complications, are the goals of new therapeutics development.

4.1 Anti-IgE

One novel therapeutic approach to allergic disease involves direct inhibition of IgE function and reactivity through the use of ''anti-IgE,'' a recombinant, humanized, monoclonal antibody (MAb; rhu-MAb-E25) with antigen specificity directed against the same site in the Fc portion of human IgE molecule that binds to FcεRI (92). Anti-IgE binds to circulating IgE, competitively inhibiting IgE binding to FcεRI (high-affinity IgE receptors) on tissue mast cells (93), and when administered parenterally, rhu-MAb-E25 disarms mast cells and basophils and inhibits mediator release. In patients with moderate asthma and demonstrable IgE-mediated hypersensitivity to aeroallergens, rhu-MAb-E25 can reduce serum IgE and reduce the mean fall in FEV_1 during both the early and late responses to allergen bronchoprovocation (94). In a phase III clinical trial, Milgrom et al. (95) showed that intravenous administration of rhu-MAb-E25 every 2 weeks for 20 weeks to patients with moderate asthma significantly reduces symptoms, allows tapering and discontinuation of inhaled corticosteroids, improves quality of life, and reduces the number of asthma exacerbations without side effects.

4.2 Interleukin-4 Antagonists

Interleukin-4 plays a critical role in immunoglobulin class-switching by B cells and the synthesis of secreted IgE. IL-4 also modulates T-helper to lymphocyte responses to antigen stimulation by promoting T helper type-2 (Th2) cytokine production (IL-4, IL-5, IL-9) and inhibiting T helper type-1 (Th1) responses (IFN-γ, TNF-β) (12,13). Neutralization of IL-4 prevents development of Th2 cells and permits differentiation of precursor Th0 cells into Th1 phenotype (96).

Several strategies are concurrently being developed to modulate IL-4 activity and, thereby, suppress atopy and immediate hypersensitivity. IL-4 activity may be neutralized by administration of specific monoclonal antibodies, by soluble IL-4 receptors, or by blockade of ligand–receptor signal transduction. By preventing IL-4 induction of IgE synthesis, these strategies may ameliorate allergic hypersensitivity responses.

4.3 Adhesion Molecule Targets

Allergic respiratory disease and allergic skin disorders are characterized by inflammation of involved tissues. Significant allergen exposure leads to late-phase allergic responses, contributing to the development of chronic inflammation and persistent symptoms. On a cellular basis, the immunopathogenesis of inflammation involves infiltration by a variety of immune cells, such as eosinophils, basophils, and lymphocytes. These leukocytes are recruited and accumulate at sites of inflammation as a result of the response to chemoattractant gradients and through the interaction between cellular adhesion molecules (CAMs) expressed by immune cells—endothelial and interstitial cells. Selectins and integrins are two families of cell adhesion molecules involved in the rolling and firm adhesion of circulating cells and the microvasculature. This interaction of adhesion molecules and their corresponding ligands facilitates transmigration between endothelial junctions.

E-selectins are expressed on vascular endothelial cells, and they bind to L-selectins on circulating leukocytes. The interaction between these two adhesion molecules initiates leukocyte ''rolling'' just before firm adhesion that is mediated by integrins. Integrins are leukocytes's surface molecules, with differential expression on lymphocytes, eosinophils, and other immune cells. Corresponding ligands are found on vascular endothelial cells and can be up-regulated in response to cytokines, such as interleukins, interferons, and tumor necrosis factor. By using in situ methods, Ohkawara et al. demonstrated increased expression of VCAM-1, E-selectin, and ICAM-1 on endothelial cells of bronchial vessels in patients with symptomatic asthma (97).

Monoclonal antibodies (MAb) have been developed against adhesion molecules, their receptors, and members from the selectin families. In a primate model of airway reactivity, anti-ICAM-1 treatment abrogated eosinophil influx after allergen challenge and blocked subsequent development of bronchial hyperreactivity (98). Other animal models of airway hypersensitivity, in which antiadhesion molecule antibody treatment has been used, have been more mixed in their results. In rats with allergic airways, anti-VLA-4 (anti-very late activation antigen-4) treatment blocked early- and late-phase allergic responses (99), anti-LFA-1 (anti-CD11a/CD18) inhibited only early responses. In a sheep with allergen-induced hypersensitivity, anti-VLA-4 abrogated the development of airway hyperreactivity without inhibiting leukocyte recruitment (100), and L-selectin blockade reduced or prevented early- and late-phase increases in airway resistance after challenge with antigen (101). Anti-VLA-4 and antiselectin therapies have been particularly interesting because of their preferential effects on eosinophil accumulation in response to antigen and the seemingly important role of eosinophils in atopic disease (102).

4.4 Phosphodiesterase Inhibitors

Theophylline is a phosphodiesterase inhibitor and has been used for the treatment of asthma for decades. In addition to its bronchodilator effects, it has many other pharmacological actions and has been applied to many other respiratory disorders. At high serum concentrations, theophylline attenuates airway responsiveness to a variety of stimuli, including histamine, methacholine, allergen, and exercise (103,104). The effects of theophylline are not confined to airway smooth muscle, and both in vitro and in vivo studies have identified immunomodulatory and anti-inflammatory effects (105,106). Theophylline also possesses a narrow therapeutic index, however, and it has been associated with significant toxicity, including arrhythmias, nausea, vomiting, seizures, and CNS stimulation.

There are now seven recognized families of cyclic nucleotide phosphodiesterase (PDE) isozymes, and each of these isozyme families (PDE_1, PDE_2, PDE_3 . . . PDE_7) has subtypes and splice variants, each with a particular tissue distribution. Theophylline is a nonspecific PDE inhibitor and affects all PDE isoenzymes indiscriminately. Isozyme-selective PDE inhibitors, are being developed to segregate the beneficial effects on airway smooth muscle and leukocytes, from the detrimental effects on the nervous system (107).

Cyclic nucleotides such as cAMP and cGMP are biochemical second messengers that mediate physiological responses to cellular signals. The receptor-mediated binding of many hormones, neuropeptides, medications, and other mediators activates adenylyl cyclase or guanylyl cyclase, which cleaves ATP or GTP, respectively, to form cAMP and cGMP, respectively. Both cAMP and cGMP activate cytosolic protein kinases, which phosphorylate key proteins, altering cellular activity. Phosphodiesterases inactivate cyclic nucleotides by hydrolyzing the 3′-phosphoester bond to form the inactive 5′-nucleotide monophosphate products (5′-AMP and 5′-GMP, respectively). By regulating cellular content of cAMP and cGMP, PDEs modulate the biological responses mediated by these second messengers.

PDE_3 and PDE_4 are the predominant isozymes found in human airway epithelial cells and also seem to regulate airway smooth-muscle tone (108). In animal models, PGE_4 inhibitors can experimentally reverse induced bronchoconstriction, but they have not been able to affect resting airway tone. When given before bronchoprovocation with histamine, PDE_3 inhibitors can also block bronchoconstriction (109). Administration of rolipram, a specific PDE_4 inhibitor, before antigen challenge in atopic monkeys, did not inhibit acute bronchoconstriction, but it did increase cAMP in bronchoalveolar lavage fluid, and reduce IL-8, TNF release, and acute inflammatory responses. When these monkeys were treated with rolipram before repeated allergen exposure, eosinophil infiltration of airways and the development of airway hyperresponsiveness to methacholine were attenuated (110).

The PDE_4 inhibitors effect eosinophil function through numerous mechanisms, including inhibition of chemoattractant release, mediator release, adhesion, differentiation, and activation (107). The pharmacological effects of PDE_4 inhibitors on airway inflammation have been demonstrated in numerous species and animal models. However, early human trials investigating PDE_3 and PDE_4 inhibitors have been unimpressive because of dose-limiting side effects, such as headache, hypotension, nausea, and vomiting (111,112). Second-generation PDE_4 inhibitors appear more promising, and one compound, CDP840 blunts late asthmatic responses after allergen challenge (113).

5 PHARMACOGENETICS

Unraveling the genetics of asthma may help delineate factors determining both susceptibility to disease and clinical phenotype. *Pharmacogenetics* is ‘‘the study of genetic variation underlying differential response to drugs’’ (114). In the future, assessing the effects of polymorphic variation on receptor and enzyme function may help clinicians predict drug responsiveness based on genotyping of select gene products. In Alzheimer's disease, for example, it has been recognized that an apolipoprotein E allele (apo E4), marks an increase risk of developing clinical disease and predicts a poor response to tacrine treatment (115,116). Certainly not all variations in drug response can be attributed to genetic differences, as factors such as age, diet, concomitant medication usage, and overall health, affect clinical drug responses and are not related to genetics. Nevertheless, genetic polymorphisms may affect drug metabolism, drug targets, or receptors, ultimately determining drug efficacy and toxicity.

Beyond considerations of inherited polymorphisms in drug metabolism enzymes, a couple of areas deserve particular attention in asthma. The leukotrienes are a family of lipoxygenated eicosanoids derived from arachidonic acid, possessing several physiological actions relevant in asthma and airway inflammation (117,118). Drug treatments are available to inhibit their production (5-lipoxygenase inhibitors) or function (receptor antagonists), reducing bronchoconstriction and inflammation (119,120). 5-Lipoxygenase (5-LO) catalyzes the transformation of arachidonic acid to leukotriene-A_4 (LTA_4), from which the cysteinyl leukotrienes, LTC_4, LTD_4, and LTE_4 are generated. Alterations in the transcriptional regulation of the 5-LO gene may be important for functional expression and subsequent clinical asthmatic phenotype (121,122). Silverman et al. (121) identified naturally occurring 5-LO promoter mutations that alter transcription factor binding and activity. Although the functional consequences of these mutations appeared small, the investigators speculated the effects might be compounded in the setting of pharmacological leukotriene antagonism.

Another area of considerable interest is the highly polymorphic β_2-adrenergic receptor (β_2AR). Certain polymorphisms have been strongly associated with certain asthma phenotypes. Turki et al. (123) report a correlation between a β_2AR polymorphism, Gly16, and nocturnal asthma phenotype. Using site-directed mutagenesis, alterations in the aminoterminus of the β_2AR has been shown to modulate receptor regulation and trafficking (45). The inherited polymorphisms of the β_2AR may also modify drug responsiveness, as in β_2AR polymorphism, Ile164 appears to disrupt G protein coupling, blocking stimulation of adenylyl cyclase (124). Without increases in intracellular cAMP, β_2AR-mediated bronchodilation cannot occur. Liggett hypothesizes that polymorphisms of the β_2AR may partly explain the clinical phenomenon of tachyphylaxis, seen in some, but not all, patients using β_2-agonists on a regular or repetitive basis. Pharmacogenetics may allow a biological explanation for some of the individual variation seen in clinical disease and response to therapy.

6 SUMMARY

Treatment of moderate to severe atopic disease may require multidrug regimens, reflecting the multifaceted nature of allergic inflammation. Furthermore, despite the central role of Th2 inflammation in allergic rhinitis (15), asthma (14), and atopic dermatitis (11), specific mediator antagonists may not be uniformly successful in the treatment of all atopic disorders. For example, antihistamines are very effective treatment for the symptoms of allergic rhinitis (41), but have minimal benefit in the treatment of asthma (42–44). Current research efforts are ongoing to identify and develop therapies aimed at critical junctures in the immunopathological process. For example, animal studies have suggested that IL-4 and IL-13 are two cytokines that are pivotal in the generation of airway allergic inflammation.

Blocking the action of these cytokines may markedly decrease the allergic inflammation (17,125).

REFERENCES

1. Trepka MJ, Heinrich J, Wichmann HE. The epidemiology of atopic diseases in Germany: an East–West comparison. Rev Environ Health 1996; 11:119–131.
2. Sporik R, Holgate ST, Platts–Mills TA, Cogswell JJ. Exposure to house-dust mite allergen (Der p I) and the development of asthma in childhood. A prospective study. N Engl J Med 1990; 323:502–507.
3. Hide DW, Matthews S, Tariq S, Arshad SH. Allergen avoidance in infancy and allergy at 4 years of age. Allergy 1996; 51:89–93.
4. Shirakawa T, Enomoto T, Shimazu S, Hopkin JM. The inverse association between tuberculin responses and atopic disorder. Science 1997; 275:77–79.
5. Bodner C, Godden D, Seaton A. Family size, childhood infections and atopic diseases. The Aberdeen WHEASE Group. Thorax 1998; 53:28–32.
6. Shaheen SO, Aaby P, Hall AJ, Barker DJ, Heyes CB, Shiell AW, Goudiaby A. Measles and atopy in Guinea–Bissau. Lancet 1996; 347:1792–1796.
7. Matricardi PM, Rosmini F, Ferrigno L, Nisini R, Rapicetta M, Chionne P, Stroffolini T, Pasquini P, D'Amelio R. Cross sectional retrospective study of prevalence of atopy among Italian military students with antibodies against hepatitis A virus. Br Med J 1997; 314:999–1003.
8. Alm JS, Swartz J, Lilja G, Scheynius A, Pershagen G. Atopy in children of families with an anthroposophic lifestyle. Lancet 1999; 353:1485–1488.
9. Peterson B, Saxon A. Global increases in allergic respiratory disease: the possible role of diesel exhaust particles. Ann Allergy Asthma Immunol 1996; 77:263–268; quiz 269–270.
10. Sly RM. Changing prevalence of allergic rhinitis and asthma. Ann Allergy Asthma Immunol 1999; 82:233–248; quiz 248–252.
11. Leung DY. Pathogenesis of atopic dermatitis. J Allergy Clin Immunol 1999; 104:S99–S108.
12. Mosmann TR, Coffman RL. TH1 and TH2 cells: different patterns of lymphokine secretion lead to different functional properties. Annu Rev Immunol 1989; 7:145–173.
13. Swain SL, Weinberg AD, English M, Huston G. IL-4 directs the development of Th2-like helper effectors. J Immunol 1990; 145:3796–3806.
14. Robinson DS, Hamid Q, Ying S, Tsicopoulos A, Barkans J, Bentley AM, Corrigan C, Durham SR, Kay AB. Predominant TH2-like bronchoalveolar T-lymphocyte population in atopic asthma. N Engl J Med 1992; 326:298–304.
15. Durham SR, Ying S, Varney VA, Jacobson MR, Sudderick RM, Mackay IS, Kay AB, Hamid QA. Cytokine messenger RNA expression for IL-3, IL-4, IL-5, and granulocyte/macrophage-colony-stimulating factor in the nasal mucosa after local allergen provocation: relationship to tissue eosinophilia. J Immunol 1992; 148:2390–2394.
16. Corry DB, Grunig G, Hadeiba H, Kurup VP, Warnock ML, Sheppard D, Rennick DM, Locksley RM. Requirements for allergen-induced airway hyperreactivity in T and B cell-deficient mice. Mol Med 1998; 4:344–355.
17. Grunig G, Warnock M, Wakil AE, Venkayya R, Brombacher F, Rennick DM, Sheppard D, Mohrs M, Donaldson DD, Locksley RM, Corry DB. Requirement for IL-13 independently of IL-4 in experimental asthma. Science 1998; 282:2261–2263.
18. Wise JT, Baginski TJ, Mobley JL. An adoptive transfer model of allergic lung inflammation in mice is mediated by $CD4^{+}CD62LlowCD25^{+}$ T cells. J Immunol 1999; 162:5592–5600.
19. Busse WW. Inflammation in asthma: the cornerstone of the disease and target of therapy. J Allergy Clin Immunol 1998; 102:S17–S22.
20. Casale TB, Baraniuk JN. Neurogenic control of inflammation and airway function. In: Mid-

dleton E, Jr, Reed CE, Ellis EF, Adkinson NF, Jr, Yunginger JW, Busse WW, eds. Allergy Principles and Practice. 5th ed. St. Louis: Mosby, 1998:183–203.
21. Polito AJ, Proud D. Epithelia cells as regulators of airway inflammation. J Allergy Clin Immunol 1998; 102:714–718.
22. Gizycki MJ, Adelroth E, Rogers AV, O'Byrne PM, Jeffery PK. Myofibroblast involvement in the allergen-induced late response in mild atopic asthma. Am J Respir Cell Mol Biol 1997; 16:664–673.
23. Doucet C, Brouty–Boye D, Pottin–Clemenceau C, Canonica GW, Jasmin C, Azzarone B. Interleukin (IL) 4 and IL-13 act on human lung fibroblasts. Implication in asthma. J Clin Invest 1998; 101:2129–2139.
24. Maune S, Werner JA, Sticherling M, Schroder JM. Fibroblasts obtained from human nasal, laryngeal and tracheal mucosa produce the chemokine RANTES. Otolaryngol Pol 1997; 51: 3–10.
25. Nonaka M, Pawankar R, Saji F, Yagi T. Distinct expression of RANTES and GM-CSF by lipopolysaccharide in human nasal fibroblasts but not in other airway fibroblasts. Int Arch Allergy Immunol 1999; 119:314–321.
26. Ghaffar O, Hamid Q, Renzi PM, Allakhverdi Z, Molet S, Hogg JC, Shore SA, Luster AD, Lamkhioued B. Constitutive and cytokine-stimulated expression of eotaxin by human airway smooth muscle cells. Am J Respir Crit Care Med 1999; 159:1933–1942.
27. Hirst SJ, Lee TH. Airway smooth muscle as a target of glucocorticoid action in the treatment of asthma. Am J Respir Crit Care Med 1998; 158:S201–S206.
28. Kassel O, Schmidlin F, Duvernelle C, Gasser B, Massard G, Frossard N. Human bronchial smooth muscle cells in culture produce stem cell factor. Eur Respir J 1999; 13:951–954.
29. Tonnel AB, Gosset P, Molet S, Tillie–Leblond I, Jeannin P, Joseph M. Interactions between endothelial cells and effector cells in allergic inflammation. Ann N Y Acad Sci 1996; 796: 9–20.
30. Goldie RG, Henry PJ. Endothelins and asthma. Life Sci 1999; 65:1–15.
31. Curran AD. The role of nitric oxide in the development of asthma. Int Arch Allergy Immunol 1996; 111:1–4.
32. Wardlaw AJ. Molecular basis for selective eosinophil trafficking in asthma: a multistep paradigm. J Allergy Clin Immunol 1999; 104:917–926.
33. Barnes PJ, Pedersen S, Busse WW. Efficacy and safety of inhaled corticosteroids. New developments. Am J Respir Crit Care Med 1998; 157:S1–S53.
34. Boushey HA. Effects of inhaled corticosteroids on the consequences of asthma. J Allergy Clin Immunol 1998; 102:S5–S16.
35. Kelly HW. Establishing a therapeutic index for the inhaled corticosteroids: part I. Pharmacokinetic/pharmacodynamic comparison of the inhaled corticosteroids. J Allergy Clin Immunol 1998; 102:S36–S51.
36. Guidelines for the diagnosis and management of asthma. Bethesda, MD: NIH/NHLBI, 1997.
37. Barnes PJ. Anti-inflammatory actions of glucocorticoids: molecular mechanisms. Clin Sci (Colch) 1998; 94:557–572.
38. Karin M. New twists in gene regulation by glucocorticoid receptor: is DNA binding dispensable? Cell 1998; 93:487–490.
39. Heck S, Bender K, Kullmann M, Gottlicher M, Herrlich P, Cato AC. I-kappaB alpha-independent downregulation of NF-kappaB activity by glucocorticoid receptor. Embo J 1997; 16: 4698–4707.
40. Barnes PJ. Molecular mechanisms of steroid action in asthma. J Allergy Clin Immunol 1996; 97:159–168.
41. Simons FER. Antihistamines. In: Middleton E, Jr, Reed CE, Ellis EF, Adkinson NF, Jr, Yunginger JW, Busse WW, eds. Allergy Principles and Practice. 5th ed. St. Louis: Mosby, 1998:612–637.
42. Menardo JL, Horak F, Danzig MR, Czarlewski W. A review of loratadine in the treatment

of patients with allergic bronchial asthma. Clin Ther 1997; 19:1278–1293; discussion 1523–1274.

43. Bentley AM, Walker S, Hanotte F, De Vos C, Durham SR. A comparison of the effects of oral cetirizine and inhaled beclomethasone on early and late asthmatic responses to allergen and the associated increase in airways hyperresponsiveness. Clin Exp Allergy 1996; 26:909–917.
44. Spector SL, Nicodemus CF, Corren J, Schanker HM, Rachelefsky GS, Katz RM, Siegel SC. Comparison of the bronchodilatory effects of cetirizine, albuterol, and both together versus placebo in patients with mild-to-moderate asthma. J Allergy Clin Immunol 1995; 96:174–181.
45. Green SA, Nelson HS. Adrenergic agents. In: Middleton E, Jr, Reed CE, Ellis EF, Adkinson NF, Jr, Yunginger JW, Busse WW, eds. Allergy Principles and Practice. 5th ed. St. Louis: Mosby, 1998:571–576.
46. Nelson HS. beta-Adrenergic therapy. In: Middleton E, Jr, Reed CE, Ellis EF, Adkinson NF, Jr, Yunginger JW, Busse WW, eds. Allergy Principles and Practice. 5th ed. St. Louis: Mosby, 1998:577–588.
47. Drazen JM, Israel E, Boushey HA, Chinchilli VM, Fahy JV, Fish JE, Lazarus SC, Lemanske RF, Martin RJ, Peters SP, Sorkness C, Szefler SJ. Comparison of regularly scheduled with as-needed use of albuterol in mild asthma. Asthma Clinical Research Network. N Engl J Med 1996; 335:841–847.
48. Nelson HS. Clinical experience with levalbuterol. J Allergy Clin Immunol 1999; 104:S77–S84.
49. Turner MO, Johnston PR, Pizzichini E, Pizzichini MM, Hussack PA, Hargreave FE. Anti-inflammatory effects of salmeterol compared with beclomethasone in eosinophilic mild exacerbations of asthma: a randomized, placebo controlled trial. Can Respir J 1998; 5:261–268.
50. McIvor RA, Pizzichini E, Turner MO, Hussack P, Hargreave FE, Sears MR. Potential masking effects of salmeterol on airway inflammation in asthma. Am J Respir Crit Care Med 1998; 158:924–930.
51. Fryer AD, Costello RW, Jacoby DB. Cholinergic mechanisms and anticholinergic therapy in respiratory diseases. In: Middleton E, Jr, Reed CE, Ellis EF, Adkinson NF, Jr, Yunginger JW, Busse WW, eds. Allergy Principles and Practice. 5th ed. St. Louis: Mosby, 1998:668–677.
52. Norris AA, Holgate ST. Cromolyn sodium and nedocromil sodium. In: Middleton E, Jr, Reed CE, Ellis EF, Adkinson NF, Jr, Yunginger JW, Busse WW, eds. Allergy Principles and Practice. 5th ed. St. Louis: Mosby, 1998:661–667.
53. Loh RK, Jabara HH, Geha RS. Mechanisms of inhibition of IgE synthesis by nedocromil sodium: nedocromil sodium inhibits deletional switch recombination in human B cells. J Allergy Clin Immunol 1996; 97:1141–1150.
54. Loh RK, Jabara HH, Geha RS. Disodium cromoglycate inhibits S mu→S epsilon deletional switch recombination and IgE synthesis in human B cells. J Exp Med 1994; 180:663–671.
55. Creticos PS. Effects of nedocromil sodium on inflammation and symptoms in therapeutic studies. J Allergy Clin Immunol 1996; 98:S143–S149; discussion S149–S150.
56. Joss JD, Craig TJ. Seasonal allergic conjunctivitis: overview and treatment update. J Am Osteopath Assoc 1999; 99:S13–S18.
57. Hoshino M, Nakamuras Y, Shin Z, Fukushima Y. Effects of ketotifen on symptoms and on bronchial mucosa in patients with atopic asthma. Allergy 1997; 52:814–820.
58. Croce J, Negreiros EB, Mazzei JA, Isturiz G. A double-blind, placebo-controlled comparison of sodium cromoglycate and ketotifen in the treatment of childhood asthma. Allergy 1995; 50:524–527.
59. Rabe KF, Dent G. Theophylline and airway inflammation. Clin Exp Allergy 1998; 28(suppl 3):35–41.
60. Weinberger M, Hendeles L, Theophylline and phosphodiesterase inhibitors. In: Middleton

E, Jr, Reed CE, Ellis EF, Adkinson NF, Jr, Yunginger JW, Busse WW, eds. Allergy Principles and Practice. 5th ed. St. Louis: Mosby, 1998:589–611.

61. Serafin WE. Drugs used in the treatment of asthma. In: Hardman JG, Limbird LE, Molinoff PB, Ruddon RW, Gilman AG, eds. The Pharmacological Basis of Therapeutics. New York: McGraw-Hill, 1996:659–682.
62. Markham A, Faulds D, Theophylline. A review of its potential steroid sparing effects in asthma. Drugs 1998; 56:1081–1091.
63. Drazen JM, Israel E, O'Byrne PM. Treatment of asthma with drugs modifying the leukotriene pathway. N Engl J Med 1999; 340:197–206.
64. McGill KA, Busse WW. Zileuton. Lancet 1996; 348:519–524.
65. Stevenson DD, Hankammer MA, Mathison DA, Christiansen SC, Simon RA. Aspirin desensitization treatment of aspirin-sensitive patients with rhinosinusitis–asthma: long-term outcomes. J Allergy Clin Immunol 1996; 98:751–758.
66. Szczeklik A, Stevenson DD. Aspirin-induced asthma: advances in pathogenesis and management. J Allergy Clin Immunol 1999; 104:5–13.
67. Malmstrom K, Rodriguez–Gomez G, Guerra J, Villaran C, Pineiro A, Wei LX, Seidenberg BC, Reiss TF. Oral montelukast, inhaled beclomethasone, and placebo for chronic asthma. A randomized, controlled trial. Montelukast/Beclomethasone Study Group. Ann Intern Med 1999; 130:487–495.
68. Villaran C, O'Neill SJ, Helbling A, van Noord JA, Lee TH, Chuchalin AG, Langley SJ, Gunawardena KA, Suskovic S, Laurenzi M, Jasan J, Menten J, Leff JA. Montelukast versus salmeterol in patients with asthma and exercise-induced bronchoconstriction. Montelukast/ Salmeterol Exercise Study Group. J Allergy Clin Immunol 1999; 104:547–553.
69. Schwartz HJ, Petty T, Dube LM, Swanson LJ, Lancaster JF. A randomized controlled trial comparing zileuton with theophylline in moderate asthma. The Zileuton Study Group. Arch Intern Med 1998; 158:141–148.
70. Pullerits T, Praks L, Skoogh BE, Ani R, Lotvall J. Randomized placebo-controlled study comparing a leukotriene receptor antagonist and a nasal glucocorticoid in seasonal allergic rhinitis. Am J Respir Crit Care Med 1999; 159:1814–1818.
71. Aaron SD, Dales RE, Pham B. Management of steroid-dependent asthma with methotrexate: a meta-analysis of randomized clinical trials. Respir Med 1998; 92:1059–1065.
72. Marin MG. Low-dose methotrexate spares steroid usage in steroid-dependent asthmatic patients: a meta-analysis. Chest 1997; 112:29–33.
73. Letko E, Bhol K, Pinar V, Foster CS, Ahmed AR. Tacrolimus (FK 506). Ann Allergy Asthma Immunol 1999; 83:179–189; quiz 189–190.
74. Diasio RB, LoBuglio AF. Immunomodulators: immunosuppressive agents and immunostimulants. In: Hardman JG, Limbird LE, Molinoff PB, Ruddon RW, Gilman AG, eds. The Pharmacological Basis of Therapeutics. New York: McGraw-Hill, 1996:1291–1305.
75. Lock SH, Kay AB, Barnes NC. Double-blind, placebo-controlled study of cyclosporin A as a corticosteroid-sparing agent in corticosteroid-dependent asthma. Am J Respir Crit Care Med 1996; 153:509–514.
76. Alexander AG, Barnes NC, Kay AB. Trial of cyclosporin in corticosteroid-dependent chronic severe asthma. Lancet 1992; 339:324–328.
77. Nizankowska E, Soja J, Pinis G, Bochenek G, Sladek K, Domagala B, Pajak A, Szczeklik A. Treatment of steroid-dependent bronchial asthma with cyclosporin. Eur Respir J 1995; 8:1091–1099.
78. Fleischer AB, Jr. Treatment of atopic dermatitis: role of tacrolimus ointment as a topical noncorticosteroidal therapy. J Allergy Clin Immunol 1999; 104:S126–130.
79. Boguniewicz M, Fiedler VC, Raimer S, Lawrence ID, Leung DY, Hanifin JM. A randomized, vehicle-controlled trial of tacrolimus ointment for treatment of atopic dermatitis in children. Pediatric Tacrolimus Study Group. J Allergy Clin Immunol 1998; 102:637–644.
80. Ruzicka T, Bieber T, Schopf E, Rubins A, Dobozy A, Bos JD, Jablonska S, Ahmed I,

Thestrup–Pedersen K, Daniel F, Finzi A, Reitamo S. A short-term trial of tacrolimus ointment for atopic dermatitis. European Tacrolimus Multicenter Atopic Dermatitis Study Group. N Engl J Med 1997; 337:816–821.
81. Bieber T. Topical tacrolimus (FK 506): a new milestone in the management of atopic dermatitis. J Allergy Clin Immunol 1998; 102:555–557.
82. Fish JE, Peters SP, Chambers CV, McGeady SJ, Epstein KR, Boushey HA, Cherniack RM, Chinchilli VM, Drazen JM, Fahy JV, Hurd SS, Israel E, Lazarus SC, Lemanske RF, Martin RJ, Mauger EA, Sorkness C, Szefler SJ. An evaluation of colchicine as an alternative to inhaled corticosteriods in moderate asthma. National Heart, Lung, and Blood Institute's Asthma Clinical Research Network. Am J Respir Crit Care Med 1997; 156:1165–1171.
83. Ballow M. Mechanisms of action of intravenous immune serum globulin in autoimmune and inflammatory diseases. J Allergy Clin Immunol 1997; 100:151–157.
84. Rabinovitch N, Gelfand EW, Leung DY. The role of immunoglobulin therapy in allergic diseases. Allergy 1999; 54:662–668.
85. Mobini N, Sarela A, Ahmed AR. Intravenous immunoglobulins in the therapy of autoimmune and systemic inflammatory disorders. Ann Allergy Asthma Immunol 1995; 74:119–128; quiz 128–133.
86. Niggemann B, Leupold W, Schuster A, Schuster R, v. Berg A, Grubl A, v. d. Hardt H, Eibl MM, Wahn U. Prospective, double-blind, placebo-controlled, multicentre study on the effect of high-dose, intravenous immunoglobulin in children and adolescents with severe bronchial asthma. Clin Exp Allergy 1998; 28:205–210.
87. Kishiyama JL, Valacer D, Cunningham–Rundles C, Sperber K, Richmond GW, Abramson S, Glovsky M, Stiehm R, Stocks J, Rosenberg L, Shames RS, Corn B, Shearer WT, Bacot B, DiMaio M, Tonetta S, Adelman DC. A multicenter, randomized, double-blind, placebo-controlled trial of high-dose intravenous immunoglobulin for oral corticosteroid-dependent asthma. Clin Immunol 1999; 91:126–133.
88. Salmun LM, Barlan I, Wolf HM, Eibl M, Twarog FJ, Geha RS, Schneider LC. Effect of intravenous immunoglobulin on steroid consumption in patients with severe asthma: a double-blind, placebo-controlled, randomized trial. J Allergy Clin Immunol 1999; 103:810–815.
89. Renal insufficiency and failure associated with immune globulin intravenous therapy—United States, 1985–1998. MMWR Morb Mortal Wkly Rep. 1999; 48:518–521.
90. Outbreak of hepatitis C associated with intravenous immunoglobulin administration—United States, October 1993–June 1994. MMWR Morb Mortal Wkly Rep 1994; 43:505–509.
91. Availability of immune globulin intravenous for treatment of immune deficient patients—United States, 1997–1998. MMWR Morb Mort Wkly Rep 1999; 48:159–162.
92. Presta LG, Lahr SJ, Shields RL, Porter JP, Gorman CM, Fendly BM, Jardieu PM. Humanization of an antibody directed against IgE. J Immunol 1993; 151:2623–2632.
93. Saban R, Haak–Frendscho M, Zine M, Ridgway J, Gorman C, Presta LG, Bjorling D, Saban M, Jardieu P. Human FcERI–IgG and humanized anti-IgE monoclonal antibody MaE11 block passive sensitization of human and rhesus monkey lung. J Allergy Clin Immunol 1994; 94:836–843.
94. Fahy JV, Fleming HE, Wong HH, Liu JT, Su JQ, Reimann J, Fick RB, Jr, Boushey HA. The effect of an anti-IgE monoclonal antibody on the early- and late-phase responses to allergen inhalation in asthmatic subjects. Am J Respir Crit Care Med 1997; 155:1828–1834.
95. Milgrom H, Fick RB, Jr, Su JQ, Reimann JD, Bush RK, Watrous ML, Metzger WJ. Treatment of allergic asthma with monoclonal anti-IgE antibody. rhuMAb-E25 Study Group. N Engl J Med 1999; 341:1966–1973.
96. Abehsira–Amar O, Gibert M, Joliy M, Theze J, Jankovic DL. IL-4 plays a dominant role in the differential development of Th0 into Th1 and Th2 cells. J Immunol 1992; 148:3820–3829.
97. Ohkawara Y, Yamauchi K, Maruyama N, Hoshi H, Ohno I, Honma M, Tanno Y, Tamura G, Shirato K, Ohtani H. In situ expression of the cell adhesion molecules in bronchial tissues

from asthmatics with air flow limitation: in vivo evidence of VCAM–1/VLA-4 interaction in selective eosinophil infiltration. Am J Respir Cell Mol Biol 1995; 12:4–12.
98. Wegner CD, Gundel RH, Reilly P, Haynes N, Letts LG, Rothlein R. Intercellular adhesion molecule-1 (ICAM-1) in the pathogenesis of asthma. Science 1990; 247:456–459.
99. Rabb HA, Olivenstein R, Issekutz TB, Renzi PM, Martin JG. The role of the leukocyte adhesion molecules VLA-4, LFA-1, and Mac-1 in allergic airway responses in the rat. Am J Respir Crit Care Med 1994; 149:1186–1191.
100. Abraham WM, Sielczak MW, Ahmed A, Cortes A, Lauredo IT, Kim J, Pepinsky B, Benjamin CD, Leone DR, Lobb RR, et al. alpha 4-Integrins mediate antigen-induced late bronchial responses and prolonged airway hyperresponsiveness in sheep. J Clin Invest 1994; 93:776–787.
101. Abraham WM, Ahmed A, Sabater JR, Lauredo IT, Botvinnikova Y, Bjercke RJ, Hu X, Revelle BM, Kogan TP, Scott IL, Dixon RA, Yeh ET, Beck PJ. Selectin blockade prevents antigen-induced late bronchial responses and airway hyperresponsiveness in allergic sheep. Am J Respir Crit Care Med 1999; 159:1205–1214.
102. Broide DH, Sullivan S, Gifford T, Sriramarao P. Inhibition of pulmonary eosinophilia in P-selectin- and ICAM-1-deficient mice. Am J Respir Cell Mol Biol 1998; 18:218–225.
103. Magnussen H, Reuss G, Jorres R. Theophylline has a dose-related effect on the airway response to inhaled histamine and methacholine in asthmatics. Am Rev Respir Dis 1987; 136: 1163–1167.
104. Hendeles L, Harman E, Huang D, O'Brien R, Blake K, Delafuente J. Theophylline attenuation of airway responses to allergen: comparison with cromolyn metered-dose inhaler. J Allergy Clin Immunol 1995; 95:505–514.
105. Scordamaglia A, Ciprandi G, Ruffoni S, Caria M, Paolieri F, Venuti D, Canonica GW. Theophylline and the immune response: in vitro and in vivo effects. Clin Immunol Immunopathol 1988; 48:238–246.
106. Kidney J, Dominguez M, Taylor PM, Rose M, Chung KF, Barnes PJ. Immunomodulation by theophylline in asthma. Demonstration by withdrawal of therapy. Am J Respir Crit Care Med 1995; 151:1907–1914.
107. Torphy TJ. Phosphodiesterase isozymes: molecular targets for novel antiasthma agents. Am J Respir Crit Care Med 1998; 157:351–370.
108. Torphy TJ, Undem BJ, Cieslinski LB, Luttmann MA, Reeves ML, Hay DW. Identification, characterization and functional role of phosphodiesterase isozymes in human airway smooth muscle. J Pharmacol Exp Ther 1993; 265:1213–1223.
109. Underwood DC, Kotzer CJ, Bochnowicz S, Osborn RR, Luttmann MA, Hay DW, Torphy TJ. Comparison of phosphodiesterase III, IV and dual III/IV inhibitors on bronchospasm and pulmonary eosinophil influx in guinea pigs. J Pharmacol Exp Ther 1994; 270:250–259.
110. Turner CR, Andresen CJ, Smith WB, Watson JW. Effects of rolipram on responses to acute and chronic antigen exposure in monkeys. Am J Respir Crit Care Med 1994; 149:1153–1159.
111. Leeman M, Lejeune P, Melot C, Naeije R. Reduction in pulmonary hypertension and in airway resistances by enoximone (MDL 17,043) in decompensated COPD. Chest 1987; 91: 662–666.
112. Fujimura M, Kamio Y, Saito M, Hashimoto T, Matsuda T. Bronchodilator and bronchoprotective effects of cilostazol in humans in vivo. Am J Respir Crit Care Med 1995; 151:222–225.
113. Harbinson PL, MacLeod D, Hawksworth R, O'Toole S, Sullivan PJ, Heath P, Kilfeather S, Page CP, Costello J, Holgate ST, Lee TH. The effect of a novel orally active selective PDE_4 isoenzyme inhibitor (CDP840) on allergen-induced responses in asthmatic subjects. Eur Respir J 1997; 10:1008–1014.
114. Kleyn PW, Vesell ES. Genetic variation as a guide to drug development. Science 1998; 281: 1820–1821.

115. Poirier J, Davignon J, Bouthillier D, Kogan S, Bertrand P, Gauthier S. Apolipoprotein E polymorphism and Alzheimer's disease. Lancet 1993; 342:697–699.
116. Corder EH, Saunders AM, Strittmatter WJ, Schmechel DE, Gaskell PC, Small GW, Roses AD, Haines JL, Pericak–Vance MA. Gene dose of apolipoprotein E type 4 allele and the risk of Alzheimer's disease in late onset families. Science 1993; 261:921–923.
117. Dahlen SE, Hedqvist P, Hammarstrom S, Samuelsson B. Leukotrienes are potent constrictors of human bronchi. Nature 1980; 288:484–486.
118. Weiss JW, Drazen JM, Coles N, McFadden ER, Jr, Weller PF, Corey EJ, Lewis RA, Austen KF. Bronchoconstrictor effects of leukotriene C in humans. Science 1982; 216:196–198.
119. Spector SL, Smith LJ, Glass M. Effects of 6 weeks of therapy with oral doses of ICI 204,219, a leukotriene D_4 receptor antagonist, in subjects with bronchial asthma. ACCOLATE Asthma Trialists Group. Am J Respir Crit Care Med 1994; 150:618–623.
120. Israel E, Dermarkarian R, Rosenberg M, Sperling R, Taylor G, Rubin P, Drazen JM. The effects of a 5-lipoxygenase inhibitor on asthma induced by cold, dry air. N Engl J Med 1990; 323:1740–1744.
121. Silverman E, In KH, Yandava C, Drazen JM. Pharmacogenetics of the 5-lipoxygenase pathway in asthma. Clin Exp Allergy 1998; 28(suppl 5):164–170; discussion 171–163.
122. Drazen JM, Yandava CN, Dube L, Szczerback N, Hippensteel R, Pillari A, Israel E, Schork N, Silverman ES, Katz DA, Drajesk J. Pharmacogenetic association between ALOX5 promoter genotype and the response to anti-asthma treatment. Nat Genet 1999; 22:168–170.
123. Turki J, Pak J, Green SA, Martin RJ, Liggett SB. Genetic polymorphisms of the beta 2-adrenergic receptor in nocturnal and nonnocturnal asthma. Evidence that Gly16 correlates with the nocturnal phenotype. J Clin Invest 1995; 95:1635–1641.
124. Liggett SB. Pharmacogenetics of relevant targets in asthma. Clin Exp Allergy 1998; 28(suppl 1):77–79; discussion 80–71.
125. Akimoto T, Numata F, Tamura M, Takata Y, Higashida N, Takashi T, Takeda K, Akira S. Abrogation of bronchial eosinophilic inflammation and airway hyperreactivity in signal transducers and activators of transcription (STAT)6-deficient mice. J Exp Med 1998; 187: 1537–1542.
126. Johnson MJ. Pharmacodynamics and pharmacokinetics of inhaled glucocorticoids. J Allergy Clin Immunol 1996; 97:169–176.
127. Johnson MJ. Development of fluticasone propionate and comparison with other inhaled corticosteroids. J Allergy Clin Immunol 1998; 101:S434–S439.
128. Derendorf H, Hochhaus G, Meibohm B, Möllmann H, Barth J. Pharmacokinetics and pharmacodynamics of inhaled corticosteroids. J Allergy Clin Immunol 1998; 101:S440–S446.

23

Synthetic and Genetically Engineered Allergen Derivatives for Specific Immunotherapy of Type I Allergy

RUDOLF VALENTA, SUSANNE VRTALA, MARGIT FOCKE-TEJKL, ANNA TWARDOSZ, INES SWOBODA, AGNES BUGAJSKA-SCHRETTER, SUSANNE SPITZAUER, and DIETRICH KRAFT

Vienna General Hospital (AKH), University of Vienna Medical School, Vienna, Austria

1 INTRODUCTION

Specific immunotherapy, which represents one of the few curative approaches toward treatment of type I allergy, is based on the systemic administration of allergens. Although specific immunotherapy has been practiced for almost 90 years, and numerous clinical studies demonstrate clinical efficacy of this treatment, the underlying immunological mechanisms are not completely understood. Major disadvantages of immunotherapy are that the administration of allergens can cause anaphylactic side effects and that treatment is performed with allergen extracts consisting of a difficult-to-standardize mixture of allergenic and nonallergenic components and, therefore, cannot be applied according to the patients sensitization profile. During the last decade an increasing number of recombinant allergen molecules have become available that can now be used for component-resolved diagnosis (CRD) of type I allergy and to study, at a molecular level, the immunological mechanisms underlying type I allergy. Based on epitope and structural analyses of biologically active recombinant allergen molecules, synthetic and genetically engineered hypoallergenic versions thereof are currently being developed for safe and component-resolved immunotherapy (CRIT). This chapter reports recent advances in the development of synthetic and genetically engineered allergen derivatives and compares these strategies with modifications that were previously applied to increase the safety of allergen extracts for immunotherapy. We further summarize experiences gained from clinical studies performed with synthetic and genetically modified allergen-derivatives in humans. Finally, we discuss perspectives on how the use of genetically engineered or synthetic hypoallergenic allergen derivatives may improve specific immunotherapy.

Type I allergy, a genetically influenced hypersensitivity disease, is caused by the formation of IgE antibodies against harmless antigens (i.e., allergens) (1,2). IgE recognition of allergens leads to both immediate and delayed symptoms of atopy. The immediate symptoms are due to allergen-induced cross-linking of IgE bound to high-affinity receptors on mast cells and basophils and the subsequent release of biological mediators (e.g., histamine and leukotrienes) (3,4). On the other hand, IgE-mediated presentation of allergens through low- and high-affinity receptors for IgE on antigen-presenting cells (APC) can induce strong T-cell activation accompanied by the release of proinflammatory as well as chemoattractive cytokines and, thereby, also contributes to the late symptoms in atopy (5,6). The central role of IgE antibodies for the pathogenesis of atopic disease is also emphasized by the fact that allergen contact represents a potent inducer for the production of allergen-specific IgE (7). Furthermore, increased levels of IgE antibodies lead to increased expression of the high-affinity receptor for IgE on effector cells (8–11). Although not definitively proved, there is strong evidence that during an established IgE response, increases of allergen-specific IgE antibodies result from the allergen-induced activation of already committed, memory IgE^+ B cells, rather than from de novo sensitization and subsequent class switching (12–14). For the latter reason it appears quite unlikely that factors that antagonize the class switch to IgE (e.g., interleukin-4 [IL-4] antagonists) can be used to down-regulate specific IgE antibody responses in adult allergic patients.

Even though the symptoms of type I allergy can be controlled by pharmacotherapy (i.e., using immunosuppressive and anti-inflammatory agents), there are only a few causative therapy approaches toward type I allergy. These approaches comprise (1) allergen-specific immunotherapy, (2) attempts to reduce the levels of IgE antibodies, (3) interference with the interaction of IgE with its receptors, and (4) specific blockade of IgE-mediated signal transduction. The latter three approaches may be suited for polysensitized patients who are allergic to numerous different allergen sources and who suffer from severe forms of atopy. If patients are sensitized against fewer allergens (oligo-, monosensitized patients), allergen-specific immunotherapy may be considered as the curative approach. Allergen-specific immunotherapy is based on the administration of allergens to induce a state of unresponsiveness (15). Since the introduction of specific immunotherapy by Noon and Freeman in 1911 (16), numerous clinical studies have documented the clinical efficacy of immunotherapy, but there is some controversy over the immunological mechanisms underlying this treatment (17,18). Classic studies initially demonstrated that allergen-specific immunotherapy induces ''blocking IgG antibodies'' that protect patients by inhibiting IgE-mediated effector cell activation and mediator release (19–26). Several other immunological changes were observed in context with successful immunotherapy. They include reduction of mediator concentrations and numbers of effector cells (mast cells, eosinophils) in the target organs of atopy (27–29), inhibition of the recruitment of T cells and eosinophils to sites of allergen contact (27–31), induction of suppressor cells (32), decreases of IL-4 production by T cells and increases of Th1-type cells in peripheral blood of treated patients (33–36), and induction of allergen-specific IgG responses against new epitopes (37).

Major disadvantages of allergen-specific immunotherapy are that the administration of allergens can cause severe anaphylactic side effects and that treatment is performed with allergen extracts consisting of difficult-to-standardize mixtures of allergens and other undefined materials (15,17). To reduce the rate of anaphylactic side effects during treatment and to increase immunogenicity, allergen extracts were bound to immunological adjuvants (38,39). In addition to adsorbing allergen extracts to adjuvants, which should prevent systemic spreading of allergens, attempts were made to reduce anaphylactic side effects by modification of allergens. Proteolytic digestion of allergen extracts yielded peptides that either failed to bind IgE antibodies, but induced T-cell responses, or represented IgE-binding haptens incapable of cross-linking effector cell-bound IgE (40–45). Chemical modification (e.g., polymerization and thus denaturation of allergens by aldehyde treatment) yielded allergoids that retained immunogenicity, but had lost allergenic activity (46–63). Another approach for the attenuation of allergen extracts was the coupling of methoxypolyethylene glycol (mPEG) to allergens, a treatment that reduced the allergenic activity of the extract and seemed to inactivate those cells that were able to bind to the mPEG-modified allergens (64–73).

Indeed, formaldehyde-polymerized allergen extracts (allergoids) represent safe preparations for allergen-specific immunotherapy and are nowadays used for routine treatment of patients. However, the use of natural allergen extracts does not allow treatment according to the patients sensitization profile, and therapy-induced sensitizations to extract components that were not recognized before immunotherapy were reported (37,74). Recent advances in the field of molecular allergen characterization and the ability to produce defined allergen molecules by recombinant DNA technology give hope that, in the near future, immunotherapy with recombinant or synthetic allergens performed according to a patient's precise sensitization pattern will be possible (75–79).

2 PRODUCTION OF RECOMBINANT ALLERGENS FOR DIAGNOSIS AND THERAPY OF TYPE I ALLERGY

Almost a decade ago, research groups who started to work on the molecular characterization of allergens by recombinant DNA technology focused on major allergens from frequently recognized allergen sources (e.g., mite, venom, birch, and grass pollen) (75). Their major goal was to reveal the molecular nature of frequently recognized allergens, to determine B-cell as well as T-cell epitopes and to produce recombinant allergens suitable to investigate immunological mechanisms underlying type I allergy. However, when it turned out that a few recombinant allergens accounted for the serological and in vivo diagnosis of type I allergy by natural allergen extracts, recombinant allergens were also considered for diagnostic and therapeutic purposes (80,81,75). The selection of allergens that should be produced as recombinant molecules for diagnostic purposes, therefore, may be based on the following consideration: Attempts should be made to produce recombinant allergen panels that equal and thus can substitute for allergen extracts from those allergen sources that frequently sensitize patients and contain most of the IgE epitopes that are also present in cross-reactive allergen sources. For example, almost 40% of allergic patients are sensitized to grass pollen, and almost 25% are sensitized to birch pollen, indicating that both allergen sources are recognized with high prevalence; therefore, they represent important allergen sources. Furthermore, birch pollen allergens contain most of the epitopes present in pollens of other early flowering trees belonging to the order Fagales (e.g., alder, hazel, oak, hornbeam) (82). Likewise, recombinant timothy grass pollen allergens resemble most of the IgE epitopes present in a variety of grass and corn species (83). From studies on prevalence of IgE recognition and representation of IgE epitopes, the most important allergen sources can be selected for the cloning work (Fig. 1).

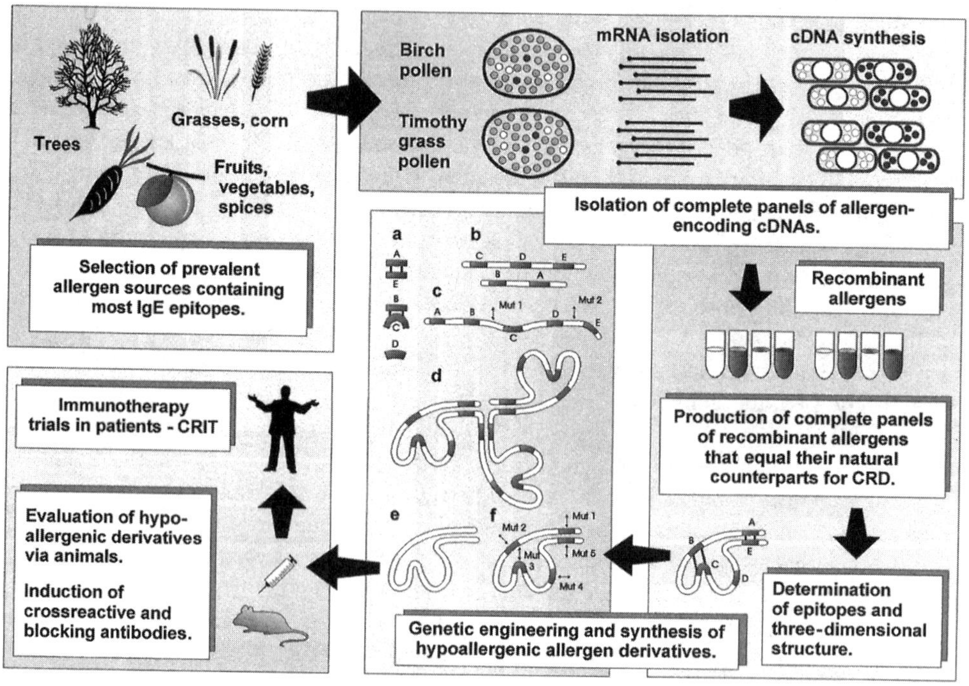

Figure 1 The key steps leading to the production of recombinant allergens for component-resolved diagnosis (CRD) of type 1 allergy and to the development of synthetic and genetically modified hypoallergenic allergen derivatives for component-resolved immunotherapy (CRIT).

The prevalence of IgE recognition should be determined with sera from different populations to exclude variations in recognition owing to different sensitization patterns in these various populations (82,84). Whether a given allergen source contains most of the relevant IgE epitopes present in related allergen sources can be determined by quantitative IgE inhibition experiments (82,83). When a given allergen extract or allergen (e.g., birch pollen extract, major birch pollen allergen, Bet v 1) completely inhibits IgE reactivity to a cross-reactive allergen extract or allergen (e.g., apple extract, major apple allergen, Mal d 1), it may be assumed that patients were originally sensitized against the first allergen source or allergen (birch pollen, Bet v 1) and because of IgE antibody cross-reactivity can exhibit symptoms after contact with the second allergen source or allergen (apple, Mal d 1) (85). Such IgE competition experiments identified pollen allergens as the primary sensitizing cause of many forms of plant or food allergy (85). Once a particular allergen source has been identified as an important elicitor of type I allergy and thus as suitable for the production of recombinant allergens, corresponding mRNA has to be isolated and converted into complementary DNA by reverse transcription (see Fig. 1). The pool of cDNA molecules is subjected to a selection procedure that identifies those cDNAs that code for allergens. Although several allergen-encoding cDNAs were isolated by DNA-based techniques (polymerase chain reaction [PCR], hybridization) we found that the construction of expression cDNA libraries, from which allergen-encoding cDNAs can be selected directly with serum IgE antibodies yielded recombinant allergens with high IgE-binding capacity and biological activity. Recombinant allergens that equal their natural counterparts in terms of IgE-binding capacity, T-cell reactivity, induction of basophil histamine release, and in vivo activity can be produced in suitable expression systems (see Fig. 1). Many recombinant allergens were produced as folded and active proteins in bacteria, whereas a few others required expression in eukaryotic cells. As soon as a panel of recombinant allergens has been produced that resembles the IgE epitopes present in the corresponding natural allergen extract, a mixture of these allergens can be used for diagnostic-screening tests (79). The individual recombinant allergens, however, can also be used to determine the IgE-reactivity profile of a given patient toward the allergenic components in a particular allergen source. The concept of using purified recombinant allergens for the determination of the patients sensitivity profile has been termed component-resolved diagnosis (CRD) (79).

3 THE CONCEPT OF COMPONENT-RESOLVED DIAGNOSIS: BASIS FOR COMPONENT-RESOLVED IMMUNOTHERAPY

Diagnosis of type I allergy is based on the detection of specific IgE antibodies in serum and on provocation testing (skin testing, nasal, ocular, bronchial, or oral provocation). Both forms of diagnosis use allergen extracts that are prepared from the allergen sources mainly by aqueous extraction. Therefore, allergen extracts consist of a difficult-to-standardize mixture of allergenic and nonallergenic moieties. The amounts of certain allergens may vary depending on the methods of extraction, variations of allergen expression, activity of proteases and other enzymes. Therefore, it is impossible to control the ratios of individual allergens in a given extract. The presence of certain major allergens in a given extract can be determined with specific antibody probes, but antibodies for rare allergens may not be available. Sensitivity to a given allergen extract (IgE reactivity, biological response) will not provide information regarding the disease-eliciting allergens. If the allergenic components of a given extract have been produced as pure recombinant allergen molecules, it is possible to determine the precise IgE-reactivity–sensitization profile of the patient by serology and provocation testing, respectively (75–77,79). The identification of the disease-eliciting allergens is relevant because allergen sources may contain allergens that are expressed only in a few closely related allergen sources (e.g., grass and corn species). In exclusive sensitization to such components, patients will exhibit symptoms to only a few allergen sources. However, if a patient reacts with highly cross-reactive allergens with conserved biological functions (e.g., profilin an ubiquitous actin-binding protein), the person will experience allergic symptoms on contact with a great variety of unrelated allergen sources (86,87). Sensitivity to cross-reactive marker allergens can thus be used to explain and predict sensitization to multiple allergen sources containing structurally and immunologically related allergens. By IgE-inhibition experiments it is possible to identify among cross-reactive allergens the molecule that contains most of the IgE epitopes and that, therefore, may represent the originally sensitizing agent. In this context it was demonstrated that cross-reactive pollen allergens contain most of the IgE epitopes present in plant-derived food, suggesting that many forms of plant food allergy are caused by primary sensitization to cross-reactive pollen allergens (85).

Recombinant allergen components can be used to define the disease-eliciting agents and may also be used to monitor the IgE reactivity profile of patients during the natural course of allergic disease and in response to therapy (88,37,79). Although the levels of allergen-specific IgE may vary, depending on allergen exposure (7), there is good evidence that the IgE recognition profile of adult allergic patients does not change in the natural

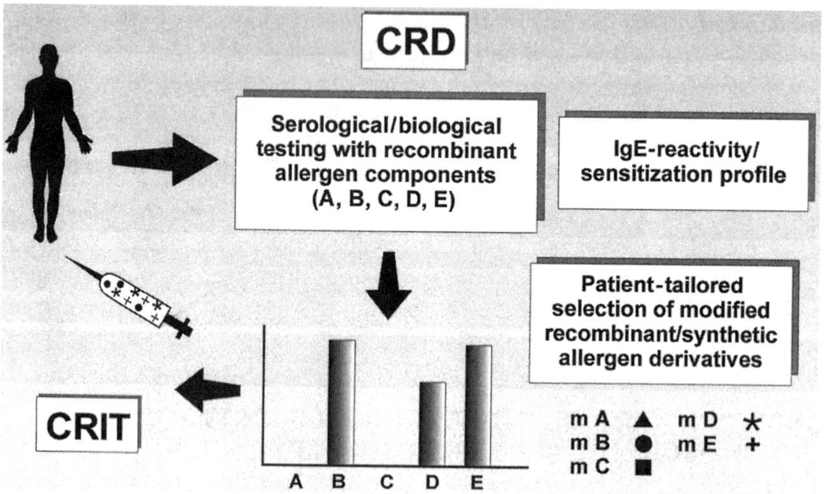

Figure 2 Component-resolved diagnosis (CRD) with recombinant allergens to determine the allergic patients IgE reactivity or sensitivity profile: the basis for component-resolved immunotherapy (CRIT) with modified recombinant or synthetic allergen derivatives.

course of disease (88). This indicates that the IgE reactivity–sensitization profile determined by component-resolved diagnosis (CRD) can be used to select the allergens for component-resolved immunotherapy (CRIT) (Fig. 2). Component-resolved immunotherapy (CRIT) would treat the patient exactly according to the individual sensitization profile and, thereby, excludes the risk of therapy-induced sensitization against new allergens. Because most recombinant allergens equal their natural counterparts in their immunological and biological properties, they can induce anaphylactic side effects when used for immunotherapy. Therefore, strategies have to be developed that allow the production of recombinant allergens with reduced allergenic activity for safe forms of CRIT (Table 1).

Table 1 Strategies for the Production of Synthetic and Genetically Modified Hypoallergenic Allergen Derivatives

Peptide chemistry	Recombinant DNA technology
1. T-cell epitope-containing peptides	1. Recombinant IgE-binding haptens
2. B-cell epitope-derived peptides and peptides derived from surface-exposed areas	2. Recombinant allergen fragments
3. Mimotopes	3. Recombinant allergen isoforms or mutants Mutations in the IgE epitopes (exchange or deletion of amino acids) Mutations that affect conformational IgE epitopes
	4. Recombinant allergen-deletion variants
	5. Recombinant allergen oligomers

4 STRATEGIES FOR THE PRODUCTION OF SYNTHETIC AND GENETICALLY MODIFIED HYPOALLERGENIC ALLERGEN DERIVATIVES

In the past, several technologies have been applied to reduce the allergenic activity of allergen extracts: 1) Proteolytic digestion of allergen extracts yielded low molecular weight haptenic fragments that failed to cross-link effector–cell-bound IgE and consequently failed to elicit mediator release (40–45). Such IgE-binding haptens were successfully used for the passive treatment of penicillin and dextran allergy as well as for active immunotherapy of allergy against bee venom and plant products (89–91,41,44,45). 2) Reduction of the allergenic activity by treatment of allergen extracts with formaldehyde represents a frequently used way to modify allergens. Exposure to formaldehyde yielded high molecular weight allergen polymers (allergoids) with a greatly reduced allergenic activity, but retained immunogenicity (46,47,49,50). When injected into experimental animal, allergoids were able to induce antibodies that inhibited the native allergen-mediated release of histamine and to induce a preferential Th1 immunity (51,62,63). A series of clinical studies documented the clinical efficacy and safety of polymerized allergen extracts (48,52–54,56–61). 3) A third strategy that has been used to modify allergen extracts is the coupling of mPEG with allergens (64). The addition of mPEG seemed to have a dual beneficial effect, as it reduced the allergenic activity of the allergens and inactivated key cells of atopy (e.g., IgE-secreting B cells, or mast cells) (64,66–68). Several clinical immunotherapy studies documented the clinical efficacy and safety of mPEG-modified allergen extracts (69–73).

In the last decade the molecular nature of many important allergens has been revealed by recombinant DNA technology (75–77). The availability of DNA and amino acid sequence data has facilitated the determination of B-cell as well as T-cell epitopes. In addition, data on the three-dimensional structure of allergens allow the rationale design of allergy vaccines and competitors for the allergen–IgE interaction (78). From the knowledge obtained through the molecular characterization of allergens, several strategies for the production of hypoallergenic synthetic and genetically modified allergen derivatives can be applied (see Fig. 1 and Table 1). Table 1 summarizes strategies that have been used for the production of hypoallergenic allergen derivatives, and Table 2 gives an overview of the characteristics of synthetic and genetically engineered allergen derivatives produced to date. It should be born in mind, however, that in addition to the investigation of the allergenic properties of an allergen derivative, it is equally important to demonstrate that this derivative is immunogenic in animal systems. Parameters that can be tested are whether the hypoallergenic derivative can induce IgG antibodies that recognize the wild-type allergen and whether the induced antibodies block IgE binding to the wild-type allergen and prevent IgE-mediated effects on cells in allergic patients (126).

4.1 T-Cell Epitope-Containing Peptides

Short T-cell epitope-containing synthetic peptides mostly lack IgE-binding capacity and allergenic activity. In addition, T-cell peptides can either induce proliferation or anergy–tolerance of T cells, depending on the dose and mode of administration (127–131). The concept of using T-cell peptides of allergens for immunotherapy is thus based on the assumption that T-cell peptides will not cause immediate allergic reactions and may down-regulate the activity of allergen-specific Th2 cells. Peptides containing T-cell epitopes of

Table 2 Synthetic and Genetically Modified Allergen Derivatives[a]

Allergen	Source	Type of modification	Reduced IgE reactivity	Reduced allergenic reactivity[b]	T-cell epitopes present	Immunogenicity	Clinical studies	Refs.
Bet v 1	Birch	Fragment	+	HR, ST	+	+	+	92–97
Bet v 1	Birch	Isoform	+	ST, CP	+	nd	+	98,99
Bet v 1	Birch	Mutant	+	ST	+	nd	nd	100
Bet v 1	Birch	Oligomer	+	HR, ST	+	+	+	93–95,97,101,102
Bet v 1	Birch	Mimotope	nd	nd	–	+	nd	103
Bet v 2	Birch	Hapten	nd	nd	nd	nd	nd	104
Bet v 4	Birch	Fragment	+	nd	nd	nd	nd	105
Bet v 4	Birch	Mutant	+	nd	nd	nd	nd	106
Aln g 4	Alder	Fragment	+	nd	nd	nd	nd	107
Bra r 1	Rape	Mutant	+	nd	nd	+	nd	108
Lol p 1	Rye grass	Deletion	+	HR	nd	nd	nd	109
Lol p 5	Rye grass	Mutant	+	HR	+	nd	nd	110,111
Phl p 1	Timothy grass	Hapten	–	HR	nd	nd	nd	112
Phl p 1	Timothy grass	Fragment peptide	+	HR, ST	+	+	nd	88,113
Phl p 5	Timothy grass	Mutant, deletion	+	HR, ST	+	nd	nd	114
Phl p 6	Timothy grass	Deletion variant	+	nd	nd	nd	nd	115
Der p 2	Mite	Mutant	+	ST	nd	nd	nd	116,117
Der f 2	Mite	Mutant	+	HR, ST	+	nd	nd	118
Lep d 2	Mite	Mutant	+	ST	+	nd	nd	119
Fel d 1	Cat	Peptide	nd	nd	+	nd	+	120–122
Bos d 2	Cow	Fragments	+	ST	+	nd	nd	123,124
PLA 2	Honey bee	Peptide	nd	ST	+	nd	+	125

[a] Allergen derivatives, sources, type of modification, immunological characteristics, clinical studies, and references are displayed.
[b] nd, not done; HR, histamine release; ST, skin testing; CP, conjunctival provocation.

the major cat allergen, Fel d 1, and of the bee venom allergen, phospholipase A_2, were therefore evaluated in first clinical immunotherapy trials in patients (120–122,125). Administration of Fel d 1-derived peptides did not lead to significant clinical improvement and substantial changes in sensitivity to Fel d 1 (122). Moreover, some Fel d 1 peptide-treated patients reported more allergic rhinitis and asthma symptoms as well as pruritus than the placebo-treated individuals. By contrast, promising results were reported for an immunotherapy study performed with phospholipase A_2-derived T-cell peptides. Patients treated with phospholipase A_2-derived peptides showed clinical improvement, signs of T-cell anergy, and increases in phospholipase A_2-specific IgG4 antibodies (125). The induction of peptide-specific anergy in the phospholipase A_2-specific T cells, as well as the increased production of phospholipase A_2-specific IgG4 antibodies, were attributed to the action of IL-10 (131).

4.2 IgE-Binding Haptens, Mimotopes

Almost two decades ago it was demonstrated that proteolytically digested allergen extracts can retain their IgE-binding capacity and exhibit reduced allergenic activity (40,42,43). Proteolytical fragmentation of allergens thus creates IgE-binding haptens containing only one binding site for one IgE antibody. Therefore, IgE-binding haptens cannot cross-link effector cell-bound IgE antibodies and fail to induce release of mediators. When applied in soluble form, IgE-binding haptens will saturate effector cells and prevent cell activation by subsequent contact with a complete allergen. In fact, low molecular weight dextran- and penicillin-derived haptens were successfully used for the treatment of penicillin and dextran allergy (89–91). Also, low molecular weight allergen fragments obtained by proteolytic digestion of allergen extracts can be used for active immunotherapy (41,44,45). Since cDNAs coding for allergens have become available, it is possible to use new technologies for the production of allergens fragments. Expression libraries were constructed from randomly fragmented allergen-encoding cDNAs, and small IgE-reactive recombinant allergen fragments were isolated (112,132,133). IgE-binding haptens could be characterized for the major timothy grass pollen allergen, Phl p 1 (112), and for a highly cross-reactive birch pollen allergen, birch profilin (104) (see Fig. 1a, D). However, IgE competition studies performed with sequential IgE epitopes derived from Phl p 1 indicated that discontinuous IgE epitopes may also account for a substantial proportion of the allergens IgE-binding capacity (88) (see Fig. 1a, A–E, B–C). Such discontinuous IgE-binding structures need to be defined by more complicated technologies (e.g., determination of the three-dimensional structure of the allergen) or may be mimicked by molecules (mimotopes) obtained from peptide libraries (78,103). However, the question arises whether it is necessary to exactly rebuild IgE epitopes to obtain immunogens suitable for focusing a protective IgG response toward IgE epitopes. Indeed, there is now increasing evidence that allergen fragments without or with low IgE-binding capacity can be used as immunogens to focus blocking IgG responses toward those parts of an allergen that are recognized by IgE.

4.3 Recombinant Allergen Fragments, Immunogenic Peptides Derived from B-cell Epitopes or Surface-Exposed Areas

The concept of using allergen fragments without IgE-binding capacity for specific immunotherapy is based on the assumption that the fragments contain amino acid sequence motifs that are part of IgE epitopes and, when used for immunization, can induce blocking IgG responses against IgE epitopes (134). Allergen fragments without IgE-binding capacity owing to change or loss of their fold can be obtained by expression of recombinant allergen fragments in heterologous host organisms, or by production as synthetic peptides (see Fig. 1b). Recombinant allergen fragments with reduced allergenic activity were produced for the major birch pollen allergen, Bet v 1 (92); a major cow dander allergen, Bos d 2 (123); the two EF-hand alder pollen allergen, Aln g 4 (107); and for the major grass pollen allergen, Phl p 6 (115). B-cell epitope-derived peptides can be produced either on the basis of the experimentally determined IgE epitopes or on the three-dimensional structure of the allergen molecule. From the three-dimensional structure of an allergen, it is possible to discriminate areas that are solvent-exposed and, thus, can interact with antibodies from areas that are buried and thus available for antibody binding (78). Likewise it is possible to use experimentally determined IgE epitopes of allergens as a basis for the production of B-cell epitope-derived vaccines. Synthetic Phl p 1-derived peptides were produced that had reduced allergenic activity, but that did induce blocking antibodies in vivo (88,113).

4.4 Recombinant Allergen Isoforms or Mutants

Isoforms of allergens that differ from each other by only a few amino acids can exhibit a greatly varying IgE-binding capacity (98). Furthermore, allergens can exist as conformational variants with strongly reduced IgE-binding activity (135). Allergens that contain calcium-binding motifs and can bind calcium by these EF-hand domains can occur as calcium-bound forms with high IgE-binding capacity and as calcium-free (apoforms) forms with reduced IgE-binding activity (136). Also, binding of IgG antibodies to allergens containing conformational IgE epitopes can expose these epitopes, most likely by a conformational change, and thus create versions with elevated IgE-binding capacity (137–140). Given the foregoing observations, strategies have been developed that use in vitro mutagenesis of allergen-encoding cDNAs as a technique to generate hypoallergenic mutants with reduced IgE-binding capacity. Such mutations may either affect amino acids within the IgE epitopes that are directly involved in the interaction with IgE antibodies (see Fig. 1f), or change the allergen conformation and, thereby, destroy discontinuous IgE epitopes (see Fig. 1c). There is good evidence that point mutations within the IgE epitopes reduced the IgE-binding capacity of the major grass pollen allergens Lol p 5 and Phl p 5, as well as of the major birch pollen allergen, Bet v 1 (100,110,111,114). Deletions of several amino acids and thus of portions of the IgE epitopes reduced the IgE-binding capacities of the major grass pollen allergen Phl p 5 (114) (see Fig. 1e). However, remains to be answered whether deletion of IgE-reactive areas from a molecule will create an immunogen that can still induce blocking IgG antibody responses against the IgE epitopes of the wild-type allergen.

The production of stable apoforms of EF-hand calcium-binding allergens represents an example for mutations that destroy discontinuous IgE epitopes by changes of the allergen conformation (106,108). Although correct disulfide bond formation of recombinant proteins produced in the cytoplasma of *Escherichia coli* is unlikely, it has been proposed that the exchange of cysteine residues in major mite allergens reduced their IgE reactivity through lack of disulfide bond formation in the mutated protein versions (116,118,119).

4.5 Recombinant Allergen Oligomers

When we produced recombinant oligomers (dimers, trimers) (see Fig. 1d) of the major birch pollen allergen, Bet v 1, the oligomers had a greatly reduced activity for basophil histamine release, but retained their IgE-binding capacity when compared with the recombinant Bet v 1 monomer (101,102). rBet v 1 trimer induced strong lymphoproliferative responses in peripheral blood mononuclear cells (PBMC) of birch pollen allergic patients and contained the relevant Bet v 1-specific T-cell epitopes (102). In addition, rBet v 1 trimer showed more than a 100-fold reduced activity to induce immediate-type skin reactions that rBet v 1 monomer and induced less activation of eosinophils and cytokine releases when evaluated in a skin blister model (93–97). Circular dichroism analysis indicated structural differences between the trimer and monomer (102). One possible explanation for the striking finding that the Bet v 1 trimer, despite IgE reactivity, exhibited a strongly allergenic activity could be that the oligomerization process has caused a reorientation of IgE epitopes which, although being recognized by IgE antibodies, may be less effective in cross-linking effector cell-bound IgE. Two clinical skin test studies demonstrated a strongly reduced allergenic activity of recombinant Bet v 1 trimer and no late-phase reactions were observed (93–95). Moreover, immunization of mice and rabbits with rBet v 1 trimer induced high titers of IgG antibodies that inhibited allergic patients IgE binding to the Bet v 1 wild-type molecule (102). Oligomerization of hypoallergenic allergen derivatives by recombinant DNA technology, therefore, may also be considered as a possible way to increase the immunogenicity of an allergy vaccine.

4.6 Allergen Gene Vaccination, Immunostimulatory DNA Sequences

Genetic vaccination with plasmid DNA encoding a given antigen has potential to induce an antigen-specific Th1 immune response that may antagonize Th2 responses in a mouse model (141,142). As demonstrated by adoptive cell transfer experiments, it seems that the immune response elicited by DNA vaccinations is dependent on $CD8^+$ cells (142,143). Although several other studies showed that it was possible to induce immune responses against latex, peanut, and birch pollen allergens in mice, it is still unclear whether allergen gene vaccination will have beneficial effects (144–146). In this context, it is worth noting that first gene vaccination trials performed in the field of malaria and HIV have shown only limited success (147–150).

Immunostimulatory DNA sequences represent another approach to use DNA to modulate an allergic immune response (151). This approach is based on the notion that certain DNA sequences that generally consist of a central nonmethylated CG dinucleotide, surrounded by less highly conserved sequences (termed CpG motifs) can induce strong Th1 immune responses. Immunostimulatory DNA sequences (ISS), therefore, may represent promising adjuvants for immunotherapy, but a potential risk of inducing autoimmune responses with ISS has to be excluded.

5 CLINICAL EXPERIENCES WITH SYNTHETIC AND GENETICALLY ENGINEERED HYPOALLERGENIC ALLERGEN DERIVATIVES

Results obtained from clinical immunotherapy studies with synthetic peptides representing T-cell epitopes of the major cat allergen Fel d 1 were not promising. It was reported that peptide immunotherapy neither reduced immediate- or late-phase skin reactivity to cat extract, nor did it modify cat antigen-specific cytokine production significantly (122). The occasionally observed systemic reactions observed during peptide treatment may likely result from IgE-independent activation of T cells by the peptides (152). Only one study performed in five patients provided evidence that immunotherapy with T-cell epitope-containing peptides derived from the bee venom allergen, phospholipase, induced peripheral T-cell anergy and improved clinical symptoms (125).

Genetically engineered hypoallergenic allergen derivatives have so far not been used in clinical immunotherapy trials, but certain of them have been characterized relative to their potential to induce immediate- and late-phase skin reactions (see Table 2). Skin test experiments demonstrating reduced allergenic activity of several genetically modified allergens were performed, but systematic skin test studies are, as yet, available only for hypoallergenic derivatives of the major birch pollen allergen, Bet v 1 (93–95,97,99). Recombinant Bet v 1 monomer, trimer, and fragments were applied by skin-prick and intradermal injection to 23 birch pollen allergic patients, 12 allergic patients without birch pollen allergy, and 8 nonatopic individuals in a Swedish study (93). The birch pollen allergic patients tolerated an approximately 100-fold dose of rBet v 1 trimer and rBet v 1 fragments versus the Bet v 1 wild-type molecule. No late-phase reactions and no false-positive reactions were observed in this study. Another skin test study performing detailed titration studies with Bet v 1 wild-type and the recombinant hypoallergenic Bet v 1 derivatives in a population of 36 birch pollen allergic patients in France before, during, and after the birch pollen season (94,95). In agreement with the Swedish study, a more than 100-fold reduced allergenic activity of the recombinant Bet v 1 derivatives was found, which remained low even during and after seasonal allergen contact. Another clinical study compared late-phase responses and eosinophil activation induced by Bet v 1 and genetically modified rBet v 1 in a skin blister model (97). The hypoallergenic recombinant Bet v 1 derivatives (fragments, trimer) induced lower levels of histamine, ECP, and GM–CSF than the Bet v 1 wild-type molecule, and recombinant Bet v 1 trimer elicited the lowest levels of IL-4 (97).

The skin test results obtained for hypoallergenic rBet v 1 derivatives document the strongly reduced capacity of these molecules to elicit immediate as well as late allergic reactions in patients. Clinical immunotherapy studies now need to be performed with recombinant hypoallergenic Bet v 1 derivatives to evaluate safety and efficacy of such a treatment.

6 WHAT MAY BE EXPECTED FROM COMPONENT-RESOLVED IMMUNOTHERAPY PERFORMED WITH HYPOALLERGENIC ALLERGEN DERIVATIVES?

The concept of component-resolved immunotherapy with hypoallergenic allergen derivatives is illustrated in Figure 2. In a first step the IgE reactivity and sensitization profile of the patient needs to be established by testing with defined recombinant allergen molecules (CRD; component-resolved diagnosis) (79,153,154). Because it was found that serum IgE levels and sensitivity toward a given allergen molecule are not always correlated, it may be necessary to select the allergen molecules for therapy according to the IgE-reactivity and sensitization profile (155). Component-resolved immunotherapy (CRIT) can then be performed using adjuvant-bound, modified recombinant or synthetic allergen derivatives with low allergenic activity (m A-m E). When one analyzes the results of numerous immunotherapy studies, it appears that injection immunotherapy with adjuvant-bound allergen extracts or chemically modified allergen extracts represents an effective and relatively safe form of immunotherapy (15,17). Therefore, we suggest continuing to improve injection immunotherapy with adjuvant-bound allergen extracts by utilizing recombinant and synthetic hypoallergenic allergen derivatives instead of natural extracts. Two advantages may be envisaged: First, it will be possible to perform therapy according to the patient's reactivity profile. Second, hypoallergenic and thus safe molecules can be produced in a defined and reproducible manner.

The selection of patients by component-resolved diagnosis (CRD) will allow the indications and contraindications for immunotherapy to be assessed in a more precise manner. Patient-tailored treatment with defined molecules should have the obvious advantage over extract-based treatment in that therapy-induced sensitization against previously unrecognized extract components cannot occur (37,74). Furthermore, insufficient therapy because of the lack of or the presence of low amounts of certain allergens in a given extract or because of the inhomogeneous or insufficient coupling of certain extract components to the adjuvant, will be unlikely.

The second major advantage is that peptide chemistry and recombinant DNA technology can be used to produce well-defined hypoallergenic allergen derivatives. Whereas chemical modification of allergen extracts is difficult to control, synthetic and genetically engineered hypoallergenic allergen molecules of consistent properties and quality can be produced by the new technologies. Owing to their greatly reduced allergenic activity, it will be possible to inject much higher doses of the synthetic or genetically engineered allergens with reduced risk of anaphylactic side effects. High-dose immunization will likely allow a reduction in the number of injections and thus make specific immunotherapy comparable with vaccination. It is expected that immunization with high doses of hypoallergenic allergen derivatives will induce a preferential allergen-specific IgG response which will be supported by an allergen-specific Th1 immune response (156–158). Moreover, the use of defined, modified molecules will direct IgG responses exactly to IgE epitopes and thus give rise to a protective immune response. Poor efficacy of immunotherapy owing to production of IgG antibodies that recognize epitopes other than those of IgE or due to induction of IgG, which may enhance IgE recognition of allergens (138,140), or perhaps induce super-cross-linking of effector cell-bound allergens can be minimized by evaluation of the allergen derivatives in suitable animal models (126).

IgG antibodies that block the IgE recognition of allergens may contribute to clinical improvement by several mechanisms: (1) Blocking IgG will prevent allergen-induced cross-linking of effector cell-bound IgE and thus reduce immediate reactions after allergen contact (37,138,88). (2) Therapy-induced IgG can also reduce IgE-mediated allergen presentation to T cells and, thus, T-cell activation (159). It is also possible that blocking antibodies prevent allergen-induced activation of eosinophils, and thereby may reduce late-phase reactions. (3) If blocking IgG antibodies can prevent binding of allergens to specific Ig ϵ memory B cells, they also may reduce rises in allergen-specific IgE levels induced by allergen contact and may contribute to a reduction of total allergen-specific IgE levels. The reduction of IgE levels may then also lead to reduced expression of FcϵRI on effector cells of atopy and, perhaps on antigen-presenting cells (8–11).

Immunotherapy studies performed with defined hypoallergenic molecules will now allow investigators to reexamine the old concept of blocking antibodies. These studies will also tell us whether immunotherapy with synthetic and genetically engineered hypoallergenic allergen derivatives is safe and effective.

ACKNOWLEDGMENTS

We thank Anton Jäger for graphic work. This study was supported by grant Y078GEN of the Austrian Science Fund, by the ICP program of the Austrian Federal Ministry for Education, Science and Culture and by a grant from Pharmacia Diagnostics AB, Uppsala, Sweden.

REFERENCES

1. Kay AB. Allergy and Allergic Diseases. Oxford, England: Blackwell Science, 1997.
2. Lockey RF, Bukantz SC, ed. Allergen Immunotherapy. 2nd ed. New York: Marcel Dekker, 1998.
3. Ravetch JV, Kinet JP. Fc receptors. Annu Rev Immunol 1991; 9:457–492.
4. Beaven MA, Metzger H. Signal transduction by Fc receptors: the Fc epsilon RI case. Immunol Today 1993; 14:222–226.
5. Bieber T. Fc epsilon RI on antigen-presenting cells. Curr Opin Immunol 1996; 8:773–777.
6. Stingl G, Maurer D. IgE-mediated allergen presentation via Fc epsilon RI on antigen-presenting cells. Int Arch Allergy Immunol 1997; 113:24–29.
7. Henderson LL, Larson JB, Gleich GJ. Maximal rise in IgE antibody following ragweed pollination season. J Allergy Clin Immunol 1975; 55:10–15.
8. MacGlashan DW Jr, Bochner BS, Adelman DC, Jardieu PM, Togias A, Lichtenstein LM. Serum IgE level drives basophil and mast cell IgE receptor display. Int Arch Allergy Immunol 1997; 113:45–47.
9. MacGlashan D, McKenzie–White J, Chichester K, Bochner BS, Davis FM, Schroeder JT, Lichtenstein LM. In vitro regulation of Fc epsilon RI alpha expression on human basophils by IgE antibody. Blood 1998; 91:1633–1643.
10. Saini SS, MacGlashan DW, Sterbinsky SA, Togias A, Adelman DC, Lichtenstein LM, Bochner BS. Down-regulation of human basophil IgE and Fc epsilon RI alpha surface densities and mediator release by anti-IgE infusions is reversible in vitro and in vivo. J Immunol 1999; 162:5624–5630.
11. MacGlashan D, Lichtenstein LM, McKenzie–White J, Chichester K, Henry AJ, Sutton BJ, Gould HJ. Upregulation of Fc epsilon RI on human basophils by IgE antibody is mediated by interaction of IgE with Fc epsilon RI. J Allergy Clin Immunol 1999; 104:492–498.
12. Romagnani S, Maggi E, del Prete GF, Troncone R, Ricci M. In vitro production of IgE by human blood mononuclear cells. Clin Exp Immunol 1980; 42:167–174.
13. Steinberger P, Bohle B, di Padova F, Wrann M, Liehl E, Scheiner O, Kraft D, Valenta R. Allergen-specific IgE production of committed B cells from allergic patients in vitro. J Allergy Clin Immunol 1995; 96:209–218.
14. Dolecek C, Steinberger P, Susani M, Kraft D, Valenta R, Boltz–Nitulescu G. Effects of IL-4 and IL-13 on total and allergen specific IgE production by cultured PBMC from allergic patients determined with recombinant allergens. Clin Exp Allergy 1995; 25:879–889.
15. Bousquet J, Lockey R, Malling HJ, the WHO panel members. Allergen immunotherapy: therapeutic vaccines for allergic diseases. A WHO position paper. J Allergy Clin Immunol 1998; 102:558–562.
16. Noon L. Prophylactic inoculation against hayfever. Lancet 1911; 1:1572–1573.
17. Bousquet J, Lockey R, Malling HJ. WHO position paper. Allergen immunotherapy: therapeutic vaccines for allergic diseases. Allergy 1998; 53:1–42.
18. Durham SR, Till SJ. Immunological changes associated with allergen immunotherapy. J Allergy Clin Immunol 1998; 102:157–164.
19. Cooke R, Barnard J, Hebald S, Stull A. Serological evidence on immunity with co-existing sensitization in a type of human allergy, hay fever. J Exp Med 1935; 62:733–750.
20. Loveless MH. Immunological studies of pollinosis: I. The presence of two antibodies related to the same pollen antigen in the serum of treated hay fever patients. J Immunol 1940; 38: 25–50.
21. Loveless MH. Immunological studies on pollinosis. IV. The relationship between thermostable antibody in the circulation and clinical immunity. J Immunol 1943; 47:165–180.
22. Sobotka AK, Valentine MD, Ishizaka K, Lichtenstein LM. Measurement of IgG blocking antibodies: development and application of a radioimmunoassay. J Immunol 1976; 117:84–90.

23. Adkinson NF, Sobotka AK, Lichtenstein LM. Evaluation of the quantity and affinity of human IgG ''blocking'' antibodies. J Immunol 1979; 122:965–972.
24. Gleich GJ, Zimmermann EM, Gleich MC, Yunginger JW. Measurement of IgG blocking antibodies by interference in the radioallergosorbent test. J Immunol 1981; 126:575–579.
25. Aalberse RC, Gaag R, Leeuwen J. Serologic aspects of IgG_4 antibodies. I. Prolonged immunization results in an IgG_4-restricted response. J Immunol 1983; 130:722–726.
26. Lichtenstein LM, Holtzman NA, Burnett LS. A quantitative in vitro study of the chromatographic distribution and immunoglobulin characteristics of human blocking antibody. J Immunol 1986; 101:317–324.
27. Furin MM, Norman PS, Creticos PS, Proud D, Kagey–Sobotka A, Lichtenstein LM, Naclerio RM. Immunotherapy decreases antigen-induced eosinophil migration into the nasal cavity. J Allergy Clin Immunol 1991; 88:27–32.
28. Otsuka H, Mezawa A, Ohnishi M, Okubo K, Sehi H, Okuda M. Changes in nasal metachromatic cells during allergen immunotherapy. Clin Exp Allergy 1991; 21:115–120.
29. Creticos PS, Adkinson NF Jr, Kagey–Sobotka A, Proud D, Meier HL, Naclerio RM, Lichtenstein LM, Norman PS. Nasal challenge with ragweed in hay fever patients: effect of immunotherapy. J Clin Invest 1985; 76:2247–2253.
30. Rak S, Rowhagen O, Venge P. The effect of immunotherapy on bronchial hyper-responsiveness and eosinophil cationic protein in pollen allergic patients. J Allergy Clin Immunol 1998; 82:470–480.
31. Durham SR, Ying S, Varney VA, Jacobson MR, Sudderick RM, Mackay IS, Kay AB, Hamid QA. Grass pollen immunotherapy inhibits allergen-induced infiltration of $CD4^+$ T lymphocytes and eosinophils in the nasal mucosa and increases the number of cells expressing messenger RNA for interferon-γ. J Allergy Clin Immunol 1996; 97:1356–1365.
32. Rocklin RE, Sheffer A, Greineder DK, Melmon KL. Generation of antigen-specific supressor cells during allergy desensitization. N Engl J Med 1980; 302:1213–1219.
33. Secrist H, Chelen CJ, Wen Y, Marshall JD, Umetsu DT. Allergen immunotherapy decreases interleukin 4 production in $CD4^+$ T cells from allergic individuals. J Exp Med 1993; 178: 2123–2130.
34. Jutel M, Pichler WJ, Skrbic D, Urwyler A, Dahinden C, Müller UR. Bee venom immunotherapy results in decrease of IL-4 and IL-5 and increase of IFN-γ secretion in specific allergen-stimulated T cell cultures. J Immunol 1995; 154:4187–4194.
35. O'Brien RM, Byron KA, Varigos GA, Thomas WR. House dust mite immunotherapy results in a decrease in Der p 2-specific IFN-γ and IL-4 expression by circulation T lymphocytes. Clin Exp Allergy 1997; 27:46–51.
36. Ebner C, Siemann U, Bohle B, Willheim M, Wiedermann U, Schenk S, Klotz F, Ebner H, Kraft D, Scheiner O. Immunological changes during specific immunotherapy of grass pollen allergy: reduced lymphoproliferative responses to allergen and shift from TH_2 to TH_1 in T-cell clones specific for Phl p 1, a major grass pollen allergen. Clin Exp Allergy 1997; 27: 1007–1015.
37. Ball T, Sperr WR, Valent P, Lidholm J, Spitzauer S, Ebner C, Kraft D, Valenta R. Induction of antibody responses to new B cell epitopes indicates vaccination character of allergen immunotherapy. Eur J Immunol 1999; 29:2026–2036.
38. Sledge RF. Treatment of hay-fever with alum-precipitated pollen. US Naval Med Bull 1938; 36:18.
39. Wheeler AW, Drachenberg KJ. New routes and formulations for allergen-specific immunotherapy. Allergy 1997; 52:602–612.
40. Attallah NA, Sehon AH. Isolation of haptenic material from ragweed pollen. Immunochemistry 1969; 6:609–619.
41. Malley A, Periman F. Induction of both reaginic and blocking antibodies with a low molecular weight fraction of timothy pollen extract. J Allergy 1969; 43:59–64.
42. Malley A, Baecher L, Mackler B, Periman F. Further characterization of a low-molecular

weight allergen fragment isolated from the green pea. Clin Exp Immunol 1976; 25:159–164.
43. Chakrabarty S, Ekramoddoullah AK, Kisil FT, Sehon AH. Allergens of Kentucky Blue Grass pollen. II. Isolation of hapten-like components from Kentucky Blue Grass pollen by preparative isoelectrofocussing. Int Arch Allergy Appl Immunol 1980; 63:369–382.
44. Litwin A, Pesce AJ, Michael JG. Regulation of the immuneresponse to allergens by immunosuppressive allergenic fragments. I. Peptic fragments of honey bee venom phospholipase A_2. Int Arch Allergy Appl Immunol 1988; 87:361–366.
45. Litwin A, Pesce AJ, Fischer T, Michael M, Michael JG. Regulation of the human immune response to ragweed pollen by immunotherapy. A controlled trial comparing the effect of immunosuppressive peptic fragments of short ragweed with standard treatment. Clin Exp Allergy 1991; 21:457–465.
46. Marsh DG, Lichtenstein LM, Campbell DH. Studies on 'allergoids' prepared from naturally occurring allergens. I. Assay of allergenicity and antigenicity of formalinized rye group I component. Immunology 1970; 18:705–722.
47. Marsh DG, Norman PS, Roebber M, Lichtenstein LM. Studies of allergoids from naturally occurring allergens. III. Preparation of ragweed pollen allergoids by aldehyde modification in two steps. J Allergy Clin Immunol 1981; 68:449–459.
48. Metzger WJ, Patterson R, Zeiss R, Irons JS, Pruzansky JJ, Suszko IM, Levitz D. Comparison of polymerized and unpolymerized antigen E for immunotherapy of ragweed allergy. N Engl J Med 1976; 295:1160–1164.
49. Moran DM, Wheeler AW. Chemical modification of crude timothy grass pollen extract. I. Antigenicity and immunogenicity changes following amino group modification. Int Arch Allergy Appl Immunol 1976; 50:693–708.
50. Wheeler AW, Jenkins PM, Moran DM. Chemical modification of crude timothy grass pollen extract. II. Class and specifity of antibodies induced by chemically modified timothy grass pollen extract. Int Arch Allergy Appl Immunol 1976; 50:709–728.
51. Wegner F, Fenkes A, Stemmann EA, Reinhardt D. Influence of preseasonal treatment with L-tyrosine-adsorbed allergoids on IgE-mediated histamine release from basophils of children suffering from allergic diseases. Agents Actions 1981; 11:111–113.
52. Grammer LC, Zeiss CR, Suszko IM, Shaughnessy MA, Patterson R. A double-blind, placebo-controlled trial of polymerized whole ragweed for immunotherapy of ragweed allergy. J Allergy Clin Immunol 1982; 69:494–499.
53. Grammer LC, Shaughnessy MA, Suszko IM, Shaughnessy JJ, Patterson R. A double-blind histamine placebo-controlled trial of polymerized whole grass for immunotherapy of grass allergy. J Allergy Clin Immunol 1983; 72:448–453.
54. Grammer LC, Shaughnessy MA, Patterson R. Modified forms of allergen immunotherapy. J Allergy Clin Immunol 1985; 76:397–401.
55. Maasch HJ, Marsh DG. Standardized extracts modified allergens–allergoids. Clin Rev Allergy 1987; 5:89–106.
56. Metzger WJ, Dorminey HC, Richerson HB, Weiler JM, Donnelly A, Moran D. Clinical and immunologic evaluation of glutaraldehyde-modified tyrosine-adsorbed short ragweed extract: a double-blind, placebo-controlled trial. J Allergy Clin Immunol 1981; 68:442–448.
57. Meriney DK, Kothari H, Chinoy P, Grieco MH. The clinical and immunological efficacy of immunotherapy with modified ragweed extract (allergoid) for ragweed hay fever. Allergy 1986; 56:34–38.
58. Norman PS, Lichtenstein LM, Marsh DG. Studies on allergoids from naturally occurring allergens. IV. Efficacy and safety of long-term allergoid treatment of ragweed hay fever. J Allergy Clin Immunol 1981; 68:460–470.
59. Norman PS, Lichtenstein LM, Kagey–Sobotka A, Marsh DG. Controlled evaluation of allergoid in the immunotherapy of ragweed hay fever. J Allergy Clin Immunol 1982; 70:248–260.

60. Norman PS, Creticos PS, Marsh DG. Frequency of booster injections of allergoids. J Allergy Clin Immunol 1990; 85:88–94.
61. Whil JA, Pilstrom L, Maasch HJ. Studies on allergen and allergoid preparations from purified timothy (*Phleum pratense*) pollen extracts. III. Comparative investigations by skin prick tests and nasal provocation tests. Int Arch Allergy Appl Immunol 1985; 76:162–167.
62. HayGlass KT, Stefura BP. Anti-interferon gamma treatment blocks the ability of glutaraldehyde-polymerized allergens to inhibit specific IgE responses. J Exp Med 1991; 173:279–285.
63. Yang X, Gieni RS, Mosman TR, HayGlass KT. Chemically modified antigen preferentially elicits induction of Th1-like cytokine synthesis patterns in vivo. J Exp Med 1993; 178:349–353.
64. Lee WY, Sehon AH. Abrogation of reaginic antibodies with modified allergens. Nature 1977; 267:618–619.
65. King TP, Kochoumian L, Chiorazzi N. Immunological properties of conjugates of ragweed pollen antigen E with methoxypolyethylene glycol or a copolymer of D-glutamic acid and D-lysine. J Exp Med 1979; 149:424–435.
66. Sehon AH. Suppression of IgE antibodies with conjugates of haptens or allergens and synthetic hydrophilic polymers. Ann NY Acad Sci 1982; 392:55–70.
67. Sehon AH. Carl Prausnitz Memorial Lecture. Suppression of antibody responses by chemically modified antigens. Int Arch Allergy Appl Immunol 1991; 94:11–20.
68. Wie SI, Wie CW, Lee WY, Filion LG, Sehon AH, Akerblom E. Suppression of reaginic antibodies with modified allergens. III. Preparation of tolerogenic conjugates of common allergens with monomethoxypolyethylene glycols of different molecular weights by the mixed anhydride method. Int Arch Allergy Appl Immunol 1981; 64:84–99.
69. Nordvall SL, Uhlin T, Ohman S, Bjorkander J, Malling HJ, Weeke B, Dreborg S, Lanner A, Einarsson R. IgG and IgE antibody patterns after immunotherapy with monomethoxy polyethyleneglycol modified honey bee venom. Allergy 1986; 41:89–94.
70. Mosbech H, Dreborg S, Pahlman I, Stahl–Skov P, Steringer I, Weeke B. Modification of house dust mite allergens by monomethoxypolyethylene glycol. Allergenicity measured by in vitro and in vivo methods. Int Arch Allergy Appl Immunol 1988; 85:145–149.
71. Mosbech H, Dreborg S, Frolund L, Ljungstedt–Pahlman I, Svendsen UG, Soborg M, Taudorf E, Weeke B. Hyposensitization in asthmatics with mPEG modified and unmodified house dust mite extract. II. Effect evaluated by challenges with allergen and histamine. Allergy 1989; 44:499–509.
72. Mosbech H, Djurup R, Dreborg S, Kaergaard–Poulsen L, Stahl–Skov P, Steringer I. Hyposensitization in asthmatics with mPEG-modified and unmodified house dust mite extract. III. Effect on mite-specific immunological parameters and correlation to changes in mite-sensitivity and symptoms. Allergy 1990; 45:130–141.
73. Schäfer T, Przybilla B, Galosi A, Burow G, Ljungstedt–Pahlman I, Dreborg S, Ring J. Two-year double blind trial of a monomethoxy polyethylene glycol (mPEG) modified grass pollen extract at different dose levels. Ann Allergy 1992; 68:334–339.
74. Van Ree R, van Leeuwen WA, Dieges PH, van Wijk RG, De Jong N, Brewczyski PZ, Kroon AM, Schilte PP, Tan KY, Simon–Licht IF, Roberts AM, Stapel SO, Aalberse RC. Measurement of IgE antibodies against purified grass pollen allergens (Lol p 1, 2, 3 and 5) during immunotherapy. Clin Exp Allergy 1997; 27:68–74.
75. Valenta R, Kraft D. Recombinant allergens for diagnosis and therapy of allergic diseases. Curr Opin Immunol 1995; 7:751–756.
76. Valenta R, Steinberger P, Duchêne M, Kraft D. Immunological and structural similarities among allergens: prerequisite for a specific and component-based therapy of allergy. Immunol Cell Biol 1996; 74:187–194.
77. Valenta R, Vrtala S, Laffer S, Spitzauer S, Kraft D. Recombinant allergens. Allergy 1998; 53:552–561.

78. Valenta R, Almo S, Ball T, Dolecek C, Steinberger P, Laffer S, Eibensteiner P, Flicker S, Vrtala S, Spitzauer S, Valent P, Denepoux S, Kraft D, Banchereau J, Lebecque S. The immunoglobulin E–allergen interaction: a target for therapy of type I allergic diseases. Int Arch Allergy Immunol 1998; 116:167–176.
79. Valenta R, Lidholm J, Niederberger V, Hayek B, Kraft D, Grönlund H. The recombinant allergen-based concept of component resolved diagnosis and immunotherapy (CRD and CRIT). Clin Exp Allergy 1999; 29:896–904.
80. Valenta R, Duchêne M, Vrtala S, Birkner T, Ebner C, Hirschwehr R, Breitenbach M, Rumpold H, Scheiner O, Kraft D. Recombinant allergens for immunoblot diagnosis of tree-pollen allergy. J Allergy Clin Immunol 1991; 88:889–894.
81. Valenta R, Vrtala S, Ebner C, Kraft D, Scheiner O. Diagnosis of grass pollen allergy with recombinant timothy grass (*Phleum pratense*) pollen allergens. Int Arch Allergy Immunol 1992; 97:287–294.
82. Niederberger V, Pauli G, Grönlund H, Fröschl R, Rumpold H, Kraft D, Valenta R, Spitzauer S. Recombinant birch pollen allergens (rBet v 1, rBet v 2) contain most of the IgE epitopes present in birch, alder, hornbeam, hazel, and oak pollen. A quantitative IgE inhibition study using sera from different populations. J Allergy Clin Immunol 1998; 102:579–591.
83. Niederberger V, Laffer S, Fröschl R, Kraft D, Rumpold H, Kapiotis S, Valenta R, Spitzauer S. IgE antibodies to recombinant pollen allergens (Phl p 1, Phl p 2, Phl p 5, and Bet v 2) account for a high percentage of grass pollen-specific IgE. J Allergy Clin Immunol 1998; 101:258–264.
84. Laffer S, Spitzauer S, Susani M, Pairleitner H, Schweiger C, Grönlund H, Menz G, Pauli G, Ishii T, Nolte H, Ebner C, Sehon AH, Kraft D, Eichler HG, Valenta R. Comparison of recombinant timothy grass pollen allergens with natural extract for diagnosis of grass pollen allergy in different populations. J Allergy Clin Immunol 1996; 98:652–658.
85. Kazemi–Shirazi L, Pauli G, Purohit A, Spitzauer S, Fröschl R, Hoffmann–Sommergruber K, Breiteneder H, Scheiner O, Kraft D, Valenta R. Quantitative IgE inhibition experiments with purified recombinant allergens indicate pollen-derived allergens as the sensitizing agents responsible for many forms of plant food allergy. J Allergy Clin Immunol 2000; 105:116–125.
86. Valenta R, Duchêne M, Pettenburger K, Sillaber C, Valent P, Bettelheim P, Breitenbach M, Rumpold H, Kraft D, Scheiner O. Identification of profilin as a novel pollen allergen: IgE autoreactivity in sensitized individuals. Science 1991; 253:557–560.
87. Valenta R, Duchêne M, Ebner C, Valent P, Sillaber C, Deviller P, Ferreira F, Tejkl M, Edelmann H, Kraft D, Scheiner O. Profilins constitute a novel family of functional plant pan-allergens. J Exp Med 1992; 175:377–385.
88. Ball T, Fuchs T, Sperr WR, Valent P, Vangelista L, Kraft D, Valenta R. B cell epitopes of the major timothy grass pollen allergen, Phl p 1, revealed by gene fragmentation as candidates for immunotherapy. FASEB J 1999; 13:1277–1290.
89. DeWeck AL, Schneider CH. Specific inhibition of allergic reactions to penicillin in man by a monovalent hapten. I. Experimental immunological and toxicologic studies. Int Arch Allergy Appl Immunol 1972; 42:782–797.
90. Hedin H, Richter W. Pathomechanism of dextran-induced anaphylactoid/anaphylactic reactions in man. Int Arch Allergy Appl Immunol 1982; 68:122–126.
91. Richter W, Hedin H, Kraft D, Messmer K. Anaphylactoid reactions after dextran II. Experimental studies in animals on the principle of hapten inhibition. Beitr Infusionsther Klin Ernähr 1981; 8:54–65.
92. Vrtala S, Hirtenlehner K, Vangelista L, Pastore A, Eichler HG, Sperr WR, Valent P, Ebner C, Kraft D, Valenta R. Conversion of the major birch pollen allergen, Bet v 1, into two nonanaphylactic T cell epitope-containing fragments; candidates for a novel form of specific immunotherapy. J Clin Invest 1997; 99:1673–1681.
93. Van Hage–Hamsten, Kronqvist M, Zetterström O, Johansson E, Niederberger V, Vrtala S, Grönlund H, Grönneberg R, Valenta R. Skin test evaluation of genetically engineered hypoal-

lergenic derivatives of the major birch pollen allergen, Bet v 1. Results obtained with a mix of two recombinant Bet v 1 fragments and rBet v 1 trimer in a Swedish population before the birch pollen season. J Allergy Clin Immunol 1999; 104:969–977.

94. Pauli G, Purohit A, Oster JP, Vrtala S, Niederberger V, Kraft D, Valenta R. Clinical evaluation of genetically engineered hypoallergenic rBet v 1 derivatives. Int Arch Allergy Immunol 1999; 118:216–217.
95. Pauli G, Purohit A, Oster JP, de Blay F, Vrtala S, Niederberger V, Kraft D, Valenta R. Clinical evaluation of genetically engineered hypoallergenic rBet v 1 derivatives by skin prick and intradermal testing: results obtained in a French population. Clin Exp Allergy 2000; 30:1076–1084.
96. Vrtala S, Akdis CA, Budak F, Akdis M, Blaser K, Kraft D, Valenta R. T cell epitope-containing hypoallergenic recombinant fragments of the major birch pollen allergen, Bet v 1, induce blocking antibodies. J Immunol 2000; 165:6653–6659.
97. Nopp A, Halldén G, Lundahl J, Johansson E, Vrtala S, Valenta R, Grönneberg R, van Hage–Hamsten M. Genetically engineered hypoallergenic derivatives of the major birch pollen allergen, Bet v 1, induce less eosinophilic activity in skin chamber fluids collected from birch pollen allergic patients than rBet v 1 wild type. J Allergy Clin Immunol 2000; 106:101–109.
98. Ferreira F, Hirtenlehner K, Jilek A, Godnik–Cvar J, Breiteneder H, Grimm R, Hoffmann–Sommergruber K, Scheiner O, Kraft D, Breitenbach M, Rheinberger HJ, Ebner C. Dissection of immunoglobulin E and T lymphocyte reactivity of isoforms of the major birch pollen allergen Bet v 1: potential use of hypoallergenic isoforms for immunotherapy. J Exp Med 1996; 183:599–609.
99. Arquint O, Helbing A, Crameri R, Ferreira F, Breitenbach M, Pichler WJ. Reduced in vivo allergenicity of Bet v 1d isoform, a natural component of birch pollen. J Allergy Clin Immunol 1999; 104:1239–1243.
100. Ferreira F, Ebner C, Kramer B, Casari G, Briza P, Kungl AJ, Grimm R, Jahn–Schmid B, Breiteneder H, Kraft D, Breitenbach M, Rheinberger H, Scheiner O. Modulation of IgE reactivity of allergens by site-directed mutagenesis: potential use of hypo-allergenic variants for immunotherapy. FASEB J 1998; 12:231–242.
101. Vrtala S, Hirtenlehner K, Susani M, Hufnagl P, Binder BR, Vangelista L, Pastore A, Sperr WR, Valent P, Ebner C, Kraft D, Valenta R. Genetic engineering of recombinant hypoallergenic oligomers of the major birch pollen allergen, Bet v 1: candidates for specific immunotherapy. Int Arch Allergy Immunol 1999; 118:218–219.
102. Vrtala S, Hirtenlehner K, Susani M, Akdis M, Akdis CA, Blaser K, Hufnagl P, Binder BR, Vangelista L, Pastore A, Sperr WR, Valent P, Ebner C, Kraft D, Valenta R. Genetic engineering of a vaccine against birch pollen allergy. Submitted.
103. Jensen–Jarolim E, Leitner A, Kalchhauser H, Zurcher A, Ganglberger E, Bohle B, Scheiner O, Boltz–Nitulescu G, Breiteneder H. Peptide mimotopes displayed by phage inhibit antibody binding to Bet v 1, the major birch pollen allergen, and induce specific IgG response in mice. FASEB J 1998; 12:1635–1642.
104. Fedorov AA, Ball T, Mahoney NM, Valenta R, Almo SC. The molecular basis for allergen crossreactivity: crystal structure and IgE epitope mapping of birch pollen profilin. Structure 1997; 5:33–45.
105. Twardosz A, Hayek B, Seiberler S, Vangelista L, Elfman L, Grönlund H, Kraft D, Valenta R. Molecular characterization, expression in *Escherichia coli* and epitope analysis of a two EF-hand calcium-binding birch pollen allergen, Bet v 4. Biochem Biophys Res Commun 1997; 239:197–204.
106. Engel E, Richter K, Obermeyer G, Briza P, Kungl AJ, Simon B, Auer M, Ebner C, Rheinberger H, Breitenbach M, Ferreira F. Immunological and biological properties of Bet v 4, a novel birch pollen allergen with two EF-hand calcium-binding domains. J Biol Chem 1997; 272:28630–28637.

107. Hayek B, Vangelista L, Pastore A, Sperr WR, Valent P, Vrtala S, Niederberger V, Twardosz A, Kraft D, Valenta R. Molecular and immunologic characterization of a highly cross-reactive two EF-hand calcium-binding alder pollen allergen, Aln g 4: structural basis for calcium-modulated IgE recognition. J Immunol 1998; 161:7031–7039.
108. Okada T, Swoboda I, Bhalla PL, Toriyama K, Singh MB. Engineering of hypoallergenic mutants of the *Brassica* pollen allergen, Bra r 1, for immunotherapy. FEBS Lett 1998; 434: 255–260.
109. Tamborini E, Faccini S, Lidholm J, Svensson M, Brandazza A, Longhi R, Grönlund H, Sidoli A, Arosio A. Biochemical and immunological characterization of recombinant allergen Lol p 1. Eur J Biochem 1997; 249:886–894.
110. Singh MB, de Weerd N, Bhalla PL. Genetically engineered plant allergens with reduced anaphylactic activity. Int Arch Allergy Immunol 1999; 119:75–85.
111. Swoboda I, de Weerd N, Bhalla PL, Niederberger V, Sperr WR, Valent P, Kahlert H, Fiebig H, Ebner C, Spitzauer S, Valenta R, Singh MB. Hypoallergenic forms of the ryegrass pollen allergen Lol p 5 as candidates for immunotherapy. Int Arch Allergy Immunol 2001; 124: 380–382.
112. Ball T, Vrtala S, Sperr WR, Valent P, Susani M, Kraft D, Valenta R. Isolation of an immunodominant IgE-hapten from an epitope expression cDNA library; dissection of the allergic effector reaction. J Biol Chem 1994; 269:28323–28328.
113. Focke M, Ball T, Mahler V, Kraft D, Valenta R. B-cell epitope-derived peptides of the major grass pollen allergen, Phl p 1, for immunotherapy [abstr]. Allergy 1999; 54:19.
114. Schramm G, Kahlert H, Suck R, Weber B, Stuwe HT, Müller WD, Bufe A, Becker WM, Schlaak MW, Jäger L, Cromwell O, Fiebig H. ''Allergen engineering'': Variants of the timothy grass pollen allergen Phl p 5b with reduced IgE-binding capacity but conserved T cell reactivity. J Immunol 1999; 162:2406–2414.
115. Vrtala S, Fischer S, Grote M, Vangelista L, Pastore A, Sperr WR, Valent P, Reichelt R, Kraft D, Valenta R. Molecular, immunological, and structural characterization of Phl p 6, a major allergen and P-particle-associated protein from timothy grass (*Phleum pratense*) pollen. J Immunol 1999; 163:5489–5496.
116. Smith AM, Chapman MD. Reduction in IgE binding to allergen variants generated by site-directed mutagenesis: contribution of disulfide bonds to the antigenic structure of the major house dust mite allergen Der p 1. Mol Immunol 1996; 33:399–405.
117. Smith AM, Chapman MD, Taketomi EA, Platts–Mills TAE, Sung SSJ. Recombinant allergens for immunotherapy: a Der p 2 variant with reduced IgE reactivity retains T-cell epitopes. J Allergy Clin Immunol 1998; 101:423–425.
118. Takai T, Yokota T, Yasue M, Nishiyama C, Yuuki T, Mori A, Okudaira H, Okumura Y. Engineering of the major house dust mite allergen Der f 2 for allergen-specific immunotherapy. Nat Biotechnol 1997; 15:754–758.
119. Olsson S, van Hage–Hamsten M, Whitley P. Contribution of disulphide bonds to antigenicity of Lep d 2, the major allergen of the dust mite *Lepidoplyphus destructor*. Mol Immunol 1998; 35:1017–1023.
120. Norman PS, Ohman JL Jr, Long AA, Creticos PS, Gefter MA, Shaked Z, Wood, RA, Eggleston PA, Hafner KB, Rao P, Lichtenstein LM, Jones NH, Nicodemus CF. Treatment of cat allergy with T-cell reactive peptides. Am J Respir Crit Care Med 1996; 154:1623–1628.
121. Norman PS, Nicodemus CF, Creticos PS, Wood RA, Eggleston PA, Lichtenstein LM, Kagey–Sobotka A, Proud D. Clinical and immunologic effects of component peptides in Allervax cat. Allergy—a disease of modern society. Int Arch Allergy Immunol 1997; 113:224–226.
122. Simons FE, Imada M, Li Y, Watson WT, HayGlass KT. Fel d 1 peptides: effect on skin tests and cytokine synthesis in cat-allergic human subjects. Int Immunol 1996; 8:1937–1945.
123. Zeiler T, Taivainen A, Rytkonen M, Rautiainen J, Karjalainen H, Mantyjarvi R, Tuomisto L, Virtanen T. Recombinant allergen fragments as candidate preparations for allergen immunotherapy. J Allergy Clin Immunol 1997; 100:721–727.

124. Kauppinen J, Zeiler T, Rautiainen J, Rytkonen–Nissinen M, Taivainen A, Mantyjarvi R, Virtanen T. Mutant derivatives of the main respiratory allergen of cow are less allergenic than the intact molecule. Clin Exp Allergy 1999; 29:989–996.
125. Müller U, Akdis CA, Fricker M, Akdis M, Blesken T, Bettens F, Blaser K. Successful immunotherapy with T-cell epitope peptides of bee venom phospholipase A_2 induces specific T-cell anergy in patients allergic to bee venom. J Allergy Clin Immunol 1998; 101:747–754.
126. Vrtala S, Ball T, Spitzauer S, Pandjaitan B, Suphioglu C, Knox B, Sperr WR, Valent P, Kraft D, Valenta R. Immunization with purified natural and recombinant allergens induces mouse IgG1 antibodies that recognize similar epitopes as human IgE and inhibit the human IgE–allergen interaction and allergen-induced basophil degranulation. J Immunol 1998, 160: 6137–6144.
127. Rothbard JB. Synthetic peptides as vaccines. Biotechnology 1992; 20:451–465.
128. Norman PS. Therapeutic potential of peptides in allergic disease. Ann Allergy 1993; 71: 330–333.
129. Akdis CA, Akdis M, Blesken T, Wyman D, Alkan SS, Müller U, Blaser K. Epitope-specific T cell tolerance to phosholipase A_2 in bee venom immunotherapy and recovery by IL-2 and IL-15 in vitro. J Clin Invest 1996; 98:1676–1683.
130. Rolland J, O'Hehir R. Immunotherapy of allergy: anergy, deletion, and immune deviation. Curr Opin Immunol 1998; 10:640–645.
131. Akdis CA, Blaser K. IL-10-induced anergy in peripheral T cell and reactivation by microenvironmental cytokines: two key steps in specific immunotherapy. FASEB J 1999; 13:603–609.
132. Greene WK, Cyster JG, Chua KY, O'Brien RM, Thomas WR. IgE and IgG binding of peptides expressed from fragments of cDNA encoding the major house dust mite allergen Der p 1. J Immunol 1991; 147:3768–3773.
133. Ong EK, Knox RB, Singh MB. Mapping of the antigenic and allergenic epitopes of Lol p 5b using gene fragmentation. Mol Immunol 1995; 32:295–302.
134. Valenta R, Vrtala S, Focke–Tejkl M, Bugajska–Schretter A, Ball T, Twardosz A, Spitzauer S, Grönlund H, Kraft D. Genetically engineered and synthetic allergen derivatives: candidates for vaccination against type I allergy. Biol Chem 1999; 380:815–824.
135. Seiberler S, Scheiner O, Kraft D, Lonsdale D, Valenta R. Characterization of a birch pollen allergen, Bet v 3, representing a novel class of Ca^{2+} binding proteins: specific expression in mature pollen and dependence of patients IgE binding on protein-bound Ca^{2+} EMBO J 1994; 13:3481–3486.
136. Valenta R, Hayek B, Seiberler S, Bugajska–Schretter A, Niederberger V, Twardosz A, Natter S, Vangelista L, Pastore A, Spitzauer S, Kraft D. Calcium-binding allergens: from plants to man. Int Arch Allergy Immunol 1998; 117:160–166.
137. Laffer S, Vangelista L, Steinberger P, Kraft D, Pastore A, Valenta R. Molecular characterization of Bip 1, a monoclonal antibody that modulates IgE binding to birch pollen allergen, Bet v 1. J Immunol 1996; 157:4953–4962.
138. Visco V, Dolecek C, Denepoux S, LeMao J, Guret C, Rousset F, Guinnepain MT, Kraft D, Valenta R, Weyer A, Banchereau J, Lebecque S. Human IgG monoclonal antibodies that modulate the binding of specific IgE to birch pollen Bet v 1. J Immunol 1996; 157:956–962.
139. Lebeque S, Dolecek C, Laffer S, Visco V, Denepoux S, Pin JJ, Guret C, Boltz–Nitulescu G, Weyer A, Valenta R. Immunologic characterization of monoclonal antibodies that modulate human IgE binding to the major birch pollen allergen Bet v 1. J Allergy Clin Immunol 1997; 99:374–384.
140. Denepoux S, Eibensteiner PB, Steinberger P, Vrtala S, Visco V, Weyer A, Kraft D, Banchereau J, Valenta R, Lebecque S. Molecular characterization of human IgG monoclonal antibodies specific for the major birch pollen allergen Bet v 1. Anti-allergen IgG can enhance the anaphylactic reaction. FEBS Lett 2000; 465:39–46.

141. Raz E, Tighe H, Sato Y, Corr M, Dudler JA, Roman M, Swain SL, Spiegelberg HL, Carson DA. Preferential induction of a Th1 immune response and inhibition of specific IgE antibody formation by plasmid DNA immunization. Proc Natl Acad Sci USA 1996; 93:5141–5145.
142. Hsu CH, Chua KY, Tao MH, Lai YL, Wu HD, Huang SK, Hsieh KH. Immuno-prophylaxis of allergen-induced immunoglobulin E synthesis and airway hyperresponsiveness in vivo by genetic immunization. Nat Med 1996; 2:540–544.
143. Hsu CH, Chua KY, Tao MH, Huang SK, Hsieh KH. Inhibition of specific IgE response in vivo by allergen–gene transfer. Int Immunol 1996; 8:1405–1411.
144. Slater JE, Paupore E, Zhang YT, Colberg–Poley AM. The latex allergen Hev b 5 transcript is widely distributed after subcutaneous injection in BALB/c mice of its DNA vaccine. J Allergy Clin Immunol 1998; 102:469–475.
145. Hartl A, Kiesslich J, Weiss R, Bernhaupt A, Mostbock S, Scheiblhofer S, Ebner C, Ferreira F, Thalhammer J. Immune responses after immunization with plasmid DNA encoding Bet v 1, the major allergen of birch pollen. J Allergy Clin Immunol 1999; 103:107–113.
146. Roy K, Mao HQ, Huang SK, Leong KW. Oral gene delivery with chitosan–DNA nanoparticales generates immunologic protection in a murine model of peanut allergy. Nat Med 1999; 5:387–391.
147. Bagarazzi ML, Boyer JD, Ugen KE, Javadian MA, Chattergoon M, Shah A, Bennett M, Ciccarelli R, Carrano R, Coney L, Weiner DB. Safety and immunogenicity of HIV-1 DNA constructs in chimpanzees. Vaccine 1998; 16:1836–1841.
148. Ugen KE, Nyland SB, Boyer JD, Vidal C, Lera L, Rasheid S, Chattergoon M, Bagarazzi ML, Ciccarelli R, Higgins T, Baine Y, Ginsberg R, Macgregor RR, Weiner DB. DNA vaccination with HIV-1 expressing constructs elicits immune responses in humans. Vaccine 1998; 16:1818–1821.
149. Ockenhouse CF, Sun PF, Lanar DE, Wellede BT, Hall BT, Kester K, Stoute JA, Magill A, Krzych U, Farley L, Wirtz RA, Sadoff JC, Kaslow DC, Kumar S, Church LW, Crutcher JM, Wizel B, Hoffman S, Lalvani A, Hill AV, Tine JA, Guito KP, de Taisne C, Anders R, Ballou WR.. Phase I/II a safety, immunogenicity, and efficacy trial of NYVAC-Pf7, a pox-vectored, multiantigen, multistage vaccine candidate for *Plasmodium falciparum* malaria. J Infect Dis 1998; 177:1664–1673.
150. Wang R, Doolan DL, Le TP, Hedstrom RC, Coonan KM, Charoenvit Y, Jones TR, Hobart P, Margalith M, Ng J, Weiss WR, Sedegah M, de Taisne C, Norman JA, Hoffman SL. Induction of antigen-specific cytotoxic T lymphocytes in humans by a malaria DNA vaccine. Science 1998; 282:476–480.
151. Van Uden J, Raz E. Immunostimulatory DNA and applications to allergic disease. J Allergy Clin Immunol 1999; 104:902–910.
152. Haselden BM, Kay AB, Larché M. Immunoglobulin E-independent major histocompatibility complex-restricted T cell peptide epitope-induced late asthmatic reactions. J Exp Med 1999; 189:1885–1894.
153. Menz G, Dolecek C, Schoenheit–Kenn U, Ferreira F, Moser M, Schneider T, Suter M, Boltz–Nitulescu G, Ebner C, Kraft D, Valenta R. Serological and skin test diagnosis of birch pollen allergy with recombinant Bet v 1, the major birch pollen allergen. Clin Exp Allergy 1996; 26:50–60.
154. Pauli G, Oster JP, Deviller P, Heiss S, Bessot JC, Susani M, Ferreira F, Kraft D, Valenta R. Skin testing with recombinant allergens rBet v 1 and birch profilin, rBet v 2: diagnostic value for birch pollen and associated allergies. J Allergy Clin Immunol 1996; 97:1100–1109.
155. Heiss S, Mahler V, Steiner R, Spitzauer S, Schweiger C, Kraft D, Valenta R. Component-resolved diagnosis (CRD) of type 1 allergy with recombinant grass and tree pollen allergens by skin testing. J Invest Dermatol 1999, 113:830–837.
156. Kolbe L, Heusser C, Kolsch E. Antigen dose dependent regulation of B epsilon-memory cell expression. Int Arch Allergy Immunol 1991; 95:202–206.

157. Secrist H, DeKruyff RH, Umetsu DT. Interleukin 4 production by $CD4^+$ T cells from allergic individuals is modulated by antigen concentration and antigen-presenting cell type. J Exp Med 1995; 181:1081–1089.
158. Akdis CA, Blesken T, Wymann D, Akdis M, Blaser K. Differential regulation of human T cell cytokine patterns and IgE and IgG4 responses by conformational antigen variants. Eur J Immunol 1998; 28:914–925.
159. Van Neerven RJ, Wikborg T, Lund G, Jacobsen B, Brinch–Nielsen A, Arnved J, Ipsen H. Blocking antibodies induced by specific allergy vaccination prevent the activation of $CD4^+$ T cells by inhibiting serum–IgE-facilitated allergen presentation. J Immunol 1999; 163: 2944–2952.

24

Anti-IgE Antibody Therapy

DONALD MacGLASHAN, JR.

Johns Hopkins University School of Medicine, Baltimore, Maryland

1 INTRODUCTION

The defining feature of immediate hypersensitivity reactions is the presence of antigen-specific IgE antibodies. In the classic description of the reaction, the IgE is bound to tissue mast cells and reexposure to antigen triggers these cells to secrete a variety of mediators. Therapeutic targets to ameliorate the disease include everything from the immune response responsible for IgE generation to the end-organ response to secreted mediators. Since the identification of IgE in the 1960s, investigators have sought ways to suppress the levels of IgE antibody, recognizing that its complete elimination would, by definition, eliminate immediate hypersensitivity reactions. There have been, and continue to be, many approaches to achieving this goal, but there is one that has reached the final stages of phase III trials, monoclonal anti-IgE antibody. This antibody is specifically engineered to bind with high affinity to free IgE on an epitope that is not accessible when IgE is bound to its high-affinity receptor (and incidentally, to the low-affinity receptor as well). As a consequence, this antibody can not cause aggregation of mast cell- or basophil-bound IgE; therefore, it cannot trigger mediator release. However, it can bind to free IgE and prevent it from binding to the mast cell or basophil, thereby preventing these cells from responding to antigenic stimulation (1–4). Thus, although IgE has not been actually eliminated from circulation, it no longer participates in the binding reaction that confers antigenic reactivity to mast cells, basophils, or other cells that possess the high- or low-affinity receptor (Fig. 1).

1.1 Characteristics of the Problem

For any therapeutic approach that seeks to reduce circulating IgE levels, it is necessary to consider the sensitivity of the system to antigenic stimulation. There remain many

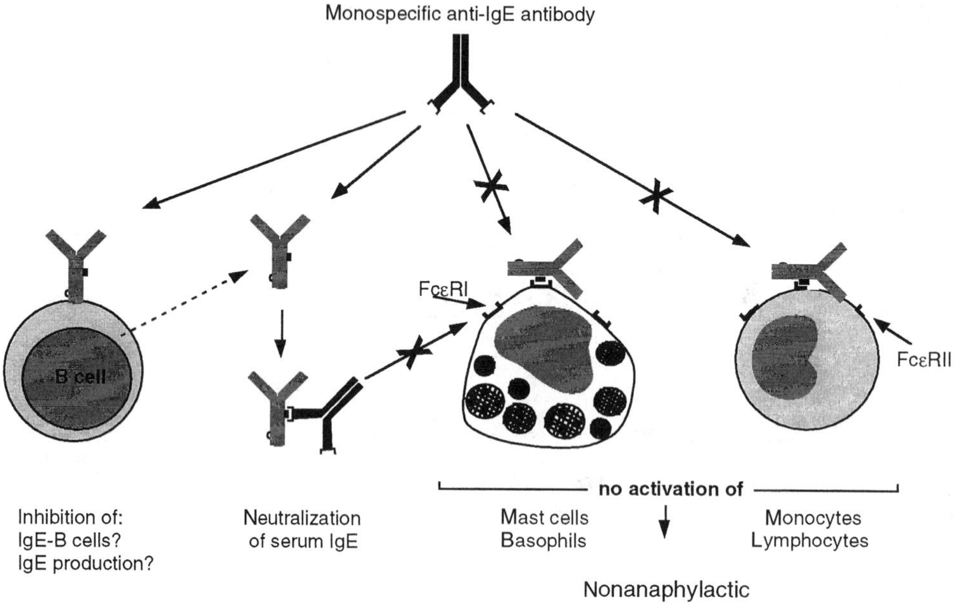

Figure 1 Characteristics of current humanized monoclonal anti-IgE antibodies.

unknown influences on the patient's response to antigenic exposure, but there is enough quantitative information concerning one aspect of the IgE-mediated reaction to make some predictions about therapeutic requirements.

The quantitative and qualitative biology of IgE-driven responses for cells other than mast cells or basophils is poorly characterized, but there are many studies of basophils (and sometimes mast cells) that provide useful predictions concerning therapeutic efficacy. If suppression of the mast cell and basophil response—by decreasing free circulating IgE—could be considered the primary target, then several questions arise.

1. How sensitive is the basophil or mast cell? In other words, how many FcεRI receptors need to be activated to drive mediator release?
2. How many receptors are typically expressed on these cells?
3. How much mediator release is needed to result in clinical symptoms that are annoying, disabling, or dangerous to the patient?

1.2 Mast Cell and Basophil Sensitivity

The answers to the first two questions are reasonably well known, whereas the answer to the third is only partially known. Measurements of basophil or mast cell sensitivity are rarely made, and it represents a relatively new parameter of their function to be studied (5,6). Previous studies have expressed this parameter as the number of antigen-specific IgE molecules (per basophil) required to induce 50% of the cells' maximum response. The maximum response itself is a parameter independent of cellular sensitivity (6), so the sensitivity parameter is expressed as a fraction of the maximum response, rather than a fraction of complete histamine release. In general, basophils require approximately 2,000 antigen-specific IgE molecules per cell to obtain 50% of the maximal response, although within the general population, this number varies from 500 to 30,000 (6). In atopic patients, basophils express approximately 250,000 high-affinity receptors for which the majority, more than 95%, are occupied with IgE antibody (6,7). As will be seen, a critical factor in the next calculation is the ratio of antigen-specific IgE to total IgE because the cell surface display of bound IgE is a reflection of the ratio as it exists for the circulating free IgE. For example, for a typical ragweed allergic donor, up to 50% of the circulating IgE is specific for various antigens associated with ragweed pollen. This means that up to 50% of the cell-bound IgE is also specific for ragweed antigens. To further the example, a patient with 250,000 FcεRI, per cell will, therefore, have up to 125,000 ragweed-specific IgE molecules on the basophil plasma membrane. If the half-maximal response of the cell occurs at 2,000 molecules, the full response will occur with only 10,000 molecules. Thus, these basophils have cell surface densities tenfold greater than is necessary to trigger maximum release.

Question 3 must now be answered; how much mediator release leads to full expression of a patient's disease? This is not well known. However, using guinea pig airway to provide some insight into this question, stimulation that leads to only 2% histamine release is sufficient to induce maximal contraction of the airway smooth muscle (8). The important caveat to this statement is that percentage of histamine release is based on the whole-airway tissue histamine content, which may not accurately reflect the proportion of cells that are actually exposed to antigenic stimulation. Nevertheless, this is the best information available and, taken at face value it suggests that very little histamine release is necessary to obtain significant changes in tissue function. Therefore, to reduce histamine release to values less than 2% requires a significant reduction in cell surface IgE antibody. In the foregoing example, less than 2% histamine release occurs only when antigen-specific IgE densities are less than 200–500 molecules per cell.

1.3 Changes Required in IgE Titer

Continuing with the foregoing example, cell surface IgE levels must be reduced from 250,000/cell to 500/cell to significantly suppress end-organ responses. Without factoring in the affinity of IgE for its receptor, a 500-fold reduction in IgE is required. However, IgE binds with very high affinity to its receptor, so the equilibrium binding curve must be followed. The data in the literature on this association–dissociation constant is probably not an accurate reflection of the affinity. But, even with this data, 50% occupancy occurs at 10 ng/mL of free-circulating IgE concentrations (9–11). Thus, the actual reduction in free IgE in an atopic patient would need to be 2,000- to 10,000-fold, provided that there were no changes in receptor expression. Fortunately, receptor expression follows IgE concentration.

1.4 Receptor Down-Regulation

It was noted in 1979 that there was a good correlation between serum IgE concentration and the number of receptors per basophil (12). This log–linear relation has now been verified in more recent studies both in basophils and in monocytes, which express far lower densities of the receptor (13). Recent studies in both human and mouse have more directly demonstrated that expression of FcεRI is tied to concentration of IgE and that IgE induces these changes by interaction with FcεRI itself (7,14–19). Thus, when IgE concentration decreases, so too does expression of FcεRI. The relation changes the calculation made in the foregoing. Instead of 2,000-fold changes in IgE, only 100-fold changes are predicted to be necessary.

2 THE ANTI-IgE APPROACH

2.1 Description of the Reagents

Two anti-IgE antibodies that fit the foregoing description have been used in clinical trials. One of the antibodies, E25, is currently undergoing the final stages of phase III trials. The two humanized antibodies that have been used in clinical trials were engineered to minimize the presence of immunogenic mouse sequences. One of the antibodies, E25, was engineered to exclude the complement-binding site, whereas CGP 51901 contains this site, but has not been observed to activate complement. In early studies, the antibodies were administered by intravenous injection but, based on some data from these early studies, subcutaneous injection was equally effective (20), and recent unpublished phase III trials have used this mode of administration. Once injected, the antibodies form immune complexes with circulating IgE appear to be limited in size (21,22). Depending on the relative concentrations of the two components, immune complexes range from cyclic trimers to hexamers of IgE and anti-IgE. Probably as a result of the small size of the complexes, they are not associated with cells expressing Fcγ receptors; therefore, they do not interact significantly with the reticuloendothelial system. The complexes, anti-IgE antibody, or both, remain associated with the blood compartment, with no preferential association with tissues, including kidney (for a study period of 1–96 hr in cynomolgus monkeys) (21–23). Elimination is primarily through urinary excretion.

2.2 Concerns Related to Depleting IgE

For any therapeutic approach that seeks to decrease free IgE antibody levels in serum and tissue, there will be concerns that relate to the speculated protective effects of IgE antibody. Because serum IgE levels are markedly elevated in patients with parasitic infections, it has long been hypothesized that IgE antibody provides protection in these diseases. Depending on the model under study, in vitro or animal studies provide support or refute a role for IgE in parasite rejection, and a variety of correlative or epidemiological studies in humans present a similar confusing picture (24–26). However, parasite-specific IgE often accounts for only a small fraction of the total IgE, leading to the alternative hypothesis that the large rise in IgE is indirectly driven by the parasite so that the antiparasitic functions of IgE are effectively diluted as the ratio of specific to nonspecific IgE falls. Whatever the basis of the association, studies of a mouse model of *Schistosoma mansoni* infections, using a polyclonal antimouse IgE, demonstrated that reduction of IgE to nondetectable levels resulted in decreased worm burden and egg production in the infected animals (27). It is not immediately clear how to reconcile these results with studies in IgE knockout mice that indicate that the absence of IgE leads to increased worm burdens (28). Clearly, the precise role of IgE in human parasitic diseases is not understood, and it will only be through long-term monitoring of patients who receive any type of IgE-reducing therapy, that definitive answers will be obtained.

The IgE antibody has also been considered to have a protective role in the development of respiratory tract infections (29). It has been nearly 25 years since this view was expressed, but there has been no further evidence to support such a viewpoint. In an anecdotal report, Levy and co-workers (30) described a healthy patient with an isolated deficiency of IgE, with no abnormalities of other immunoglobulins. She had no identified increase in the incidence of infections. In the clinical trials of anti-IgE antibody thus far reported, no increased incidence of infections has been observed.

2.3 Concerns Related to Antibody Therapies

With long-term administration of humanized antibodies comes concern that eventually there will be an immune response to the humanized antibody. Thus far, rhuMAb-E25 has not induced a detectable antibody response in humans. The E25 antibody has been engineered to eliminate the complement-binding site, and there has been no incidence or evidence of complement activation. There has also been no evidence of immune complex-mediated tissue damage (e.g., nephrotoxicity) and, in the long-term phase I study, there was no evidence of increased sinopulmonary or other infections. However, treatment of atopy may require a prolonged course of therapy, so that these concerns may not become manifest for some time. Only empirical observations for long-term administration will clarify these issues.

3 RESULTS FROM CLINICAL STUDIES

With one exception, published clinical trials of E25 have focused on its efficacy in assisting in the treatment of asthma. The decision to target asthma is multifaceted, but includes the belief that this disease is often more life-threatening, disabling, and dependent on oral and inhaled steroids, the side effects of which can be damaging. On the other hand, asthma is a complex disease with a dependence on IgE-mediated reactions that is not always evident. Consequently, the proof-of-concept aspect to studies with anti-IgE antibody (i.e., that eliminating IgE will eliminate immediate hypersensitivity diseases) is less directly addressed when the drug is used to treat asthma. Nevertheless, all asthma trials have produced positive results, which is an indication that even this disease has a strong component related to atopy, at least as a trigger. The only trial for seasonal rhinitis was made early in the clinical testing phase of E25, when administration of the drug was not yet optimized. However, even this study yielded some useful insights.

3.1 Rhinitis Study

For the trial of E25 in patients with seasonal allergic rhinitis (20), E25 was administered on the basis of body weight, and a population of 240 individuals was divided into four groups in a placebo-controlled, randomized, parallel group design. Each of the groups received treatments beginning 1 month before the ragweed season and every 2 weeks thereafter, for a total of eight doses. Dosing including placebo, subcutaneous antibody, at 0.15 mg/kg, the same dose intravenously, and a higher dose of 0.5 mg/kg intravenously. As will be seen in the following, these doses are not very high, and in patients receiving 0.15 mg/kg, free IgE levels were not suppressed more than 60%. Even at 0.5 mg/kg, suppression of free circulating IgE levels averaged only 70% (in only a few patients did such levels become undetectable; i.e., $\leq$24 ng/mL). There were no statistically significant effects on symptoms of allergic rhinitis. This study suggested that subcutaneous and intravenous administrations should be equivalent in efficacy. In addition, it was possible to tease out of the data indications for what doses of antibody might be effective and from these observations the approach to dosing was changed to account for the amount of circulating IgE before treatment. These data provided valuable information for the phase I safety assessment of high doses of E25 given for a 1-year period.

3.2 Asthma Studies

Three E25 trials using persons with asthma have been published and all three suggest that E25 has statistically significant effects on the course of the disease. The first two trials also used a dosing scheme that was dependent only on body weight. However, in both cases, the dose of anti-IgE antibody was higher than that used in the rhinitis trial (either 0.5 or 1 mg/kg). Both studies used a similar design and focused on patients with mild to moderate asthma. Parallel group, randomized, placebo-controlled studies of mild atopic asthmatics was performed by Boulet and his colleagues (31) and Fahy et al. (32).

In the study by Boulet et al. (31), the patients were receiving only β_2-adrenergic agonists on an as-needed basis. Six doses of anti-IgE antibody (rhuMAb-E25) were administered intravenously, 2 weeks apart, with an initial dose of 2 mg/kg and subsequent doses of 1 mg/kg. Serum IgE levels in the actively treated group were reduced to approximately 10% of their starting levels (and to those of the placebo group). Two clinical endpoints were examined: 1) the PC_{15} to allergen bronchial challenges, four times before treatment, two during, and two after the end of treatment; and 2) methacholine bronchoprovocation challenges before, during, and after treatment. Skin test results to relevant allergens were also examined. Most notable in these studies was that by day 27 of the treatment, there was a reduction in the airway responsiveness to allergen challenge, measured as a fourfold increase in the PC_{15}. This change persisted throughout treatment. Modest, but statistically significant changes in the methacholine reactivity were reported. Notably, there were no changes in skin test reactivity to the relevant allergens. The implications of this observation will be further explored later.

In the study performed by Fahy and colleagues, patients with mild asthma were treated with weekly intravenous 0.5 mg/kg doses of E25 for 9 weeks. Pretrial serum IgE levels were 500 IU/mL or less (1100 ng/mL). Airway responsiveness was assessed by bronchial allergen challenges and methacholine reactivity (in this case, the effect of prior allergen on methacholine reactivity was assessed by also performing methacholine bronchoprovocation 24 hr after allergen challenge). Both the early and late decrements in FEV_1 to inhaled allergen were attenuated by anti-IgE (Fig. 2). Skin tests, sputum induction and serum IgE levels were monitored. Free serum IgE levels were undetectable by the end of the study in six of the nine patients who received E25. Measurement of free serum IgE in serum where there is both free E25 and immune complexes of IgE and E25 is difficult. Typically, IgE assays are sensitive to 0.1–0.25 ng/mL of IgE. In early studies of E25, the assessment of free IgE was restricted to levels above 25 ng/mL of IgE. More recently (e.g., in the phase I trial, discussed in the following, and the most recent asthma trial), minimum detectable levels were 3–5 ng/mL.

The most recently published trial of E25 focused on moderate to severe asthmatics (33). The dosing of anti-IgE antibody was modified to reflect knowledge obtained from the phase I, open-label, 1-year toxicology trial to be presented later. Anti-IgE was administered on the basis of both body weight and the concentration of circulating IgE before treatment. Because the antibody reduces free circulating IgE by stoichiometrically binding to it, it was decided to adjust dosing to account for the wide variation in baseline values of plasma IgE. This study had three phases; a 4-week run-in phase; an 8-week treatment phase; and an 8-week treatment phase during which oral or inhaled steroid use was tapered.

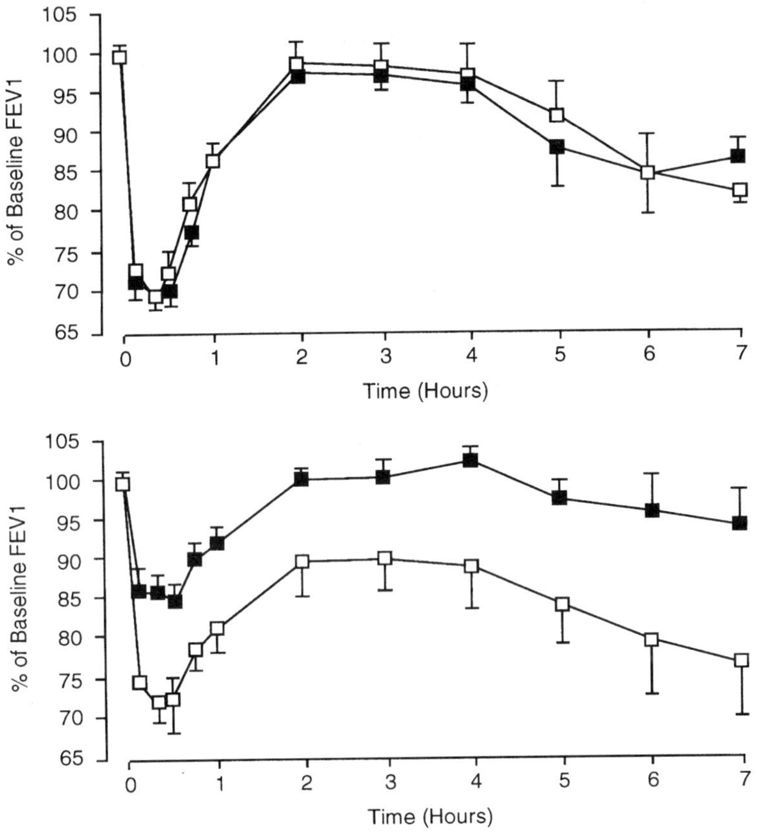

Figure 2 In asthmatics, treatment with rhuMAb-E25 anti-IgE antibody reduced both the early and late response to inhaled allergen challenge. The pulmonary function parameter, FEV_1, as a percentage of the baseline FEV_1 before challenge, is shown on the ordinate. The data shown in the top panel represents results (mean ± SD) from nine patients treated with placebo: open squares are the results before treatment; closed squares are the results after treatment. The bottom panel shows results for nine patients treated with E25 (before and after). (From Ref. 32.)

The primary outcome measure was a quality of life index, but a variety of other indices of efficacy were examined. The study population of 317 were divided into those receiving placebo, and two groups receiving either 5.8 or 2.5 μg/kg (body weight) per nanogram per milliliter of plasma IgE. In those treated with E25, free circulating IgE levels decreased 97 and 95% with high- or low-dose anti-IgE, respectively (a change from 1000 ng/mL to 10–18 ng/mL). Statistically significant changes in several indices occurred in both low- and high-dose treatment groups, although changes were generally more marked in the high-dose group. For the high-dose group, symptom scores, inhaled β-agonist use, and quality of life indices were different from placebo treatment. Most notably these indices changed in the first 8 weeks of treatment, and the change was maintained during the final 8 weeks when steroid use was tapered. For this parameter, there was greater withdrawal from both inhaled and oral steroids in those patients receiving E25. Discontinuation of steroids occurred in 33–43% of the treated patients versus 17% of placebo-treated patients. Reductions of steroid use greater than 50% occurred in 57–78% of E25-treated patients versus 33% of those treated with placebo. Thus, patients treated with E25 experienced an improvement in symptoms while simultaneously decreasing their steroid use. Interestingly, compared with placebo there were no statistically significant changes in FEV_1, but peak flow measurements did increase significantly in patients being treated with high-dose E25 ($\Delta = 30.7$ L/min from a baseline of 378 L/min).

3.3 Adverse Events

One of the major concerns for the anti-IgE antibody approach is the potential for inducing anaphylactic reactions. In the variety of clinical trials of either CGP51901 or E25, the most common side effect has been the development of a small number of urticarial reactions, all of which occurred with the initial administration and were easily managed with appropriate intervention. For example, in the phase I toxicology trial, discussed later, 4 out of 47 patients reported such reactions. These patients were negative to skin testing with E25 and were given an additional dose of intravenous E25. One patient experienced a reaction and withdrew from the study. Similar reactions are recognized with other initial infusions of a variety of monoclonal antibodies, and in this context, no evidence of mast cell–basophil mediator release or complement activation was found during the E25 or CGP51901 reactions. If the dose of antibody is high, spreading the initial infusion out over several days, reduces the incidence of urticaria. In the asthma study by Milgrom et al. (33), there was no statistically different incidence of these mild urticarial reactions (5.3%) and equivalent numbers of patients from placebo and E25-treated groups withdrew from the study for various reasons. The overall rate of urticarial reactions for E25 antibody is now reported to be approximately 2%.

4 BIOLOGICAL CHANGES DURING THERAPY

An open-label, phase I safety trial of rhuMAb-E25 examined the safety of high doses of the antibody, given every 2 weeks for nearly 1 year to 47 subjects with perennial allergic rhinitis and positive skin-prick tests to dust mites. The dosing took into account the baseline serum IgE levels, and the subjects were stratified according to the baseline IgE; high (251–550 IU/mL) and low (85–250 IU/mL). The dose of E25 was either 0.15 mg/kg/IU/mL or 0.03 mg/kg/IU/mL given intravenously.

Free and total IgE levels were monitored and skin test titrations made before treatment and after 182 days. Some subjects were also examined by nasal provocation. For 15 patients, an extensive evaluation of several characteristics of peripheral blood basophils was made before treatment, 90 days into treatment, at the point just before treatment termination and at the end of a monitoring period that extended up to 1 year posttermination (7,16). The point at which the last assessment was made was determined by the return of free serum IgE levels above 50% of the pretreatment levels or 1 year, which ever occurred sooner.

For the basophil parameters, the response of the cells to stimulation with goat polyclonal anti-IgE antibody, *Dermatophagoides farinae* (DF) antigen or the bacterial peptide, fmet-leu-phe (FMLP) was examined. FMLP was used as an internal control: this stimulus activates basophils through a mechanism not dependent on FcεRI and yet remains a physiological means of assessing general basophil secretory functions. In addition, the cell surface density of FcεRI, both occupied and unoccupied, was examined by two techniques, so-called acetate stripping (where IgE is stripped from washed enriched basophils of known number and measured by radioimmunoadsorbant test to calculate absolute cell surface IgE density) or by flow cytometry (which gives a relative assessment of cell surface IgE densities with a sensitivity that is somewhat poorer than the acetate strip method when the basophil purity is low). The relation of the changes in surface FcεRI/IgE and response to antigenic challenge was evaluated in the context of what was happening in vivo. Because the phase I trial included no placebo controls, two mild atopic donors were followed during the same time frame, but they did not receive any treatment. Although this number of controls was small, extensive previous experience examining several basophil parameters longitudinally suggested that no gross changes in receptor expression would occur and changes in histamine secretion vary only modestly (6,34,35).

For the entire group, free circulating IgE levels dropped approximately 100-fold within 24 hr of the first dose of E25 and remained at this low level throughout the first 180 days of treatment (from a baseline of ≈400 ng/mL to an average of 4 ng/mL throughout the first 180 days). For a group of three individuals, the kinetics of FcεRI expression on basophils was monitored every day for the first week of treatment and decreased with an initial half-life of approximately 3 days. Within 5 weeks of treatment, the expression of FcεRI on the basophils of approximately 75% of subjects had decreased to below detection by flow cytometry. By 10 weeks, FcεRI expression on basophils of all but one subject was undetectable by flow cytometry. The acetate-stripping method is more sensitive, and a 12-week–time point measurement showed that average cell surface expression had decreased from a pretreatment level of 220,000/cell to 8,000/cell. The decrease in cell surface IgE was greater, from a similar starting point of ≈220,000 to less than 2,200 (most often below the detection of this assay). This difference between FcεRI and IgE is because not only had the expression of FcεRI decreased, but also the equilibrium at this concentration of free IgE (≈5 ng/mL) meant that less than 25% of the available receptors were occupied.

After 180 days of treatment, the dosing regimen was altered: 3- to 20-fold less E25 was administered every 2 weeks. The next series of measurements for the various basophil parameters occurred just before E25 termination at 1 year. Because the E25 doses were lower, there was a modest rise in free IgE that amounted to a threefold increase at the 1-year time point. Along with this rise in free IgE, the expression of FcεRI rose from the mean of 8,000/basophil at 12 weeks to 35,000 at 52 weeks (Fig. 3). Following the termination of E25 treatment, free IgE levels and the expression of FcεRI on basophils rose somewhat linearly with a doubling every 3 weeks. The final termination date for the study depended on reaching 50% of pretreatment levels of free IgE. This occurred for most subjects within 6 months, but there were a few who were terminated because they had reached the 1-year posttermination point without yet reaching 50% of pretreatment IgE levels. At the end of the study, however, for all subjects, the expression of basophil FcεRI was within statistical equivalence of pretreatment levels.

The variability in the effects of E25 treatment on basophil function proved useful in developing a predictive model (discussed in the following). The median response of the subjects' basophils to stimulation with DF antigen was 10% of the pretreatment response. The response to stimulation with polyclonal anti-IgE antibody (which should cross-link or aggregate all available cell surface IgE) was decreased to 50% of pretreatment levels. These results were consistent with our previous understanding about the relation between cell surface IgE density and histamine release. With IgE densities hovering just below 1500/basophil, the antigen-specific IgE density was probably well below 300 molecules per basophil. The secretion response should be quite low at this point if the cells were challenged with antigen. On the other hand, 1500 molecules of IgE per basophil,

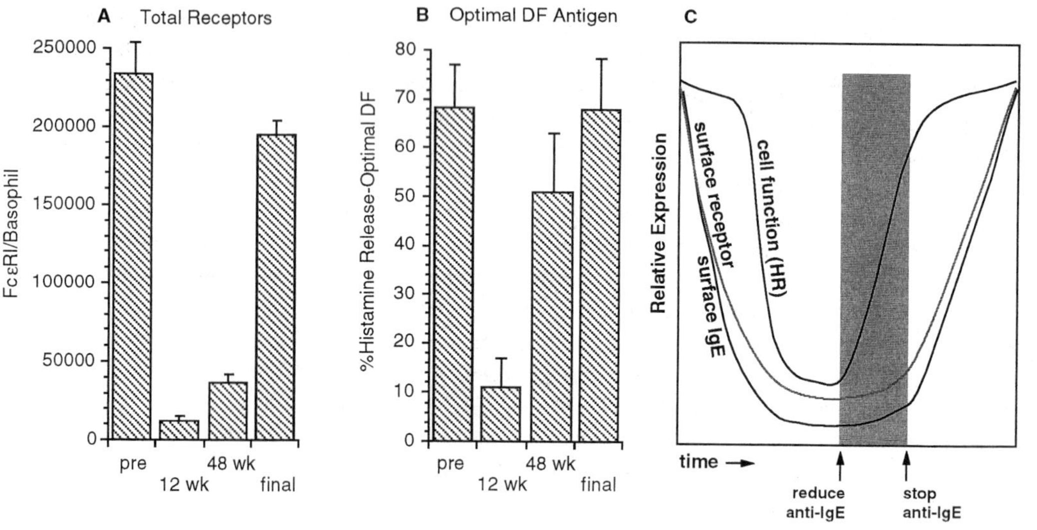

Figure 3 Synopsis of the changes in expression of FcεRI and the in vitro function of peripheral blood basophils from a subpopulation of 15 patients in the year-long phase I trial of rhuMAb-E25: (A) the levels of FcεRI expression, before treatment, 12 weeks into treatment, 48 weeks into treatment (just before cessation of treatment), and a final measurement occurring 4–12 months after treatment was stopped; (B) the in vitro histamine release response for the same four periods of measurement; (C) the characteristics of the changes that we expect represent what is happening during treatment. The *x*-axis is not strictly linear in time. The gray region represents the time during which the amount of E25 administered was decreased 3- to 20-fold, leading to a small increase in free serum IgE, a small increase in the expression of basophil FcεRI and, therefore, cell surface IgE. Consequently, the function of the cell changes more dramatically.

stimulated with anti-IgE antibody, would be approximately the EC_{50} for secretion. The response to FMLP did not change over the course of the study and neither did the responses or FcεRI expression levels of the two nontreated subjects included in the study. These results were notable for supporting prior estimates concerning the relation between cell surface expression of FcεRI (and, therefore, IgE) and the functional responses of the cell.

An important observation came from the comparison between data obtained at 90 days versus that obtained after 52 weeks. During the period between 90 and 360 days (probably owing to the shift in dosing beginning at 180 days), both free circulating IgE and FcεRI expression increased only modestly. In contrast, the functional response of the cells became nearly the same as that before treatment. These results were also consistent with our understanding of the quantitative relations. When free IgE was suppressed $\approx$100-fold, receptor expression was decreased on average 26-fold and cell surface IgE fell below the EC_{50} for secretion. But as evidenced by the results for anti-IgE antibody, the functional response was hovering close to the EC_{50} point. One would have predicted that from this starting point, small rises in FcεRI/IgE would have a dramatic effect on secretion, and the results suggest that they did. At the conclusion of the posttermination period (nearly 1 year after the last dose of E25 for some subjects), both anti-IgE and DF antigen-driven secretion had returned to pretreatment levels (see Fig. 3).

The antigen-driven response of basophils was markedly decreased after 90 days of treatment. Likewise, skin tests also demonstrated a marked suppression of mast cell secretion (36). On average, the titration of antigen required for wheal-and-flare indicated a need for 32-fold more antigen. Dosing of antigen in the test tube versus dosing for skin tests can not be easily compared. In the test tube, secretion is examined at concentrations of antigen that are both optimal and suboptimal. In general, both experimental and theoretical studies demonstrate that the concentration of antigen that is optimal for secretion is not a function of cell surface IgE density. Therefore, one cannot overcome apparent suppression of the secretory response by using more antigen if the concentration is already at the predetermined optimum (an increase in antigen concentration simply moves into the supraoptimal region of its biphasic dose–response curve). The concentration of antigen in the skin is unknown and could very well be suboptimal for many cells. Furthermore, additional antigen may simply recruit a larger region of mast cells, giving the appearance of overcoming some suppression. It is unclear what the response of individual mast cells are under these circumstances.

The in vivo results suggested that suppression of the density of cell surface antigen-specific IgE was just sufficient to blunt the antigen-driven response for most donors. Furthermore, the marked increase in antigen-induced histamine release with only a modest increase in receptor expression (and, therefore, antigen-specific IgE) reinforced the perception that the dosing was marginally adequate. The notion that suppression of the response was teetering on a point between nearly normal function and marked inhibition suggests a new prediction concerning the efficacy of the therapy. As long as the dosing of anti-IgE is just sufficient to suppress function, efficacy will depend on the ratio of antigen-specific to total IgE. This comes about because the lower the ratio, the less likely the cell will have enough cell surface IgE to mount a normal response to antigen stimulation. Such a correlation was found in the phase I trial. There was a good correlation between the ratio of DF-specific to total IgE before treatment and the ratio of histamine release induced by DF antigen for the 12-week treatment response/pretreatment response. Although the number of data points is few for a correlation of this kind, the trend indicates that if the starting specific/total IgE ratio is too high, suppression of the functional response is minimal. If suppression of free circulating IgE were far more complete, then the specific/total ratio would not be contributory because cells would not possess enough IgE (total or specific) to mount a secretory response.

Consequently, these results suggest a somewhat paradoxical prediction that those patients with a multiplicity of antigen sensitivities might respond better to this therapy than those with single specificities (where the specific/total ratio may be high). However, there are important caveats to this prediction, and they have as a basis the same concerns noted previously about administering E25 without consideration for the circulating level of IgE. If one gives enough antibody to suppress IgE for any individual, these issues are moot, but practical considerations will not allow this possibility.

The important issue is that free circulating IgE be suppressed to levels probably below 5–10 ng/mL. If a patient begins with 100 ng/mL of IgE for which 50% is specific for some one antigen, E25 given at doses used for more typically atopic individuals would still work, despite the high specific/total ratio, because the starting IgE level is low. Conversely, even a very low specific/total ratio may not allow a standard dosing of E25 to work if IgE levels begin at more than 10,000 ng/mL. For a typical atopic patient, with IgE levels in the 500–1000 ng/mL range, the kinds of dosing schedules being suggested should have some effect, although success will probably depend on some of the less well-studied aspects of basophil–mast cell secretion, biology, or modulation. For example, the relative sensitivity of a subject's basophils to IgE-mediated stimulation varies significantly. One patient's basophils may require only 300 molecules of cell surface IgE to mount a normal response, whereas another's basophils may require 30,000 (6). The cause of the sensitivity difference is currently unknown, but could affect the success of any therapy that seeks to suppress circulating free IgE.

5 SUMMARY

From the published studies of E25, it is now clear that this approach to treating atopic disease can be successful. But there remain many issues, both practical and biological. For the study of atopic disease, a potentially excellent new tool has been provided that could allow IgE to be effectively eliminated, given the correct-dosing regimen, and provide the investigator with a means to ask questions about the role of IgE in the expression of a particular disease. No place is this more evident than in the study of asthma for which a long-standing debate revolves around the precise contribution of atopy to the genesis and maintenance of this disease. Furthermore, use of the drug may finally resolve questions about the role of IgE in parasitic rejection. From the perspective of the patient, at a minimum, the drug provides a proof-of-concept for all potential therapies seeking to reduce circulating IgE levels. With proper consideration of dosing, the drug appears as if it could provide remarkable improvement in the course of atopic disease. Some concerns still revolve around the improvement roles IgE may play in parasitic diseases, the cost of therapy, and that very long-term treatment effects have yet to be studied.

REFERENCES

1. Chang TW, Davis FM, Sun N–C, Sun CRY, MacGlashan DW Jr, Hamilton RG. Monoclonal antibodies specific for human IgE-producing B cells: a potential therapeutic for IgE-mediated allergic diseases. Biotechnology 1990; 8:122–126.
2. Jardieu P. Anti-IgE therapy. Curr Opin Immunol 1995; 7:779–782.
3. Presta LG, Lahr SJ, Shields RL, et al. Humanization of an antibody directed against IgE. J Immunol 1993; 151:2623–2632.
4. Saban R, Haak–Frendscho M, Zine M, Presta LG, Bjorling DE, Jardieu P. Human anti-IgE monoclonal antibody blocks passive sensitization of human and rhesus monkey bladder. J Urol 1997; 157:689–693.
5. MacGlashan DW Jr, Peters SP, Warner J, Lichtenstein LM. Characteristics of human basophil sulfidopeptide leukotriene release: releasability defined as the ability of the basophil to respond to dimeric cross-links. J Immunol 1986; 136:2231–2239.
6. MacGlashan DW Jr. Releasability of human basophils: cellular sensitivity and maximal histamine release are independent variables. J Allergy Clin Immunol 1993; 91:605–615.
7. MacGlashan DW Jr, Bochner BS, Adelman DC, et al. Down-regulation of FcεRI expression on human basophils during in vivo treatment of atopic patients with anti-IgE antibody. J Immunol 1997; 158:1438–1445.
8. Undem BJ, Pickett WC, Adams GK. Antigen-induced sulfidopeptide leukotriene release from the guinea pig superfused trachea. Eur J Pharmacol 1987; 142:31–37.
9. Ishizaka T, Helm B, Hakimi J, Niebyl J, Ishizaka K, Gould H. Biological properties of a recombinant human immunoglobulin epsilon-chain fragment. Proc Natl Acad Sci USA 1986; 83:8323–8327.
10. Miller L, Blank U, Metzger H, Kinet JP. Expression of high-affinity binding of human immunoglobulin E by transfected cells. Science 1989; 244:334–337.

11. Hakimi J, Seals C, Kondas JA, Pettine L, Danho W, Kochan J. The alpha subunit of the human IgE receptor (FcεRI) is sufficient for high affinity IgE binding. J Biol Chem 1990; 265:22079–22081.
12. Malveaux FJ, Conroy MC, Adkinson NFJ, Lichtenstein LM. IgE receptors on human basophils. Relationship to serum IgE concentration. J Clin Invest 1978; 62:176–181.
13. Sihra BS, Kon OM, Grant JA, Kay AB. Expression of high-affinity IgE receptors (Fc epsilon RI) on peripheral blood basophils, monocytes, and eosinophils in atopic and nonatopic subjects: relationship to total serum IgE concentrations. J Allergy Clin Immunol 1997; 99:699–706.
14. Hsu C, MacGlashan JDW Jr. IgE antibody up-regulates high affinity IgE binding on murine bone marrow derived mast cells. Immunol Lett 1996; 52:129–134.
15. MacGlashan DW Jr, White JM, Schroeder JT, Bochner BS, Lichtenstein LM. Regulation of FcεRI expression on human basophils by IgE antibody. J Allergy Clin Immunol 1997; 99:S103.
16. Saini SS, MacGlashan DW Jr, Sterbinsky SA, et al. Down-regulation of human basophil IgE and FcεRIa surface densities and mediator release by anti-IgE infusions is reversible in vitro and in vivo. J Immunol 1999; 162:5623–5630.
17. Yamaguchi M, Sayama K, Yano K, et al. IgE enhances Fc epsilon receptor I expression and IgE-dependent release of histamine and lipid mediators from human umbilical cord blood-derived mast cells: synergistic effect of IL-4 and IgE on human mast cell Fc epsilon receptor I expression and mediator release. J Immunol 1999; 162:5455–5465.
18. Lantz CS, Yamaguchi M, Oettgen HC, et al. IgE regulates mouse basophil FcεRI expression in vivo. J Immunol 1997; 158:2517–2521.
19. Yamaguchi M, Lantz CS, Oettgen HC, et al. IgE enhances mouse mast cell FcεRI expression in vitro and in vivo: evidence for a novel amplification mechanism in IgE-dependent reactions. J Exp Med 1997; 185:663–672.
20. Casale T, Bernstein I, Busse W, et al. Use of an anti-IgE humanized monoclonal antibody in ragweed-induced allergic rhinitis. J Allergy Clin Immunol 1997; 100:110–121.
21. Fox JA, Hotaling TE, Struble C, Ruppel J, Bates DJ, Schoenhoff MB. Tissue distribution and complex formation with IgE of an anti-IgE antibody after intravenous administration in cynomolgus monkeys. J Pharmacol Exp Ther 1996; 279:1000–1008.
22. Liu J, Lester P, Builder S, Shire SJ. Characterization of complex formation by humanized anti-IgE monoclonal antibody and monoclonal human IgE. Biochemistry 1995; 34:10474–10482.
23. Racine–Poon A, Botta L, Chang TW, et al. Efficacy, pharmacodynamics, and pharmacokinetics of CGP 51901, an anti-immunoglobulin E chimeric monoclonal antibody, in patients with seasonal allergic rhinitis. Clin Pharmacol Ther 1997; 62:675–690.
24. Akue JP, Hommel M, Devaney E. High levels of parasite-specific IgG1 correlate with the amicrofilaremic state in *Loa loa* infection. J Infect Dis 1997; 175:158–163.
25. Ogilvie BM, Parrott DM. The immunological consequences of nematode infection. Ciba Found Symp 1977; 46:183–201.
26. Butterworth AE. Immunological aspects of human schistosomiasis. Br Med Bull 1998; 54:357–368.
27. Amiri P, Haak–Frendscho M, Robbins K, McKerrow JH, Stewart T, Jardieu P. Anti-immunoglobulin E treatment decreases worm burden and egg production in *Schistosoma mansoni*-infected normal and interferon gamma knockout mice. J Exp Med 1994; 180:43–51.
28. King CL, Xianli J, Malhotra I, Liu S, Mahmoud AA, Oettgen HC. Mice with a targeted deletion of the IgE gene have increased worm burdens and reduced granulomatous inflammation following primary infection with *Schistosoma mansoni*. J Immunol 1997; 158:294–300.
29. Cain WA, Amman AJ, Hong R, Ishizaka K, Good RA. IgE deficiency associated with chronic sinopulmonary infection. J Clin Invest 1969; 48:12a–13a.

30. Levy D, Chen J. Healthy IgE-deficient person. N Engl J Med 1970; 283:541–542.
31. Boulet L, Chapman K, Cote J, et al. Inhibitory effects of an anti-IgE antibody E25 on allergen-induced early asthmatic responses. Am J Respir Crit Care Med 1997; 155:1835–1840.
32. Fahy J, Fleming H, Wong H, et al. The effect of an anti-IgE monoclonal antibody on the early- and late-phase responses to allergen inhalation in asthmatic subjects. Am J Respir Crit Care Med 1997; 155:1828–1834.
33. Milgrom H, Fick RB, Su JQ, et al. Treatment of allergic asthma with monoclonal anti-IgE antibody. N Engl J Med 1999; 341:1966–1973.
34. Knol EF, Koenderman L, Mul FPJ, Verhoeven AJ, Roos D. Differential activation of human basophils by anti-IgE and formyl-methionyl-leucyl-phenylalanine. Indications for protein kinase C-dependent and -independent activation pathways. Eur J Immunol 1991; 21:881–885.
35. Nguyen KL, Gillis S, MacGlashan DW Jr. A comparative study of releasing and nonreleasing human basophils: nonreleasing basophils lack an early component of the signal transduction pathway that follows IgE cross-linking. J Allergy Clin Immunol 1990; 85:1020–1029.
36. Togias A, Corren J, Shapiro G, et al. Anti-IgE treatment reduces skin test (ST) reactivity. J Allergy Clin Immunol 1998; 101:S171.

25

Allergen Injection Immunotherapy

EVA-MARIA VARGA

Universitätsklinik für Kinder- und Jugendheilkunde, Graz, Austria

STEPHEN R. DURHAM

Imperial College School of Medicine, National Heart & Lung Institute, and Royal Brompton Hospital, London, England

1 INTRODUCTION

Allergen injection immunotherapy for the treatment of IgE-mediated diseases was started in the United Kingdom by Noon in 1911. Since then it has been widely used worldwide as an effective treatment of allergic diseases. However, it has been over only the last three decades that insight into the immunological basis of allergic disease and the mechanisms of immunotherapy has emerged. Research in this area not only provides fundamental knowledge of allergy itself, but also may lead to the development of more highly targeted forms of treatment.

Allergen injection immunotherapy (AII) involves subcutaneous administration of increasing doses of allergen extract to improve symptoms and requirements for medication after natural reexposure to this allergen. Immunotherapy reduces immediate allergen-induced symptoms and concentrations of inflammatory mediators in the target organs affected. A further characteristic is its ability to attenuate late-phase responses. This has been shown in the nose, lung, and skin. Furthermore, allergen immunotherapy may act by modifying the T-lymphocyte response to subsequent natural allergen exposure.

This chapter will focus on the use of allergen injection immunotherapy for the treatment of allergy to aeroallergens and insect stings. An overview of recent studies documenting clinical efficacy will be followed by consideration of the mechanisms of immunotherapy from changes in antibody levels to altered T-lymphocyte responses and T-cell anergy.

Allergen injection immunotherapy has been highly effective in selected patients with clear evidence of IgE-mediated diseases (1,2). However, efficacy must always be balanced against possible side effects. Atopic allergic individuals have allergen-specific IgE antibodies bound to high-affinity receptors for IgE (FcεRI) on the surface of mast cells, basophils, and other inflammatory cells. Allergen cross-links adjacent IgE molecules on the surface of these cells to cause cell activation and release of inflammatory mediators that result in signs and symptoms in the target organ. For example, within 15 min of nasal allergen exposure, symptoms of nasal discharge, congestion, and itchiness are accompanied by the release of histamine, tryptase, and membrane lipid-derived mediators, including prostaglandin (PG) D_2 and leukotriene (LT)C_4, and possibly, platelet-activating factor (PAF). Mast cells and basophils also produce cytokines including interleukin (IL)-4 and IL-5. IL-4 induces synthesis of a sterile ε-germline gene transcript by B cells, the critical first step in heavy-chain switching in favor of IgE antibody production. Interleukin 5, as well as IL-3 and granulocyte–macrophage colony-stimulating factor (GM–CSF) promote eosinophil maturation, recruitment, activation, and prolonged survival, features characteristic of the late phase of an allergic reaction. T-lymphocytes are also recruited during allergic late-phase reactions and produce a range of cytokines and chemokines that contribute to the perpetuation of the inflammatory cascade.

Allergen injection immunotherapy profoundly influences every step of this inflammatory process. In contrast, antiallergic drugs, such as antihistamines, although highly potent, intervene at only one level of the ongoing allergic reaction. Corticosteroids act at many different levels and, although highly effective, represent a symptomatic treatment that needs to be taken long-term and, in contrast to allergen immunotherapy, does not have the potential to modify allergic disease over an extended period.

2 CLINICAL EFFICACY

By using the term ''therapeutic vaccine'' a recent WHO report (3) emphasized the prophylactic role of allergen immunotherapy. Allergen immunotherapy is indicated in selected patients with IgE-mediated disease. For optimal results standardized allergen vaccines containing an adequate amount of major allergen (generally 5–20 μg in monthly maintenance injections) should be given for a sufficient duration of time (usually 3–5 years). The use of allergen immunotherapy in children, at the onset of allergic disease, may have added potential to influence the natural course of allergic disease (4).

Clinical efficacy of allergen immunotherapy has been reported in many studies of seasonal rhinitis (3). For example, in one study, grass pollen immunotherapy was used in patients with severe summer hayfever uncontrolled by antiallergic drugs (5). Results showed a highly significant 60% decrease in diary records of symptoms and a 70% decrease in rescue medication use during the pollen season (Fig. 1). Clinical improvement was accompanied by a reduction in immediate conjunctival and skin responses as well as a decrease in nasal sensitivity to allergen challenge. In addition, grass pollen immunotherapy significantly inhibited the allergen-induced late-phase (6–24 hr) skin response (Fig. 2). During 4 years of follow-up (6) clinical improvement was maintained and accompanied by a further sustained decrease in immediate conjunctival allergen sensitivity and in the size of the allergen-induced late cutaneous response. Allergen immunotherapy has also been effective in mite-sensitive patients (4,7,8), although less so than for pollinosis. This may relate to the heterogeneous nature of perennial rhinitis and asthma in which allergy to mites may be only one of the determinants.

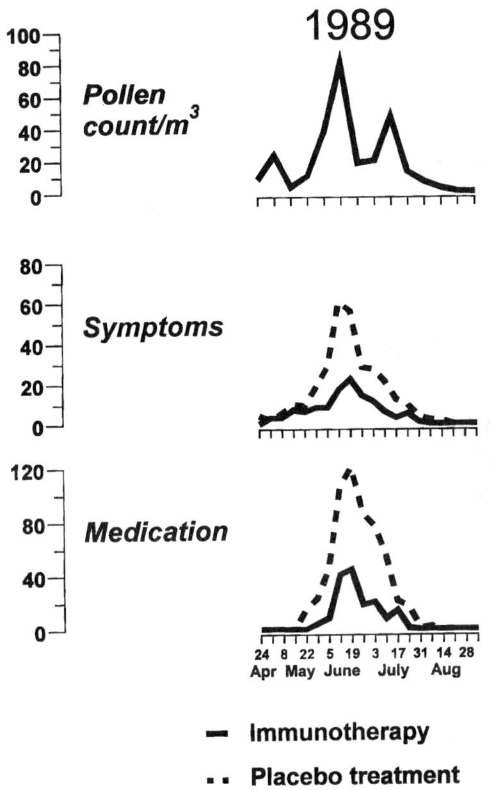

Figure 1 Median weekly pollen counts, symptom, and medication scores following 1 year of a double-blind placebo-controlled trial of grass pollen immunotherapy: Analysis of the area under the curve with the Mann-Whitney U-test revealed significant differences in symptoms ($p < 0.01$) and medication scores ($p < 0.01$) between immunotherapy-treated and placebo groups.

In patients with insect sting allergy, venom immunotherapy has been highly effective (9,10). Although complete loss of immediate skin sensitivity to venom is rare, several studies have shown that following 3–5 years of treatment, venom immunotherapy may be safely discontinued (11,12), although a follow-up study indicated a recurrence rate for systemic reactions of 5–15% after 5–10 years (11a). In one study in 30 venom-sensitive patients, immunotherapy was discontinued after at least 5 years of treatment, regardless of diagnostic test results. After 12 months without therapy, live sting challenge caused no systemic reaction in 29 patients (13). Another study reported reactions at resting over a 4-year observation period in 12.5% of 200 patients who had received 3–5 years of venom immunotherapy (14).

Depending on the up-dosing regimen being used, clinical efficacy of allergen injection immunotherapy becomes evident within months and is maintained during continuation of treatment (6). However, few studies have addressed the question of long-term effects, once immunotherapy is discontinued (15). In a trial of grass pollen-sensitive patients who had received immunotherapy for 2½ years, Mosbech et al. (16) reported persistent reductions in symptom and medication scores 6 years after discontinuation of treatment. However, allergic rhinitis may improve spontaneously with time, and this study did not include

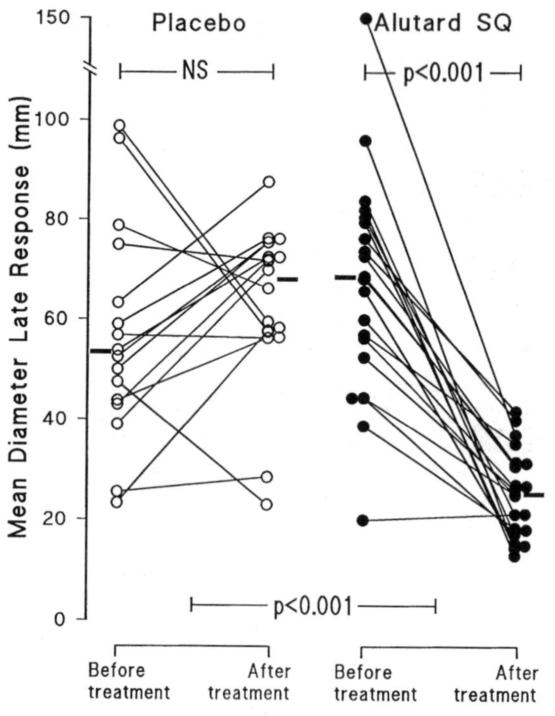

Figure 2 The diameter of the late skin response after intradermal 30 BU grass pollen extract before and after 9 months treatment in placebo- (open circles) and immunotherapy- treated (Alutard SQ ALK Denmark) (closed circles) patients. Median values are represented by the solid bars. NS, not significant. (From Ref. 34.)

a control group for the natural history of the disease. In a recent trial of the discontinuation of immunotherapy for grass pollen allergy (17) our group has reported persistently reduced scores for seasonal symptoms and the use of rescue antiallergic drugs compared with placebo 3 years after withdrawal of treatment. In parallel with prolonged clinical remission, persistent alterations of immunological reactivity were reflected in suppression of the allergen-induced late skin response and associated T-lymphocyte recruitment and cytokine production.

Despite that numerous studies have unanimously stated the clinical efficacy of allergen immunotherapy, the mechanisms by which it exerts its beneficial effects are still not fully understood.

3 MECHANISMS

3.1 Allergen-Specific Antibodies

Earlier studies focused primarily on changes in allergen-specific serum IgE and IgG antibody concentrations (18). Although pollen immunotherapy reportedly (19) blunts the seasonal increase in allergen-specific serum IgE, such IgE levels initially rise, decline gradually, and become normal during a prolonged treatment period. Furthermore, the time of clinical improvement and reduced target-organ sensitivity does not coincide with reduced IgE levels. Moreover, basophil histamine release decreases at a time when IgE levels increase (20). It can be speculated that either local changes in IgE production in the target organ or functional changes in IgE might be responsible, but this remains to be tested.

The ''blocking antibody'' theory postulates that increases in allergen-specific IgG antibodies after immunotherapy compete with IgE for allergen binding, thereby blocking activation of mast cells (21,22), basophils, and possibly other cells expressing surface IgE receptors. In support of this theory, a study of allergen injection immunotherapy in ragweed-sensitive patients, found an increased IgG/IgE-binding ratio that correlated significantly with a fall in symptom scores (23). In venom immunotherapy an early increase in IgG levels protected against insect stings in a population of patients, but had no predictive value in individual patients (24). In our own studies, patients undergoing grass pollen immunotherapy, demonstrated a 10-fold increase in allergen-specific IgG4 within months of immunotherapy, with further increases up to 100-fold. In contrast, IgG4 levels in placebo-treated patients remained almost unchanged.

Visco et al. (25) have recently shown that human IgG antibodies block IgE binding to Bet v 1 the major birch pollen allergen and inhibit Bet v 1-induced histamine release. Some recent studies have questioned the blocking antibody theory, focusing more on other properties of IgG immunoglobulins. There is evidence that IgG antibodies induced by immunotherapy can recognize different epitopes from IgE antibodies (26) and may prevent aggregation of FcεRI-bound IgE through steric hindrance, rather than direct competition for allergen-binding sites. Another possibility is that allergen–IgG complexes bound on cell surfaces may alter antigen procession and impair the ability of antigen-presenting cells (APC) to costimulate T cells through the CD28 molecule (27), resulting in a state of T-cell anergy.

3.2 Effector Cells

Many studies have shown that immunotherapy may influence inflammatory cell recruitment, activation, and mediator release during early- and late-phase allergic reactions after allergen challenge and during naturally occurring disease. In ragweed-sensitive patients (28) concentrations of histamine, *N*-p-tosyl-L-arginine methylester (TAME) esterase activity, and PGD_2 in nasal lavage fluid obtained after challenge with ragweed pollen grains were markedly decreased following immunotherapy. This was in contrast to a control group of untreated patients in whom an allergen–dose-dependent increase in the concentration of these mediators could be observed.

The transepithelial migration of tryptase-positive mast cells is a characteristic feature of current symptomatic seasonal and perennial allergic rhinitis (29,30). Nasal scrapings obtained from mite-sensitive children before and after house dust mite immunotherapy (31) demonstrated a significant reduction in the number of metachromatic cells, presumed mast cells in the nasal epithelium. Interestingly, cell numbers were reduced only in the subgroup of patients who responded to treatment. The number of mast cells in the skin was decreased after 9 months during successful grass pollen immunotherapy (32). A significant decrease in both tryptase-only and tryptase-positive, chymase-positive mast cell numbers was observed in pollen-treated compared with placebo-treated patients (Fig. 3). Furthermore, reductions in the numbers of mast cells in the skin correlated with the clinical response to treatment as reflected by diary symptom and medication scores during the pollen season.

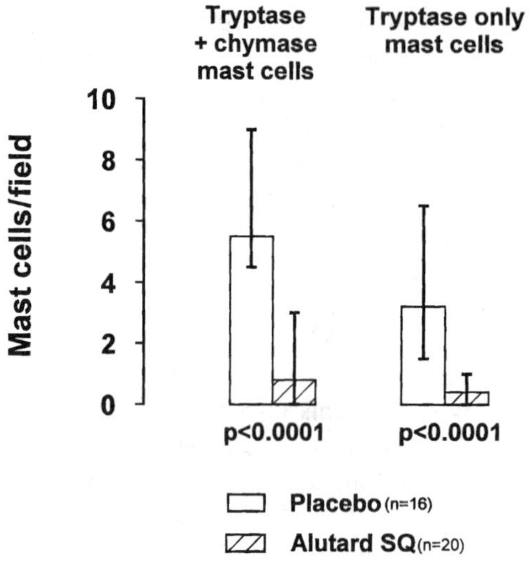

Figure 3 Cutaneous mast cell numbers before and after 9 months of subcutaneous immunotherapy (Alutard SQ) or placebo (histamine) treatment: Tryptase- plus chymase-containing mast cells (connective tissue type) and tryptase–only-containing mast cells (mucosal type) are expressed as median values ± interquartile ranges. Levels of statistical significance refer to between-group comparisons (Mann Whitney U-test).

A characteristic feature of immunotherapy is its ability to inhibit late-phase allergic reactions in the target organs affected. In grass pollen-sensitive patients, inhibition of the allergen-induced late-phase cutaneous response following 1 year of immunotherapy, was accompanied by only a modest reduction in eosinophil cell numbers (33,34) in the skin. In a study of birch pollen allergic asthmatics (35), nonspecific bronchial hyperresponsiveness, eosinophil cell counts in bronchial biopsies, and concentrations of eosinophil cationic (ECP) protein in bronchoalveolar lavage samples were assessed. All these parameters were markedly reduced during the birch pollen season only in the immunotherapy-treated, but not in the placebo-treated, patients.

In ragweed-sensitive patients, immunotherapy reduced the percentage of eosinophils in nasal washings obtained 24 hr following allergen challenge (36). This reduction correlated with the dose used for maintenance immunotherapy. In a double-blind placebo controlled study by our own group (37), local nasal provocation with grass pollen (and a control challenge) were performed after a 12-month double-blind trial of immunotherapy. Apart from inhibiting both immediate and late nasal symptoms, immunotherapy also inhibited the associated infiltration of the nasal mucosa by total (major basic protein-containing) and ‘‘activated’’ (cationic protein-containing) eosinophils (Fig. 4).

3.3 Modulation of T Lymphocytes and Cytokine Production

Whereas the early-phase allergic reaction is characterised by degranulation of mast cells and release of proinflammatory mediators, usually resolving within the first 2 hr after allergen exposure, the more prolonged late-phase reaction lasts up to 48 hr. It is accompanied by recruitment of inflammatory cells, such as eosinophils and particularly activated T-lymphocytes to the site of allergen exposure. Such late-phase reactions may represent a model for more chronic allergic inflammation in the mucosae of atopic subjects.

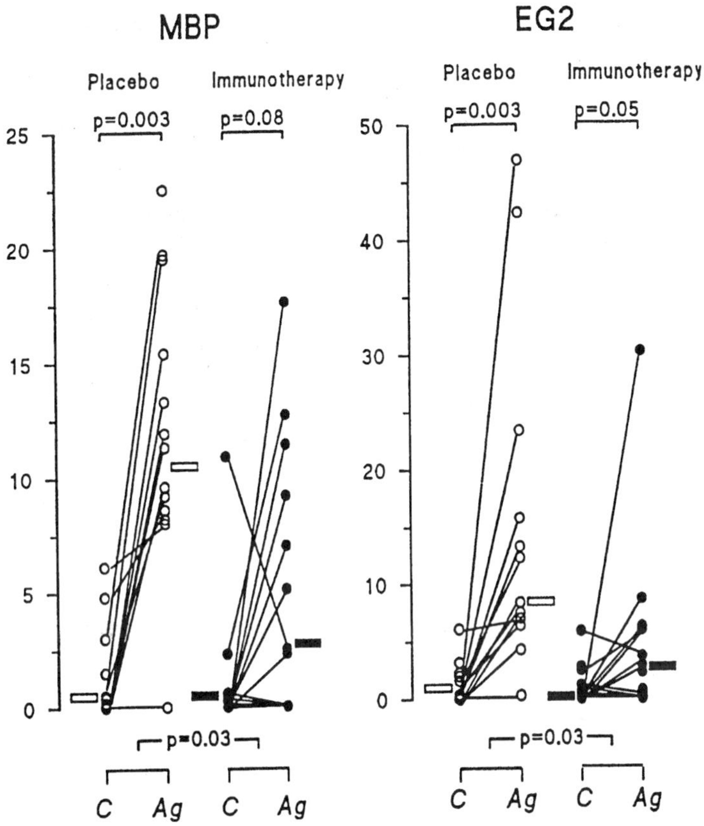

Figure 4 Cellular infiltration with total (MBP^+) and "activated" ($EG2^+$) eosinophils 24 hr after nasal provocation with allergen and control (allergen diluent) solution: Horizontal bars represent median cell counts. The differences between counts 24 hr after allergen challenge minus control counts for placebo-treated (open circles) and immunotherapy-treated (closed circles) patients are compared by using the Mann-Whitney U-test. Levels of statistical significance are shown. Within-group comparisons were performed with the Wilcoxon test. (From Ref. 37.)

Following murine studies (38), studies in humans (39,40) have confirmed that T-helper (Th) T cells can be broadly subdivided into two phenotypes based on the cytokines they produce. Th1-type cells produce predominantly interferon (IFN)-γ (an activator of macrophages), whereas Th2-type cells produce IL-4 and IL-5. Although this functional dichotomy in humans is not so clearcut, studies have suggested that allergen-specific T cells from atopic subjects are biased toward the secretion of Th2-type cytokines. This is in contrast to allergen-specific T cells from nonatopic subjects (39) or T cells that respond to bacterial antigens (40) that are biased in favor of production of Th1-type cytokines such as IFN-γ. Biopsy studies of both the upper and lower airways of allergic patients have shown increases in the number of cells expressing mRNA encoding Th2-type cytokines following allergen exposure (41,42).

It seems logical that immunotherapy may improve clinical symptoms by inducing altered T-cell responses to allergen exposure possibly by modifying or reducing the amount of cytokines they produce. For example, inhibition of IL-4 and IL-5 production would result in altered allergen-specific IgE antibody production by B cells and diminished recruitment, activation, and survival of eosinophils. Allergen-specific T cells from nonatopic subjects are characterized by Th0- or Th1-type cytokine production. Alterations of the Th2/Th1 balance in favor of type-1 cytokine responses by immunotherapy might occur either by immune deviation of Th2 responses to "protective" Th1 responses or by inducing unresponsiveness of Th0/Th2 responses (anergy). Several studies support this view. Lack et al. (43), in a study of rush immunotherapy in house dust mite allergic children, have reported increased INF-γ production by peripheral blood $CD4^+$ T cells. Reduced proliferation to allergen and parallel increases in anti-DPT IgG4 levels were also found. A close inverse relation between IFN-γ levels and cutaneous sensitivity to allergen was observed. In a study by Secrist et al. (44), allergic patients received immunotherapy with either house dust mite or grass pollen allergen over a mean period of 5 years. $CD4^+$ T-cell lines cultured from peripheral blood were stimulated with allergen and expanded in the presence of IL-2. Immunotherapy resulted in a significant reduction in IL-4 production (Fig. 5) that was accompanied by a reduction in allergen-specific IgE levels and a decrease in the allergen-induced late-phase skin response. However, the levels of IFN-γ were equivalent in treated and untreated patients, as was allergen-induced T-cell proliferation. Jutel et al. (45) measured peripheral blood mononuclear cell proliferation in bee venom-sensitive patients before and at time intervals after rush immunotherapy. Cell cultures were stimulated with the major bee venom allergen phospholipase A_2 and nonspecifically with mito-

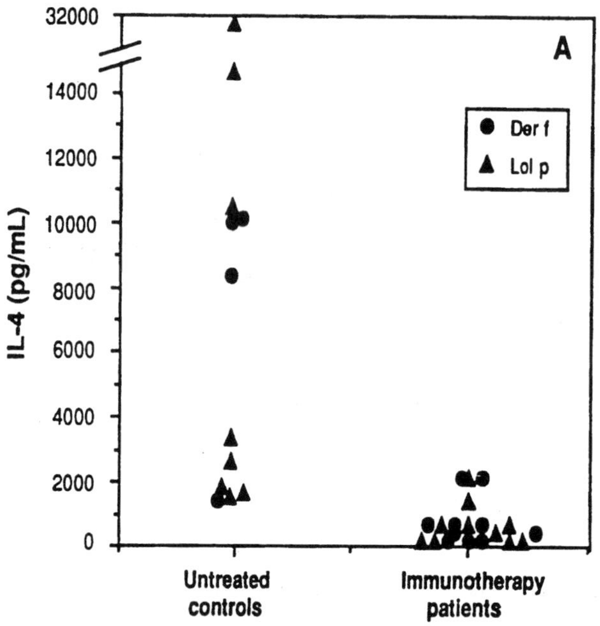

Figure 5 IL-4 production in response to allergen: CD8-depleted cells were stimulated with allergen on day 0, and restimulated on day 7 with the same allergen. On day 14, the cultures were harvested, and the cytokine profiles of cells determined. Mean IL-4 production was 7919 ± 2480 pg/mL in the untreated control groups and 477 ± 169 pg/mL in the immunotherapy treated group ($p < 0.02$; Mann-Whitney U-test). (From Ref. 44.)

gen. Whereas T-cell proliferation was modestly reduced, a decrease in IL-4 and an increase in IFN-γ was observed on day 6 of culture.

In contrast, in another study (46), IL-5 production from cultured peripheral blood mononuclear cells, did not reveal any differences between hayfever patients who had received prolonged courses of immunotherapy and untreated hayfever controls.

Local T-cell responses after allergen provocation in the nasal mucosa and in skin have also been reported following immunotherapy (34,37). In addition to attenuating allergen-induced early- and late-phase responses in the nose, 12 months of grass pollen immunotherapy reduced the number of $CD4^+$ T-helper cells in biopsies of the nasal mucosa (37). Using in situ hybridization, the numbers of cells expressing mRNA for IFN-γ at 24 hr after nasal allergen challenge increased significantly in the group of immunotherapy-treated patients (Fig. 6) whereas in placebo-treated patients there was no change. This increased IFN-γ expression in actively treated patients correlated inversely with symptom and medication scores during the grass pollen season. These findings in the nose were confirmed by results from a study of allergen-induced late-phase cutaneous responses that examined cellular infiltration and cytokine mRNA expression following 9 months of im-

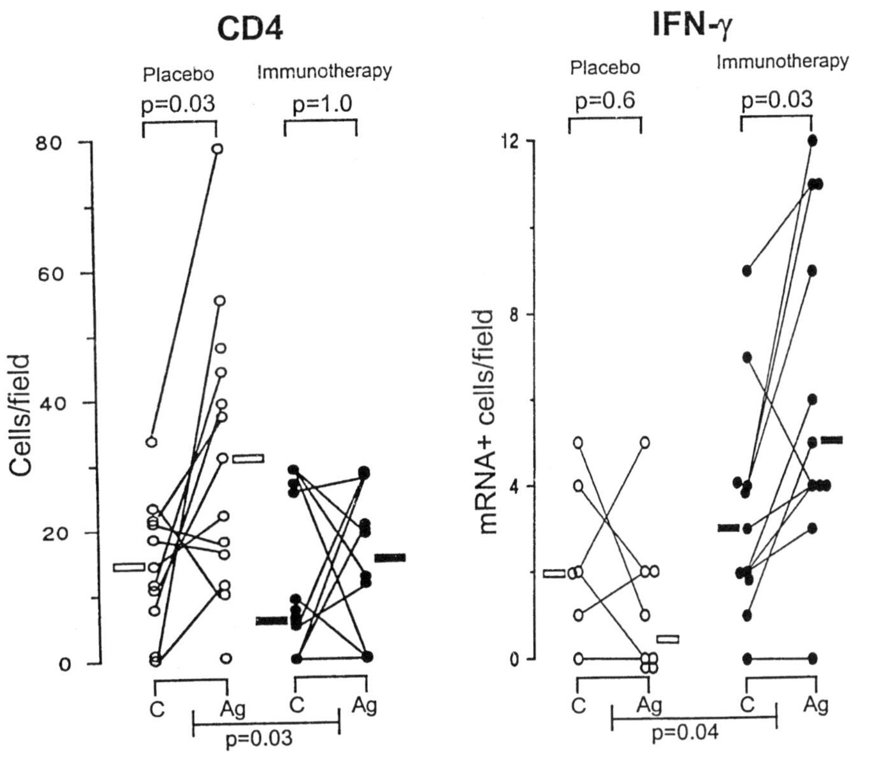

Figure 6 Cellular infiltration with $CD4^+$ T lymphocytes and in situ hybridization with an antisense riboprobe against mRNA for IFN-γ. The differences in cell counts (24 hr after allergen challenge minus control counts) for placebo-treated (open circles) and immunotherapy-treated (closed circles) patients were compared by using the Mann-Whitney U-test; within-group comparison by using the Wilcoxon test. (From Ref. 37.)

munotherapy (34). Clinical improvement was accompanied by a decrease in the late skin response size, and analysis of skin biopsies revealed significant reductions in $CD4^+$ T cells and a trend for reduced eosinophil cell numbers. Although in situ hybridization demonstrated equivalent expression of the Th2-type cytokines IL-4 and IL-5 in both active- and placebo-treated patients, significant increases in IFN-γ and IL-2 mRNA-expressing cells were observed in the immunotherapy-treated group only. Expression of these Th1-type cytokines was paralleled by corresponding increases in $HLA\text{-}DR^+$ and $CD25^+$ (IL-2 receptor) cells. These studies provide evidence for induction of a predominatly Th1-type cytokine response following successful immunotherapy. Furthermore, inhibition of late cutaneous responses following grass pollen immunotherapy, was associated with significant local increases in IL-12 mRNA-expressing cells following allergen challenge (47). As IL-12 is a potent inducer of Th1-type T-cell differentiation (48), these findings suggest that increased IFN-γ production by T-cells in the target organ may be regulated by exposure to local cytokines such as IL-12.

Taken together these studies suggest that immunotherapy-induced changes in circulating antibody levels and alterations in inflammatory cell function within the blood and target organs may occur indirectly as a consequence of either immune deviation in favor of Th1 responses or by induction of T-cell tolerance. Therefore, it is of particular interest to ascertain whether these alterations in immunological reactivity persist once immunotherapy is discontinued.

To address this issue we performed a double-blind placebo-controlled trial of withdrawal of immunotherapy in grass pollen hayfever patients (17). Patients who had received grass pollen immunotherapy for 3–4 years were randomized to continue either with active treatment or receive placebo injections for a further 3 years. A matched immunotherapy-naive group of hayfever sufferers was followed in parallel to control for the natural course of the disease. Cutaneous biopsies obtained at 24 hr after allergen challenge were examined for T-cell infiltration and for the number of cells expressing mRNA for IL-4. Both immunotherapy-treated groups expressed significantly lower symptom and medication scores compared with the untreated group whether or not immunotherapy had been withdrawn for 3 years. Although there was a tendency for the immediate skin response to return, the late cutaneous response following intradermal 10 SQ grass pollen challenge remained virtually completely inhibited in both actively treated groups (Fig. 7). Furthermore, immunotherapy resulted in a significant reduction in allergen-induced local increases in total $(CD3^+)$ T-cell numbers and marked decreases in the number of cells expressing IL-4 mRNA, compared with the matched untreated hayfever control group (see Fig. 7). Again, these altered responses were detected whether or not immunotherapy had been withdrawn 3 years earlier.

Taken together these data provide evidence that 3–4 years of allergen immunotherapy results in persistent clinical improvement, a sustained inhibition of the late skin response and persistent alterations in immunological reactivity that last for several years after withdrawal of therapy.

Other possible mechanisms of immunotherapy include the induction of allergen-specific suppressor T cells, T-cell unresponsiveness, or both.

3.4 Cytotoxic Suppressor T Cells, T-Cell Anergy

In animal models of aeroallergen sensitization (49,50), specific suppressor T cells were able to down-regulate allergen-specific T-cell responses in vivo and in vitro. In a study

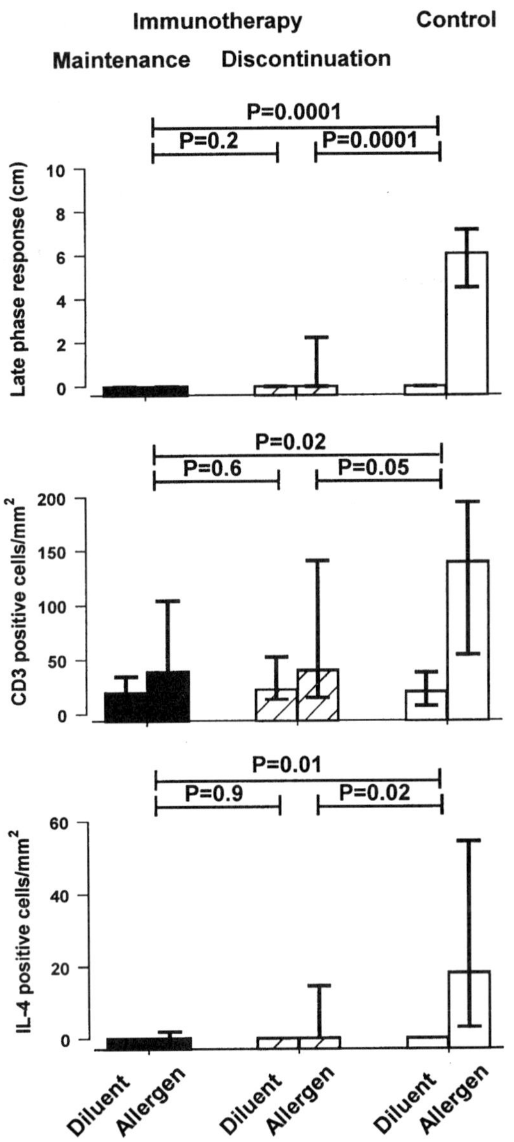

Figure 7 Late skin responses and numbers of $CD3^+$ T cells and cells containing IL-4 mRNA in skin biopsy specimens obtained 24 hr after intradermal injection of allergen or diluent: Cell counts per square millimeter are expressed as medians and interquartile ranges. Maintenance group: 7 yr of grass pollen IT, discontinuation group: 4 yr IT (3 yr withdrawal), control: IT-naive group. Levels of statistical significance (p-values) refer to between-group comparisons (Mann Whitney U-test).

of immunotherapy for ragweed allergic rhinitis, Rocklin et al. (51), by using a suppressor cell assay, observed increased suppressive activity of mononuclear cells to ragweed antigen. These cells, presumed to be T cells, exerted their suppressive activity only after 6 and 12 months of immunotherapy, but failed to do so in untreated hayfever patients or healthy controls. These suppressor cells were characterized by surface histamine receptors and by reversal of their suppressive activity when exposed to histamine. Similarly, following immunotherapy with rye grass. Nagaya (52) reported the induction of a subpopulation of suppressor–cytotoxic T cells, which suppressed T-cell proliferation following culture in rye grass allergen.

Various mechanisms could result in allergen-specific T-cell responsiveness following allergen immunotherapy. First, there is evidence of activation-induced programmed cell death (apoptosis) of T cells (53), which may be prevented by costimulation of T cells by CD28 (54). Induction of surface-bound IgG antibodies on monocytes, the production of which is facilitated by a cytokine milieu in favor of IFN-γ, impairs CD28 costimulated antigen-presentation to T cells (27). It can be speculated that this may represent a way to selectively delete Th2-type T cells.

In vitro induction of anergy of helper CD4 T-cell clones has been demonstrated following stimulation with supraoptimal concentrations of immunogenic peptides derived from allergen proteins and bacterial superantigens (55). This T-cell unresponsiveness is allergen-specific and reversible by addition of IL-2. It is attractive to speculate that allergen immunotherapy may act, at least in part, by establishing a state of anergy of allergen-specific T cells.

Ebner et al., in a trial of grass pollen immunotherapy (56), reported markedly reduced T-cell proliferative responses and a decline in the numbers of allergen-specific T-

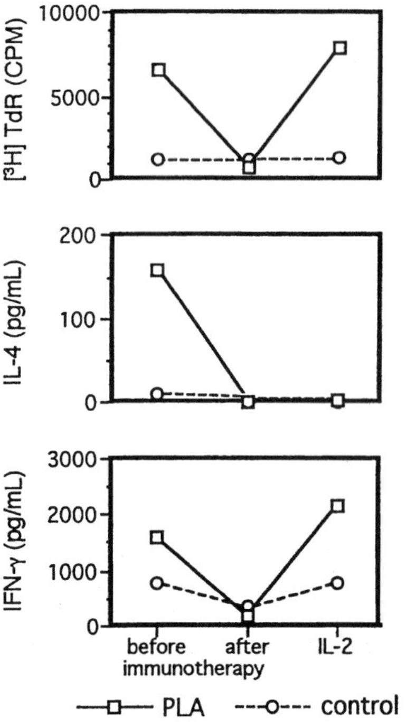

Figure 8 Differential recovery of bee venom allergen (phospholipase A; PLA)-induced proliferation and IFN-γ and IL-4 production in vitro: After immunotherapy, PLA-induced T-cell proliferation and IL-4 and IFN-γ production were inhibited. Addition of IL-2 to cultures restored proliferation and IFN-γ production but not IL-4 production. Data shown are representative of four such experiments. (From Ref. 57.)

cell clones that could be derived during treatment. Those allergen-specific T-cell clones that remained, showed deviation towards a Th1-type as compared with those before treatment. Consistent with the foregoing study and previous in vitro and in vivo models of T-cell anergy, Akdis et al. (57), following a trial of ultrarush immunotherapy with bee venom, reported markedly reduced T-cell proliferative responses to bee venom allergen, which could be restored by addition of IL-2 or IL-15. Furthermore, not only was T-cell proliferation restored after addition of IL-2, but this was also accompanied by selective production of IL-2 and IFN-γ without any production of IL-4, IL-5, or IL-13 (Fig. 8).

Anergized T cells can be reactivated to produce either Th1- or Th2-type cytokines depending on the cytokine microenvironment. Thus, the success or failure of allergen immunotherapy, may be directed by regulatory cytokines. In bee venom allergic individuals receiving rush venom immunotherapy this state of allergen-specific T-cell anergy was fully established by 4 weeks and occurred in parallel to increases in IL-10 production by circulating T lymphocytes, B cells, and monocytes (58). In a recent review (59) Akdis and Blaser emphasized the pluripotent role of IL-10, not only as an inhibitor of both Th1- and Th2-type T-cell cytokine production and proliferation, but also as an inhibitor of effector cells, such as mast cells, basophils, and eosinophils. Evidence for impaired B7.1/CD28 costimulation through IL-10 or action of IL-10 on the cytokine gene transcription level comes from several studies in humans (60,61). By "reestablishing" a normal

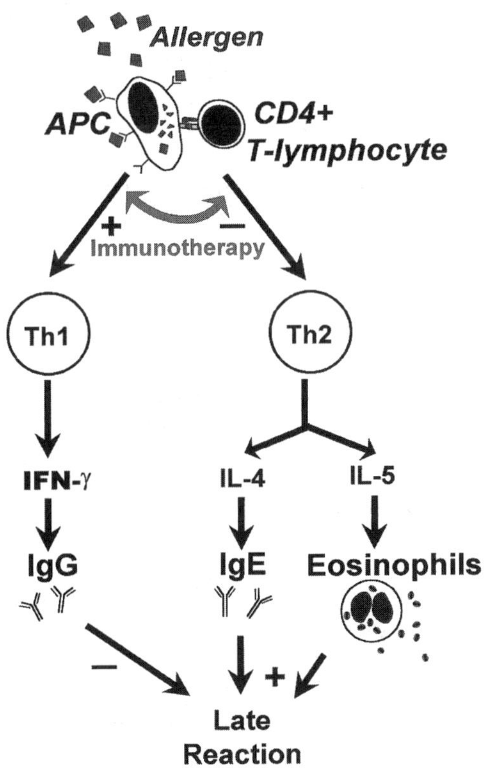

Figure 9 Hypothesis of mechanisms of immunotherapy: shift in favor of a Th1-type response may occur either as a consequence of selective down-regulation (anergy) of the Th2-response (possibly mediated by IL-10) or immunodeviation under the influence of IL-12.

IgE/IgG ratio the effects of IL-10 may possibly lead to the allergic status reverting to ''normal.'' Therefore, it is reasonable to speculate that the success of allergen immunotherapy depends on the amount of IL-10 produced. It may also explain why polysensitized individuals with high levels of Th2-type cytokines, show less response to immunotherapy. These findings also support the earlier introduction of allergen immunotherapy in the treatment of allergic diseases, especially in childhood allergic disease in which sensitization to only a limited number of allergens is common. Immunotherapy, if introduced early, could prevent new sensitizations by establishing a balanced cytokine milieu, approaching the ''normal,'' healthy state.

A hypothesis that attempts to interrelate alternative mechanisms of T-cell modulation following successful immunotherapy is indicated in Figure 9. Research into the development of more targeted forms of treatment is currently being undertaken. This includes evaluation of allergen immunotherapy administration by alternative routes, including oral, sublingual, and intranasal. Anti-IgE antibodies that prevent binding of IgE to FcεRI represent a more broad and novel approach to therapy, although the clinical efficacy and possible long-term consequences are still unknown. Other therapeutic targets include the pro-allergic cytokines IL-4 and IL-5. The recent development of ''nonstimulatory'' allergen peptides, representing distinct T-cell epitopes, may circumvent IgE-dependent activation of mast cells, but still anergize allergen-specific T cells, thereby minimizing the risk of anaphylaxis during immunotherapy.

These alternative strategies provide an optimistic outlook for the future treatment of allergic patients.

ACKNOWLEDGMENTS

We acknowledge the Austrian Science Fund, which funded E. M. Varga, and the National Asthma Campaign, Medical Research Council UK and ALK Abello (Denmark and Austria), for financial support.

REFERENCES

1. Frew AJ. Injection immunotherapy. British Society for Allergy and Clinical Immunology Working Party. Br Med J 1993; 307:919–923.
2. Malling H, Weese B. Position paper of the European Academy of Allergy and Clinical Immunology. Allergy 1993; 48(suppl 14):9–35.
3. Bousquet J, Lockey RF, Malling H–J. WHO Position Paper Allergen Immunotherapy: therapeutic vaccines for allergic diseases. Allergy 1998; 44(suppl 53).
4. Des Roches A, Paradis L, Menardo J–L, Bouges S, Daures J–P, Bousquet J. Immunotherapy with a standardized *Dermatophagoides pteronyssinus* extract. VI. Specific immunotherapy prevents the onset of new sensitizations in children. J Allergy Clin Immunol 1997; 99(4):450–453.
5. Varney VA, Gaga M, Frew AJ, Aber VR, Kay AB, Durham SR. Usefulness of immunotherapy in patients with severe summer hayfever uncontrolled by antiallergic drugs. Br Med J 1991; 302:265–269.
6. Walker SM, Varney VA, Gaga M, et al. Grass pollen immunotherapy: efficacy and safety during a 4-year follow-up study. Allergy 1995; 50:405–413.
7. Ewan PW, Alexander MM, Snape C, Ind PW, Agrell B, Dreborg S. Effective hyposensitization in allergic rhinitis using a potent partially purified extract of house dust mite. Clin Allergy 1988; 18:501–508.

8. Abramson M, Puy R, Weiner J. Immunotherapy in asthma: an updated systematic review. Allergy 1999; 54:1022–1041.
9. Müller U, Helbling A, Berchtold E. Immunotherapy with honeybee venom and yellow jacket venom is different regarding efficacy and safety. J Allergy Clin Immunol 1992; 89:529–535.
10. Müller U, Berchtold E, Helbling A. Honeybee venom allergy: results of a sting challenge 1 year after stopping successful venom immunotherapy in 86 patients. J Allergy Clin Immunol 1991; 87:702–709.
11. Golden DB, Kwiterovich KA, Kagey–Sobotka A, Valentine MD, Lichtenstein LM. Discontinuing venom immunotherapy. Outcome after five years. J Allergy Clin Immunol 1996; 97:579–587.
11a. Golden DBK, Kagey–Sabotka A, Lichtenstein LM. Survey of patients after discontinuing venom immunotherapy. J Allergy Clin Immunol 2000; 105:385–390.
12. Bousquet J, Knani J, Velasquez G, Menardo JL, Guilloux L, Michel FB. Evolution of sensitivity to Hymenoptera venom in 200 allergic patients followed for up to 3 years. J Allergy Clin Immunol 1989; 84:944–950.
13. Golden DBK, Addison B, Gadde J, Kagey–Sobotka A, Valentine MD, Lichtenstein LM. Prospective observations on stopping prolonged venom immunotherapy. J Allergy Clin Immunol 1989; 84:162–167.
14. Lerch E, Muller UR. Long-term protection after stopping venom immunotherapy. J Allergy Clin Immunol 1998; 101:606–612.
15. Grammer LC, Shaughnessy MA, Suszko IM, Shaughnessy JJ, Patterson R. Persistence of efficacy after a brief course of polymerized ragweed allergen: a controlled study. J Allergy Clin Immunol 1984; 73:484–489.
16. Mosbech H, Osterballe O. Does the effect of immunotherapy last after termination of treatment? Follow-up study in patients with grass pollen rhinitis. Allergy 1988; 43:523–529.
17. Durham SR, Walker SM, Varga EM, Jacobson MR, O'Brien F, Noble W, Till SJ, Hamid QA, Nouri–Aria K. Long-term clinical efficacy of grass pollen immunotherapy. N Engl J Med 1999; 341:468–475.
18. Lichtenstein L, Ishizaka K, Norman P, Sobotka A, Hill B. IgE antibody measurements in ragweed hay fever. Relationship to clinical severity and the results of immunotherapy. J Clin Invest 1973; 52:477–482.
19. Gleich GJ, Zimmermann EM, Henderson LL, Yunginger JW. Effect of immunotherapy on immunoglobulin E and immunoglobulin G antibodies to ragweed antigens: a six-year prospective study. J Allergy Clin Immunol 1982, 70:261–271.
20. Malling HJ, Skov PS, Permin H, Norn S, Weeke B. Basophil histamine release and humoral changes during immunotherapy. Dissociation between basophil-bound specific IgE, serum value, and cell sensitivity. Allergy 1982; 70:187–190.
21. Star M, Weinstock M. Studies in pollen allergy. III. The relationship between blocking antibody levels, and symptomatic relief following hyposensitization with Allpyral in hayfever subjects. Int Arch Allergy 1970; 38:514–521.
22. Golden DB, Meyers DA, Kagey–Sobotka A, Valentine MD, Lichtenstein LM. Clinical relevance of the venom-specific immunoglobulin G antibody level during immunotherapy. J Allergy Clin Immunol 1982; 69:489–493.
23. Zeiss CR, Metzger WJ, Levitz D. Quantitative relationship between IgE antibody and blocking antibodies specific for antigen E in patients given immunotherapy with ragweed antigen E. Clin Exp Immunol 1977; 28:250–255.
24. Golden DB, Meyers DA, Kagey–Sobotka A, Valentine MD, Lichtenstein LM. Clinical relevance of the venom specific immunoglobulin G antibody level during immunotherapy. J Allergy Clin Immunol 1982; 69:489–493.
25. Visco V, Dolecek C, Denepoux S, et al. Human IgG monoclonal antibodies that modulate the binding of specific IgE to birch pollen Bet v 1. J Immunol 1996; 157:956–962.
26. Aalberse RC, Van Milligen F, Tan KY, Stapel SO. Allergen-specific IgG4 in atopic disease. Allergy 1993; 48:559–569.

27. Barey S, Wettendorf M, Leo O, et al. FcR-cross-linking on monocytes results in impaired T cell stimulatory capacity. Int Immunol 1995; 7:179–189.
28. Creticos PS, Adkinson NF Jr, Kagey–Sobotka A, et al. Nasal challenge with ragweed pollen in hay fever patients. Effect of immunotherapy. J Clin Invest 1985; 76:2247–2253.
29. Bentley AM, Jacobson MR, Cumberworth V, et al. Immunohistology of the nasal mucosa in seasonal allergic rhinitis: increases in activated eosinophils and epithelial mast cells. J Allergy Clin Immunol 1992; 89:877–883.
30. Varga EM, Jacobson MR, Till SJ, Masuyama K, O'Brien F, Rak S, Lund V, Scadding GK, Hamid QA, Durham SR. Cellular infiltration and cytokine mRNA expression in perennial allergic rhinitis. Allergy 1999; 54:338–345.
31. Otsuka H, Mezawa A, Ohnishi M, Okubo K, Seki H, Okuda M. Changes in nasal metachromatic cells during allergen immunotherapy. Clin Exp Allergy 1991; 21:115–119.
32. Durham SR, Varney VA, Gaga M, Jacobson MR, Varga EM, Frew AJ, Kay AB. Grass pollen immunotherapy decreases the number of mast cells in the skin. Clin Exp Allergy 1999; 29: 1490–1496.
33. Nish WA, Charlesworth EN, Davis TL, et al. The effect of immunotherapy on the cutaneous late phase response to antigen. J Allergy Clin Immunol 1994; 93:484–493.
34. Varney VA, Hamid QA, Gaga M, et al. Influence of grass pollen immunotherapy on cellular infiltration and cytokine mRNA expression during allergen-induced late-phase cutaneous responses. J Clin Invest 1993; 92:644–651.
35. Rak S, Lowhagen O, Venge P. The effect of immunotherapy on bronchial hyperresponsiveness and eosinophil cationic protein in pollen-allergic patients. J Allergy Clin Immunol 1988; 82: 470–480.
36. Furin MJ, Norman PS, Creticos PS, et al. Immunotherapy decreases antigen-induced eosinophil cell migration into the nasal cavity. J Allergy Clin Immunol 1991; 88:27–32.
37. Durham SR, Ying S, Varney VA, et al. Grass pollen immunotherapy inhibits allergen-induced infiltration of $CD4^+$ T lymphocytes and eosinophils in the nasal mucosa and increases the number of cells expressing messenger RNA for interferon-γ. J Allergy Clin Immunol 1996; 97:1356–1365.
38. Mossman TR, Coffman RL. Th1 and Th2 cells: different patterns of lymphokine secretion lead to different functional properties. Annu Rev Immunol 1989; 7:145–173.
39. Wierenga EA, Snoek M, de Groot C, et al. Evidence for compartmentalization of functional subsets of $CD2^+$ T lymphocytes in atopic patients. J Immunol 1990; 144:4651–4656.
40. Del Prete GF, De Carli M, Mastromauro C, et al. Purified protein derivative of *Mycobacterium tuberculosis* and excretory-secretory antigen (s) of *Toxocara canis* expanded in vitro human T cells with stable and opposite (type 1 T helper or type 2 T helper) profiles of cytokine production. J Clin Invest 1991; 88:344–350.
41. Bentley AM, Meng Q, Robinson DS, Hamid Q, Kay AB, Durham SR. Increases in activated T lymphocytes, eosinophils, and cytokine mRNA expression for interleukin-5 and granulocyte/macrophage colony-stimulating factor in bronchial biopsies after allergen inhalation challenge in atopic asthmatics. Am J Respir Cell Mol Biol 1993; 8:35.
42. Robinson D, Hamid Q, Bentley A, Ying S, Kay AB, Durham SR. Activation of $CD4^+$ T cells, increased Th2-type cytokine mRNA expression, and eosinophil recruitment in bronchoalveloar lavage after allergen inhalation challenge in patients with atopic asthma. J Allergy Clin Immunol 1993; 92:313.
43. Lack G, Nelson HS, Amran D, Oshiba A, Jung T, Bradley KL, Giclas PC, Gelfand EW. Rush immunotherapy results in allergen-specific alterations in lymphocyte function and interferon-gamma production in $CD4^+$ T cells. J Allergy Clin Immunol 1997; 99:530–538.
44. Secrist H, Chelen CJ, Wen Y, Marshall JD, Umetsu DT. Allergen immunotherapy decreases interleukin 4 production in $CD4^+$ T cells from allergic individuals. J Exp Med 1993; 178: 2123–2130.
45. Jutel M, Pichler WJ, Skrbic D, Urwyler A, Dahinden C, Müller UR. Bee venom immunother-

apy results in decrease of IL-4 and IL-5 and increase of IFN-γ secretion in specific allergen-stimulated T cell cultures. J Immunol 1995; 154:4187–4194.

46. Till S, Walker S, Dickason R, et al. IL-5 production by allergen-stimulated T cells following grass pollen immunotherapy for seasonal allergic rhinitis. Clin Exp Immunol 1997; 110:114–121.
47. Hamid QA, Schotman E, Jacobson MR, Walker SM, Durham SR. Increases in IL-12 messenger RNA$^+$ cells accompany inhibition of allergen-induced late skin responses after successful grass pollen immunotherapy. J Allergy Clin Immunol 1997; 99:254–260.
48. Manetti R, Parronchi P, Giudizi MG, et al. Natural killer cell stimulatory factor (interleukin 12) induces T helper type 1(Th)-specific immune responses and inhibits the development of IL-4 producing Th cells. J Exp Med 1993; 177:1199–1204.
49. Mc Menamin C, Holt PG. The natural immune response to inhaled soluble protein antigens involves major histocompatibility complex (MHC) class I-restricted CD8$^+$ T cell-mediated but class II-restricted CD4$^+$ T-cell dependent immune deviation resulting in selective suppression of immunoglobulin E production. J Exp Med 193; 178:889–899.
50. Renz H, Lack G, Saloga J, et al. Inhibition of IgE production and normalization of airways responsiveness by sensitized CD8$^+$ T cells in a mouse model of allergen-induced sensitization. J Immunol 1994; 152:351–360.
51. Rocklin RE, Sheffer AL, Greineder DL, Melmon KM. Generation of antigen-specific suppressor cells during allergy desensitization. N Engl J Med 1980; 302:1213–1219.
52. Nagaya Hiroshi. Induction of antigen-specific suppressor cells in patients with hayfever receiving immunotherapy. J Allergy Clin Immunol 1985; 75:388–394.
53. Kabelitz D, Pohl T, Pechhold K. Activation-induced cell death (apoptosis) of mature peripheral T lymphocytes. Immunol Today 1993; 14:338–339.
54. Radvanyi LG, Shi Y, Vaziri H, Sharma A, Dhala R, Mills GB, Miller RG. CD28 costimulation inhibits TCR-induced apoptosis during a primary T cell response. J Immunol 1996; 156(5): 1788–1798.
55. O'Hehir RE, Yssel H, Verma S, et al. Clonal analysis of differential lymphokine production in peptide and superantigen induced T cell anergy. Int Immunol 1991, 8:819–826.
56. Ebner C, Siemann U, Bole B, et al. Immunological changes during specific immunotherapy of grass pollen allergy: reduced lymphoproliferative responses to allergen and shift from Th2 to Th1 in T cell clones specific for Phl p 1, a major grass pollen allergen. Clin Exp Allergy 1997; 27:1007–1015.
57. Akdis CA, Akdis M, Blesken T, et al. Epitope-specific T cell tolerance to phospholipase A_2 in bee venom immunotherapy and recovery by IL-2 and IL-15 in vitro. J Clin Invest 1996; 98:1676–1683.
58. Akdis CA, Blesken T, Akdis M, Wüthrich B, Blaser K. The role of IL-10 in specific immunotherapy. J Clin Invest 1998; 102:98–106.
59. Akdis CA, Blaser K. IL-10 induced anergy in peripheral T cell and reactivation by microenvironmental cytokines: two key steps in specific immunotherapy. FASEB J 1999; 13:603–609.
60. Schandane L, Alonso–Vega C, Willems F, Gerard C, Delvaux A, Velu T, Devos R, de Boer M, Goldman M. B7/Cd28-dependent IL-5 production by human resting T cells is inhibited by IL-10. J Immunol 1994; 152:4368–4374.
61. Wang P, Wu P, Siegel MI, Egan RW, Billah MM. IL-10 inhibits transcription of cytokine genes in human peripheral blood mononuclear cells. J Immunol 1994; 153:811–816.

26

DNA Immunomodulation of Asthma

JOEL N. KLINE and ZUHAIR K. BALLAS

University of Iowa College of Medicine, Iowa City, Iowa

1 INTRODUCTION

Few developments in the history of immunology rival Jenner's use of cowpox to confer immunity against smallpox (1). One can safely state that Jenner's experiments were the forerunners of what is now referred to as immunomodulation or, more generally, biological response modification. Many vaccines have been developed since, but most are centered around modifications of the same basic idea: administer an attenuated, killed, or related pathogen to a naïve population to induce protective immunity (2,3). More recently, peptides (which bypass the antigen-presenting process) have been used as immunogens, with limited success. With the advent of molecular biology techniques, the potential for biological response modification has expanded to encompass selective targeting of certain genes. Recent technical advances have conferred the capacity of regulating the ''dose'' of a given gene from total inactivation (knockout) to expression in every cell (transgenic). Between these two ends of the spectrum, one can determine where, or when, a certain gene can be expressed by controlling the promotor region or by using an antibiotic selection marker, respectively (4,5). Regulation of the gene dose is readily accomplished in mice by manipulating the embryonic stem cell; this is clearly not feasible in humans.

Several techniques have been used to manipulate already expressed genes and to replace an absent or mutated gene. Antisense oligonucleotides have been used to regulate gene translation. Antisense oligonucleotides are single-stranded nucleic acids designed to hybridize with mRNA of a given gene, thereby causing translational arrest and subsequent depletion of the protein product (6–9). For a missing or mutated gene or gene product, DNA (gene) therapy has been introduced. Perhaps the most straightforward, and successful, approach to gene therapy has been the introduction of adenosine deaminase (ADA) gene in patients with the ADA-deficient type of severe combined immunodeficiency (SCID) (10). ADA-deficient SCID patients have a mutation in their ADA gene that renders the gene nonfunctional. This results in the accumulation of deoxyadenosine products, which are toxic to T and B lymphocytes. Because ADA deficiency is most detrimental to lymphocytes and lymphocytes are long-lived, Blaese et al. (10) transfected the ADA gene in the lymphocytes of patients with ADA deficiency and reinjected the lymphocytes into the patients, leading to a significant expression of the ADA enzyme. Other attempts at gene therapy have been less successful. The gene therapy trials that received most attention, although they had limited success, were those for cystic fibrosis (CF) (11–14). These trials illustrate the difficulties inherent in gene modulation in an organ-based disease, such as CF (as opposed to a lymphocyte-based disease, such as ADA deficiency) or asthma. CF is a well-defined disease with a well-defined single genetic defect with one organ as the major disease site. It would thus appear that CF is an ideal disease for gene therapy. The problems arise from several aspects of gene therapy, including the choice of vector, the immunogenicity of the vector, the delivery of the vector (regional vs. systemic), and the persistence of the administered gene. If gene therapy of CF, a single-gene disease, has been so disappointing, one can imagine the difficulties inherent in the gene therapy of a disease wherein multiple genes are affected. How about a disease in which the putative genes are overactive, rather than deficient or mutated? How about a disease that is heterogeneous, involves several cells, including circulating cells (lymphocytes and eosinophils), and stationary cells (pulmonary epithelial cells and mast cells)? In other words: how about using gene therapy for asthma?

Asthma is a heterogeneous disease with two common end results: reversible airway obstruction and airway inflammation (15–17). Several mechanisms influence airway caliber, including neurogenic mechanisms, adrenergic receptors, and chemical mediators. Asthmatic inflammation is predominantly eosinophilic. The eosinophilic infiltrate, however, is the end product of an intricate interplay between mast cells, T lymphocytes, cytokines, chemokines, and bronchial epithelial cells (see Chap. 15). Although the exact cascade of events is not fully delineated, it is now clear that T lymphocytes play a central role. Of the T lymphocytes, Th2 cells are believed to be the most important by virtue of their elaboration of interleukin (IL)-4, IL-5, and IL-13 (18–21). One has to point out that Th2-type cytokines can also be secreted by mast cells, activated eosinophils, natural killer (NK) cells, and the newly described NKT cells (22–25). Of the Th2 cytokines, IL-4 and IL-13 have been clearly shown to favor IgE synthesis: IL-13 has a direct inflammatory effect on the bronchial tree, and IL-5 prolongs eosinophil survival (26–28). As described in Chapter 2, initiation of mast cell mediator release (by binding of an allergen to its specific IgE) triggers a cascade of events, including the elaboration of chemokines and the expression of adhesion molecules, which results in the recruitment of inflammatory cells. When the inflammatory cells arrive at the bronchi, they also secrete various cytokines, thus establishing an almost autonomous loop. Therefore, it is not surprising that proper control of asthma cannot be obtained without controlling the inflammation cascade. Any therapy, and certainly any DNA-based therapy, is doomed to failure unless these issues are taken in consideration.

We have thus far painted a rather grim, albeit realistic, picture of a daunting task for DNA-based therapies, especially for asthma. However, some rather ingenious approaches have been devised for DNA-based modulation of asthma. One can classify these approaches into the following categories: (1) control of bronchial reactivity; (2) direct introduction of specific cytokines; (3) global induction of Th1, and suppression of Th2 cytokines.

2 CONTROL OF BRONCHIAL REACTIVITY

Purine nucleosides have an interesting history. Guanosine, substituted at the 8 position with a thiol or bromine group, is a potent stimulator of T cells, B cells, macrophages, NK cells, and cytokine secretion (29–31). Adenosine, on the other hand, induces a transient contraction of guinea pig tracheal smooth muscle (32,33). It also induces bronchoconstriction when inhaled by asthmatics, but not normal individuals, in a manner similar to histamine or methacholine bronchoprovocation (34–39). These effects of adenosine can be duplicated by AMP (which is rapidly changed to adenosine by 5′-nucleotidase). The bronchoconstriction induced by adenosine or AMP cannot be duplicated by inosine, an adenosine metabolite, or by guanosine (a closely related purine), suggesting the existence of adenosine-specific receptors. Indeed, it is now known that there are at least four adenosine-specific receptors: A1, A2A, A2B, and A3 (40,41). The A1 receptor is almost nonexistent in normal lung tissue, but is abundant in asthmatic lungs. Indeed, because adenosine receptors are expressed on mast cells, binding of adenosine to mast cells enhances FcεRI-dependent mast cell degranulation and the release of bronchoconstricting mediators (42–45). It has been suggested that the ability of theophylline to inhibit adenosine-mediated mast cell activation may be its primary physiological effect, as it can do so at doses much smaller than those needed to inhibit mast cell phosphodiesterase (39,46,47). In addition to acting on mast cells and smooth muscle, adenosine may act on neural pathways and other inflammatory cells. Ali et al., using a rabbit asthma model, demonstrated a dose-dependent bronchoconstriction induced by aerosolized adenosine that could be inhibited by theophylline (48,49). Nyce and Metzger (50) designed an antisense oligodeoxynucleotide (ODN) aimed at the human adenosine A1 receptor mRNA. Antisense ODNs are single-stranded nucleic acids (with a phosphorothioate backbone, used to enhance in vivo stability) designed to specifically hybridize to the mRNA of the protein of interest, thereby preventing RNA translation. This results in decreased synthesis of the targeted protein (adenosine A1 receptor in this case); the normal turnover of the protein results in a net and significant reduction in the number of molecules expressed. Because there is a considerable homology between the human and rabbit A1 receptor, Nyce and Metzger (50) tested their antisense ODN in a rabbit asthma model. They delivered the antisense DNA by aerosol to the lungs of allergic rabbits. This resulted in a significant decrease (on the order of 50–60%) in adenosine-induced, allergen-induced, and methacholine-induced bronchoconstriction. Moreover, the antisense ODNs caused nearly 75% decrease in A1 receptor density on bronchial smooth muscle, with no effect on adenosine A2 receptor density, thus demonstrating specificity. These effects appeared to last for 7–10 days. This elegant study illumines the advantages of antisense therapy. It is specific and can be delivered directly to the organ of interest. Because asthma is a multifactorial disease, one could target more than one mRNA at the same time. One can envisage an antisense cocktail directed, for example, against adenosine receptor, adhesion molecules, chemokines, and eosinophil cationic protein (ECP). Drawbacks of this approach include that it is not clear how frequently one needs to administer the ODN to obtain long-lasting effects, what are the long-term side effects, and whether other, not yet described, receptors will be induced with the blockade or elimination of primary physiological pathways. Indeed, the redundancy of pathways, molecules, and receptors reduces the likelihood of long-term benefit.

3 MODULATION OF SPECIFIC CYTOKINES

As detailed in Chapter 15, Th2 cytokines are believed to be pivotal in asthma. Because Th1 and Th2 responses are counterregulatory, it is reasonable to assume that one can modulate the disease by delivering Th1 cytokine genes (e.g., IL-12 or interferon [IFN]-γ) into the lung. Hogan et al. (51), using a murine asthma model, found that mucosal gene transfer (vaccinia virus vector) of IL-12 into the lung inhibited local Th2 cytokine production, prevented the development of allergic diseases, and inhibited bronchial hyperreactivity. Interestingly, these effects appeared to be mediated through the induction of IFN-γ secretion, for no protective effect was seen in IFN-γ knockout mice. It is thus not surprising that Li et al. (52) showed that local delivery of IFN-γ gene, using a plasmid expression vector, in mouse lungs resulted in IFN-γ expression in the airway epithelium, decreased Th2 cytokine expression, and decreased airway hyperreactivity. Dow et al. (53) compared the systemic versus pulmonary delivery of IFN-γ genes, using plasmid expression vector and cationic liposomes, in a murine asthma model. These authors found that both local and systemic administration of IFN-γ gene decreased airway eosinophilia and airway hyperreactivity. Interestingly, systemic, but not intratracheal, delivery of IFN-γ resulted in a significant decline in serum IgE levels. Both modes of delivery appeared to be superior to treatment with recombinant IFN-γ. The reasons for these discrepancies are unclear, but may be dependent on the pharmacokinetics of the metabolism and production of IFN-γ.

These studies clearly demonstrate that local gene delivery is feasible and is superior to simple administration of the protein product. Issues that remain to be explored include the duration of gene expression and the cell types in which the gene is expressed. A significant issue is the use of any viral vector for gene delivery. The first dose, while delivering the gene of interest, may immunize the host against the viral vector. If the vector induces expression of Th1 cytokines, then these cytokines should enhance the immune response against the vector. Subsequent doses may be not only ineffective (owing to neutralization), but also may be detrimental owing to killing of the transfected cells by cytotoxic T lymphocytes specific to the viral vector. In asthma, a second dose may lead to more inflammation.

Another approach at modulating cytokines utilizes the fact that NF-κB is a common "upstream" pathway for many cytokines and chemokines. NF-κB has been implicated in the regulation of several cytokines and chemokines including tumor necrosis factor (TNF)-α, IL-1β, IL-2, IL-6, IL-12, IL-8, macrophage inflammatory peptide (MIP)-1, RANTES, granulocyte colony-stimulating factor (G-CSF), granulocyte–macrophage colony stimulating factor (GM-CSF), and IFN-β. Inhibition of NF-κB could theoretically help in asthma by controlling chemokines believed to play a central role in asthma (e.g., regulated on activation, normal T-cell expressed and secreted; RANTES). NF-κB is present in the cytoplasm, where it is rendered inactive by binding to IκB. Proinflammatory signals lead to proteolysis of IκB, thereby activating NF-κB, which then migrates to the nucleus where it binds to sites in the promoter regions of the genes of several cytokines, chemokines, and adhesion molecules (54–56). It is believed that corticosteroids bind a cytoplasmic receptor (the glucocorticoid receptor; GR) resulting in repression of NF-κB activation. Mathieu et al. (57) reasoned that overexpression of GR in a cell may inhibit

NF-κB and may render the cell more susceptible to the corticosteroid effects. They (57) transfected human lung epithelial cells with a GR-expression vector and found that this resulted in decreased expression of NF-κB and decreased production of RANTES, in vitro. It remains to be seen whether this would be feasible in vivo. Even if this approach is feasible, it is nonspecific. A potential drawback of this approach is that minimizing or abolishing a wide range of inflammatory mediators may be detrimental to the host.

4 "GLOBAL" INDUCTION OF Th1, AND SUPPRESSION OF Th2, CYTOKINES

It is evident from the foregoing discussion that selective targeting of one cytokine or one receptor, while exerting some therapeutic effect, will not be sufficient for a clinically significant modulation of asthma. It would be ideal if one could find one therapeutic modality that can fundamentally change the underlying basis of eosinophilic inflammation. There is now considerable evidence-based acceptance that the balance between Th1 and Th2 may be at the foundation of the eosinophilic inflammation seen in asthma. Theoretically, skewing this balance towards Th1, and suppressing Th2, should have a clinically significant therapeutic effect in asthma. How can one accomplish this? A clue can be found in the epidemiological studies of asthma. Data suggest that exposure to bacteria may provide a protective influence against the development of asthma and atopic disorders; as a corollary, a decline in childhood infections could contribute to the increasing prevalence and severity of asthma in the industrialized world. In one series of studies, von Mutius and colleagues have examined the prevalence of asthma and atopy in former East Germany and former West Germany (58). Despite the worse air pollution and lower standard of living that characterized East Germany, these investigators demonstrated that asthma and atopy are significantly more prevalent in former West Germany than in the former East Germany. This difference was associated with an increased percentage of children exposed to earlier childhood infections in group daycare situations. These data are supported by other studies, such as those that have correlated numbers of older siblings (and thus earlier exposure to childhood infections) with protection against atopic disorders (59). In a related investigation, Shirakawa and coinvestigators have convincingly demonstrated an inverse association between strength of tuberculin skin response (purified protein derivative; PPD) and atopy (60). Mycobacterial infection, or vaccination with BCG (bacille Calmette–Guerin), induces a strong Th1 response. The implication of the studies of Shirakawa et al. is that mycobacterial infection, hence a strong Th1 response, during childhood may prevent the development or expression of atopy and asthma (60). These studies support the concept that bacterial infection may be protective in asthma. One can invoke several mechanisms by which bacteria could be helpful (or harmful) in asthma. One possibility is that it is the bacterial DNA, rather than any other component of the bacteria, that may be inducing the protective effect. As alluded to earlier, purine nucleosides exert significant effects in an immune response. It has recently become appreciated that bacterial DNA differs from mammalian DNA by two key features. First, bacterial DNA has the expected 1:16 frequency of CG base pairs (because these have a phosphodiester backbone, they are referred to as CpG), whereas mammalian DNA appears to have a markedly decreased frequency (1:50–1:100). Moreover, when CpGs are present in mammalian DNA, the cytosines are typically methylated, whereas they are unmethylated in bacterial DNA.

Although it had previously been recognized that bacterial DNA was immunostimulatory and caused a variety of effects, including induction of NK cell activity (61) and stimulation of lymphocyte proliferation (62–64), Krieg and colleagues first identified the role of CpG motifs in inducing these responses (65). This activity is markedly reduced or abolished by methylation of the DNA. Moreover, the immunostimulatory effects of bacterial DNA can be reproduced using oligonucleotides (short stretches of synthesized single-stranded DNA) that contain one or more CpG motifs. CpG DNA has very specific effects on the pattern of inflammation, inducing release of IFN-γ from NK cells (66); IFN-α and IL-12 from macrophages, dendritic cells, and other mononuclear phagocytes (67–69); and IL-18 from T lymphocytes (70). The result of CpG stimulation is thus to skew immune responses to a strongly Th1-type inflammation; this subsequently has been shown to promote protective vaccine-induced antibody responses (71) as well as resistance to bacterial pathogens, such as *Listeria monocytogenes* (72).

These properties of CpG oligodeoxynucleotides (ODN) would make it ideal for the treatment of asthma. We have been engaged in examining the ability of CpG ODN to abolish eosinophilic inflammation and bronchial hyperreactivity in a murine asthma model (73). Murine asthma models are now well established for use in research of human asthma pathophysiology. However, these models typically result in the development of peribronchial as well as perivascular inflammation, whereas human asthma is associated with only peribronchial inflammation, a potentially significant difference. Employing a schistosome egg–egg antigen murine model of asthma, we used an active ODN that includes two CpG motifs (TCCAT*GACGTT*CCT*GACGTT*) and a control ODN that was identical except for rearrangement of the CpG motifs (TCCATGA*GCT*TCCTGA*GTCT*).

We first examined the effect of CpG ODN on the development of airway inflammation and found that the marked airway eosinophilia induced in this asthma model was almost entirely abrogated by pretreatment with CpG, but not with control, ODN (Table 1). This protection was also reflected in the histopathology; the pronounced peribronchial and perivascular cellular infiltrate characteristic of asthmatic inflammation was markedly reduced in the CpG-treated mice (Fig. 1). We next evaluated the pulmonary cytokine response induced in this model and by the treatment with CpG ODN. As expected, the mice sensitized and then challenged to schistosome egg proteins release high levels of IL-4 and low levels of IFN-γ and IL-12 into the lung lavage fluid (see Table 1). Mice treated with CpG ODN at the time of sensitization demonstrate pulmonary induction of both Th1 cytokines, which is not seen in the mice treated with the control ODN.

Bronchial hyperreactivity, a characteristic trait of asthma, was also successfully reduced by treatment with CpG ODN. Asthmatic mice develop marked bronchial hyperreactivity to inhaled methacholine (Fig. 2), which was almost completely abrogated by treatment with CpG ODN, but not with control ODN.

Finally, we were able to demonstrate that CpG DNA was effective in preventing eosinophilic airway inflammation in sensitized mice. Treatment with CpG ODN led to a marked reduction in the development of subsequent antigen-induced airway eosinophilia (73).

Because we found that the induction of Th1-type cytokines was associated with the protection conferred by CpG ODN in this model of asthma, we next examined whether IFN-γ or IL-12 was required for this protection (74). We found that in the absence of either IFN-γ or IL-12, CpG ODN were still able to prevent the induction of antigen-induced airway eosinophilia and bronchial hyperreactivity to inhaled methacholine. A dose–response study of the effects of decreasing amounts of CpG ODN demonstrated, however, that in the absence of IFN-γ, IL-12, or both Th1 cytokines, greater amounts of CpG ODN were required to obtain the same level of suppression of eosinophilia (Fig. 3).

Table 1 Effects of CpG DNA on Airway Eosinophilia and Cytokine Release

Treatment group	BAL eosinophils	BAL IL-4	BAL IFN-γ	BAL IL-12
Saline control	$0.0 \pm 0.3 \times 10^6$ cells	4.5 ± 1.1 pg/mL[b]	15.1 ± 7.3 pg/mL	0.7 ± 0.2 ng/mL
Asthma	$3.2 \pm 0.5 \times 10^6$ cells[a]	118.1 ± 32.5 pg/mL[a]	23.5 ± 18.4 pg/mL	1.7 ± 0.4 ng/mL
CpG ODN	$0.3 \pm 0.2 \times 10^6$ cells[b]	23.7 ± 2.9 pg/mL[b]	417.6 ± 132 pg/mL[a,b]	5.9 ± 1.9 ng/mL[a,b]
Control ODN	$2.8 \pm 0.9 \times 10^6$ cells[a]	84.6 ± 19.7 pg/mL[a]	118.9 ± 87.1 pg/mL[a]	2.1 ± 0.8 ng/mL

All values mean +SEM, $n = 4$ in each group.
[a] $p < 0.05$ vs. saline control group.
[b] $p < 0.05$ vs. asthma group.

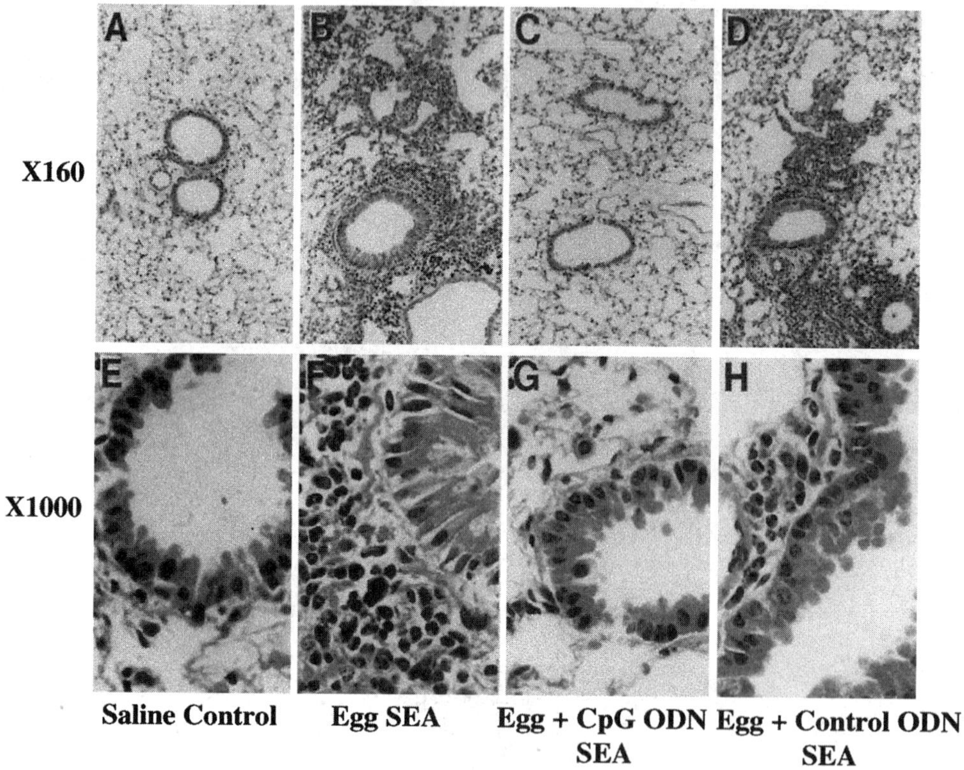

Figure 1 CpG ODN prevent peribronchial eosinophilia in a murine model of asthma: C57BL/6 mice were exposed to schistosome eggs with or without ODN (day 0) or saline alone and then challenged in the airways with schistosome egg antigen (SEA) on days 7 and 14. These sections are representative of at least four individual mice in each group. (A, E) saline control; (B, F) schistosome egg, SEA; (C, G) schistosome egg + CpG ODN, SEA; (D, H) schistosome egg plus control ODN, SEA (A–D 25×, E–H 1000×). Significant peribronchial eosinophilic inflammation and epithelial activation, which is induced by SEA in mice sensitized to schistosome eggs, is markedly diminished by coadministration of CpG ODN, but not by control ODN. (From Ref. 73.)

Thus, both Th1 cytokines appear to contribute to the effect of CpG, although neither is absolutely necessary.

Other investigators have confirmed and extended our initial findings that CpG ODN are effective in modulating murine models of asthma (Table 2). Broide and colleagues, using the ovalbumin model of murine asthma, found a marked inhibition of IL-5 and induction of IFN-γ by CpG DNA (75). This study also importantly reported that treatment with CpG DNA (administered either systemically or by mucosal delivery) led to diminished eosinophilia in all compartments; not only bronchoalveolar washings, but also parenchymal lung, peripheral blood, and bone marrow eosinophilia were reduced. Moreover, a single treatment with CpG DNA was as effective in inhibiting airway eosinophilia as seven consecutive daily injections of corticosteroids, providing an efficacy equivalent to the gold standard of anti-inflammatory agents. Finally, they also noted that CpG DNA was effective in preventing airway eosinophilia even when administered at time points subsequent to allergen sensitization.

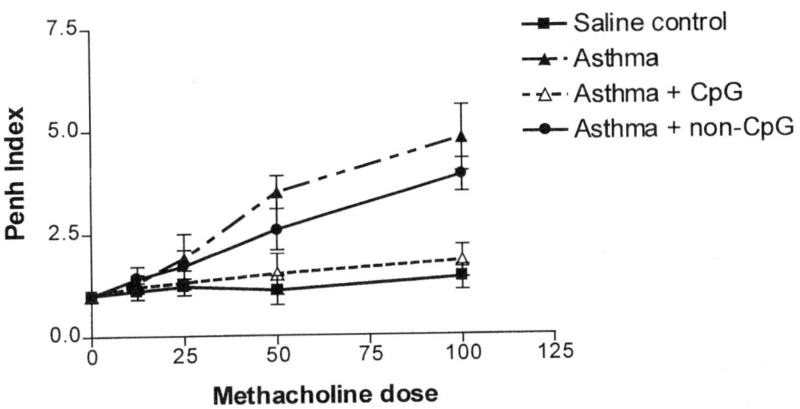

Figure 2 CpG ODN inhibits the development of bronchial hyperresponsiveness to inhaled methacholine in a murine model of asthma: C57BL/6 mice were treated as described in Figure 1; 24 hr after the second exposure to SEA, the mice were placed in whole-body plethysmographs and underwent methacholine challenge (between 12.5 and 100 mg/mL). Penh Index is a calculated measure of bronchospasm. The mice sensitized to schistosome eggs without ODN or in the presence of non-CpG (control) ODN exhibited significant bronchial reactivity to inhaled methacholine, compared with control mice or mice exposed to schistosome eggs in the presence of CpG ODN. (From Ref. 73.)

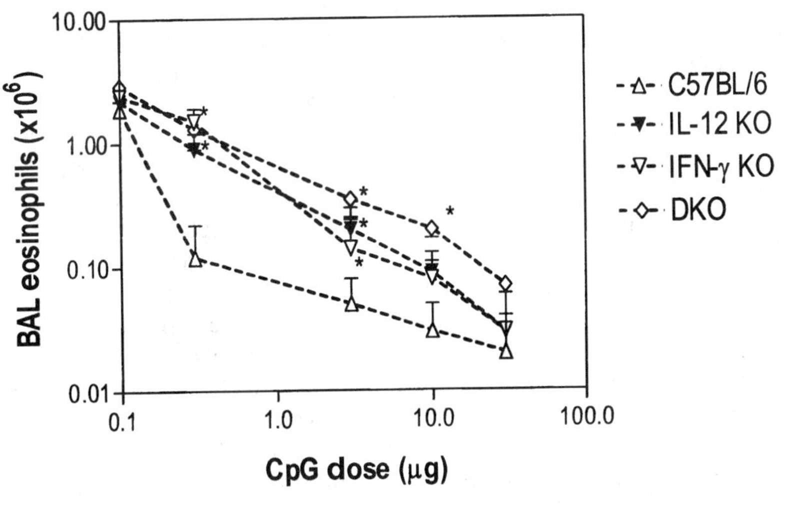

Figure 3 In the absence of IFN-γ or IL-12, mice are relatively deficient in response to CpG ODN: Varying amounts of CpG ODN (0.3, 3, 10, or 30 μg) were administered to wild-type C57BL/6, IFN-γ KO, IL-12 KO, and DKO (IFN-γ/IL-12 KO) mice at the time of sensitization to schistosome eggs. All mice that received 30 μg and the wild-type mice that received 10 μg of CpG ODN were fully protected against airway eosinophilia. There was no difference in airway eosinophilia among any of the groups that received no CpG ODN (not shown). A significant difference in the development of airway eosinophilia was seen between the wild-type and the knockout (KO) mouse groups that received between 0.3 and 10 μg of CpG ODN. *$p < 0.01$, versus wild-type C57BL/6 group; $n = 4$ mice in each group. (From Ref. 74.)

Table 2 Reported Effects of CpG DNA in Murine Models of Asthma

	Investigator		
Asthma model attributes or CpG effects	Kline	Broide	Sur
Antigen	Schistosome	Ovalbumin	Ragweed
Mouse strain	C57BL/6	BALB/c	BALB/c
CpG DNA prevents airway eosinophilia	Yes	Yes	Yes
CpG DNA prevents bronchial hyperreactivity	Yes	Yes	Yes
CpG DNA prevents induction of IgE	Yes	Yes	Yes
CpG DNA prevents systemic eosinophilia	nd	Yes	nd
CpG DNA inhibits Th2 cytokines	Yes	Yes	Yes
CpG DNA induces Th1 cytokines	Yes	Yes	Yes
CpG DNA is effective with mucosal administration	nd	Yes	Yes
CpG DNA is effective even when given after sensitization	Yes	Yes	Yes
CpG DNA effective up to 6 wk postadministration	nd	nd	Yes
CpG DNA effects require IFN-γ	No	nd	Yes
CpG DNA as effective as daily steroid injection	nd	Yes	nd

nd, not determined.

In a more recent manuscript, Sur et al. used a ragweed model of murine asthma to examine the effects of CpG DNA on airway inflammation (76). The novel aspect of this study was the focus on long-term prevention of inflammation. In addition to confirming that CpG DNA is effective in inducing Th1 and suppressing Th2 responses (including immunoglobulin responses) and preventing the eosinophilia and bronchial hyperreactivity of asthma, these investigators examined the late effects of CpG treatment. They repeated antigen challenges up to 65 days following treatment, and found that CpG was effective in preventing eosinophilia as late as 6 weeks after its administration. Unlike our studies, in this model CpG DNA was ineffective in preventing eosinophilic inflammation in IFN-γ knockout mice, suggesting that IFN-γ may be central in the response to CpG.

Thus, studies by our group and others have demonstrated that CpG DNA can effectively block the development of airway eosinophilia, bronchial hyperreactivity, and Th2-type antibody responses against the sensitizing antigen. CpG DNA is effective even when administered subsequent to sensitization, and appears to be at least as effective as daily corticosteroids in preventing asthmatic airway inflammation. These responses to CpG DNA are associated with the induction of Th1-type cytokines, including IFN-γ, IL-12, and IL-18. The potential benefits of CpG ODN extend beyond their effects on eosinophilia. CpG can also induce B-cell proliferation and increased immunoglobulin secretion. One can thus speculate that CpG may result in accelerated clinical response, because by suppressing Th2 cytokine, the isotype of the antibodies made would switch toward IgG; the B-cell stimulatory effects of CpG would minimize the time needed for the accumulation of significant amounts of antigen-specific IgG. CpG might, therefore, have another role as an adjuvant to allergen immunotherapy.

A theoretical concern about using CpG is that Th1 responses are associated with autoimmune diseases. Indeed, the balance between Th1 and Th2 is needed for the equilibrium between tolerance and immunity. To date, there have been no significant adverse effects associated with CpG, but most of the studies have been in animals and have been acute rather than chronic. Human trials are underway and prolonged administration of CpG in murine tumor immunotherapy models appears to be well tolerated (Ballas, unpublished observations).

5 SUMMARY

This is an exciting time in the chronology of asthma and allergic diseases. Although the pharmacopeia for treatment of these diseases has advanced greatly, most of our current therapies are aimed at the symptoms, rather than the underlying mechanism. Immunotherapy remains the only therapeutic modality that addresses the underlying mechanism, albeit by effects are still not fully understood. The approaches summarized in this chapter, alone or in combination, may yet allow one to reverse the atopic state. Meanwhile, other innovative DNA-based approaches are being developed, including the use of allergen DNA with or without CpG. Because most of the Th2 cytokines are on chromosome 5, the completion of the human genome project may open whole new venues of research aimed at controlling these cytokines at the chromosomal level.

REFERENCES

1. Bonnabeau RC Jr. Edward Jenner and the advent of vaccination. Minn Med 1983; 66:331–333.
2. Baxby D. The Jenner bicentenary: the introduction and early distribution of smallpox vaccine. FEMS Immunol Med Microbiol 1996; 16:1–10.
3. Brown F. From Jenner to genes—the new vaccines. Lancet 1990; 335:587–590.
4. Wehner JM, Bowers BJ. Use of transgenics, null mutants, and antisense approaches to study ethanol's actions. Alcohol Clin Exp Res 1995; 19:811–820.
5. Lo D. Animal models of human disease. Transgenic and knockout models of autoimmunity: building a better disease? Clin Immunol Immunopathol 1996; 79:96–104.
6. Branch AD. A hitchhiker's guide to antisense and nonantisense biochemical pathways. Hepatology 1996; 24:1517–1529.
7. Inouye M, Mao JR, Shimamoto T, Inouye S. In vivo production of oligodeoxyribonucleotides of specific sequences: application to antisense DNA Ciba Found Symp 1997; 209:224–233.
8. Galderisi U, Cascino A, Giordano A. Antisense oligonucleotides as therapeutic agents. J Cell Physiol 1999; 181:251–257.
9. Weiss B, Davidkova G, Zhou LW. Antisense RNA gene therapy for studying and modulating biological processes. Cell Mol Life Sci 1999; 55:334–358.
10. Blaese RM, Culver KW. Gene therapy for primary immunodeficiency disease. Immunodefic Rev 1992; 3:329–349.
11. McElvaney NG. Is gene therapy in cystic fibrosis a realistic expectation? Curr Opin Pulm Med 1996; 2:466–471.
12. Boucher RC. Status of gene therapy for cystic fibrosis lung disease [comment]. J Clin Invest 1999; 103:441–445.
13. Graham SM. Gene therapy for cystic fibrosis: perspectives for the otolaryngologist. Clin Otolaryngol 1998; 23:481–483.
14. Welsh MJ. The development of gene transfer for cystic fibrosis. Adv Intern Med 1995; 40: 429–444.
15. Hegele RG. Role of viruses in the onset of asthma and allergy: lessons from animal models. Clin Exp Allergy 1999; 29(suppl 2):78–81.
16. Fish JE, Peters SP. Airway remodeling and persistent airway obstruction in asthma. J Allergy Clin Immunol 1999; 104:509–516.
17. Pearlman DS. Pathophysiology of the inflammatory response. J Allergy Clin Immunol 1999; 104:S132–S137.

18. Gelfand EW. Essential role of T lymphocytes in the development of allergen-driven airway hyperresponsiveness. Allergy Asthma Proc 1998; 19:365–369.
19. Elias JA, Zhu Z, Chupp G, Homer RJ. Airway remodeling in asthma. J Clin Invest 1999; 104: 1001–1006.
20. Wills–Karp M. Immunologic basis of antigen-induced airway hyperresponsiveness. Annu Rev Immunol 1999; 17:255–281.
21. Chung KF, Barnes PJ. Cytokines in asthma. Thorax 1999; 54:825–857.
22. Warren HS, Kinnear BF, Phillips JH, Lanier LL. Production of IL-5 by human NK cells and regulation of IL-5 secretion by IL-4, IL-10, and IL-12. J Immunol 1995; 154:5144–5152.
23. Coffman RL, Mocci S, O'Garra A. The stability and reversibility of Th1 and Th2 populations. Curr Top Microbiol Immunol 1999; 238:1–12.
24. Galli SJ, Maurer M, Lantz CS. Mast cells as sentinels of innate immunity. Curr Opin Immunol 1999; 11:53–59.
25. Lucey DR. Evolution of the type-1 (Th1)–type-2 (Th2) cytokine paradigm. Infect Dis Clin North Am 1999; 13:1–9, v.
26. Wills–Karp M, Luyimbazi J, Xu X, Schofield B, Neben TY, Karp CL, Donaldson DD. Interleukin-13: central mediator of allergic asthma. Science 1998; 282:2258–2261.
27. Zhu Z, Homer RJ, Wang Z, Chen Q, Geba GP, Wang J, Zhang Y, Elias JA. Pulmonary expression of interleukin-13 causes inflammation, mucus hypersecretion, subepithelial fibrosis, physiologic abnormalities, and eotaxin production. J Clin Invest 1999; 103:779–788.
28. Lalani T, Simmons RK, Ahmed AR. Biology of IL-5 in health and disease. Ann Allergy Asthma Immunol 1999; 82:317–332; quiz 332–313.
29. Goodman MG. Cellular and biochemical studies of substituted guanine ribonucleoside immunostimulants. Immunopharmacology 1991; 21:51–68.
30. Feldbush TL, Ballas ZK. Lymphokine-like activity of 8-mercaptoguanosine: induction of T and B cell differentiation. J Immunol 1985; 134:3204–3211.
31. Thompson RA, Ballas ZK. Lymphokine-activated killer (LAK) cells. V. 8-Mercaptoguanosine as an IL-2-sparing agent in LAK generation. J Immunol 1990; 145:3524–3531.
32. Larsson K, Sollevi A. Influence of infused adenosine on bronchial tone and bronchial reactivity in asthma. Chest 1988; 93:280–284.
33. Karlsson JA. Purines and sensory neuropeptides in human asthma. Bull Eur Physiopathol Respir 1987; 23:95s–101s.
34. Aalbers R, Kaufman HF, Groen H, Koeter GH, de Monchy JG. Allergen-induced changes in adenosine 5′-monophosphate bronchial responsiveness: effect of nedocromil sodium. Ann Allergy 1992; 69:339–345.
35. Holgate ST, Church MK, Polosa R. Adenosine: a positive modulator of airway inflammation in asthma. Ann NY Acad Sci 1991; 629:227–236.
36. Holgate ST. Experimental models in asthma. Clin Exp Allergy 1999; 29(suppl 3):82–86.
37. Ng WH, Polosa R, Church MK. Adenosine bronchoconstriction in asthma: investigations into its possible mechanism of action. Br J Clin Pharmacol 1990; 30:89S–98S.
38. Mann JS, Holgate ST, Renwick AG, Cushley MJ. Airway effects of purine nucleosides and nucleotides and release with bronchial provocation in asthma. J Appl Physiol 1986; 61:1667–1676.
39. Mann JS, Holgate ST. Specific antagonism of adenosine-induced bronchoconstriction in asthma by oral theophylline. Br J Clin Pharmacol 1985; 19:685–692.
40. Stiles GL. Adenosine receptors. J Biol Chem 1992; 267:6451–6454.
41. Olah ME, Stiles GL. Adenosine receptors. Annu Rev Physiol 1992; 54:211–225.
42. Forsythe P, McGarvey LP, Heaney LG, MacMahon J, Ennis M. Adenosine induces histamine release from human bronchoalveolar lavage mast cells. Clin Sci (Colch) 1999; 96:349–355.
43. Polosa R, Ng WH, Crimi N, Vancheri C, Holgate ST, Church MK, Mistretta A. Release of mast-cell-derived mediators after endobronchial adenosine challenge in asthma. Am J Respir Crit Care Med 1995; 151:624–629.

44. Polosa R, Holgate ST. Adenosine bronchoprovocation: a promising marker of allergic inflammation in asthma? Thorax 1997; 52:919–923.
45. Rafferty P, Beasley R, Southgate P, Holgate S. The role of histamine in allergen and adenosine-induced bronchoconstriction. Int Arch Allergy Appl Immunol 1987; 82:292–294.
46. Mann JS, Cushley MJ, Holgate ST. Adenosine-induced bronchoconstriction in asthma. Role of parasympathetic stimulation and adrenergic inhibition. Am Rev Respir Dis 1985; 132:1–6.
47. Cushley MJ, Tattersfield AE, Holgate ST. Adenosine-induced bronchoconstriction in asthma. Antagonism by inhaled theophylline. Am Rev Respir Dis 1984; 129:380–384.
48. Ali S, Mustafa SJ, Metzger WJ. Adenosine-induced bronchoconstriction in an allergic rabbit model: antagonism by theophylline aerosol. Agents Actions 1992; 37:165–167.
49. Ali S, Mustafa SJ, Metzger WJ. Adenosine receptor-mediated bronchoconstriction and bronchial hyperresponsiveness in allergic rabbit model. Am J Physiol 1994; 266:L271–L277.
50. Nyce JW, Metzger WJ. DNA antisense therapy for asthma in an animal model. Nature 1997; 385:721–725.
51. Hogan SP, Foster PS, Tan X, Ramsay AJ. Mucosal IL-12 gene delivery inhibits allergic airways disease and restores local antiviral immunity. Eur J Immunol 1998; 28:413–423.
52. Li XM, Chopra RK, Chou TY, Schofield BH, Wills–Karp M, Huang SK. Mucosal IFN-gamma gene transfer inhibits pulmonary allergic responses in mice. J Immunol 1996; 157:3216–3219.
53. Dow SW, Schwarze J, Heath TD, Potter TA, Gelfand EW. Systemic and local interferon gamma gene delivery to the lungs for treatment of allergen-induced airway hyperresponsiveness in mice. Hum Gene Ther 1999; 10:1905–1914.
54. Barnes PJ, Karin M. Nuclear factor-kappaB: a pivotal transcription factor in chronic inflammatory diseases. N Engl J Med 1997; 336:1066–1071.
55. Blackwell TS, Christman JW. The role of nuclear factor-kappa B in cytokine gene regulation. Am J Respir Cell Mol Biol 1997; 17:3–9.
56. Barnes PJ. Anti-inflammatory actions of glucocorticoids: molecular mechanisms. Clin Sci (Colch) 1998; 94:557–572.
57. Mathieu M, Gougat C, Jaffuel D, Danielsen M, Godard P, Bousquet J, Demoly P. The glucocorticoid receptor gene as a candidate for gene therapy in asthma. Gene Ther 1999; 6:245–252.
58. von Mutius E, Fritzsch C, Weiland SK, Roll G, Magnussen H. Prevalence of asthma and allergic disorders among children in united Germany: a descriptive comparison. Br Med J 1992; 305:1395–1399.
59. von Mutius E, Martinez FD, Fritzsch C, Nicolai T, Reitmeir P, Thiemann HH. Skin test reactivity and number of siblings. Br Med J 1994; 308:692–695.
60. Shirakawa T, Enomoto T, Shimazu S, Hopkin JM. The inverse association between tuberculin responses and atopic disorder. Science 1997; 275:77–79.
61. Yamamoto S, Kuramoto E, Shimada S, Tokunaga T. In vitro augmentation of natural killer cell activity and production of interferon-alpha/beta and -gamma with deoxyribonucleic acid fraction from *Mycobacterium bovis* BCG. Jpn J Cancer Res 1988; 79:866–873.
62. Pisetsky DS, Reich CF. Stimulation of murine lymphocyte proliferation by a phosphorothioate oligonucleotide with antisense activity for herpes simplex virus. Life Sci 1994; 54:101–107.
63. Messina JP, Gilkeson GS, Pisetsky DS. Stimulation of in vitro murine lymphocyte proliferation by bacterial DNA. J Immunol 1991; 147:1759–1764.
64. Messina JP, Gilkeson GS, Pisetsky DS. The influence of DNA structure on the in vitro stimulation of murine lymphocytes by natural and synthetic polynucleotide antigens. Cell Immunol 1993; 147:148–157.
65. Krieg AM, Yi AK, Matson S, Waldschmidt TJ, Bishop GA, Teasdale R, Koretzky GA, Klinman DM. CpG motifs in bacterial DNA trigger direct B-cell activation. Nature 1995; 374: 546–549.
66. Cowdery JS, Chace JH, Yi AK, Krieg AM. Bacterial DNA induces NK cells to produce IFN-

gamma in vivo and increases the toxicity of lipopolysaccharides. J Immunol 1996; 156:4570–4575.

67. Ballas ZK, Rasmussen WL, Krieg AM. Induction of NK activity in murine and human cells by CpG motifs in oligodeoxynucleotides and bacterial DNA. J Immunol 1996; 157:1840–1845.
68. Halpern MD, Kurlander RJ, Pisetsky DS. Bacterial DNA induces murine interferon-gamma production by stimulation of interleukin-12 and tumor necrosis factor-alpha. Cell Immunol 1996; 167:72–78.
69. Klinman DM, Yi AK, Beaucage SL, Conover J, Krieg AM. CpG motifs present in bacteria DNA rapidly induce lymphocytes to secrete interleukin 6, interleukin 12, and interferon gamma. Proc Natl Acad Sci USA 1996; 93:2879–2883.
70. Roman M, Martin–Orozco E, Goodman JS, Nguyen M–D, Sato Y, Ronaghy A, Kornbluth RS, Richman DD, Carson DA, Raz E. Immunostimulatory DNA sequences function as T helper-1-promoting adjuvants. Nat Med 1997; 3:849–854.
71. Krieg AM, Yi AK, Schorr J, Davis HL. The role of CpG dinucleotides in DNA vaccines. Trends Microbiol 1998; 6:23–27.
72. Krieg AM, Love–Homan L, Yi AK, Harty JT. CpG DNA induces sustained IL-12 expression in vivo and resistance to *Listeria monocytogenes* challenge. J Immunol 1998; 161:2428–2434.
73. Kline JN, Waldschmidt TJ, Businga TR, Lemish JE, Weinstock JV, Thorne PS, Krieg AM. Modulation of airway inflammation by CpG oligodeoxynucleotides in a murine model of asthma. J Immunol 1998; 160:2555–2559.
74. Kline JN, Krieg AM, Waldschmidt TJ, Ballas ZK, Jain V, Businga TR. CpG oligodeoxynucleotides do not require Th1 cytokines to prevent eosinophilic airway inflammation in a murine model of asthma. J Allergy Clin Immunol 1999; 104:1258–1264.
75. Broide D, Schwarze J, Tighe H, Gifford T, Nguyen MD, Malek S, Van Uden J, Martin–Orozco E, Gelfand EW, Raz E. Immunostimulatory DNA sequences inhibit IL-5, eosinophilic inflammation, and airway hyperresponsiveness in mice. J Immunol 1998; 161:7054–7062.
76. Sur S, Wild JS, Choudhury BK, Sur N, Alam R, Klinman DM. Long term prevention of allergic lung inflammation in a mouse model of asthma by CpG oligodeoxynucleotides. J Immunol 1999; 162:6284–6293.

27

Mechanisms of Allergic Disease and the Implications for Therapeutic Interventions

LAWRENCE B. SCHWARTZ

Virginia Commonwealth University, Richmond, Virginia

This concluding chapter summarizes my perspective of the in-depth contributions to *Inflammatory Mechanisms in Allergic Diseases*. Each of the chapters noted in the following contains more detailed information.

Immediate hypersensitivity is the foundation of the field of allergy and immunology. The immediate hypersensitivity response to a single allergen challenge occurs in two phases—early and late—but these phases often overlap, particularly with a prolonged, natural exposure to an allergen. Vasoactive and spasmogenic responses, of rapid onset and short duration, are primordial elements defining the pathophysiology of the atopic disorders. The underlying biology of this appendage of the immune response remains elusive. Primary components of the effector arm of this response include mast cells, basophils (Chap. 2), and IgE (Chaps. 8 and 9). Various types of cells, particularly T lymphocytes (Chap. 5), and factors, including interleukin (IL)-4/13 and CD40L, stem cell factor (SCF), and IL-3, are needed to produce and sustain these primary participants. Underpinning allergic inflammation is the activation of Th2 lymphocytes (Chap. 5), apparently the default preference for immunity at birth. During infancy, certain microbial insults typically activate Th1 and inhibit Th2 lymphocytes. Ungoverned, the Th2 pathway enhances IgE production (Chap. 8). Mediators important to the early phase of an immediate hypersensitivity response include histamine and selected vasoactive metabolites of arachidonic acid (Chap. 10) or related lipids. Subservience to IgE appears to relegate mast cells and basophils to effector roles within the domain of acquired immunity. Modes for directly activating either mast cells, basophils, or both cell types, including neuropeptides, complement anaphylatoxins, cytokines, chemokines, or microbial molecules, unleash these cells from the restraints of acquired immunity and facilitate their ingress into the domain of innate immunity. Such direct activation avoids antigen processing and presentation to Th2 cells, the need for Th2 lymphocytes to court antigen-specific B cells and instruct them to switch to IgE production, and arming mast cells and basophils with IgE. How important a role mast cells and basophils play in innate immunity may affect the safety of therapeutic interventions aimed at these cells and their mediators.

The characteristic phlogistic features of the experimental late-phase response to allergen challenge and of chronic allergic disease further extends the scope of immediate hypersensitivity and provides new therapeutic challenges. These features vary somewhat with the target organ, but they uniformly involve the recruitment and nurturing of leukocytes (Chap. 6), particularly of eosinophils (Chap. 3) and basophils, and sometimes of neutrophils (Chap. 4). Inflammation (pain, swelling, redness, and warmth, with leukocyte recruitment), a term with which most physicians are comfortable, is an integral component in the definitions of asthma and atopic dermatitis, but similar to a complex human emotion, escapes precise definition. An inflammatory cascade is initiated when mast cells and basophils produce and secrete mediators, including cytokines and chemokines (Chap. 11), leading to the recruitment of other cells that, in turn, produce their own distinct but overlapping patterns of mediators, and in the process, activating organ-resident epithelial cells, fibroblasts, endothelial cells, smooth-muscle cells, and glandular cells to produce their own patterns of mediators and functional responses in the context of the organ involved. Attempts to abrogate allergic inflammation evoke the reflex administration of topical or systemic glucocorticoids, followed by more corticosteroid therapy if the initial dose proves inadequate. Eosinophils disappear from the treated site, typically by apoptosis, but may reflect only the patina of inflammation. Careful dissection of the inflammatory response reveals that some components are impervious to corticosteroids, and significant variations of responsiveness to these anti-inflammatory agents exist among different individuals. Consequently, allergic inflammation is not reflected by a single marker, nor is it quenched by a single pharmacological intervention.

A cellular response, whether to an activator or suppressor, a chemotactic agent or an inducer of apoptosis, proceeds from signals transmitted inside the responding cell. Current molecular techniques have facilitated a detailed understanding of the proximal, intermediate, and distal molecules involved, including those that interact with cell surface or internal receptors, those altering the expression of genes, and those affecting differentiation, proliferation, survival, and degranulation of a cell. Signaling through the high-affinity receptor for IgE (Chap. 9) is central to immediate hypersensitivity, not only in mast cells and basophils, but also in other cell types that may express this receptor, including antigen-processing cells, such as Langerhans cells, monocytes, and eosinophils.

The capacity for allergic inflammatory disease to result in sustained alterations to the structure and function of a particular organ is now recognized, and it is often referred to as tissue remodeling. The impact is great. Dysfunction may persist long after the inflammatory or allergic components of the disease have withered. Airway remodeling in asthma, most likely initiated, augmented, or driven by inflammation-related moieties (Chaps. 15 and 21), may be a major cause of chronic obstructive pulmonary disease (COPD); prevention and reversal of remodeling become important therapeutic targets. Extracellular matrix (Chap. 7), produced by resident cells that have been altered by inflammation, provides a structural framework that optimizes organ function. A thickened, fibrotic basement membrane of an airway widens the airway wall and, thereby, enhances bronchial hyperreactivity. This tissue remodeling may depend on imbalances between opposing processes. What determines the balance between fibrosis and fibrolysis, scarring and repairing, processes with disparate outcomes that employ some of the same components? Will transforming growth factor (TGF)-β stimulate fibrosis by direct effects on fibroblasts, or diminish fibrosis by attenuating inflammation? Will mast cell tryptase promote fibrosis by stimulating procollagen production, or enhance fibrolysis by activating prostromelysin that, in turn, activates procollagenase?

Signs of inflammation associated with immediate hypersensitivity characterize many of the disorders within the provenance of physicians trained in allergy and immunology. Allergic rhinitis (Chap. 12) reveals leaky postcapillary venules; dilated venous sinusoids; intraepithelial mast cells; recruited eosinophils, basophils, and Th2 lymphocytes; activated epithelial and endothelial cells and mucosal–glandular hyperreactivity to allergens, cholinergics, and irritants. Nasal polyps, inundated with eosinophils, occur in a subpopulation of subjects with allergic rhinitis and reflect profound tissue remodeling (Chap. 13), somewhat analogous to remodeling in the lower airway. Inflammation of the sinuses elicited by viruses, bacteria, and fungi (Chaps. 13 and 21), may require treatment of the inflammatory process, the microbe, both or neither; illustrating the need for better data to guide clinicians. In other cases, inflammation of the sinuses may prove to be nonmicrobial in nature, analogous to inflammatory bowel disease (Chap. 13). In the lower airway, the increasing incidence of atopic asthma and the associated societal disease burden highlight the need for better therapeutic interventions to prevent and to treat this disorder, goals more achievable with a better understanding of its pathogenesis (Chaps. 15 and 21).

In the eye (Chap. 14), seasonal and perennial allergic conjunctivitis often shows signs of inflammation without obvious tissue remodeling, whereas atopic keratoconjunctivitis, typically associated with atopic dermatitis, and vernal keratoconjunctivitis, remodels ocular tissue into cataracts and keratoconus. In the skin, both urticaria and angioedema (Chap. 17), and atopic dermatitis (Chap. 16) manifest components of immediate hypersensitivity, but tissue remodeling is evident only in the latter condition. Although antigen-specific IgE-mediated reactions can occur in each, autoimmune IgG that cross-links FcεRI may drive the majority of chronic urticaria cases, whereas the force driving atopic dermatitis, genetically influenced and involving Th2 (Th1 to a lesser extent) lymphocytes, remains an enigma.

Systemic anaphylaxis (Chap. 18), sometimes fatal owing to cardiovascular collapse or respiratory obstruction, is primarily thought of as the early exigent phase of an immediate hypersensitivity response, but local or systemic inflammation present before or during the event may influence clinical severity. Hypersensitivity reactions to drugs, although sometimes accounted for by classic antigen–IgE-mediated reactions, more often involve other forms of hypersensitivity (Chap. 19), typically requiring haptenization of the drug or its metabolite to a carrier. In some cases the MHC–peptide complex can be directly haptenized and presented to T cells. In toxic epidermal necrolysis, homotypic contacts between keratinocytes lead to their apoptosis when Fas ligand is induced on these cells, and is prevented by intravenous immunoglobulin G (IVIG) that contains antibodies that neutralize the Fas–Fas ligand pathway.

Inflammation of blood vessels, vasculitis, also is accounted for by different types of hypersensitivity, although typically not immediate hypersensitivity (Chap. 20). When remodeling of vessels occurs, perfusion is impaired, the consequences being dictated by the organ system involved. The inflammatory process may be propelled by foreign antigen, autoantibody, or microbial-derived superantigens. Immune complexes require Fcγ receptors to elicit inflammation, which is augmented by complement activation. T cells appear to be critical effector cells in some of the vasculitides, particularly when granulomas predominate.

The therapy of allergic disorders is at a crossroad. Most major advances have targeted various effector mechanisms (Chap. 22):

1. Mediator antagonists against histamine and sulfidopeptide leukotrienes
2. Neural pathway modulators, including α- and β_2-adrenergic agonists and cholinergic antagonists
3. Methylxanthines with modest bronchodilating and anti-inflammatory properties
4. Anti-inflammatory agents with weak (sodium cromoglycate and nedocromil) or strong (glucocorticoids) potencies

Although these interventions may reduce symptoms, none are curative, and their influence on tissue remodeling is unproved. Newer agents, anti-inflammatory phosphodiesterase (types 3 and 4) inhibitors, adhesion molecule antagonists, and cytokine (e.g., IL-4) antagonists may extend pharmacological efficacy. Therapy aimed at neutralizing IgE (anti-IgE MAb) (Chaps. 22 and 24) should reduce the IgE-mediated component of asthma and other atopic diseases, but does not appear to alter the underlying atopic state, because the disease recurs when therapy is discontinued. Conventional immunotherapy with intact allergens (Chap. 25), when effective, is associated with up-regulation of Th1 and down-regulation of Th2-mediated hypersensitivity. However, side effects from injecting strong allergens and including nonallergenic components together with allergenic proteins may limit the effectiveness and scope of immunotherapy. Consequently, conventional immunotherapy is contraindicated when atopic asthma is moderate or severe. New immunomodulatory strategies aim to either shift the Th2-dominated immune response to one that is Th1-dominated, or to simply down-regulate the Th2 pathway.

Three novel therapeutic approaches may substantially alter the treatment of allergic disorders.

1. Allergenic peptides can be genetically engineered to reduce side effects and increase efficacy (Chap. 23), opening the future possibility of immunotherapeutic agents that are safer and more effective than those currently available.
2. Immunostimulatory oligonucleotides, containing the CpG motif characteristic of microbial organisms, to which the natural exposure has diminished with good hygiene and vaccinations, are microbial danger signals capable of shifting default Th2 to Th1 immunity (Chap. 26). Administration of such nucleotides early in life may prevent Th2-dependent atopy from developing, or later in life might switch ongoing Th2-mediated hypersensitivity to the Th1 pathway. Whether the latter outcome eliminates or reduces the disease burden, or simply shifts the type of hypersensitivity from immediate to either immune complex- or cell-mediated will need to be carefully assessed.
3. Science has ascended to the genomic era. Understanding why different individuals respond differently to potential antigens and to various therapeutic interventions is now tangible. Polymorphisms known to occur in the genes for 5-lipoxygenase and the β_2-adrenergic receptor appear to influence how an asthmatic patient will respond to a leukotriene antagonist or a β_2-receptor agonist. Pharmacogenomics (Chap. 22), now in its infancy, may permit optimal individualization of therapy. One corollary to the abundant genetic variation already exposed

is that a single panacea for the treatment of disorders involving immediate hypersensitivity is dubious.

Credulous opportunities for therapeutic intervention arise with each new layer of understanding of the network of allergic inflammation and tissue remodeling. The veiled relations between environmental and genetic factors gradually evaporates. New markers of disease activity appear. I trust that the extensive knowledge and insights revealed by the contributors to *Inflammatory Mechanisms in Allergic Diseases* will help readers embrace these new findings and concepts with circumspect optimism.

Index

About the Editors

BURTON ZWEIMAN is Professor of Medicine and Neurology at the University of Pennsylvania School of Medicine, Philadelphia. The author, coauthor, editor, or coeditor of numerous publications, he was President of the American Academy of Allergy, Asthma and Immunology (1994) and the American Board of Allergy and Immunology (1979), as well as editor of the *Journal of Allergy and Clinical Immunology* (1988–1993). He received the A.B. degree (1952) in chemistry and the M.D. degree (1956) in medicine from the University of Pennsylvania, Philadelphia.

LAWRENCE B. SCHWARTZ is the Charles and Evelyn Thomas Professor of Medicine and Chair of the Division of Rheumatology, Allergy and Immunology at Virginia Commonwealth University, Richmond. The author, coauthor, editor, or coeditor of numerous publications, he is a Fellow of the American Academy of Allergy, Asthma and Immunology and the American College of Allergy, Asthma and Immunology, as well as a member of the European Society of Allergy and Clinical Immunology and the American Association of Immunologists, among others. The President of the American Board of Allergy and Immunology (2001), he received the B.S. degree (1970) from the University of Illinois, Urbana, and the M.D. (1976) and Ph.D. (1976) degrees from Washington University, St. Louis, Missouri.

ISBN 0-8247-0540-8

90000

9 780824 705404